The Childbearing Family
A NURSING PERSPECTIVE

The Childbearing Family
A NURSING PERSPECTIVE

SECOND
EDITION

Mary Ann Miller, R.N., M.S.N.
Assistant Professor, Graduate Program in Maternal-Child Nursing, College of Nursing, University of Delaware, Newark

Dorothy A. Brooten, Ph.D., F.A.A.N.
Chairperson, Health Care of Women and the Childbearing Family Section, School of Nursing, The University of Pennsylvania, Philadelphia

Illustrated by Donna Nicolo, B.S.N.

LITTLE, BROWN
AND COMPANY,
BOSTON/TORONTO

TO *Elizabeth Miller,* without whom half of this book would not have been possible

TO *Gary Brooten,* whose love and support were so important in making the other half possible

TO *Lisa Brooten* and *Lars Brooten,* now two young adults whose maturity and understanding have provided their mother with both joy and satisfaction in combining parenthood and career

Contents

Preface

This second edition of *The Childbearing Family: A Nursing Perspective* reflects the continued expansion and complexity of today's nursing practice. During the 6 years since the first edition was published, particularly with the advent of perinatal and neonatal nursing as subspecialties, many more nurses have assumed roles in which they have been required to make increasingly sophisticated judgments based on careful health assessments of their clients. The trend toward consumer participation in health care decisions has also brought an additional dimension to the planning, implementation, and evaluation of client care. Nurse researchers have attended to both of these factors in their investigation of problems relevant to reproductive health care.

Throughout this edition, we emphasize the findings of nursing research to support the rationale for nursing care. Our focus remains on the nursing process applied to the care of the childbearing family. The content is organized to provide a basic foundation in this area of nursing practice and to provide understanding as well as a challenge for students and also for current practitioners. Therefore, after appropriate chapters, readers are presented with clinical situations and assessment guides to stimulate the formation of their own nursing care plans.

Part 1, Family Health and Reproduction, presents the history of, and current trends in, the care of the childbearing family, considers the reproductive health care of women, including concepts of sexuality (especially during pregnancy), contraception, infertility, and abortion; and thoroughly reviews the female and male reproductive systems. In the remainder of the text (Parts 2 through 5), the physiologic and psychosocial bases of the entire reproductive process are discussed, reflecting the latest developments in the care of childbearing families. The importance of the family concept (especially the role of the father) and the nursing process are emphasized throughout the text.

We would like to pay special tribute to Donna Nicolo, whose illustrations continue to receive much critical acclaim. We would also like to acknowledge the efforts of many others who helped in the preparation of this second edition: Betty Armstrong and Lisa Brooten, for typing the manuscript; the public relations departments of Thomas Jefferson University Hospital and Pennsylvania Hospital; Booth Maternity Center; representatives of Mead Johnson Laboratories; and the publishers and authors who gave their permissions for selected illustrations and tables. The Little, Brown and Company editors who worked on this edition were Ann West and Carol Snarey.

M. A. M.
D. A. B.

PART 1 FAMILY HEALTH AND REPRODUCTION

Chapter 1 Trends in Childbearing

Broadly interpreted, *obstetrics* refers to all aspects of reproduction and the childbearing process—conception and contraception, pregnancy, labor, the postpartum period, and whatever pathology may be involved. It extends from an understanding of intrauterine development to an appreciation of the consequences of world population growth. The practice of health care personnel working within this discipline is aimed at the ideal that every pregnancy end in a healthy mother, baby, and family unit. Since this is not always a possibility, health care personnel try to prevent deviations from health or at least recognize them at an early stage and prevent undesirable consequences or minimize their ill effects as much as possible. As a result, they promote the optimal physical and emotional well-being for each member of the family unit.

HISTORICAL PERSPECTIVE

To appreciate the present trends in childbearing, one should have some understanding of their historic precedents. The term *obstetrics* is derived from the Latin verb *obstare*, meaning to protect or to stand by. *Obstetrix* referred to the midwife or the woman who stood by the expectant mother and gave her aid. Actually *midwifery*, rather than *obstetrics*, was the more widely used term until the latter part of the nineteenth century in both the United States and Great Britain. In England today the two words are used synonymously.

Historically, most women were delivered with the assistance of midwives whose knowledge was based purely on experience. When complications developed, medicine men or priests were called upon to pray over the mother. It is not surprising that childbirth was associated with mystery and superstition.

In the ancient Greek, Roman, Hindu, and Egyptian cultures, Hippocrates and others began to write the theory of obstetrics. Although medieval times saw a decline in the process of obstetrical knowledge and practice, midwives continued to perform deliveries. Women gave birth while sitting on special stools or obstetrical chairs (Fig. 1-1).

From the seventeenth to nineteenth centuries further advances were made in the science of obstetrics. The first modern cesarean operation was performed, puerperal fever was described, and obstetrical forceps and the use of chloroform as an anesthetic were introduced. Even greater strides have been made in the twentieth century. Between 1900 and 1910, antepartal care became an organized part of the medical and nursing supervision of mothers. Statistics began to be compiled and groups were established to study and to remedy high infant and maternal mortality. In 1912 the Children's Bureau was established by the U.S. government to conduct research and provide education to promote the health and welfare of children of all ages. In the 1920s, the Frontier Nursing Service was established in Kentucky and the Margaret Sanger Research Bureau was founded for planned parenthood and infertility research and assistance.

During the 1930s, a part of the Social Security Act, administered by the Children's Bureau, extended services for infant care to local areas. Maternity clinics, prenatal classes, premature care centers, and "well baby" clinics were established. Public health nursing services were provided for pregnant women. Improvements during the 1940s and 1950s, which had a dramatic effect in

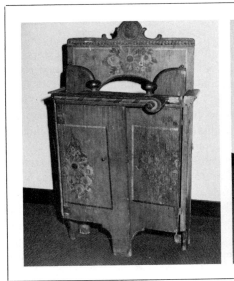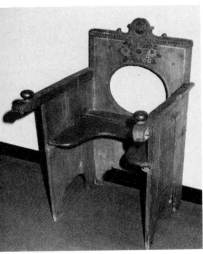

Figure 1-1. Birth chair used by early midwives. The chair was folded and carried on the midwife's back as she went from house to house assisting with deliveries. (Courtesy of Thomas Jefferson University, Philadelphia, Pa.)

lowering maternal mortality, included the development of blood transfusions, antibiotics, the increased number of hospital deliveries, and the rising standards of hospital care.

MATERNAL AND INFANT CARE PROGRAMS

In the past decade the number of neighborhood prenatal clinics has increased, high-risk clinics have been established, and programs have been developed for pregnant women who are unable to afford health care. In 1963 in the United States, Maternal and Infant Care (MIC) programs were funded under Title V of the Social Security Act, with the purpose of providing health care to high-risk pregnant women and, following delivery, to their newborn infants. The projects have been set up in large and medium-sized cities and in rural areas where there are few doctors in private practice or where clinics are overcrowded. Federal funding meets up to 75 percent of the operating costs. The woman, depending on her financial situation and overall physical condition, receives care without cost or pays only a portion of it.

Populations served by these programs have reported decreases in maternal and infant mortality, in premature births, in low birth weight babies, and in the number of pregnant women delivering without prenatal care. The number of women returning for postpartum and family planning visits has increased, as has the number of women seeking prenatal care early in pregnancy.

Communities, in addition to establishing MIC programs, have developed increasing numbers of neighborhood health centers. These centers include on their staffs nonprofessionals from the community, who are able to contribute the community's perspective when the needs of the consumers are considered and appropriate services are planned.

Other factors have also resulted in better services for pregnant women and reduced mortality and morbidity for them and their babies. Improved methods of anesthesia and analgesia, more sophisticated use of x-ray and ultrasonic diagnostic tools, and generally improved standards of living and sanitation have all played a part in these advances. Better education of health personnel has resulted in specialized training for physicians and nurses. Nurse midwives, as well as clinical nurse specialists, are being increasingly utilized.

VITAL STATISTICS
Birth Rate and Fertility Rate

Statistics often provide clues regarding the magnitude of certain problems or trends in population growth. The birth rate is always of interest to those predicting the need for obstetrical personnel. This rate has shown rather steady decreases until the middle of the last decade (Table 1-1). There is evidence to suggest that the decline in the birth rate in the United States is approaching a true reversal [21]. This is based on the rapidly rising proportion of young women who have not yet had any children as well as on a slight increase in their fertility [18]. Provisional data reported by the National Center for Health Statistics indicate that 1981 was the fifth consecutive year in which the number of births increased in the United States. The birth rate was at its highest level since 1971 [16].

Since 1963 family planning programs throughout the United States have undergone tremendous expansion, improved methods of contraception have been developed, and abortion has become legalized. Due to these factors and perhaps also because of socioeconomic improvement and better health care, the population of women having children has changed in character. Until recently, fertility rates for white and nonwhite women have decreased but the decline has been greater for the nonwhite population. Even though the fertility of nonwhite women is still higher than that of white women, the decline has reduced the proportion of births to both white and nonwhite women at unfavorable ages and parities and increased their average interpregnancy intervals. It is estimated that these demographic changes were responsible for 27 percent of the decrease in infant mortality from 1965 to 1972. Provisional data for 1980 show a reversal in the decline in fertility rates.

Although childbearing rates remain highest for women under the age of 30, the increase in the rate of births by women in this group has been relatively small. The largest increases in births have been observed for women aged 30 to 34 and 35 to 39. This trend can be expected to continue through the 1980s as women born

Table 1-1. Birth Rate in the United States per 1,000 Population

Year	Birth Rate
1940	19.4
1945	20.4
1950	24.1
1955	25.0
1960	23.7
1965	19.4
1970	18.4
1975	14.8
1977	15.4
1979	15.8
1981	16.9*

* Provisional data.
Sources: From U.S. National Center for Health Statistics. *Vital Statistics of the United States.* Hyattsville, Md., 1981; and U.S. National Center for Health Statistics. Births, marriages, divorces, and deaths for 1981. *Monthly Vital Statistics Report* 30(12):3, 1982. DPHS Publication (PHS) 82-1120.

in the post–World War II years enter these age groups [16]. For these older women the projected increase in the proportion of births is 37 percent, and the projected increase in the absolute number of births is 46 percent [3].

Changes in maternal age distribution play an important part in the incidence of certain pregnancy-related problems, such as hypertensive disorders and Down's syndrome (which is more frequent among women aged 35 years or older). Such changes have broad implications for provision of health services [3]. They will probably result in an increased demand for amniocentesis for prenatal chromosomal diagnosis as well as for other services for women at risk during pregnancy.

Maternal Mortality   A statistic of particular concern is that of maternal mortality (Table 1-2). Since the 1940s there has been a marked decrease in maternal mortality in the United States, Canada, and most of Western Europe. Over the past 20 years maternal deaths in the United States have declined 80 percent. Many factors are responsible for the tremendous fall in the maternal death rate. Most of them have already been mentioned: use of blood transfusions, antibiotics, better standard of living, better education of health practitioners, and more widely available antepartal care.

Maternal deaths resulting from the childbearing process (pregnancy, delivery, post partum) are stated in terms of the number of deaths per 100,000 live births (Table 1-3). Many of these deaths are caused by hypertensive disorders of pregnancy, hemorrhage, or infection. Heart disease is not officially recognized as a statistical category among the causes of maternal mortality, but it is related to a significant number of maternal deaths. Maternal mortality varies with the age of the woman. Increased age is also often related to the number of previous pregnancies; the effects of the two appear to be additive. The increased incidence of hypertension and a greater tendency to uterine hemorrhage are causative factors. Maternal mortality also tends to be greater among very young pregnant women, who are more subject to a variety of complications. The optimal age for childbearing seems to be between 20 and 24 years of age.

One of the most serious problems in maternity care in the United States is the markedly higher maternal mortality among nonwhite women and those in rural areas. These women often receive care that is inferior in quantity as well as quality. Since few health personnel choose to practice in rural and poverty areas, deliveries may not be properly attended. Pregnant women who live in urban poverty areas may have their care provided in great measure by large institutions, and that care may be fragmented and depersonalized as a result. This may, in itself, discourage early and regular attendance, although there may also be problems with lack of transportation, inadequate baby-sitting arrangements, fear, lack of understanding about the necessity of care, or long waiting periods.

Table 1-2. Maternal Mortality in the United States (per 100,000 Live Births) from Deliveries and Complications of Pregnancy, Childbirth, and the Puerperium

Deaths	1940	1950	1960	1965	1970	1977	1978
Maternal deaths	376.0	83.3	37.1	31.6	21.5	11.2	9.6
White deaths	319.8	61.1	26.0	21.0	14.4	7.7	6.4
Nonwhite deaths	773.5	221.6	97.9	83.7	55.9	26.0	23.0

Sources: Modified from U.S. National Center for Health Statistics. *Vital Statistics of the United States.* Hyattsville, Md., 1981; U.S. National Center for Health Statistics. Maternal mortality. *Monthly Vital Statistics Report* 29(6):4, 1980. DPHS Publication No. (PHS) 80-1120.

Lower socioeconomic status may be accompanied by poor living standards, poor nutrition, or increased stress, any of which can increase a woman's chances of a complicated pregnancy. It does not take much thought to conclude that many of the above factors can be easily remedied by interested health personnel.

Perinatal and Infant Mortality

Perinatal mortality is the sum of the fetal and neonatal death rates, or the number of stillborn infants and neonatal deaths per 1,000 total births.

A fetal death (or stillbirth) is said to have occurred when the period of gestation is 20 weeks or more or the fetus weighs 500 grams or more and is born without any sign of life—no heartbeat, respiration, or movement. (The loss of a fetus up to 20 weeks of gestation or weighing less than 500 grams is referred to as a spontaneous abortion—see Chap. 18.) This death rate, which is related to the quality of care before and during birth, has been reduced somewhat (Table 1-4). Improvements in prenatal care, fetal diagnosis, and fetal monitoring have contributed to the reduction in the fetal death rate.

Neonatal death rates are relatively high, although significant reductions have occurred (Table 1-5). More than half of the neonatal deaths (deaths of live-born infants up to 28 days of age) occur during the first day of life, which emphasizes the importance of careful observation and accurate assessment of the newborn's condition. Premature birth remains the most frequent cause of neonatal death; central nervous system injuries, whether from hypoxia or trauma, and congenital malformations are also significant factors.

The infant death rate (calculated per 1,000 live births) includes deaths of infants under 1 year of age, exclusive of fetal deaths. This rate is decreasing gradually, as can be seen in Table 1-6. Most infant deaths occur during the neonatal period.

Table 1-3. Maternal Mortality in the United States (per 100,000 Live Births) by Age, Race, and Cause of Death

For over a decade the infant and perinatal mortality rates have decreased in the United States. Postneonatal mortality has declined more than has fetal and

Age/Cause	1957–1958			1967–1968			1978		
	White	Nonwhite	Total	White	Nonwhite	Total	White	Nonwhite	Total
All ages	26.9	108.3	39.2	18.1	66.6	26.3	6.4	23.0	9.6
Under 20	18.0	60.0	27.5	13.0	35.3	19.2	5.0	11.5	7.0
20–24	13.0	55.5	19.5	10.1	45.5	15.4	5.2	19.3	7.9
25–29	20.0	98.5	30.0	13.5	66.0	20.3	6.4	25.7	9.2
30–34	37.5	180.5	56.5	28.7	109.8	41.3	12.9	52.0	18.8
35–39	66.5	272.0	94.5	51.2	179.0	72.7	25.7	93.0	38.9
40–44	109.5	382.5	147.5	100.1	250.2	126.8	53.5	110.9	66.3
All causes	26.9	108.3	39.2	18.1	66.6	26.3	6.4	23.0	9.6
Infection	3.0	8.5	4.0	3.4	7.2	4.0	1.3	4.0	1.8
Preeclampsia/ eclampsia	6.5	31.5	10.0	3.0	13.5	4.8	1.5	3.2	1.9
Hemorrhage	5.5	19.5	7.5	2.7	7.3	3.5	0.6	2.9	1.1
Ectopic pregnancy	1.5	10.5	3.0	1.0	7.4	2.1	0.5	3.7	1.1
Abortion	3.0	21.0	6.0	2.3	13.4	4.2	0.1	1.8	0.5
Other	7.5	19.5	9.0	5.7	18.0	7.8	2.2	7.2	3.2

Sources: From *Statistical Bulletin of the Metropolitan LIfe Insurance Co.*, vol. 53. New York, June 1972; U.S. National Center for Health Statistics. *Vital Statistics of the United States.* Hyattsville, Md., 1981; U.S. National Center for Health Statistics. Maternal mortality. *Monthly Vital Statistics Report* 29(6):4–5, 1980. DPHS Publication No. (PHS) 80-1120.

Table 1-4. Fetal Mortality in the United States per 1,000 Live Births[a]

Deaths	1950	1960	1965	1970	1975	1977
Fetal deaths (stillbirths)	19.2	16.1	16.2	14.2	10.7	9.9
White deaths	17.1	14.1	13.9	12.4	—[b]	—[b]
Nonwhite deaths	32.5	26.8	27.2	22.6	—[b]	—[b]

[a] Period of gestation was 20 weeks (or 5 months), or more, or was not stated.
[b] Not available.
Source: From U.S. National Center for Health Statistics. *Vital Statistics of the United States.* Hyattsville, Md., 1981.

Table 1-5. Neonatal Mortality in the United States per 1,000 Live Births[a]

Deaths	1940	1950	1960	1965	1970	1975	1977	1981
Neonatal deaths	28.8	20.5	18.7	17.7	15.1	11.6	9.9	7.9[b]
White deaths	27.2	19.4	17.2	16.1	13.8	10.4	8.7	—[c]
Nonwhite deaths	39.7	27.5	26.9	25.4	21.4	16.8	14.7	—[c]

[a] Of infants under 28 days, exclusive of fetal deaths.
[b] Provisional data.
[c] Not available.
Sources: Modified from U.S. National Center for Health Statistics. *Vital Statistics of the United States.* Hyattsville, Md., 1981; U.S. National Center for Health Statistics. Births, marriages, divorces, and deaths for 1981. *Monthly Vital Statistics Report* 30(12):3, 1982. DPHS Publication No. (PHS) 82-1120.

Table 1-6. Infant Mortality in the United States per 1,000 Live Births[a]

Deaths	1940	1950	1960	1965	1970	1975	1977	1981
Infant deaths	47.0	29.2	26.0	24.7	20.0	16.1	14.1	11.7[b]
White deaths	43.2	26.8	22.9	21.5	17.8	14.2	12.3	—[c]
Nonwhite deaths	73.8	44.5	43.2	40.3	30.9	24.2	21.7	—[c]

[a] Of infants under 1 year, exclusive of fetal deaths.
[b] Provisional data.
[c] Not available.
Sources: From U.S. National Center for Health Statistics. *Vital Statistics of the United States.* Hyattsville, Md., 1981; U.S. National Center for Health Statistics. Births, marriages, divorces, and deaths for 1981. *Monthly Vital Statistics Report* 30(12):3, 1982. DPHS Publication (PHS) 82-1120.

neonatal mortality, but the risk of death per unit of time is still at its peak in early fetal life. The decrease in infant mortality has occurred at the same time as improvements in medical techniques, in the organization and availability of health services, and in economic conditions and standards of living, and changes in the demographic characteristics of the childbearing population of the United States.

Advances in medical techniques since 1965 have made possible improved maternity care with fetal monitoring and improved methods of newborn care in intensive care units. The greater availability of high technology services in urban areas has had a positive impact on perinatal and neonatal mortality. Improvements in the standard of living since 1963 include many elements that affect infant mortality, such as housing, nutrition, transportation, and education. Changes in the health care delivery system plus new sources of funds for medical care have made it possible for some patients to use previously unavailable services.

While these changes in medical techniques, organization and availability of health services, improved standards of living, and demographic characteristics of the childbearing population have resulted in decreased infant and perinatal mortality in the United States, the improved rates have not significantly changed the relative position of this country in comparison with others. Many problems remain.

Major causes of infant deaths in the United States include congenital malformations, sudden infant death syndrome, low birth weight and its resulting sequelae such as respiratory distress syndrome, and certain complications of pregnancy and labor, especially those involving placental insufficiency, the umbilical cord, and birth injury. These factors are often significant in neonatal morbidity: It has been estimated that for every two neonatal deaths from congenital malformations, three infants with serious malformations survive. In terms of emotional and financial cost to the family and society, the morbidity from congenital malformations is more devastating than the traumatic but brief impact of early mortality. Decreasing the incidence of congenital malformations in the newborn is clearly a high priority in health care, whether achieved by identifying and removing responsible teratogens or by offering prenatal diagnosis and selective abortion to the mothers of affected fetuses.

The birth rate of low birth weight infants has remained remarkably steady over the past 20 to 30 years in all countries in which it has been reported, even though some factors normally associated with low birth weight such as socioeconomic variables have changed positively. Currently, greater numbers of low birth weight infants are surviving, but many suffer marked neurologic and respiratory damage.

In addition to these problems, death rates remain high for fetuses of teenagers, women over 35 years of age, nonwhite women, and women in lower socioeconomic groups. Infant and perinatal mortality is also consistently higher in certain states and cities. Even though death rates in rural areas are higher, the vast majority of births and of infant and perinatal deaths occur in urban areas.

In the effort to achieve further reductions in perinatal and infant mortality rates, several directions become clear. Despite advances in medical technology, not all geographic areas have benefited from their development. However, efforts to increase access to these services through regionalization are already reducing perinatal and infant mortality. The problems of the large number of low birth weight infants with congenital anomalies and the increased fetal death rates among some groups of women require more aggressive approaches to risk assessment during pregnancy and to preventive care.

MATERNAL/NEO-
NATAL INTENSIVE
CARE UNITS

Before and after the birth, both mother and newborn are observed very carefully. Recent changes in the care of high-risk mothers and neonates have resulted in the development of intensive care units especially for them. This organized intensive care has led to a decrease in mortality among neonates and fewer serious handicapping conditions among surviving infants [13, 20]. The development of a number of medical subspecialties such as neonatology and perinatology has provided well-trained and highly skilled personnel to care for high-risk mothers and infants in these intensive care units.

Regionalization

Because such skilled personnel are limited in number and because intensive care units require rather expensive equipment, it has been recommended that the sites for such units be chosen carefully and that each unit be large enough for efficient and effective service in a wide geographic area. In the last decade the American Academy of Pediatrics, the American College of Obstetricians and Gynecologists, and other related groups have drawn up guidelines for the implementation of regional perinatal programs. A regionalization program is a cooperative effort among institutions in a specific geographic area to promote the orderly distribution of services to the public. It assures access to necessary services for all patients who require them, supports frequent consultation among professionals, establishes standards of care, and provides continuing education for health personnel. The concept of three levels of care underlies the operation of these programs [9, 10].

Level I (primary) facilities have the primary mission of providing care for mothers and newborns with uncomplicated care requirements. These hospitals are usually located in sparsely populated areas. A part of their mission is to be able to identify the high-risk client as quickly as possible so she can be referred to a center that can provide more complex care. The Level I agencies must be able to provide emergency care in the event of a sudden complication.

Level II (secondary) agencies provide care for most clients, including most of the high-risk women. These hospitals are located in cities or suburbs where most deliveries occur. Some of these agencies may even have the facilities to care for mothers and newborns with very complicated requirements, but in many cases it would not be cost-effective to maintain the broad range of services required for this purpose; such clients are usually sent to a tertiary center. Level II units have a highly trained, multidisciplinary staff and modern, well-maintained equipment.

Level III (tertiary) agencies provide care for normal as well as high-risk mothers and newborns, but they specialize in caring for those who require the most complicated care. Coordination of the entire regional program occurs at this level. It includes establishment of care standards, provision of continuing education, provision of outreach consultation, and the conduct of relevant clinical research. Regions served by Level III centers have from 8,000 to 12,000 deliveries a year.

It is recommended that Level III units have 24-hour anesthesia, obstetric, and pediatric staff coverage; have the ability to perform a cesarean delivery within 15 minutes at any hour; provide 24-hour consultation service by telephone to Level I and II units in the region; and provide the equipment and a qualified team of physicians and nurses for maternal and newborn transport from a referring hospital to the perinatal/neonatal center on a round-the-clock basis.

While the role of nursing in planning these programs has not been very evident in the past, recent efforts to involve nurses in the organization of regional perinatal nursing care have met with success [10].

GENETIC
COUNSELING

Families seek genetic counseling for a number of reasons, usually because of the birth of a child with anomalies, a family history of a genetic disorder, or infertility problems such as unexplained frequent abortion. Recent accomplishments in genetic counseling have helped to reduce infant mortality and morbidity. Refinements in chromosome studies and in biochemical and tissue culture methods have greatly improved our ability to diagnose, treat, and advise families on genetic matters. From a sample of amniotic fluid, it is possible to detect all major chromosomal abnormalities and a large number of inborn errors of metabolism. With this information, couples at risk can be better informed when they decide whether or not to have children. They may choose to conceive, have the amniotic fluid of the fetus tested for abnormalities, and then choose whether to continue the pregnancy, depending on the results. This advance has enabled couples who in the past would not have chosen to have children to go through the childbearing process.

Genetic counseling has had other benefits as well. Serious problems in interpersonal relationships between a couple are averted by informing them that a genetic trait is an unfortunate coincidence of parental genotype and is not related to habit, conduct, or misconduct. This information should help to dispel guilt feelings; the knowledge that all persons are carriers of a variety of disorders likewise lessens their anxiety. This knowledge also helps to decrease in the extended family any hostility or feelings that the couple should not bear children.

For purposes of counseling, a genetic history is taken. The age, sex, and past and present health of the father, mother, siblings, and all close relatives of the couple are recorded, and a pedigree chart is compiled. The age at death and cause of death are noted for those relatives who have died. It is also important to record how the diagnosis of cause of death was made (e.g., biopsy, clinical examination, or biochemical test) and the age of onset of the genetic disorder in each family member. (Siblings may not yet be affected because they are too young.) With this information as a base, the couple is counseled by reviewing their special problems and explaining the genetic prognosis and the alternatives open to them.

As nurses assume increasing responsibility, whether in the traditional setting or in an expanded role, they are becoming involved in situations in which families need genetic counseling. They must be aware of common genetic conditions and patterns of inheritance; the nurse's role in identification of conditions that may have a genetic basis; the resources to which families with genetic conditions can be referred; how families can actually make contact with those resources; and how nurses can effectively participate in the referral and follow-up of those families with genetic problems [12].

Once families are referred to a genetic clinic, they are put in touch with professionals who are especially knowledgeable and prepared to give the kind of support they need. Getting the family to the point where they accept this type of referral may take considerable time and energy. Portraying a positive attitude toward the family and being willing to listen and to discuss and answer their questions may give them the initial support they need to begin to work through their problem.

Birth-defect monitoring systems are in effect in Canada, Great Britain, Finland, Sweden, Norway, Hungary, and Israel. Recently, the United States established such a system. Data on more than 230 different kinds of birth defects are collected from one million births per year in 1,200 short-term hospitals in the United States. The information is computerized and reported quarterly by the Centers for Disease Control in Atlanta. This system enables the detection of any unusual pattern in the occurrence of birth defects, such as regional outbreaks that might be linked to drugs, viral infections, radiation, pollutants, or other environmental causes. Identification of such patterns minimizes the risk of these birth defects reaching epidemic proportions.

The March of Dimes Birth Defects Foundation is a valuable resource for current information on genetic counseling in general and on specific genetic counseling programs. Most of these programs include services such as necessary laboratory testing, diagnosis, social services and referrals, psychologic evaluation counseling about risks in terms of probability of occurrence of a genetic defect, and information about alternative approaches to the problem [12].

THE FAMILY CONCEPT IN CHILDBEARING

More attention is now being paid to the response of the total family to the pregnancy experience. Recently prenatal classes have been established for children to help them accept and welcome a new baby. The expectant father also is receiving the attention he deserves. He or a close friend or relative is encouraged to become involved in childbirth preparation classes. He is an essential member of the health team, giving emotional and physical support to the woman during pregnancy and labor (Fig. 1-2). He usually is encouraged to accompany the woman to the delivery room where they share in the birth of their baby. In some instances he may even participate in the actual delivery. He is encouraged to be present when the baby is fed in the hospital and to participate in the infant's care. If there are other children in the family, they may be able to visit their mother during this time. Anxiety levels are kept at a minimum for both mother and children when such visits are possible. In some birth centers or birthing rooms, children are present during the birth of a sibling.

Rooming-in is a desirable option for many families. This arrangement permits parents to see and care for their baby whenever they wish. Usually visitors are limited; the father is encouraged to help care for and feed the infant (after he washes his hands and puts on a gown). Policies regarding rooming-in vary from hospital to hospital. In some hospitals the baby remains with the mother 24 hours a day; in others he is returned to the nursery during the night. In some institutions the physical plant is specifically designed to accommodate mothers who desire rooming-in. In other hospitals existing facilities can usually be easily modified to provide the service.

Figure 1-2. Father thoughtfully supports mother during labor and awaits the birth of their child. (Courtesy of Booth Maternity Center, Philadelphia, Pa.)

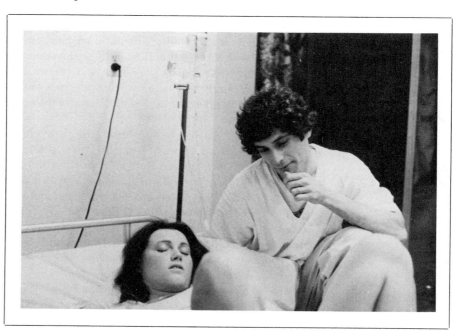

Some obstetricians are consenting to do deliveries in the home, where the mother can readily receive emotional support from the father and other family members during the birth process. Home deliveries are usually less expensive than hospital deliveries, and there is also less danger of mother and newborn acquiring hospital-borne infections. The main disadvantage of home delivery is the lack of emergency services, equipment, techniques, and educated personnel, which are available in the hospital. However, in the minds of some parents this is outweighed by the advantage of home delivery—the ability to be together in familiar surroundings during the birth of their baby. Efforts to meet the needs of these consumers have resulted in the establishment of birth centers and birthing rooms in clinical agencies where a homelike atmosphere is combined with the safety features of the hospital setting.

The current trend toward primary care nursing will undoubtedly encourage a spirit of unity as the parents and their family members relate to the same nurse throughout the childbearing process. The continuum of care begins when the nurse first meets the parents in the clinic or doctor's office and continues as she follows them through the pregnancy, labor, delivery, and postpartum period and makes home visits when necessary. This approach is similar to the continuity of care currently provided by the nurse midwife.

NURSE MIDWIFERY   The first nurse midwives in the United States were trained in England and were first employed by the Frontier Nursing Service in 1925. By 1931 the first school for nurse midwifery had opened in New York City, but professional nurse midwives did not enter the organized system of health care until 1955. The United States has been slow to acknowledge the role of nurse midwives and to utilize their services, possibly because the profession has had to outgrow the reputation of the old "granny midwives," nonprofessionals whose practice was based on experience rather than education.

The last decade has witnessed the growth of a spirit of collaboration and cooperation among health professionals. The nurse midwife is increasingly seen as the teammate of the doctor. In many instances the pregnant woman is seen initially by both the doctor and the nurse midwife. If her condition is not complicated in any way, she may choose to have the nurse midwife follow her throughout her pregnancy and labor. The nurse midwife will deliver her baby and attend to her postpartum and family planning needs, including home visits. The doctor is available for consultation throughout the childbearing process.

The nurse midwife often provides additional services for the patients, such as individual counseling and general health education, arranging for alternative positions during delivery, helping with immediate breast-feeding after birth, and urging the presence of the father or other close relative to support the mother and promote effective parenting. Parents who have had contact with a nurse midwife usually find the experience beneficial and request the same type of service again. In some groups of pregnant women cared for by nurse midwives, there has been a decrease in the rates of prematurity and neonatal deaths [8, 19].

The American College of Nurse-Midwives is the professional organization that sets the standards for quality care by midwives. It also provides guidelines and accreditation for educational programs and issues a certifying examination. In the 1950s there were five or six such programs; today there are 23 nurse midwifery programs that prepare nurses to become certified. Fourteen of them lead to a master's degree as well. (See Appendix I for a list of these programs.)

The nurse midwife is an outstanding example of the expanded role of the nurse in childbearing settings. Clinical nurse specialists with advanced preparation can provide many of the same services (excluding the actual delivery of the baby). These professionals have a broad orientation to health care and relate to families on a very personal level, characteristics increasingly being demanded by the consumer. Because of this, and because fewer physicians are choosing obstetrics as a specialty, the need for prepared nurse practitioners can only be more pressing in the future.

BIOETHICAL CONSIDERATIONS

In recent years the development of advanced health care technologies has led to a surge of interest in bioethical questions on issues that have societal consequences. Through publicity in professional and popular literature, these matters have become the concern of the general public as well as of health practitioners. This concern primarily has been expressed in a requirement for informed patient consent before undergoing therapeutic or experimental procedures. Specific areas in women's reproductive health care that have been subject to such bioethical debate have included abortion, aminocentesis/fetal diagnosis, fetal experimentation, contraception/sterilization, in vitro fertilization, maintenance of life supports for very young or defective infants, and patients' rights.

Most bioethical debates are about whether the means are proportional to the ends. Are there certain means that should never be used, regardless of how good the end is perceived to be? Are deception, invasion of privacy, not keeping promises, for example, justified by the "good" end? Who is to define the "good"? Should it be the health professional, the patient, a committee? Is the patient autonomous? If so, what is the role of the health professional? Who speaks for the patient when he is not capable of exercising his autonomy? [11]

Does the right to autonomy extend to a woman's right to put her unborn child at greater than average risk of death or damage by putting herself outside the reaches of technology? On the other hand, are health professionals justified in imposing a procedure on a woman when it is not strictly indicated? Are there instances when the needs of the woman become secondary to the needs and goals of the health care provider? How can the health professional ensure that the woman's value system determines the action to be taken? [6, 11]

Other serious ethical problems are caused by conflicts between pursuit of knowledge for its own sake and the consequences of such research, e.g., in genetic engineering. How is the new knowledge obtained and how will it be used? The issue of human rights is also hotly debated. What value is placed on human life? How far should one go in one's allegiance to bureaucratic (institutional) values when they conflict with the rights of the patient? Does the health care provider have more respect for power than principle? Is the risk of "making waves" a viable option in professional practice? [15]

With expanded roles in nursing comes increased responsibility, frequently without clear lines of authority. As nurses function independently on higher professional levels than in the past, it becomes even more imperative that they understand the importance of professional ethics. Ethics and ethical judgment are the foundation of professional integrity. Professional ethics, an extension of personal ethics, are the professional ideals that form the foundation of proper patient care [15]. Thus nurse philosophers are focusing attention on the obligation of nurses and all health professionals to identify ethical issues with which they must deal, to raise questions, and to take time to think about the implications for their own professional practice. (For more detailed discussions of bioethical issues in professional practice, consult the bibliographic references at the end of this chapter.)

INFLUENCES OF
CULTURE

Recently, increased attention has been given to the need for health professionals to understand how individuals define health, what they perceive as their health care needs, and what health care services they desire. Emphasis has been placed on determining the cultural norms that dictate how individuals respond to each of the above questions. In today's world in which a variety of ethnic backgrounds are represented in most groups of women seeking reproductive health care, cultural influences have a definite impact on the delivery of that care.

All cultures have their own belief systems for health and illness, birth and death. The most prescribed rules and rituals usually surround childbearing and childrearing. Aamodt [1] focuses on four main components of a cultural system that impact on these two specific processes. The first component, the moral and value system, prescribes conduct involving the notions of duty, desirability, and obligation. Are children desirable? What is the value placed on human life? Is one expected to take care of oneself? Is one obligated "to do what is right"? What number of children is considered the norm in the context of a particular culture?

The second component of a cultural system is the kinship system. This refers to categories of reciprocal rights, duties, and obligations of role behavior for all relationships that result from marriage and family life. Who marries whom? Who has sexual intercourse? Who takes care of the children? The third component, the knowledge and belief system, defines the processes of menstruation, conception, childbearing, and labor and delivery. Finally, the ceremonial and ritual systems provide the means for the reenactment of the relationship of the symbolic elements in the cultural system and allow for their incorporation into daily life.

Garner [7] points out that a variety of areas in childbearing need special consideration. In childbirth, culture and custom tend to dictate where and in what position a woman delivers and who supports her during delivery. During pregnancy and post partum the woman's need for dietary restrictions and other rituals may continue to direct a flexible interpretation of traditional hospital routines. Beliefs about sexual intercourse and sexual modesty may influence the approach you take when discussing such subjects as contraception and breastfeeding.

Culture is a dynamic concept. Many of its primary elements will be altered over time by variables such as education and socioeconomic status. Many third and fourth generation women will not even be aware of some of their culture's traditional beliefs. Health professionals' responsibility is to identify the woman's aspirations for health as well as what she values as good health care. Health professionals must reconcile their own values with those of the different culture so that the goals of the health care program can be mutual and efforts are not counterproductive. Problems such as ethnocentrism (belief that one's own values are superior or more desirable), cultural blindness (refusal to acknowledge that beliefs of other cultures exist), and cultural imposition (imposition of one's own value system on others) all interfere with and limit our communication with and effectiveness in working with women whose attitudes are different from our own [14].

Be inquisitive and observant. The more informed you become, the easier it will be to make the necessary adjustments in nursing care.

RESEARCH IN NURSING

Every practitioner is responsible for providing quality patient care. Improvements in its delivery can only occur as a result of a strong base of nursing research. Students in nursing, as well as practitioners, have the obligation as professionals to become actively involved in some research activity. A nurse can fulfill this obligation in different ways without actually being involved in designing projects and in collecting data. In fact, it is recognized that true competence in designing research projects most likely requires advanced study.

If nursing is to continue to grow in professional stature, it is essential that it nurture an attitude of curiosity that questions and analyzes the validity of assumptions on which our actions are based. This curiosity moves students or practitioners to question sweeping generalizations found in the professional literature, to wonder why such statements are correct (or incorrect), and to investigate the rationale behind these statements. It stimulates them to question policies that formulate routine aspects of patient care, to evaluate present approaches to it, to wonder about different, more individualized, or better approaches to patient care, and to try some of them to see what results are achieved. This curiosity causes them to want to be knowledgeable about current research in the field, to interpret the findings of such studies critically, and to share this information with their co-workers. It inspires them to be willing to apply the results of clinical research to their own practice and to identify further research problems. Nursing is already characterized by a careful assessment of patients and their environment. An exciting dimension is added when this assessment is used as a basis for developing better methods of patient care.

Many students already use scientific research procedures on a small scale when their curriculum includes independent study. Here they recognize how problems in clinical nursing can be systematically studied, and they have the opportunity to look at those problems creatively, considering a wide variety of approaches for their study and solution. They must identify and critically read relevant research in their subject area, develop a plan for investigating their problem, and implement that plan.

Comprehensive research and critical analysis of the literature naturally precede application of results of studies to clinical practice. Nurses should not doubt their ability to understand research; there is nothing magical about understanding research that has been carefully documented and clearly presented by the author. Whether it is being read with the purpose of implementing findings in practice or in order to generate new ideas for further research, it is essential for the reader to assess whether the findings are valid and reliable. A methodical, thoughtful, critical analysis of research studies should provide the reader with that assessment.

Castles [4] enumerates certain steps involved in such an approach.

1. Note the credentials of the author. They might bear some relationship to the validity of the research.
2. Look at the title. It should give a clear and comprehensive indication of what the study is about.
3. Look for the definition of the problem and the statement of the purpose. Are they clear?
4. Pay attention to the methodology used. Look at the variables. How were they controlled? Will the findings be valid? Be careful about applying the findings to a general population if the sample was nonrandom, very small, etc. Was the data collection appropriately done?
5. Look at the conclusions of the study. Do they relate to the stated purpose? Are they based on the data? Are they relevant to nursing practice? Were any limitations to the study noted?
6. Was the research published in a peer-reviewed research journal where the work was reviewed by knowledgeable peers?

Notter [17] and Abdellah and Levine [2] agree that clinical research is a top priority in today's nursing research. Childbearing is a fertile area for the generation of nursing research ideas. At a time when nursing is developing in so many new professional directions, we must depend on active and sound nursing research to provide us with the firm foundation for our growing practice.

REFERENCES

1. Aamodt, A. Culture. In A. Clark (Ed.), *Culture, Childbearing, Health Professionals.* Philadelphia: Davis, 1978.
2. Abdellah, F., and Levine, E. *Better Patient Care Through Nursing Research.* New York: Macmillan, 1965.
3. Adams, M., Oakley, G., and Marks, J. Maternal age and births in the 1980's. *Journal of the American Medical Association* 247:493, 1981.
4. Castles, M. R. A practitioner's guide to utilization of research findings. *Journal of Obstetric, Gynecologic and Neonatal Nursing* 4(1):50, 1975.
5. Eisner, V., Pratt, M., Hexter, A., Chabot, M., and Soyal, N. Improvement in infant and perinatal mortality in the United States, 1965–1973: Priorities for intervention. *American Journal of Public Health* 68:359, 1978.
6. Fromer, M. *Ethical Issues in Health Care.* St. Louis: Mosby, 1981.
7. Garner, V. Cultural Aspects of Health and Illness Behaviors in Childbearing. In L. McNall (Ed.). *Contemporary Obstetric and Gynecologic Nursing.* St. Louis: Mosby, 1980.
8. Gatewood, T. S., and Stewart, R. Obstetricians and nurse-midwives: The team approach in private practice. *American Journal of Obstetrics and Gynecology* 123:35, 1975.
9. Harrison, L. K. Making a good thing better: The regionalization of neonatal intensive care units. *Journal of Obstetric, Gynecologic and Neonatal Nursing* 4(3):49, 1975.
10. Hawkins, M. Nursing and regionalization of perinatal services. *Journal of Obstetric, Gynecologic and Neonatal Nursing* 9:215, 1980.
11. Hellegers, A. Ethical Issues in Obstetrics. In S. Aladjem (Ed.), *Obstetrical Practice.* St. Louis: Mosby, 1980.
12. Horan, M. Genetic counseling: Helping the family. *Journal of Obstetric, Gynecologic and Neonatal Nursing* 6(5):25, 1977.
13. Korones, S. *High-Risk Newborn Infants.* St. Louis: Mosby, 1981.
14. Leininger, M. *Transcultural Health Care Issues and Conditions.* Philadelphia: Davis, 1976.
15. Maurice, S., And Warrick, L. Ethics in professional nursing practice. *Journal of Obstetric, Gynecologic and Neonatal Nursing* 8:327, 1979.
16. National Center for Health Statistics. Annual summary of births, deaths, marriages and divorces: United States, 1980. *Monthly Vital Statistics Report*, September 17, 1981. DPHS Publication No. (PHS) 81-1120.
17. Notter, L. The vital significance of clinical nursing research. *Cardio-Vascular Nursing* 8:19, 1972.

18. Pritchard, J., and MacDonald, P. *Williams Obstetrics* (16th ed.). New York: Appleton-Century-Crofts, 1980.
19. Ross, M. G. Health impact of a nurse midwife program. *Nursing Research* 30:353, 1981.
20. Schlesinger, E. Neonatal intensive care: Planning for services and outcomes following care. *Journal of Pediatrics* 82:916, 1973.
21. Sklar, J., and Berkov, B. The American birth rate: Evidences of a coming rise. *Science* 189:693, 1975.

FURTHER READING

Allgaier, A. Alternative birth centers offer family-centered care. *Hospitals* 52:97, 1978.
Aubry, R. H. ACOG: Standards for Safe Childbearing. In D. Stewart and L. Stewart (Eds.), *21st Century Obstetrics Now!* Marble Hill, Mo: NAPSAC, Inc., 1977.
Birth defect monitoring system. *National Foundation—Maternal Newborn Advocate*, Vol. 2. February 1975.
Boyd, S., and Mahon, P. The family-centered cesarean delivery. *The American Journal of Maternal-Child Nursing* 5:176, 1980
Brown, M. A cross-cultural look at pregnancy, labor, and delivery. *Journal of Obstetric, Gynecologic and Neonatal Nursing* 5(5):35, 1976.
Chase, H. C., and Nelson, F. Education of mother, medical care, and condition of infant. *American Journal of Public Health* 63(Supplement):27, 1973.
Clark, A. (Ed.). *Culture, Childbearing, Health Professionals.* Philadelphia: Davis, 1978.
Devitt, N. The statistical case for elimination of the midwife: Fact vs. prejudice, 1890–1935. Part I. *Women and Health* 4:81, 1979.
Devitt, N. The statistical case for elimination of the midwife: Fact vs. prejudice, 1890–1935. Part II. *Women and Health* 4:169, 1979.
Dillon, T. Midwifery 1977. *American Journal of Obstetrics and Gynecology* 130:917, 1978.
Eppink, H. Genetic causes of abnormal fetal development and inherited disease. *Journal of Obstetric, Gynecologic and Neonatal Nursing* 6(5):14, 1977.
Estes, M. A home obstetric service with expert consultation and back-up. *Birth and the Family Journal* 3:151, 1978.
Folk superstition and birth rate. (Editorial.) *Science News* 107:104, 1975.
Griffith, S. Childbearing and the concept of culture. *Journal of Obstetric, Gynecologic and Neonatal Nursing* 11:181, 1982.
Grosso, C., Barden, M., Henry, C., and Vieau, M. The Vietnamese American family. . . and grandma makes three. *The American Journal of Maternal-Child Nursing* 6:177, 1981.
Haire, M., Davidson, K. and Boehm, F. Perinatal nursing education in Tennessee: A regional approach. *Journal of Obstetric, Gynecologic and Neonatal Nursing* 10:451, 1981.
Hansen, F. Nursing care in the neonatal intensive care unit. *Journal of Obstetric, Gynecologic and Neonatal Nursing* 11:17, 1982.
Hazell, L. A study of 300 elective home births. *Birth and the Family Journal* 1:11, 1975.
Holden, J., and Holden, L. Perinatal research laboratories. *Medical Center Quarterly Report of the University of Michigan* 1:7, Winter 1974.
Hollingsworth, A., Brown, L., and Brooten, D. The new immigrants—childbearing practices. *RN* 43:44, 1980.
Intensive care for newborns: Are there times to pull the plug? (Editorial.) *Science* 188:133, 1975.
Jones, K., Smith, D., Harvey, M., Hall, B., and Quan, L. Older paternal age and fresh gene mutation. *Obstetrical and Gynecological Survey* 30:672, 1975.
Kieffer, G. *Bioethics: A Textbook of Issues.* Reading, Mass.: Addison-Wesley, 1979.
Lubic, R., and Ernst, E. The childbearing center: An alternative to conventional care. *Nursing Outlook* 12:754, 1978.
Maloni, J. The birthing room: Some insights into parents' experiences. *American Journal of Maternal-Child Nursing* 5:314, 1980.
Maurice, S., and Warrick, L. Ethics in professional nursing practice. *Journal of Obstetric, Gynecologic and Neonatal Nursing* 8:327, 1979.
Meleis, A., and Sorrell, L. Arab American women and their birth experiences. *American Journal of Maternal-Child Nursing* 6:171, 1981.
Perez, P. Nurturing children who attend the birth of a sibling. *American Journal of Maternal-Child Nursing* 4:215, 1979.
Purtilo, A., and Cassel, C. *Ethical Dimensions in the Health Professions.* Philadelphia: Saunders, 1981.
Quilligan, E. The obstetric intensive care unit. *Hospital Practice* 7:61, 1972.
Reame, N. E., and Hafez, F. S. Hereditary defects affecting fertility. *New England Journal of Medicine* 292:675, 1975.

Rising, S. A consumer-oriented nurse-midwifery service. *Nursing Clinics of North America* 10:251, 1975.

Rising, S., and Lindell, S. The childbearing center: A nursing model. *Nursing Clinics of North America* 17:11, 1982.

Roberts, D., Farr, L., Guthrie, R., and Nelson, R. Perinatal care. *Journal of the Kansas Medical Society* 75:259, 1974.

Sahin, S. The multifaceted role of the nurse as genetic counselor. *American Journal of Maternal-Child Nursing* 1:211, 1976.

Schlesinger, E., Lowery, W., Glaser, D., Milliones, M., and Mazumdar, S. A controlled test of the use of registered nurses for prenatal care. *Health Services Reports* 88:400, 1973.

Schmeck, H. Genetic flaws can come from father. *New York Times* February 24, 1980. E, 20.

Stern, P. Solving problems of cross-cultural health teaching: The Filipino childbearing family. *Image* 13:47, 1981.

Sweet, P. Prenatal classes especially for children. *American Journal of Maternal-Child Nursing* 4:82, 1979.

Terris, M., and Glasser, M. A life table analysis of the relation of prenatal care to prematurity. *American Journal of Public Health* 64:869, 1974.

Thompson, C. Legal aspects of genetic screening. *Journal of Obstetric, Gynecologic and Neonatal Nursing* 6(5):34, 1977.

U.S. Department of Health, Education and Welfare, Public Health Service. Promoting community health. DHEW Publication (HSA) 75-5016. Washington, D.C., 1975.

Westoff, C. The decline of unplanned births in the United States. *Science* 191:38, 1976.

Chapter 2 Reproductive Health Care of Women

Since early times health care for women has been concerned with their obstetric and gynecologic needs, regardless of whether the practitioners were men or women. In the United States, from 1845 on, the majority of women's health problems, whether physical or emotional, were attributed to diseases of their reproductive organs [21]. Historically, women's reproductive function has been associated with their intellectual functioning. In the late 1800s Edward Clarke, a Harvard professor, was convinced that after puberty females should not exercise their minds without restriction, since higher education left a great number of females in poor health for life. Clarke believed that work in a factory was far less damaging to a woman than schooling, since any educated woman tended to lose her "maternal instincts and become coarse and forceful" [5].

Other physicians proposed that overstimulation of the female brain stunted growth and caused nervousness, headaches, difficult childbirth, and insanity. Another educational variable was studied by Clelia Mosher, whose research into menstruation among college women from 1890 to 1920 indicated a correlation between dress and menstrual difficulties. Tight corsets and heavy skirts interfered with respiration, deformed the body, and resulted in chronic disturbances of the pelvic organs and prolonged menstrual pain and flow [5].

Given this perspective, it is not surprising that authors of obstetrics and gynecology texts have historically and consistently viewed women as though they were bipeds with little function other than reproduction and the duty to keep their husbands happy [33]. Physicians, particularly male obstetricians, gynecologists, and psychiatrists, have defined "normal" womanhood. They have determined whether women are healthy or sick and have treated women medically so that they could be "normal" again.

CURRENT SITUATION A recent review of advertisements in obstetric and medical journals shows that advertisers for that audience persist in portraying women as victims, sexy, dumb, or miserable [26]. More women than men are portrayed in these advertisements as having psychosomatic symptoms and as suffering from psychotropic illnesses. This observation is supported by Fidell [13] in her review of sex role stereotypes in health care. She states that some physicians do hold stereotypic views of women which predispose them to make a psychogenic diagnosis. Bernstein and Kane [4] reached the same conclusion using case simulations and questionnaires in a recent survey of 253 primary-care physicians. Twenty-five percent of the physicians believed that women were likely to make excessive demands on physician time, although only 14 percent believed this likely of men ($p < .01$). Women's complaints were judged more likely to be influenced by emotional factors (65% vs. 51% in men, $p < .01$) and were identified as psychosomatic more often than were men's complaints (21% vs. 9%, $p < .01$).

This general attitude is supported by Armitage [2] who found that physicians tend to take illness more seriously in men than in women. Armitage speculates that the finding may have been the result of the physicians' increased familiarity with the women (since they made more frequent visits) or that the physician was responding to current stereotypes that regard the male as typically stoic and the female as typically hypochondriac. On the other hand, a recent report by Verbrugge [39] suggests on the basis of data from the National Ambulatory Medical Care Survey that men and women are usually treated similarly for their complaints.

REACTIONS OF WOMEN

The failure of many obstetrician/gynecologists to recognize the individuality and intellectual capacities of many of their clients has led groups of concerned women to challenge this masculine stronghold. Today more women are asserting their need to define their femininity in their own terms and to assume some control and decision-making functions regarding their obstetric and gynecologic health care. In a few instances self-help has been seen by some angry women as the only alternative to subjecting themselves to humiliation and unwanted interference at the hands of otherwise qualified physicians. They feel compelled to sacrifice the advantages of scientific medicine in order to retain their self-respect [17]. In their view they are asking for relatively few concessions on the part of health professionals: primarily a redefinition of the doctor-patient relationship, including complete explanations of medical information, avoidance of unquestioned trust, and acceptance of "relevant others" in labor and delivery [17]. In general, physicians have been slow to respond in a positive manner to these requests. In view of the fact that health professionals in obstetrics and gynecology are primary care providers for many women who otherwise never have contact with the health care system, their relationships with their clients take on added relevance. According to Marieskind [21], about 40 percent of obstetrician/gynecologists in private practice report that 50 percent of their clients rely on them as primary physicians. According to other sources, evidence exists that as high as 86 percent of women see no other health care professional on a regular basis [38, 40]. It would be almost unpardonable if even a part of this segment of the population were to be deprived of adequate health care because of physician or institutional adherence to the traditional concept of health care professional dominance and the prevailing norms of the male-female relationship.

INCENTIVES TO CHANGE

The women's health movement has been influential in causing changes in women's health care delivery in three main areas: raising consciousness, providing health-related services (self-help groups), and attempting to change established health institutions [20]. Individuals such as Friedson [14], in analyzing the physician-patient relationship, a well-established health care phenomenon, have stated that professional policy should not be the only determinant of how patients should be managed in the course of their treatment. In a plea for recognition of patients' rights, Seiden [34] comments that unless a woman has some psychiatric disorder impairing her competence for decision-making, she should be treated as the person in charge who employs medical personnel as consultants and assistants rather than dictators. The physician's focus on illness, however, has only served to increase the woman's dependence on him or her. Also contributing to the physician's power position are high status, advanced education, and, in most instances, substantial income. If the physician chooses to address the woman as "honey" while she must address the physician by title and surname, the power difference is only emphasized. The women's movement has served to publicize some of these inequities in the physician-client relationship.

Even before the women's health movement gained momentum, American childbirth procedures were questioned. Groups such as the International Childbirth Education Association pointed out that some of the procedures that disregarded women's psychologic and physiologic needs were not well grounded in scientific research but were rooted in hospital and medical tradition [31]. Researchers have historically been interested in examining determinants of patient satisfaction with health care. Results of one study [7] indicated that satisfaction was directly related to a belief in the quality of care being received, a positive staff-patient relationship, and a positive evaluation of clinic procedures, especially when time and money were involved. Even in the early research it was evident that the presence of the nurse contributed in a substantial manner to the client's satisfaction with care [7]. A report in 1957 [28], well before the influence of the women's movement, pointed out the importance of human qualities in the physician's approach to patients.

A variety of investigators have looked specifically at the problem of determining what women want in obstetric care in order to have a satisfying childbearing experience. When questioned directly about their obstetrician/gynecologists, one group of women were more concerned with the physician's patronizing or dictatorial attitudes than with his or her capabilities as a physician [19]. Scaer and Korte [32] focused on institutional aspects of obstetric care in a survey of 645 mothers. They found that the four areas of greatest concern to the women were presence of the partner in labor and delivery, help and support from the hospital staff, increased contact between baby and mother, and more liberal visiting from their other children. Repeatedly, the expectations of pregnant women have included many items related to the concept of their participation and decision-making [25]. In general, the greater the woman's sense of participation, the higher her level of satisfaction [27].

In one nursing study of the labor and delivery experience [35], the sustaining presence of the nurse was the most frequently cited element related to the woman's satisfaction with her care. The second most frequently cited measure was an explanation of what was occurring. Generally the expressed needs of the 80 women in this study by Shields were categorized as maintenance of control, realization of expectations, and maintenance of self-esteem. In Butani and Hodnett's study of 50 women [6] the same items generally were specified as determinants of client satisfaction with the childbirth experience.

CHANGES IN CARE   Consumer dissatisfaction with the traditional hospital birthing process, desire for recognition of birth as a normal family event, and desire for individualized care have led not only to changes in traditional settings, the development of in-hospital birthing rooms and birthing centers, but also to home delivery services, usually by lay midwives, or (less frequently) by physicians and nurse midwives. The issue of an out-of-hospital birth is emotionally charged, but the data to firmly support arguments either for or against it are not plentiful. It has been difficult to obtain accurate data on home births, for example, because many members of the medical community have chosen to ignore these women [11]. These physicians have brought pressure to bear on colleagues who do attend home births with threats of loss of hospital admitting privileges, expulsion from the medical society, and, occasionally, loss of license [22]. Some of the research that has been done on women having births at home has shed light on their reasons for that choice: the comfortable home environment, distrust of medical professionals, the importance of the father's active role in the process, and a desire to assume personal responsibility for one of their major life decisions [15]. Mehl and others report that in 1,146 elective home births from five home delivery services in northern California, complication rates were lower than the California average [23].

Other cooperative efforts of consumers and client-oriented health care providers have resulted in the establishment of birthing centers within and outside of hospital settings [3, 12, 18]. The more closely these centers have followed guidelines that promote client autonomy and recognize client rights, such as the American Public Health Association guidelines for alternatives in maternity care [1], the greater the level of satisfaction expressed by the maternity clients. Some institutions, not willing to go as far as establishing an alternative birth center or birthing room, have made efforts along the lines of providing birthing beds [37], establishing day-care plans with short hospital stays and subsequent home visits by a nurse [16], or increasing policy flexibility which challenges such routines as "once a C-section, always a C-section" [24].

Increased demand for consumer participation has led to a resurgence in demand for the services of nurse midwives. Historically, nurse midwives have been oriented to meet the human needs of women in childbirth for noninterference and support, in addition to needs for safety. Nurse midwives have given birthing women the personal attention that physicians have often been too rushed to provide. It has even been suggested that the elimination of midwifery in the United States in the first part of this century slowed the decline in infant and maternal mortality [9]. Where midwives have been permitted to practice, patient outcomes have improved, including an increased percentage of patients returning for prenatal and postpartum visits [29, 36], an increase in visits for methods of contraception [29], and a low rate of complications [36]. Given the acceptance of nurse midwives by women [8, 10], this group of health professionals may hold the key to the ultimate provision of safe and satisfying obstetric services to a majority of childbearing clients. For reasons of economy and power, the idea is still not well accepted by many obstetricians.

IMPLICATIONS FOR THE FUTURE

For too long the energies of health professionals have ignored the needs of the normal or low-risk childbearing family. These needs are now receiving attention as part of a consumer-based movement questioning conventional childbirth practices and seeking to develop alternative approaches. The needs of these women have been broadly identified: to be treated as adults, to be informed, to give birth with the necessary support, to have a choice in the procedures that are pressed upon them [30]. The trend toward smaller families means that couples want to make each childbirth experience meaningful and satisfying. Research on parent-infant interaction has emphasized the importance of parent participation in the childbirth experience.

The recent self-help movement in women's health care demonstrates the gap that still exists between professional provider and client. It has forced some health care professionals to face the fact that while "customary procedure" may be an adequate defense against malpractice, it no longer serves to meet the needs of consumers. Since most routine procedures are not based on research data, health professionals must accept the fact that until they are subjected to empirical study, those procedures should be negotiable.

Because only a relatively small number of consumers are vocal in expressing their disappointment with the status quo, health professionals run the risk of falling into the trap of dismissing their input. A collaborative effort between professional and client will provide the solution to some of the health care delivery problems of today. Nurses, as client advocates, will play a key role in this endeavor.

REFERENCES

1. Alternatives in maternity care. *American Journal of Public Health* 70:310, 1980.
2. Armitage, K. Response of physicians to medical complaints in men and women. *Journal of the American Medical Association* 241:2186, 1979.
3. Barton, J., et al. Alternative birthing center: Experience in a teaching obstetric service. *American Journal of Obstetrics and Gynecology* 137:377, 1980.
4. Bernstein, B., and Kane, R. Physicians' attitudes toward female patients. *Medical Care* 19:600, 1981.
5. Bullough, V., and Voght, M. Women, menstruation, and nineteenth-century medicine. *Bulletin of the History of Medicine* 42:66, 1973.
6. Butani, P., and Hodnett, D. Mothers' perceptions of their labor experiences. *Maternal-Child Nursing Journal* 9:73, 1980.
7. Caplan, E., and Sussman, M. Rank order of important variables for patient and staff satisfaction with outpatient service. *Journal of Health and Human Behavior* 7:133, 1966.
8. Corea, G. *The Hidden Malpractice.* New York: Morrow, 1977.
9. Devitt N. The statistical case for elimination of the midwife: Fact versus prejudice, 1890–1935. *Women and Health* 4:81, 1979.
10. Dillon, T. Midwifery, 1977. *American Journal of Obstetrics and Gynecology* 130:916, 1978.
11. Epstein, J., and McCartney, M. A home birth service that works. *Birth and the Family Journal* 4:71, 1977.
12. Ernst, E., and Forde, M. Maternity care: An attempt at an alternative. *Nursing Clinics of North America* 10:241, 1975.
13. Fidell, L. Sex role stereotypes and the American physician. *Psychology of Women Quarterly* 4:313, 1980.
14. Friedson, E. *Profession of Medicine.* New York: Dodd, Mead, 1971.
15. Hazell, L. A study of 300 elective home births. *Birth and Family Journal* 2:11, 1975.
16. Hickey, L. Maternity day care program offers economical, family-oriented care. *Hospitals* 51(23):85, 1977.
17. Kaiser, B., and Kaiser, I. The challenge of the women's movement to American gynecology. *American Journal of Obstetrics and Gynecology* 120:652, 1974.
18. Kerner, J., and Ferris, C. An alternative birth center in a community teaching hospital. *Obstetrics and Gynecology* 51:371, 1978.
19. Luy, M. What's behind women's wrath toward gynecologists? *Modern Medicine* 42(21):17, 1974.
20. Marieskind, H. The women's health movement. *International Journal of Health Services* 5:216, 1975.
21. Marieskind, H. *Women in the Health System.* St. Louis: Mosby, 1980.
22. Mehl, L. Delivery in the home. *Comprehensive Therapy* 4(3):18, 1978.
23. Mehl, L., et al. Outcomes of elective home births: A series of 1146 cases. *Journal of Reproductive Medicine* 19:281, 1977.
24. Merrill, B., and Gibbs, C. Planned vaginal delivery following cesarean section. *Obstetrics and Gynecology* 52:50, 1978.
25. Micklethwait, L., et al. Expectations of a pregnant woman in relation to her treatment. *British Medical Journal* 2:188, 1978.
26. Moyer, L. What obstetrical journal advertising tells about doctors and women. *Birth and Family Journal* 2:111, 1975.
27. Nunnally, D., and Aguiar, M. Patients' evaluation of their prenatal and delivery care. *Nursing Research* 23:469, 1974.
28. Reader, G., et al. What patients expect from their doctors. *Modern Hospital* 89:88, 1957.

29. Record, J., and Cohen, H. The introduction of midwifery in a prepaid group practice. *American Journal of Public Health* 62:354, 1972.
30. Riley, E. What Do Women Want—The Question of Choice in the Conduct of Labor. In T. Chard and M. Richards (Eds.), *Benefits and Hazards of the New Obstetrics*. Philadelphia: Lippincott, 1977.
31. Ruzek, S. *The Women's Health Movement*. New York: Praeger, 1978.
32. Scaer, R., and Korte, D. MOM survey: Maternity options for mothers—what do women want in maternity care? *Birth and Family Journal* 5:20, 1978.
33. Scully, D., and Bart, P. A funny thing happened on the way to the orifice: Women in the gynecology textbooks. *American Journal of Sociology* 78:1045, 1973.
34. Seiden, A. The maternal sense of mastery in primary care obstetrics. *Primary Care* 3:717, 1976.
35. Shields, E. Nursing care in labor and patient satisfaction. *Journal of Advanced Nursing* 3:535, 1978.
36. Slome, C., et al. Effectiveness of certified nurse midwives. *American Journal of Obstetrics and Gynecology* 124:177, 1976.
37. Sumner, P., et al. The labor-delivery bed-simplified obstetrics. *Journal of Reproductive Medicine* 13:158, 1974.
38. The obstetrician and gynecologist: Primary physician for women. *Journal of the American Medical Association* 231:815, 1975.
39. Verbrugge, L. Physician treatment of men and women patients. *Medical Care* 19:609, 1981.
40. Willson, J., and Burkons, D. Obstetrician-gynecologists are primary physicians to women. *American Journal of Obstetrics and Gynecology* 136:744, 1976.

FURTHER READING   Anderson, S. Childbirth as a pathological process: An American perspective. *American Journal of Maternal-Child Nursing* 2:240, 1977.

Burchell, R., and Gunn, J. The new birth experience. *Journal of Obstetric, Gynecologic and Neonatal Nursing* 9:250, 1980.

Collier, P. Health behaviors of women. *Nursing Clinics of North America* 17:121, 1982.

Derby, G. An approach to health assessment of women. *Nursing Clinics of North America* 17:127, 1982.

Devitt, N. The transition from home to hospital birth in the U.S. *Birth and the Family Journal* 4:47, 1977.

Dunbar, S., Patterson, E., Burton, C., and Stukert, G. Women's health and nursing research. *Advances in Nursing Science* 4:1, 1981.

LaGodna, G. The single rural woman: Invisible struggles. *Advances in Nursing Science* 4:17, 1981.

Lieberman, J. Childbirth practices: From darkness into light. *Journal of Obstetric, Gynecologic and Neonatal Nursing* 5(3):41, 1976.

Lovell, M. Silent but perfect "partners": Medicine's use and abuse of women. *Advances in Nursing Science* 4:25, 1981.

McGrellis, N. Labor and delivery 120 years ago. *Journal of Obstetric, Gynecologic and Neonatal Nursing* 5(3):56, 1976.

Mehl, L. Options in maternity care. *Nursing Dimensions* 7(1):26, 1979.

Stimeling, G. Will common delivery techniques soon become malpractice? *Journal of Legal Medicine* 5:20, 1975.

Wertz, R., and Wertz, D. *Lying-in: A History of Childbirth in America*. New York: Schocken, 1979.

Woods, N. Women's health: Perspectives for nursing research. *Nursing Clinics of North America* 17:113, 1982.

Chapter 3 Sexuality

An individual's awareness of his own body is never complete, since his body is constantly changing throughout life. Therefore, revision of his perception of his body image occurs often. Recognition of one's body as weak or strong, big or little, sickly or healthy, sexually alive or unresponsive is a significant part of one's total sense of identity.

Infancy is filled with experiences that help bring about a sense of the body and its capacities for pleasure and discomfort. Babies are frequently observed exploring their bodies. They learn to be comfortable with their bodies and find them a source of pleasure, especially if their parents are warm and consistent in touching and handling them.

During the preschool years, the child's basic concept of himself as a sexual being is developed. This conception is positively or negatively reinforced by the reactions he receives when he explores or exposes his body. Children at this age begin to question where babies come from, especially if a new baby is expected in the family; however, unless adults bring up the subjects of conception or intercourse, the preschooler is rarely interested in such explicit information.

As Broderick [5] notes, during these years several factors are especially important in the development of the child's sexual identity. One important element is his or her self-image as a boy or a girl, an identification constantly reinforced by adults and other children. In establishing his identity, the preschooler is always absorbing styles, mannerisms, speech patterns, attitudes, and assumptions of people surrounding him. Equally important to his identity are his experiences with adults and children of the opposite sex and his feelings about a lasting relationship with a member of the opposite sex. It is interesting to note that the majority of 5-year-olds are already committed to the idea of eventual marriage for themselves.

Another influential factor on a child's sexual identity is the child's relationship with his parents. If his parents accept his gender at birth and provide a warm, loving, and consistent environment, the child is more likely to incorporate their standards and social values than he would be if discord existed between parents, or between parents and the child. The behavioral patterns established during this period affect the child's future emotional and sexual life.

The experiences of preadolescence are an important shaping force in an individual's sexuality. There is a wide range of knowledge of sexual matters in this age group. Most children have some idea that pregnancy and childbirth are related to sexual intercourse. Girls' questions mainly involve menstruation and pregnancy, while boys ask for definitions of slang terms as well as information about pregnancy and intercourse.

Children of this age tend to group with peers of the same sex, practicing their own sexual roles before interacting comfortably with members of the opposite sex. They may privately choose a special girlfriend or boyfriend, but their choice is usually kept to themselves, giving them an opportunity to fantasize emotional involvement with this special person without fear of rejection or humiliation. While they rehearse this emotional commitment in their own imaginations, they are developing some of the social skills useful in boy-girl relations.

During adolescence there is a shift from questions about menstruation, intercourse, and conception to questions about sexual standards and social relationships between boys and girls. The younger adolescent is concerned with standards and values, whereas the older adolescent is more interested in the psychology of social relationships. Self-understanding and sensitivity to others are the key assets that can be acquired during this period.

For young men ejaculation serves as a symbol of sexual maturity, and for girls menstruation does the same. The frequent erections that a young male adolescent has may be embarrassing at times. Masturbation is his major source of sexual release; although it is a positive and gratifying experience, it also may provoke guilt and anxiety. Masturbation rates in females are generally lower. In our society, females are encouraged to be sexually stimulating to men but not necessarily to act on their own sexual needs.

Petting is one of the most common forms of sexual behavior during the late teens, when the focus is on the strategy of boy-girl relations. This period of life is more supportive to a person's sexual self-image than any other because the beginning process of courtship, which occurs most commonly in this age group, is very flattering. Relationships based on exploitation are usually rejected in favor of those based on mutual concern.

There are a few periods in the life cycle at which there are high rates of sexual activity. These are usually adolescence for the male, the early and romantic years of marriage for men and women, and, for some, later periods of highly charged extramarital affairs. Most of the time sexual activity is less intense.

Cultures that encourage women to respond sexually produce women who generally have a sexual response equal to that of men. If female sexuality is discouraged, female response tends to be weaker. Masters and Johnson [16] postulate that females have a greater capacity for sexual response than males, and that cultural restraints have been imposed in order to provide a better balance between the sexes.

Middle age can be a difficult period sexually because of decreasing sexual powers, dissatisfaction with some aspects of marriage, and unflattering physical changes. Sexual difficulties in middle age are closely related to deterioration of self-image and self-confidence.

Advancing age is seen as the end of sexuality by some, and waning sexual prowess is often confronted by ridicule. At age 60, 75 percent of men can achieve intercourse, 30 percent at age 70, and 14 to 20 percent at 80 [5]. The aging female is capable of orgasmic response indefinitely if regularly exposed to effective sexual stimulation. During menopause many women face an identity crisis as their roles as wives and mothers change when children leave home or husbands die.

RELIGIOUS INFLUENCES

Of all the factors (such as social class, ethnic background, and age) that may influence a person's concept of sexuality, religious identity may be one of the most important, since it influences almost every aspect of life.

Jewish history [3] reflects changes in attitudes toward sexual conduct, varying from restrictive to permissive, depending on the degree of orthodoxy. Jewish tradition has always prized modesty; it has also given full recognition to the sexuality of women, even ascribing to them a greater sex drive than that of men.

It praises premarital chastity but imposes no penalty for its violation. Procreation is not considered the sole function of intercourse although contraception other than for medical reasons is regarded as sinful even today by many Orthodox Jews. Abortion is generally considered acceptable when the mother's life or mental health is in jeopardy. Thus, nonpuritanical attitudes accompanied by a self-imposed discipline of sexual restraint appear to be the general trend among present-day Jewish people.

Early Christianity emphasized the monogamous family and the moral upbringing of children. Sex was often equated with sin. Women's sexuality and pleasure in sex were denied, while men were inhibited in their sexual attitudes. For both men and women, sex was associated with guilt. Sexual intercourse was considered acceptable only in marriage and only for the purpose of procreation, and many prohibitions were placed on the manner in which intercourse could take place. Even today in certain states, married couples can be convicted as criminals for using certain positions of intercourse or forms of caresses, such as oral-genital contact.

Generally, attitudes of Protestants toward sexuality [21, 28] rely less upon religious authority than those of Catholics or Jews, but this does not imply greater sexual freedom. Early Protestant church leaders saw sexual drives as basic needs and wished to create a more accepting atmosphere; however, prudery and shame became the prevailing attitudes. Luther doubted that any man or woman could be free from lust since the libido was overwhelmingly strong. Marriage then became a remedy for concupiscence. Calvin saw sex in marriage as proper and decent, not lustful. Contemporary Protestantism includes attitudes ranging from acceptance of premarital expressions of affection to disapproval of dancing and movies. Supporters of a traditional morality are in the majority and disapprove of sex outside of marriage. Divorce is permitted, however, and contraception is acceptable.

Catholicism, more than the other major religions, has definite rules regarding the sexual behavior of its followers [25]. While it does not deny the pleasures associated with sexual intercourse, it sees procreation as its main purpose. Premarital and extramarital sex are not allowed. The fundamental premise is based on a relationship between sex and marriage that involves two basic concerns: the protection of human life in every form and respect for the meaning or significance of an act as revealed in its objective "natural" structure. Any deliberate attempt to inhibit the normal structure and progress of the physiologic process initiated when a couple has intercourse constitutes an objective immoral act. Thus the rhythm and cervical mucus methods of contraception are the only acceptable ones, since they involve cooperation with nature through periodic abstinence. Pope Paul VI's position in the encyclical *Humanae Vitae*, emphasizing that the marital act must always be open to procreation, continues to be supported by current Church leadership.

During the past 20 years, a number of Catholic scholars have seriously questioned the adequacy of the Church's sexual ethics. The Council Fathers of Vatican II took these criticisms under consideration. They recognized the implications of the current population growth trend, acknowledging the need for some form of family regulation. They displayed a mature understanding of the sexual dimensions of conjugal love. This may have marked the beginning of a careful reformulation of the specifically Catholic approach to human sexuality in the light of contemporary cultural and theological developments.

The underlying philosophy remains the same, however. Since sexual relations are designed both to unite the partners as persons and to provide for the continuity of the human race through parenthood, responsible sex can be engaged in only by married couples. Their commitment to a community of life and love within which they can strive for mutual fulfillment and happiness helps them create the human environment in which children can be fittingly raised.

SOCIOECONOMIC
INFLUENCES

While religion may have significant influences on sexuality, so too may cultural and socioeconomic background. In today's middle class there is certainly much less role segregation than existed in the past. More women now maintain jobs outside the home and share childrearing with their mates. Today's ideal of marriage is a relationship between husband and wife built on happiness, communication, and mutual gratification. This is also true in the sexual sphere, where there is emphasis on the partners' recognizing each other's needs and working toward satisfaction for both.

Brenton [4] sees this shift as a challenge for today's men. He notes that the contemporary male faces sexual responsibilities far exceeding those of men in the past. Today a man must gratify both himself and his sexual partner. He must make sure he is a good lover. In addition, he must cope with the sexually liberated woman, something that can require a considerable amount of adjustment.

Many contemporary women suffer from sexual inhibition caused by their socialization, by feelings of guilt, and by overemphasis on the importance of sex in addition to the new expectations of mutuality. All of these factors may serve to intensify the problem of sexual adjustment for couples today.

In the lower socioeconomic groups, role segregation is still predominant, clearly defining what role is appropriately male or female. In general the male is still viewed as the head of the household and expects to offer little help in household tasks and childrearing. The double standard is still more firmly entrenched in the lower class than in the middle class. Further, in families of lower socioeconomic status there is a tendency for men and women to enjoy the company of and rely heavily on a close-knit group of friends and relatives of the same sex.

In some subcultures boys are expected to engage in sex with girls whenever the opportunity arises. A reputation for "making out" is very valuable within peer groups. Thus, boys must learn patterns of seduction and their ability is then judged by their peers.

Girls, on the other hand, often operate under different rules. In some subcultures girls are rated according to their degree of promiscuity. Virgins are highly valued and often protected, especially in Italian, Greek, Spanish, and Portuguese societies [22]. Girls who have sex with only one boy may have status, especially if they later marry him. More promiscuous girls are regarded as "easy lays." Overall within these subcultural groups, girls are protected from sexual stimulation, and efforts are made to conceal from them basic facts about sex and their future sexual roles.

According to research done by Rainwater [19, 20], many young black girls in the ghettos are not expected to be virginal unless they are not mature enough or unless they lack the opportunity. The fear of being taken advantage of or getting into trouble, however, may leave them with an ambivalence toward having intercourse. Having sex may also be looked on as a test or symbol of maturity. Pregnancy, however, is seen as the real measure of maturity for some young women, just as fathering a child confers maturity on some boys and young men. If the girl does become pregnant, value is placed on establishing the identity of the father since this confers a form of legitimacy on the birth. Within the black ghetto family many parents often feel helpless about adolescent sexual behavior, and, while they do not necessarily have an attitude of approval toward illegitimate birth, they are often more tolerant of it as a reality of life.

SEXUAL OUTLETS   While masturbation, oral-genital lovemaking, and erotic dreams may release sexual tension, intercourse provides the major sexual outlet for most men and women. As with any facet of a relationship, sexual intercourse becomes entwined in a complex of emotions—love, affection, and companionship, as well as physical attraction.

Historically, in some groups intercourse has been viewed as a husband's pleasure and a wife's duty. Today it is generally recognized and accepted that it should be mutually satisfying, thus enhancing intimacy and nurturing a growth of trust between partners. This approach is important, for as Kinsey and associates [13] note, many partners report pain and nervousness following intense arousal that is not followed by orgasm. Two main deterrents to reaching orgasm may be fatigue and preoccupation; therefore, an awareness of the feelings and responses of the partner is essential in lovemaking.

While biological mechanisms are involved, learning is also required to find optimal patterns of sexual gratification for both partners. It should be kept in mind that everyone at times may experience difficulties of shyness, aversion, or unresponsiveness. During pregnancy when a couple's usual technique becomes uncomfortable for either partner or is no longer satisfying, experimentation may become necessary. Preferable positions may involve them lying on their sides either face to face or with the man entering the woman from the rear.

In addition to varying positions, other techniques may be employed during pregnancy. Oral-genital contact may be used, perhaps for the first time. In talking with an expectant couple, you might mention that many couples rely on this technique more frequently during pregnancy, when their usual method is no longer satisfying. Oral-genital contact may be used to achieve orgasm, or it may be used in foreplay to arouse either partner and to maintain or effect an erection in the male.

Masturbation is another technique that is often used during pregnancy, particularly by the male partner. While its use normally begins in childhood and peaks during adolescence, masturbation is very common in the middle and later years. Better educated men, both single and married, tend to masturbate more often than those in the lower socioeconomic class. Women who have difficulty achieving orgasm are advised to try masturbation so that they may learn about their body's responses in a private and relaxed way.

Most authorities now agree that masturbation should be viewed as a normal sexual outlet. This has hardly been the view throughout history, however. To our grandparents it was a sinful perversion that caused warts, impotence, blindness, or even madness. To carry on the battle against masturbation, a public figure named Henry Varlie delivered a lecture in 1833 to an attentive audience. The 3,000 men listened as he dealt with onanism, or self-abuse, a practice as common as it was hateful and injurious. He pointed out the results—a low stature, contracted chest, weak lungs, liability to a sore throat, a tendency to colds, indigestion, depression, drowsiness, and idleness. In addition, he declared that disease, decay, and death among young men were chiefly caused by this terrible practice. Needless to say, the lecture was a success and was subsequently published in book form. Respected physicians then advocated a treatment—cold showers and exercise in the open air. While all of this hardly changed the public's masturbating practices, it did have an effect on attitudes toward them. Some people still attribute premature ejaculation, impotence, or lassitude to masturbation, but there is no proven direct relationship [2, 26].

While masturbation is considered a normal practice, it can be considered excessive if it becomes the exclusive form of sexual expression when alternatives are available. It may be used as a conscious substitute for interpersonal love and, in this way, may signify withdrawal, reinforcing timidity about forming social and sexual relationships. When used excessively it may also signify a deeper underlying problem in a relationship, perhaps a breakdown in communication or perhaps the inability of a couple to come to sexual terms with each other. During adolescence excessive masturbation may be a symptom of conflicts such as boredom, frustration, loneliness, poor self-image, school pressures, or conflicts with parents. The adolescent uses masturbation to relieve tension, but the conflicts themselves must be resolved, usually through counseling.

Before you can help others cope with their sexual needs, you should be aware of your own sexual values. Consider the influences your life experiences have had on your feelings about your own sexuality. You need to be sensitive to others' views on sex and sexuality that may be quite different from your own, and you need to respect others' rights to those views. Perhaps most of all, recognize that people's sexual needs are as important as the more obvious physical needs that are traditionally identified.

Examine your attitudes toward masturbation, premarital and extramarital intercourse, oral-genital sexual activity, and sex during pregnancy and post partum [29]. Even the most liberal among us often have strong feelings about these subjects, feelings that may affect our ability to make objective assessments about clients and to assist them as effectively as possible. Sexually knowledgeable nurses who are aware of their own feelings are less likely to be shocked by clients who reveal intimate sexual information and less likely to censure clients' behavior or the language they use to describe their sexual activity.

As a nurse, you have an ideal opportunity to counsel pregnant women and their partners about sexuality during childbearing. You have an obligation to correct misinformation the couple may have, to clear up their confusion, and to assist them with their sexual adaptation to pregnancy. Obtaining a sexual history is the first step in this process. In taking a sexual history you should communicate your comfort in talking about sex and encourage the couple to discuss sexual concerns, indicating that the topic is an appropriate part of health care during pregnancy [29]. You might begin by exploring the following areas [1, 10, 27, 29].

ASSESSMENT
Relevant Health History

What was the woman's age at menarche? Have menstrual periods been trouble-some? How many pregnancies has the woman had? Any abortions? Has the couple been satisfied with their method of contraception? How is their overall health? Has the couple had problems with intercourse in the past? Frequency? Pain? Adequate lubrication? Is either partner taking medication that might interfere with sexual performance?

Attitudinal Factors

What are the couple's feelings about masturbation, oral-genital sex? About intercourse, masturbation, and oral-genital sex during pregnancy? Do the wom-an's ideas differ from her partner's? How have the frequency and pattern of their sexual activity changed since pregnancy?

Sexual Self-concept

What are the couple's feelings about childbirth, breast-feeding, baby care? How does pregnancy make the woman feel? How does it make her partner feel? How does the couple feel about the changes in the woman's appearance? Do they feel that maternity clothes make the pregnant woman more attractive?

Couple's Relationship

Was the pregnancy planned? How will their lives be changed by having a baby? How has their life together changed already? What plans have been interrupted? How do they plan to manage the changes and interruptions?

Knowledge Level

What is their knowledge of pregnancy and its effect on sexuality? What have they been told about sex in pregnancy? What is their expectation of what is going to occur?

PLANNING AND INTERVENTION

Several nurse researchers [6, 9, 12, 14, 24] have investigated the needs and concerns expressed by women and their partners regarding their sexuality during pregnancy and the postpartum period. Their findings contain a number of common areas that deserve your attention when you plan interventions based on assessment of the sexual knowledge and activity of the pregnant woman and her partner.

Coital Positions

Couples are often concerned about the difficulty in maintaining satisfactory sexual activity when discomfort or awkwardness of position presents a barrier. Pain (dyspareunia) usually results from pressure on the woman's pregnant abdomen or from deep penile thrusting. If the woman's symphysis pubis has separated due to relaxation of supportive ligaments, she will have severe pain on pelvic motion. You might recommend a change in position. The side-by-side position is helpful in early pregnancy, especially when temporary breast tender-ness may be a problem. Couples should be encouraged to use a position where pressure is not put on the woman's breasts and to decrease breast-fondling as a part of lovemaking. Reassure them that the breast tenderness should be tempo-rary. The female superior position is helpful since no pressure is put on the woman's abdomen and she can control the depth of penetration, lifting off her partner if she becomes uncomfortable. In late pregnancy a rear entry position may be preferred, since, again, there is no pressure on the woman's abdomen which is supported on the bed. Rear entry may be accomplished "dog fashion" also.

Amount of Sexual Activity

Many couples are concerned about the changes in their desire for sexual activity during pregnancy. Research in this area has not been conclusive, although a majority of researchers have found that coital activity and incidence of orgasm are usually below the prepregnant level and decrease as pregnancy advances [7, 11, 23]. (Masters and Johnson [16] have been the only researchers to find a great increase in eroticism and sexual activity during the second and early third trimesters of pregnancy.)

It has been theorized that such changes in sexual activity occur because of many factors, such as nausea and vomiting, breast tenderness, fatigue and sleepiness in the first trimester; fear of harming the fetus of the woman (especially if a previous baby was born with an anomaly); fear of infection; feeling of loss of attractiveness; partner's loss of interest; couple's fear that the fetus can hear or see them having intercourse; and frustration with changing interest levels. Ellis [6] found that instead of intercourse many couples desired other forms of sexual activity such as touching, cuddling, stroking, and masturbation. It is essential for you to emphasize the importance of communication between the woman and her partner, so that each is aware of the other's feelings. Sometimes it can be reassuring to them to hear that these are the usual feelings that pregnant couples have.

Safety of Sexual Activity

The research that has been done has not produced conclusive evidence that coitus during pregnancy is harmful. It has demonstrated that coital response does slow fetal heart rate but there has been no evidence of fetal distress [16]. It has been postulated that prostaglandins in the male ejaculate may stimulate uterine contractions which could result in premature labor [15]. Research [8, 18, 23] has not confirmed this cause-and-effect reaction. Naeye [17] has concluded that coitus during pregnancy may result in amniotic fluid infection; however, he has not recommended coital abstinence but rather has urged that couples observe fastidious perineal cleanliness or use condoms to decrease the possibility of infection.

You should generally recommend that intercourse would be inadvisable for varying periods of time if the woman has a history of more than one spontaneous abortion, a threatened abortion in the first trimester, an impending fetal loss in the second trimester, a premature rupture of membranes, or pain or bleeding in the third trimester. You should caution against masturbation as well if orgasm for the woman is prohibited, since orgasm by masturbation is more intense than the orgasm of intercourse. Sometimes in very late pregnancy when the fetal head is engaged and the cervix is lower in the vagina, vigorous penile thrusting may cause the penis to strike the cervix, causing vaginal bleeding. In this case, advise the couple to use an alternative to intercourse for sexual satisfaction. In many instances, if you carefully explain the reasons for abstinence from intercourse, the couple's negative feelings will be greatly reduced.

Orgasmic Changes

In the last trimester orgasmic contractions may be tonic rather than rhythmic. They may be followed by cramps and backache. You could recommend that the woman's partner give her a soothing back rub following intercourse to relieve this discomfort.

First Coitus
Post Partum

It has been common practice to advise couples to refrain from intercourse for 6 weeks post partum, a longer time than is physiologically necessary. Physiologically it is possible for couples to resume intercourse by the third postpartum week, provided that lochial discharge has stopped and the episiotomy has healed. (In one study [9] the mean time in which 42 couples chose to resume intercourse was 4.4 weeks, so it is obvious that couples do not abide by advice that is unrealistic. Nevertheless, they often feel guilty about "disobeying orders.") Advise couples that for about 3 months post partum they might expect physical responses to sexual stimulation to be less rapid and less intense, and the woman's orgasms may be shorter and weaker. You should recommend the continuation of sitz baths to hasten episiotomy healing.

Postpartal
Dyspareunia

Persistent vulvar varicosities may be painful, but sitz baths or witch hazel compresses may be helpful. Sitz baths will also help the tender perineum, as mentioned above. A torn or greatly stretched perineal body may lead to a gaping vaginal orifice and decreased orgasmic response. Recommend continuation of perineal tightening (Kegel) exercises to strengthen the pubococcygeal muscle. The use of a side-by-side or female superior position for intercourse will also allow for more control by the woman. If the woman is experiencing vaginal tenderness, you might recommend that her partner insert two fingers into her vagina to identify specific areas of discomfort and to relax the pubococcygeal muscle.

Vaginal Lubrication

For up to the first 6 months post partum, vaginal lubrication may not be adequate due to lack of hormonal stimulation. You can recommend the use of a sterile, unscented, water-soluble gel or contraceptive cream or jelly to solve this problem.

Increased Pleasure

The pregnancy effect of increased vascularization may result in marked pelvic engorgement which requires several hours of resolution after sexual arousal. This may produce a pleasurable effect.

Breast Changes

The lactating woman may lose milk in involuntary spurts in response to sexual stimulation. You might recommend that during lovemaking the woman wear a bra with absorbent pads if the couple finds the release of milk distasteful. For the majority of men, the woman's enlarged breasts provide no extra sexual stimulation, although there are a number of male partners who report the opposite opinion.

Vaginal Discharge

If the couple's lovemaking is inhibited because of vaginal discharge, it is probably because they are concerned about the discomfort, the messiness, or the healing process. This does not pose a problem for the majority of men and women post partum.

Fear of Infection

If the couple expresses fear of infection, you might recommend fastidious perineal cleanliness or the use of a condom during intercourse.

Relationship Between
the Partners

Attempts to resume sexual activity may lead to relationship problems postpartally because of fatigue, sleeplessness, discomfort, or vaginal discharge. The woman may be so involved in caring for the baby that her energy level is depleted when sexual activity is suggested by her partner. The couple also may fear that the baby may waken during their lovemaking. Again, communication between the woman and her partner is essential if the relationship is to grow. If each partner is sensitized to the needs of the other, the task may be accomplished more easily. You might explain the physiology of postpartum sexual changes to them, reassuring them that they can respond to each other but that it will take a period of time. It might be helpful to recommend that the male partner give the woman extra caressing, kissing, and holding in order to arouse her. In addition you might recommend that they use alternative forms of sexual expression during this period.

With the exception of Masters and Johnson's work [16], most studies of sex during pregnancy have been retrospective, have involved only the woman, and have focused on coitus during pregnancy as a potential source of pathology. From the nursing research in this area, Swanson [24], Hames [9], and Kyndely [14] have arrived at a set of recommendations for health professionals to follow in their work with couples during pregnancy.

1. Prenatal care should include both the woman and her partner, equally and individually.
2. Education and counseling should include discussion of the normal and expected physiologic and psychologic changes of pregnancy and post partum. It should include information about birth control.
3. Male partners need male support. Recognize this and plan for it in the context of giving care.
4. Sexual activity during pregnancy should be discussed with both partners. If intercourse is prohibited, discuss the reason with the couple, specifying which sexual activities may be used as safe substitutes.
5. Instruct all couples in the use of various positions and techniques for intercourse and sexual stimulation. Inform couples that orgasm, whether through vaginal intercourse or manual stimulation, results in uterine contractions.
6. Continually assess the couple's interactions for the effects of childbearing on their family and be sensitive to their needs.
7. Inform nursing mothers that sexual arousal may cause involuntary milk leakage.
8. Inform couples that they may resume sexual activity postpartally as soon as bleeding has stopped, discomfort has disappeared, and they are psychologically ready.
9. Give the woman and her partner opportunities to ask questions.

REFERENCES

1. Adams, G. The sexual history as an integral part of the patient history. *American Journal of Maternal-Child Nursing* 1:170, 1976.
2. Alexander, J. Masturbation as a substitute. *Man and Woman* (Part 27) 2:729, 1972.
3. Borowitz, E. *Choosing a Sex Ethic (A Jewish Inquiry)*. New York: Schocken, 1969.
4. Brenton, M. *The American Male*. New York: Coward-McCann, 1966.
5. Broderick, C. Normal Sociosexual Development. In C. Broderick and J. Bernard (Eds.), *The Individual, Sex, and Society*. Baltimore: Johns Hopkins Press, 1969.
6. Ellis, D. Sexual needs and concerns of expectant parents. *Journal of Obstetric, Gynecologic and Neonatal Nursing* 9:306, 1980.
7. Falicov, C. Sexual adjustment during first pregnancy and postpartum. *American Journal of Obstetrics and Gynecology* 117:991, 1973.

8. Goodlin, R., Keller, D., and Raffin, M. Orgasm during late pregnancy. *Obstetrics and Gynecology* 38:916, 1971.
9. Hames, C. Sexual needs and interests of postpartum couples. *Journal of Obstetric, Gynecologic and Neonatal Nursing* 9:313, 1980.
10. Hogan, R. *Human Sexuality: A Nursing Perspective.* New York: Appleton-Century-Crofts, 1980.
11. Holtzman, L. Sexual practices during pregnancy. *Journal of Nurse Midwifery* 21(1):22, 1976.
12. Inglis, T. Postpartum sexuality. *Journal of Obstetric, Gynecologic and Neonatal Nursing* 9:298, 1980.
13. Kinsey, A., Pomeroy, W. B., Martin, C. E., and Gebhard, P. H. *Sexual Behavior in the Human Female.* New York: Pocket Books, 1965.
14. Kyndely, K. The sexuality of women in pregnancy and postpartum: A review. *Journal of Obstetric, Gynecologic and Neonatal Nursing* 7(1):28, 1978.
15. Mann, E., and Armstead, T. Pregnancy and Sexual Behavior. In B. Sadock, H. Kaplan, and A. Freedman (Eds.), *The Sexual Experience.* Baltimore: Williams & Wilkins, 1976.
16. Masters, W. H., and Johnson, V. E. *Human Sexual Inadequacy.* Boston: Little, Brown, 1970.
17. Naeye, R. Coitus and associated amniotic fluid infections. *New England Journal of Medicine* 301:1198, 1979.
18. Pugh, W., and Fernandez, F. Coitus in late pregnancy. *Obstetrics and Gynecology* 1:636, 1953.
19. Rainwater, L. Crucible of identity: The Negro lower-class family. *Daedalus* 95:172, 1966.
20. Rainwater, L. Sex in the Culture of Poverty. In C. Broderick and J. Bernard (Eds.), *The Individual, Sex, and Society.* Baltimore: Johns Hopkins Press, 1969.
21. Seymour, J. The Importance of Ethics—Moralistic Considerations in Counseling upon Sexual Matters. In H. L. Silverman (Ed.), *Marital Therapy.* Springfield, Ill.: Thomas, 1972.
22. Sjovall, T. The Development of Contraception: Psychodynamic Considerations. In K. Elliott (Ed.), *The Family and Its Future.* London: Churchill, 1970.
23. Solberg, D., Butler, J., and Wagner, N. Sexual behavior in pregnancy. *New England Journal of Medicine* 288:1098, 1973.
24. Swanson, J. The marital sexual relationship during pregnancy. *Journal of Obstetric, Gynecologic and Neonatal Nursing* 9:267, 1980.
25. Thomas, J. L. The Catholic Tradition for Responsibility in Sexual Ethics. In J. C. Wynn (Ed.), *Sexual Ethics and Christian Responsibility.* New York: Association Press, 1970.
26. Toner, B. Masturbation—the realities. *Man and Woman* (Part 8) 1:204, 1972.
27. Watts, R. Dimensions of sexual health. *American Journal of Nursing* 79:1568, 1979.
28. Wynn, J. C. (Ed.). *Sexual Ethics and Christian Responsibility.* New York: Association Press, 1970.
29. Zalar, M. Sexual counseling for pregnant couples. *American Journal of Maternal-Child Nursing* 1:176, 1976.

FURTHER READING

Adams, B. *The American Family.* Chicago: Markham, 1971.
Church, J. *Understanding Your Child from Birth to Three.* New York: Random House, 1973.
Cohn, S. Sexuality in pregnancy: A review of the literature. *Nursing Clinics of North America* 17:91, 1982.
Comfort, A. (Ed.). *The Joy of Sex.* New York: Crown, 1972.
Fogel, C., and Woods, N. *Health Care of Women: A Nursing Perspective.* St. Louis: Mosby, 1981.
Goode, W. J. (Ed.). *The Contemporary American Family.* Chicago: Quadrangle, 1971.
Grummon, D., and Barclay, A. (Eds.). *Sexuality: A Search for Perspective.* New York: Van Nostrand Reinhold, 1971.
Hogan, R. *Human Sexuality: A Nursing Perspective.* New York: Appleton-Century-Crofts, 1980.
Lion, E. *Human Sexuality in Nursing Process.* New York: Wiley, 1982.
McCary, J. *Human Sexuality.* Princeton, N.J.: Van Nostrand, 1967.
Mims, F., and Swenson, M. *Sexuality: A Nursing Perspective.* New York: McGraw-Hill, 1980.
Rayner, E. *Human Development.* London: Allen & Unwin, 1971.
Reiss, I. L. *The Family System in America.* New York: Holt, Rinehart, & Winston, 1971.
Reiss, I. L. *Readings on the Family System.* New York: Holt, Rinehart, & Winston, 1972.

Selby, J., and Calhoun, L. Sexuality During Pregnancy. In P. Ahmed (Ed.), *Pregnancy, Childbirth, and Parenthood.* New York: Elsevier, 1981.

Sherman, J. *On the Psychology of Women.* Springfield, Ill.: Thomas, 1971.

Tolor, A., and DiGrazia, P. Sexual attitudes and behavior patterns during and following pregnancy. *Archives of Sexual Behavior* 5:539, 1976.

Woods, N. F. *Human Sexuality in Health and Illness.* St. Louis: Mosby, 1979.

Chapter 4 Structure and Function of the Reproductive Organs

STRUCTURE OF THE FEMALE REPRODUCTIVE ORGANS

The female reproductive system consists of the external genitalia and internal organs.

External Organs

The female external genital structures are collectively called the *pudenda* or *vulva* and include the mons pubis, labia majora, labia minora, clitoris, and vestibule or pudendal cleft (Fig. 4-1).

The most anterior is the *mons pubis* or *mons veneris*, an adipose cushion shaped as an inverted triangle, lying over the anterior surface of the symphysis pubis and covered with pubic hair. Continuous with the mons, two folds of adipose tissue, the *labia majora*, extend downward and merge, forming the *posterior commissure*. The outer surface of the labia majora is covered with hair, while the inner surface appears moist and more delicate. In addition to adipose tissue, the labia majora contain connective tissue rich in elastic fibers, sebaceous glands, and many veins. These veins may become varicosed, which is an important point for the nurse to remember if shaving this area is part of preparation for delivery. In addition, hematomas may develop in the labia following the trauma of delivery. In nulliparous women the labia majora meet at the midline and thus provide some protection for underlying structures. After childbearing, they tend to gape. The labia majora correspond to the scrotum in the male.

The *labia minora* are two thin folds of connective tissue lying beneath the labia majora. Similar in appearance to mucous membrane, they contain sebaceous glands, sweat glands occasionally, a few nonstriated muscle fibers, a rich variety of nerve endings, and many blood vessels that dilate during sexual excitement. Anteriorly, the labia minora are divided into two portions: the upper, which forms the prepuce, or clitoral covering, and the lower, which joins the ventral surface of the clitoris to form the *frenulum clitoridis*. Posteriorly, the labia minora merge at the *fourchette*, located behind the posterior commissure.

The *clitoris* is a projection of erectile tissue, nerves, and blood vessels situated where the labia minora divide anteriorly. Its physiologic function is to initiate or intensify levels of sexual tension. It consists of the erectile body, which contains two corpora cavernosa, and the glans, made up of a small mass of erectile tissue fitted over the pointed end of the body and covered with very sensitive epithelium. The clitoris is the equivalent of the male penis.

The *vaginal vestibule*, or *pudendal cleft*, is that area bounded by the labia minora and extending from the clitoris to the fourchette. It is perforated by the openings of the urethra, paraurethral glands, vagina, and ducts of Bartholin's glands.

The *urethra* is situated between the clitoris and vagina. Its orifice has the appearance of a vertical slit or of an inverted V with its margins in contact with each other. The openings of the two ducts of the *paraurethral* glands (Skene's glands) are located on each side of the orifice. They are homologous to the male prostate and are particularly susceptible to gonococcal infection.

Figure 4-1. External female genitalia.

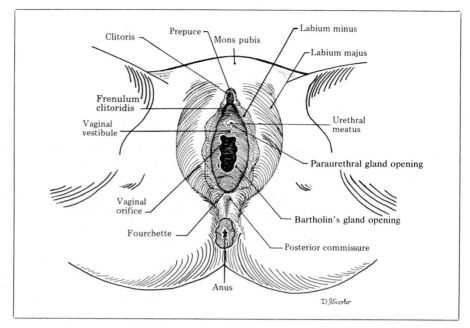

Two bean-shaped *Bartholin's glands*, similar to the bulbourethral glands in the male, open on either side of the vagina. They produce a mucoid material in response to sexual stimulation, but this is a negligible factor in *primary* vaginal lubrication. They are subject to various infections, including gonorrhea.

Bounded anteriorly by the pubis and posteriorly by the coccyx, the *perineum* has a diamond shape. It can be divided into anterior and posterior regions by a line drawn between the ischial tuberosities. The anterior section is called the urogenital diaphragm, with deep transverse perineal muscles and the urethral sphincter. The posterior portion, referred to as the pelvic diaphragm, forms a sling for the urethra, vagina, and rectum, and provides constrictor action for the vagina and rectum. It contains two main muscle groups: the coccygeal and the levator ani. The levator ani is composed of the iliococcygeal, the pubococcygeal, and puborectal muscles (Fig. 4-2).

Another structure found in the posterior portion between the vagina and anus is the *perineal body*, which provides the main support to the pelvic floor. It consists of the levator ani and a number of other muscles, the bulbocavernous, the superficial transverse perineal muscles, and the external sphincter ani, all of which meet midway at the central tendon of the perineum. This is the area most likely to be lacerated while being stretched by the descending fetal head during childbirth. (When the term *perineum* is used, it commonly refers to the region between the vagina and rectum, even though that region is only a small part of the entire perineal structure.)

The *hymen*, a thin fold of vascularized mucous membrane at the vaginal orifice, separates the internal from the external genital organs. Occasionally it is completely absent or it completely closes the lower end of the vagina, but most often it is centrally perforated. Anatomically, neither its absence nor its presence can be considered a criterion for virginity, although the intact hymen usually

Figure 4-2. Muscles of the perineum. A. Superficial perineal muscles. B. Deep perineal muscles.

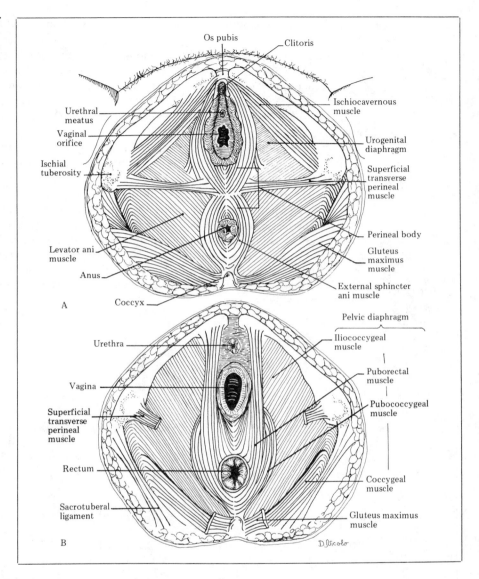

ruptures with the first intercourse. After childbearing, the remnants of the hymen form scarlike nodules.

The *vagina* is a relatively insensitive, well-vascularized musculomembranous tube that extends from the vulva to the uterus and lies between the bladder and the rectum. It functions as the excretory duct of the uterus, the female organ of copulation, and part of the birth canal during labor.

The vaginal wall has an outer fibrous coat, a middle muscular layer, and an inner mucous lining corrugated by thick transverse ridges or *rugae*. These are found in the lower part of the vagina, especially in young women, and tend to become obliterated with repeated childbirth. The mucous layer contains considerable glycogen that, when broken down into lactic acid by the action of Döderlein's bacillus, contributes to the acidity of the vagina, particularly in pregnancy (Fig. 4-3).

The vagina is directed upward and backward from the vulva, but in the supine position it is directed almost precisely posteriorly. Its posterior wall is approximately 9 centimeters (3½ inches) long, while the anterior wall is somewhat shorter. The upper portion of the posterior wall is separated from the rectum by a deep fold of peritoneum, which forms the *Douglas's cul-de-sac* (or pouch of Douglas).

The upper part of the vagina surrounding the cervix ends in a blind vault which is divided into anterior, posterior, and two lateral *fornices*. Their thin walls allow internal pelvic organs to be easily palpated. The posterior fornix is the deepest and provides surgical access to the peritoneal cavity.

Normally the walls of the vagina lie in contact with each other. The upper portion is easily distended, but the lower vagina, surrounded by the musculature of the pelvic and urogenital diaphragms, offers more resistance.

Figure 4-3.   Side view of female genitourinary anatomy.

Glands are normally absent from the vagina, and secretions from the uterus keep the canal moist. The character of the secretions varies with the phase of the menstrual cycle. Before puberty, vaginal pH ranges between 6.8 and 7.2. After

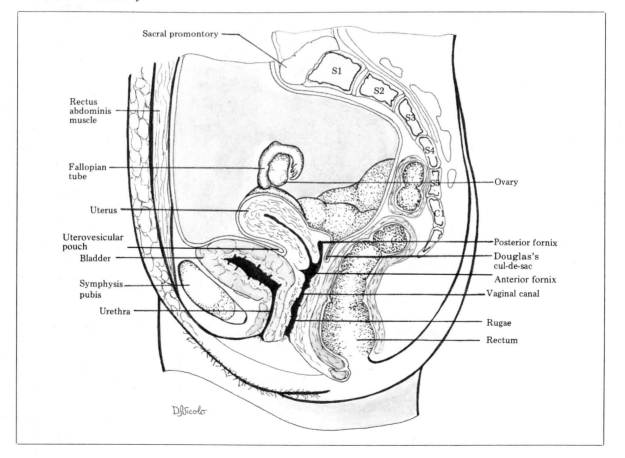

puberty, the pH is lowest in midcycle and highest premenstrually, ranging between 3.5 and 4.0. Three to 4 days before and 1 day after ovulation, cervical mucus increases in quantity and becomes less viscous; this causes it to be less resistant to penetration by spermatozoa.

The character of vaginal secretions also changes under sexual stimulation. After one-half hour of sexual stimulation without intercourse, the vaginal secretions increase and reach a pH of 4.25 to 4.5 [8, 10]. Droplets of vaginal lubricating material can then be seen throughout the rugal folds of the vagina.

Internal Organs   The female internal reproductive organs include the uterus, fallopian tubes (uterine tubes), and ovaries (Fig. 4-4).

UTERUS

The uterus, a hollow, thick-walled, muscular organ weighing approximately 60 grams (2 ounces) and located in the pelvic cavity between the bladder and the rectum, serves for the reception, retention, and nutrition of the fetus. The position of the uterus is slightly anteflexed over the bladder.

The pear-shaped upper two-thirds of the uterus is known as the *corpus* (or *body*). The uppermost portion between the insertion of the fallopian tubes is called the *fundus*. At both lateral edges, near the insertion of the fallopian tubes, are two sections called the *cornua*. Pacemakers that initiate uterine contractions and control their rhythm are most often found in these areas. (The cervix, discussed later, forms the lower third of the uterus.)

Figure 4-4. Internal female reproductive organs

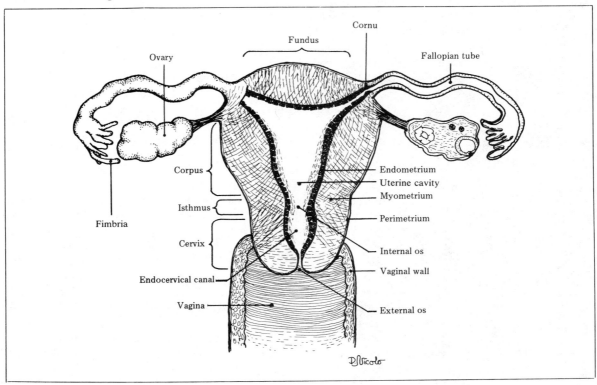

The wall of the corpus is composed of three layers: serous, muscular, and mucous. The serous coat, or *perimetrium*, is a peritoneal covering that is firmly adherent to the outside of the uterus and covers the fundus and most of the body.

The muscular coat, or *myometrium*, is composed of bundles of smooth muscle united by connective tissue containing many elastic fibers. The muscle fibers progressively decrease and the fibrous tissue increases toward the lower uterus. The cervix contains mainly fibrous tissue with a small amount of muscular and elastic tissue; thus, it is firmer and more rigid. The fundus is the most muscular part of the uterus. During pregnancy the muscle content of the upper portion of the uterus increases without a similar increase in the cervix.

The myometrium is arranged in three layers, which become more distinct in pregnancy. They include an outer hoodlike layer that covers the fundus and extends to various ligaments and a thin internal layer consisting of sphincterlike fibers around the openings of the tubes and the internal os of the cervix. Between these two lies a dense network of muscle fibers perforated in all directions by blood vessels. The main portion of the uterine wall is formed by this central layer; each of its cells interlaces with the next. After delivery, these cells contract and, as a result, constrict blood vessels.

The mucous coat, or *endometrium*, which lines the slitlike uterine cavity, is covered with columnar, partially ciliated epithelium. It is perforated by a large number of minute openings, the mouths of the uterine glands. These glands secrete a thin alkaline fluid that keeps the uterine cavity moist. The endometrium normally varies in thickness, being quite thin after menstruation. It then increases rapidly in thickness and before the next menstrual period contains many convoluted glands and numerous blood vessels.

Knowing the arrangement of the blood vessels in the endometrium is valuable in understanding certain aspects of female physiology. The uterine and ovarian arteries and their branches carry blood to the uterus. The arterial branches enter the uterine wall at a slant, become parallel to the surface, and are called *arcuate arteries*. From these, *radial arteries* branch out toward the endometrium at sharp angles. Smaller *basal arteries* branch from the radial arteries. The endometrial portions of the radial arteries have a corkscrew appearance and are called *coiled arteries*. The walls of these arteries are very sensitive to hormonal influences, especially those causing vasoconstriction. The coiled arteries are thought to play a part in menstrual bleeding (Fig. 4-5).

The position of the uterine artery is significant, since the uterine artery and the ureter are in close proximity at the level of the internal os. It is at this point that the ureter may be accidentally ligated, injured, or cut during pelvic surgery.

The *isthmus* is the lowermost portion of the uterine body and connects with the supravaginal portion of the cervix. The mucous layer of the isthmus is less complex and less affected by periodic changes of the menstrual cycle. In the last months of pregnancy, the isthmus, normally indicated by a slight uterine constriction, becomes more distinct. During labor it becomes part of the lower uterine segment.

The lower third of the uterus, cylindrical in shape and projecting into the upper portion of the vagina, is called the *cervix*. It contains a central spindle-shaped canal, the *endocervical canal*, which communicates with the uterus above and the vagina below. The supravaginal portion contains a small opening, the *internal os*;

Figure 4-5. Blood supply to the vagina, uterus, fallopian tubes, and ovaries.

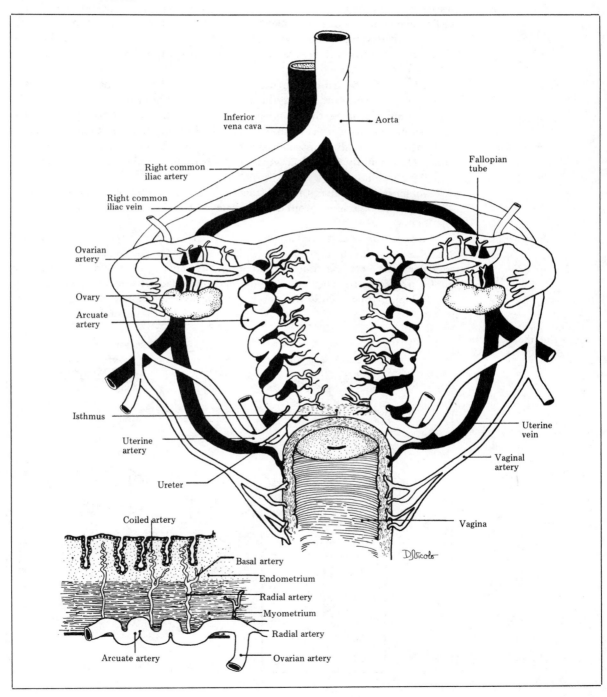

its lower portion, or vaginal part, contains the *external os*. This lower part is described as having anterior and posterior lips, both of which are usually in contact with the posterior wall of the vagina. If the lips project toward the anterior vaginal wall, the uterus may be retroverted (tipped posteriorly).

The external os varies in appearance from a small oval opening in a nulligravida to a transverse slit following childbirth. The cervix of the nulligravida feels like the tip of the nose, whereas in the gravid woman, it feels softer, like the ear lobe or lips.

The cervix is basically composed of connective tissue, some smooth muscle fibers, elastic tissue, and many blood vessels. Peripherally, the cervix contains circular muscle fibers that connect with the uterine myometrium above. The mucosa of the endocervical canal is composed of columnar epithelium. Mucous cells of this epithelium furnish the thick tenacious secretions of the cervical canal. Occasionally the endocervical glands become occluded and result in the so-called Nabothian cysts.

Ligaments.   Ligaments extend from the sides of the uterus and give it support. The principal ligaments around the uterus are the broad, round, and uterosacral ligaments (Fig. 4-6).

The *broad ligaments* are two winglike structures that extend from the lateral margins of the uterus to the pelvic walls and divide the pelvic cavity into anterior and posterior sections. Each broad ligament consists of a fold of peritoneum containing several structures. The inner two-thirds serves as an attachment for the fallopian tubes, while the outer third forms the *suspensory ligament* of the

Figure 4-6. Ligaments supporting the uterus in the pelvic cavity.

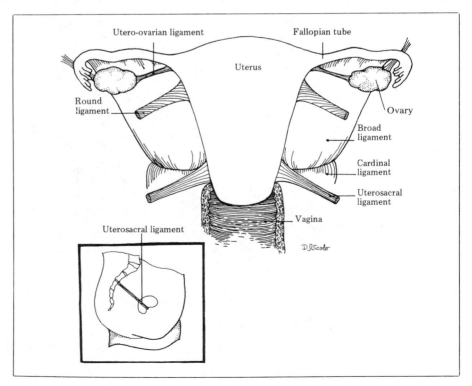

ovary and contains the ovarian blood vessels. The broad ligament allows anterior-posterior movement of the uterus but opposes lateral motion. The lower portion of this ligament is thickened; it is continuous with the connective tissue of the pelvic floor. The most dense portion, the *cardinal ligament*, is firmly united to the upper portion of the cervix and lateral margins of the uterus. It encloses the uterine vessels and ureters and offers base support to the uterus.

The *round ligaments* are fibromuscular cords which arise from the lateral surface of the uterus below the insertion of the fallopian tubes. Each runs outward and upward in a fold of peritoneum continuous with the broad ligament. They pass through the inguinal canal and terminate in the labia majora. Their function is to give support to the body of the uterus.

The *uterosacral ligaments* originate from the upper posterior portion of the cervix and insert into the fascia over the second and third sacral vertebrae. They aid in keeping the uterus in its normal position, exerting traction on the cervix and pulling it into the posterior fornix.

Ligament support causes the usual position of the uterus to be slightly anteflexed. In a standing woman, the uterus is almost horizontal, with the fundus resting on the bladder. Distention of the bladder and/or rectum can influence uterine position. While the body of the uterus is free to move anteriorly and posteriorly, the cervix is anchored by the cardinal and uterosacral ligaments.

Nerve Supply. The uterine nerve supply is derived principally from the sympathetic nervous system and also from the parasympathetic and cerebrospinal nervous systems. The sympathetic fibers maintain uterine tone by stimulating muscle contraction and promoting vasoconstriction. Stimulation from the parasympathetics has an opposing effect by inhibiting uterine muscle contraction and promoting vasodilatation. Action of the parasympathetics allows for intermittent uterine contractions.

The eleventh and twelfth thoracic nerve roots carry sensory fibers from the uterus, transmitting the pain of uterine contractions to the central nervous system. Motor fibers going to the uterus leave the spinal cord at the seventh and eighth thoracic vertebrae. The separation of the motor and sensory levels permits the use of epidural and spinal anesthesia in labor.

FALLOPIAN TUBES

The fallopian tubes (uterine tubes) are a pair of ducts, richly supplied with elastic tissue, which convey oocytes to the cavity of the uterus. Except for a distal portion, they are enclosed in a fold of peritoneum known as the *mesosalpinx*. The tubes, approximately 11 centimeters (4½ inches) long, are divided into four sections: the interstitial portion, isthmus, ampulla, and infundibulum.

The *interstitial portion* is found within the anterolateral wall of the uterus and is the most muscular section of the tube. Immediately adjacent to the interstitial segment is the straight, narrow *isthmus*. The *ampulla*, continuous with the isthmus, is the longest and widest portion of the tube; it is there that fertilization takes place. The ampulla ends in the *infundibulum*, or *fimbriated end*, the funnel-shaped outer portion of the tube that extends into the abdominal cavity. The lining of the infundibulum contains folds continuous with those of the ampulla, and it is these folds that give the end of the tube its fimbriated appearance. The longest fold reaches toward the tubal pole of the ovary. It is believed to aid in conducting the ovum from the ruptured follicle into the lumen of the tube.

The tubal structure is composed of several tissue layers (serous, muscular, mucous). The outside serous covering is peritoneum, beneath which is a tissue coat containing nerves and many blood vessels. Next, the muscle layer is divided into outer longitudinal and deeper, thicker, inner circular fibers. These undergo constant rhythmic contractions, which are weakest during pregnancy and strongest during the transport of ova. The mucous lining of the tube contains ciliated and nonciliated epithelium. The current created by the cilia in both the fallopian tubes and the uterus flows from the fimbriated ends, where the cilia are most abundant, to the exernal os of the uterus. During the menstrual cycle the mucosal lining undergoes growth associated with increased secretory activity. Occasionally diverticula extend through the mucosal lining into the muscular wall; these diverticula may possibly contribute to the development of ectopic or extrauterine pregnancies.

OVARIES

The ovaries are two small, almond-shaped organs having the dual function of ovum development and hormone production. In the adult, the organs are connected with the broad ligament of the uterus by a peritoneal fold called the *mesovarium*. The ovaries are supported by two additional ligaments running within the broad ligament. The ovarian ligament connects one pole of the ovary to the uterus, while the suspensory ligament, containing the ovarian vessels and nerves, connects the opposite pole of the ovary to the lateral pelvic wall. The ovaries receive their blood supply from the ovarian arteries, which branch off the aorta below the renal arteries.

The exterior of the ovaries varies in appearance with age. In young women it is smooth with small clear follicles; in the mature woman, more corrugated; in the elderly woman, markedly convoluted.

The ovary is composed of an outer zone, the cortex, and an inner zone, the medulla. The *cortex* varies in thickness with age, becoming thin with advancing years. It contains connective tissue cells and fibers, among which are scattered ovarian follicles in various stages of development. Of the 300,000 primary oocytes present at birth, the majority degenerate without reaching maturity. The outermost portion of the cortex, the *tunica albuginea*, appears dull and white. The ovarian *medulla*, or central portion, is composed of loose connective tissue and contains a large number of arteries and veins, nerve fibers, and a small number of smooth muscle fibers.

Breasts   The breasts are generally considered accessory glands of reproduction. Their growth and function involve the coordinated action of the nervous system, reproductive system, and hormones. The breasts are composed of a mass of glandular tissue and are supported by fibrous tissue; they contain a thick layer of fat and many blood vessels (Fig. 4-7).

The *nipple*, located near the center of the breast, contains a considerable number of muscle fibers and a rich nerve supply. The nipple is an erectile organ by virtue of muscle contraction and vascular engorgement; it becomes firmer and more prominent as a result of stimulation. Surrounding the nipple is a thin,

Figure 4-7. Breast and ductal system.

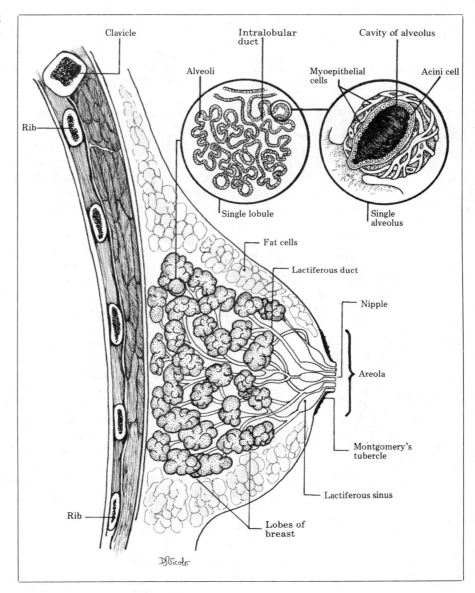

pigmented, circular area of skin, the *areola*, which contains roughened elevations that represent sebaceous glands (Montgomery's tubercles or Montgomery's glands).

Each breast contains a network of ducts, which branch into a network of alveolar units. The *alveoli* are sacs made up of a layer of secretory cells (*acini cells*) which are surrounded by a covering of myoepithelial cells that contract to force milk into the duct system in response to stimulation. A group of alveoli makes up a *lobule*, and a group of lobules makes up each of the 15 to 20 *lobes* of the breast. Covered by contractile muscle cells, intralobular ducts from the alveoli lead to lactiferous ducts and then widen to form *lactiferous sinuses* or milk reservoirs behind the areola. Then, becoming constricted once more, some 8 to 15 of the ducts open on the surface of the nipple. Lymph vessels in the breast are numerous and, for the most part, join the lymph nodes of the axilla. The majority of lymph vessels follow the lactiferous ducts and converge toward the nipple, joining a plexus under the areola.

Breast size depends largely on the amount of superficial fat but also on the amount of glandular tissue present. The amount of glandular tissue is very small in women who are not lactating. Therefore, breast size alone is not a good predictor of a woman's future ability to produce an adequate milk supply. Developments at puberty include increasing amounts of ovarian hormones, a conspicuous growth and branching of the ductal system, and extensive depositing of fat in the breasts. A characteristic differentiation of glands occurs in pregnancy. Breast tissue atrophies at the time of menopause.

FUNCTION OF THE FEMALE REPRODUCTIVE ORGANS

A woman's reproductive function has a specific beginning and end. *Puberty* represents the beginning of reproductive life, and the climacteric, or *menopause*, represents its ending. Puberty covers a time span during which many maturational changes are taking place, including a rapid change in size and shape of the body, maturation of the gonads and the reproductive tract, and the development of secondary sexual characteristics.

While a growth spurt begins at approximately 8 years of age, most growth occurs between the ages of 10 and 15, when fatty deposits develop on the hips and shoulders. The breasts and pubic hair begin to develop at about the same time, between the ages of 8 and 13, and axillary hair will develop about 2 years later. Menarche (the beginning of menstruation) usually occurs between the ages of 10 and 14, although a wider age range (9–17 years) would be considered normal. The average age of menarche in the United States is now 12½ years [13]. Over the past 100 years, the onset of menstruation in this country has been occurring at a progressively earlier age, as a result (according to some) of the better nutrition of American youth. More recent findings indicate that the decline in the age of menarche has ended [12]. There are variations in the timing of all the above processes, but the sequence remains the same. It is not known what changes initiate puberty, but current theory suggests that hypothalamic maturation is necessary. Following this, the pituitary is stimulated to release follicle-stimulating hormone (FSH) and luteinizing hormone (LH). The gonads respond by producing steroid hormones, which influence growth and development at puberty. A knowledge of the functioning of these steroid and pituitary hormones is essential to an understanding of their roles in the menstrual cycle and in reproduction.

Pituitary Hormones

The pituitary hormones include FSH, LH, and prolactin. *FSH*, a glycoprotein, is produced and secreted by the anterior pituitary in response to a releasing factor from the hypothalamus. This substance travels to the pituitary via the hypophyseal-portal system.

FSH release is influenced by the level of estrogen or by neurologic impulses from higher brain centers. In the absence of estrogen, FSH-releasing factor is uncontrolled, and FSH is secreted in larger amounts. This situation occurs after surgical removal of the ovaries or after menopause. Levels of FSH can be reduced by administration of exogenous estrogens.

Functions of FSH include stimulation of ovarian follicle growth and ovarian estrogen production. However, hormone production and ovulation will not occur unless LH is also present. The FSH level fluctuates throughout the menstrual cycle, with its peak in the middle of the cycle. The level remains low throughout pregnancy, reflecting pituitary inactivity.

LH, also a glycoprotein, is produced and secreted by the anterior pituitary by the same mechanism as that of FSH. Release of LH is regulated by feedback effects of steroid hormones (estrogen or progesterone) on the hypothalamus. Neural impulses may also affect FSH and LH gonadotropin levels by being channeled into the hypothalamus from other areas of the brain as a result of changes in the internal or external environment. Therefore, such factors as light or emotional state can influence reproductive function.

Levels of LH are low in childhood and gradually rise to a plateau at puberty. In the mature female there is a midcycle surge just before ovulation. The administration of estrogen and/or progesterone can inhibit the midcycle surges of LH and FSH; this forms the basis of action of oral contraceptives.

Early in the menstrual cycle LH, in association with FSH, causes changes in the ovarian theca and granulosa cells; these changes result in estrogen production. LH is instrumental in causing the fully developed follicle to rupture when the proper ratio of LH to FSH develops. It initiates the formation of the corpus luteum, which responds to LH by increased hormone secretion. LH is responsible for the accumulation in granulosa cells of cholesterol or cholesterol-like substances, which are apparently the precursors of progesterone.

Prolactin is a pituitary protein also known as mammotropin, or lactogenic hormone. Its secretion is controlled by the hypothalamus via releasing *and* inhibiting factors. While prolactin has not been isolated in pure form in humans, its activity stimulates milk formation in mammalian species when the breasts have been primed by prior quantities of estrogen, progesterone, and adrenal steroids. High doses of estrogen and/or progesterone will prevent the release of prolactin, whereas suckling and estrogen in low doses stimulate its release. In addition to stimulating the production of milk, prolactin facilitates breast growth through development of the lobulo-alveolar structures.

Ovarian Hormones   The ovarian hormones are estrogen and progesterone. *Estrogens*, the hormones of femininity, are responsible for the development and maintenance of female secondary sexual characteristics. Both men and women have circulating estrogens and androgens. The relative amount of androgens determines body type, breast development, hair growth, and reproductive activity. An imbalance of androgens in women can interfere with estrogen production and the response of the target organ to the hormone.

Estrogens are steroid growth hormones that have a specific effect on tissues derived from the müllerian ducts: the fallopian tubes, endometrium, the musculature of the uterine body, and the cervix. Estradiol, the most active estrogenic substance, is the principal ovarian secretory product and precursor of many urinary estrogen metabolites. In the ovary it is produced by the thecal cells of the follicle and the luteinized granulosal cells of the corpus luteum. During pregnancy estradiol is also produced by the placenta. In addition to estradiol, there are other natural estrogens, estrone and estriol, as well as a number of synthetic estrogens.

In the mature female, blood levels of estradiol and excretion of urinary metabolites have two peaks during the menstrual cycle: at ovulation (approximately day 14) and at the height of the luteal phase (approximately day 21). During the 4 to 5 days prior to the next menstrual period, estrogen secretion decreases rapidly. Estrogen levels rise progressively in pregnancy. The majority of urinary estrogen in pregnancy is estriol. Estrogens are found in the amniotic fluid and in the fetal circulation in higher concentrations than those found in the maternal circulation.

Estrogens affect a number of tissues in specific ways.

1. *Vagina*: Estrogens promote thickening and cornification of the vaginal epithelium.
2. *Cervix*: Under the influence of estrogen, the cervix increases in size and vascularity and develops mucous glands. The cervical mucus increases in quantity, increases in pH, becomes less viscous, and is more readily penetrated by spermatozoa. Microscopically, the dried mucus assumes the pattern of a fern (Fig. 4-8).
3. *Uterus*: Estrogens cause proliferation of endometrial glands and blood vessels, hypertrophy of the myometrium, and an increase in electrical and contractile activities. Estrogens increase the sensitivity of the myometrium to oxytocin and appear to cause the release of prostaglandins from the uterus.
4. *Fallopian tubes*: The fallopian tubes are dependent on estrogen for their contractility, secretion, and function, since estrogens cause the mucosal lining and musculature to develop.

Figure 4-8. Diagram of fern pattern seen on microscopic examination of cervical mucus at midcycle in normal menstruating women.

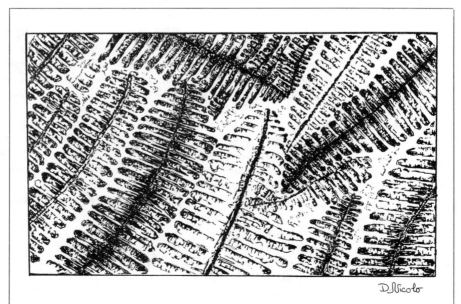

5. *Ovary*: Estradiol exerts a local effect, stimulating growth of the ovarian follicle even in the absence of FSH. It potentiates ovarian response to pituitary gonadotropins.
6. *Breasts*: Growth and development of the nipple, areola, and breast ducts occur under the influence of estrogens. The deposition of fat is enhanced.
7. *Endocrine glands*
   a. Pituitary: The effects of estrogen on the pituitary were discussed in the previous section.
   b. Thyroid: Serum thryoid-binding globulin is increased, resulting in an increased protein-bound iodine level.
   c. Adrenal: Estrogens cause a decrease in adrenal hormone metabolism but lengthen the half-life of the adrenal steroids in the blood.
8. *Skeletal system*: Increased estrogen levels in young girls lead to premature epiphyseal closure, and estrogens can have a positive influence on the calcium balance, upon which bone integrity depends.
9. *Skin*: The estrogens are responsible for an increase in skin pigmentation, particularly in the breast areola.

Progesterone has been described as the hormone of pregnancy. Unlike estrogen, it has no primary growth-initiating effect but rather affects tissues already under the influence of estrogen. Progesterone is responsible for the uterine endometrial and myometrial changes that permit and maintain implantation, and it contributes to decreased uterine contractility.

The major sources of progesterone are the corpus luteum and, in pregnancy, the placenta; it can also be produced in the adrenal gland and the ovarian follicle. The main metabolite of progesterone is pregnanediol. Its presence varies with the phase of the menstrual cycle. During the follicular phase, the urinary pregnanediol levels and blood progesterone levels are barely detectable. Progesterone blood levels peak approximately 1 week after ovulation and formation of the corpus luteum. Progestins (synthetic forms of progesterone) act synergistically with estrogen to inhibit hypothalamic stimulation of pituitary gonadotropin production and release.

Progesterone affects a number of tissues in specific ways.

1. *Vagina*: Under the influence of progesterone, the vaginal lining decreases in thickness.
2. *Cervix*: Progesterone causes the secretions of the cervix to become scanty, more viscous, and impermeable to spermatozoa. The ferning pattern is absent when the dried mucus is viewed microscopically.
3. *Uterus*: The *endometrium* changes from a proliferative to a secretory type. Changes in the uterine glands reflect increased tortuosity, glycogen deposits, and evidence of secretion. Likewise, blood vessels proliferate, becoming more tortuous and coiled. The above changes are conducive to proper nutrition for the implantation and retention of the ovum.

   The *myometrial* and *smooth muscle* contractions are milder and less frequent. This effect is believed to be caused by progesterone's ability to interfere with the electrical conductivity of myometrial cells. This action is partially responsible for the uterine ability to retain the growing fetus without expulsion prior to term.

4. *Breasts*: Progesterone causes growth of the acini cells and lobules, preparing them for lactation.
5. *Central nervous system*: Through action at the level of the hypothalamus, progesterone causes the increase in body temperature that occurs after ovulation.
6. *Renal*: Progesterone contributes to an increase in aldosterone secretion with a resulting retention of water and electrolytes. It is reported that progesterone interferes with aldosterone action at the renal tubule [9].

Reproductive Cycle   The reproductive cycle is dependent on constant harmonious interactions among the central nervous system, the pituitary gland, and the reproductive tract. In the

Figure 4-9. Hormone changes during typical menstrual cycle. (Adapted from R. C. Benson, *Current Obstetric and Gynecologic Diagnosis and Treatment* [3rd ed.]. Los Altos, Calif.: Lange, 1980.)

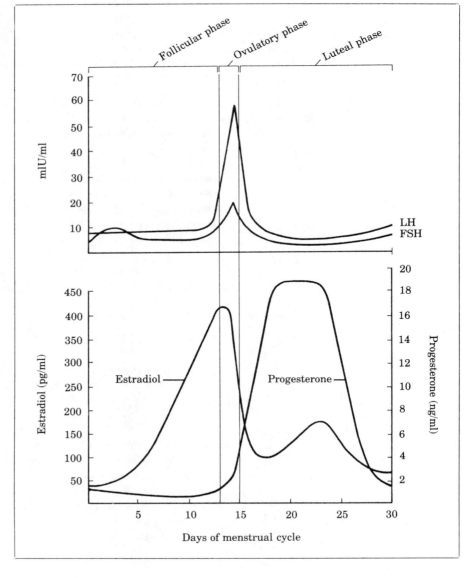

mature woman, the reproductive structures undergo a series of changes that is repeated approximately every 28 days. This 28-day cycle has three phases, as shown in Figure 4-9. The first, or *menstrual* phase, is the period of active bleeding. It is followed by the *proliferative* phase (*follicular* or *preovulatory* phase), during which the ovarian primordial follicles, which contain the oocytes, mature. This is also known as the *estrogenic* phase because estrogen is the primary female steroid produced during this period. The third, or *secretory*, phase includes the formation of the corpus luteum and its secretion of estrogen and progesterone. This is also referred to as the *luteal*, *postovulatory*, or *progestational* phase. The menstrual and proliferative phases of the cycle precede ovulation.

MENSTRUAL PHASE

The onset of vaginal bleeding designates the first day of the menstrual phase and also the first day of the 28-day menstrual cycle. During the preceding secretory phase, the endometrium has developed into three distinct layers: the zona basalis (next to the myometrium), the zona spongiosa, and the zona compacta (the outermost layer). Menstrual bleeding follows the degeneration of the spongiosa and compacta endometrial layers resulting from the congestion of blood vessels and formation of small hematomas. Approximately 4 to 24 hours before the onset of bleeding, the coiled arteries become constricted, which causes these two layers to receive an inadequate supply of blood. Following the period of vasoconstriction, the coiled arteries relax, hemorrhage ensues, and the degenerated compacta and spongiosa layers slough off. Menstrual bleeding, which is mostly arterial, lasts for 3 to 5 days. A wide variation exists in duration and amount of bleeding, although the average amount is 50 to 150 milliliters.

PROLIFERATIVE PHASE

The 9-day proliferative phase follows the period of menstrual bleeding. During this portion of the cycle, ovarian primordial follicles, which contain the oocytes, are stimulated by pituitary FSH and LH and ovulation occurs. During each cycle one mature follicle (graafian follicle) makes its way to the surface of the ovary. The follicle consists of an ovum surrounded by a layer of granulosa cells. The granulosa cells are enveloped by circles of specialized stromal cells, the *theca interna*, and a layer of less differentiated cells, the *theca externa*. It is believed that the granulosa supply the ova with nutritional stores and developmental information. The theca interna is the site of estrogen formation. Early production of estrogen is necessary to ensure a continued response to FSH by the follicle. Thus, FSH and estrogen act synergistically to prepare follicles to respond to LH. This is accomplished by increasing the activity or numbers of LH receptors in the follicle.

The increase in follicle size is accomplished by development of a fluid-filled cavity, the *antrum*, as well as by granulosa cell proliferation. As the fluid cavity enlarges, the ovum is pushed to one side, surrounded by a mass of granulosa cells, the *cumulus oophorous*, with which it is discharged at the time of rupture. While the follicle is still very small, a clear elastic membrane, the *zona pellucida*, envelops the ovum. It probably persists until after the ovum has reached the uterus. Attached to the zona pellucida is a single layer of granulosa cells, called the *corona radiata*. The corona radiata remains with the ovum after ovulation but must be separated before fertilization can take place (Fig. 4-10).

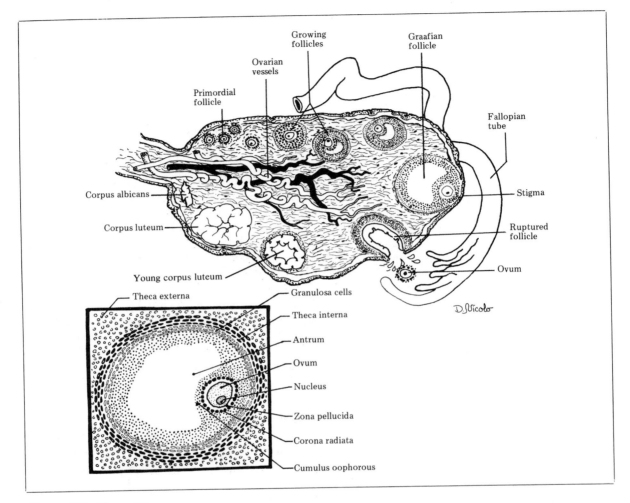

Figure 4-10. The ovary, showing maturation and release of ovum. Inset (in box) shows a developing graafian follicle.

At maturity the follicle protrudes above the surface of the ovary. The point of rupture and subsequent discharge of the ovum becomes very thin and is known as the *stigma*. Actual rupture occurs gradually and is probably caused by increased distensibility and local enzymatic destruction of the follicular wall. Usually only one follicle ruptures each month. Many follicles, however, reach the halfway point and then regress. Their thecal cells undergo change and produce androgens, which further contributes to follicular regression. Studies suggest that this midcycle increase in androgen production causes an increase in libido [11].

Estrogen secretion begins on day 1 of the menstrual cycle and reaches a peak just before the preovulatory surge of FSH and LH, which presumably triggers ovulation. The estrogen levels decline just prior to or with ovulation but increase again in the next half of the cycle. Progesterone is present at low levels prior to ovulation and is secreted by both the ovary and adrenal gland. During the proliferative phase, the endometrium responds to increased estrogen levels by general thickening of the endometrial layers and elongation and coiling of the glands.

OVULATION

There is marked variability in the length of menstrual cycles. Researchers report that 95 percent of all cycles are between 15 and 45 days long, with an average of 28 days [2]. Ovulation marks the midpoint of a 28-day cycle. Since in any cycle ovulation occurs approximately 14 days before the first day of the next menses, the secretory phase is relatively constant in length.

Ovulation can be detected in a number of ways. Approximately 25 percent of all women experience *mittelschmerz*, or pain in the lower abdomen, on or about the day of ovulation. It is thought to result from peritoneal irritation by fluid or blood escaping from the ruptured follicle. During or just after ovulation, increased levels of progesterone cause a rise in body temperature. (This temperature pattern forms the basis for the rhythm method of contraception.) Cervical mucus increases in amount and changes from an opaque to a clear substance, with decreased viscosity and clearly identified microscopic strands, which facilitate sperm transport [1]. Due to the high estrogen levels prior to ovulation, cervical mucus forms a ferning pattern microscopically. The demonstration by biopsy of a secretory endometrium is a strong indication that ovulation has occurred. Another means of determining that ovulation has occurred is the demonstration of an increase in serum progesterone.

Detection of ovulation is important in order to facilitate or avoid conception. Since the life spans of the sperm and ovum are limited, fertilization must take place within about 24 hours after ovulation if conception is to occur.

SECRETORY PHASE

The secretory phase begins around the time of ovulation. It is characterized by increased progesterone secretion, corpus luteum formation, and further endometrial development. About the middle of the secretory phase, estrogen reaches a second peak in the menstrual cycle.

The *corpus luteum*, or yellow body, is formed by the collapsed follicle. The follicle initially fills with blood that is replaced by lipid-rich luteal cells. The theca and granulosa cells left behind in the ovary proliferate and, together with the luteal cells, form the corpus luteum. The corpus luteum produces large quantities of progesterone and some estrogen. The unique feature of the corpus luteum is its limited life span, which limits the secretory phase of the menstrual cycle to a more constant period. After an average life of 10 to 14 days, the luteal cells degenerate, causing a withdrawal of estrogen and progesterone. These cells are replaced by connective tissue, forming the *corpus albicans*. If, however, fertilization occurs, the corpus luteum remains active during the first trimester of pregnancy.

During the secretory phase the endometrium becomes markedly increased in thickness and extremely vascular, succulent, and rich in glycogen. The endometrial arteries are more coiled and closer to the endometrial surface, making an ideal site for implantation and growth of the fertilized ovum.

Other signs of increased serum progesterone and corpus luteum formation include breast tenderness, fluid retention, and the symptoms of premenstrual tension.

OOGENESIS

Gametogenesis is the term applied to the process by which primordial or primitive germ cells are transformed into mature germ cells, or *gametes*. In females, primitive germ cells, called *oogonia*, are transformed through reduction division (meiosis) into the mature oocyte. The essential biological feature of gametogenesis is this reduction division or meiotic cellular division. *Meiosis*, characterized by a long and unusual prophase, results in the reduction of the diploid number of chromosomes, 46 in humans, to the haploid number of 23. Each mature oocyte contains the haploid number of chromosomes, with 22 autosomes and one sex chromosome (the X chromosome) (Fig. 4-11).

In the first of the two maturation divisions, the *primary oocyte* undergoes an early meiotic or reduction division. In the process of division, one daughter cell receives the majority of the cytoplasm plus 23 chromosomes and is called the *secondary oocyte*. The other daughter cell receives 23 chromosomes but little cytoplasm, and is referred to as the *first polar body*. This reduction division is thought to occur immediately prior to ovulation.

Figure 4-11. Maturation of female reproductive cells, resulting in formation of one mature ovum.

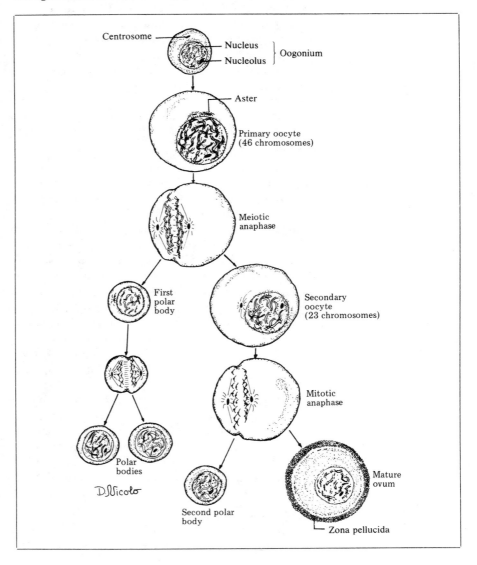

If fertilization occurs, the secondary oocyte is capable of completing a second maturation division, this one mitotic in nature. Again, both daughter cells contain 23 chromosomes. One daughter cell receives the majority of the cytoplasm and is called the *mature ovum*. The other daughter cell, which receives little cytoplasm, is called the *second polar body*.

The mature ovum differs from typical cells because of its large size and protective envelope, the zona pellucida. Another important difference is that, under ordinary circumstances, the mature ovum is incapable of further cell division because it possesses no centrosome—a deficiency that is corrected by the spermatozoon if fertilization occurs. If the secondary oocyte does not meet with a spermatozoon, it degenerates or passes through the genital passages and is cast off and lost.

STRUCTURE OF THE MALE REPRODUCTIVE ORGANS

The male reproductive organs include external and internal structures (Fig. 4-12).

External Organs

The external organs of the male consist of the penis and the scrotum. The *penis* is the male organ of copulation; it is attached to the anterior and lateral walls of the pubic arch and lies in front of the scrotum. The skin of the penis is thin, highly pigmented, and freely moveable. It is covered with hair only at the base.

Structurally, the penis is composed chiefly of cavernous (erectile) tissue, and it contains the urethra. The engorgement of cavernous tissue with blood produces a considerable enlargement of the penis and its erection. Two longitudinal columns of erectile tissue, the *corpora cavernosa*, are located laterally. They are sponge-like, contain large venous sinuses, and form the chief bulk of the organ. The *corpus spongiosum* (or *corpus cavernosum urethrae*) is the smaller third longitudinal column, which is also composed of erectile tissue. It is centrally located beneath the corpora cavernosa and contains the urethra. Toward the distal end of the penis, the corpus spongiosum expands, and, spreading toward the dorsal surface, forms a cap, the *glans penis*. This covers the conical end of the united corpora cavernosa and contains the urethral orifice. Overhanging the glans is the *prepuce*, a fold of loose skin. (This foreskin is removed in circumcision.) The penis receives its blood supply from the internal pudendal arteries and its nerve supply from the pudendal nerve and pelvic sympathetic plexus.

The *scrotum* is a pouchlike continuation of the abdominal wall located behind the penis. It is divided by a septum into two sacs, each containing and supporting one of the testes and its epididymis. The scrotum is more pigmented than the rest of the body and is covered with sparse hair. In the subcutaneous tissue of the scrotum are small muscle fibers, the *tunica dartos*, which contract with decreased temperature and give a more wrinkled appearance to the scrotum. This response causes the testes to assume a position closer to the perineum, where they absorb body heat and maintain a temperature compatible with the viability of spermatozoa. Under normal temperature conditions, the fibers are relaxed and the scrotum is pendulous and free from wrinkles. In the adult, the temperature in the scrotal sac is about 2°C (5°F) lower than that in the abdomen. This lower temperature is essential for the production of sperm. If the testes are kept at an elevated temperature for long periods of time (as with prolonged high fever or undescended testes), sterility may result.

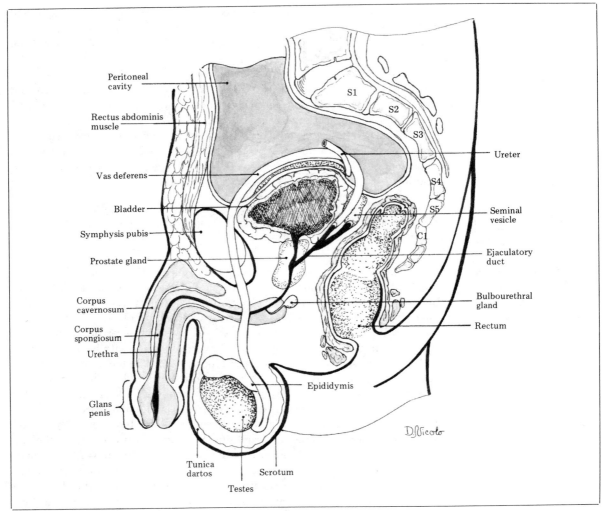

Figure 4-12. Side view
of male genitourinary
anatomy.

A serous membrane, the *tunica vaginalis*, lines the walls of the scrotal sac. It resembles the peritoneum in structure and appearance. The scrotum, like the penis, receives its blood supply from the internal pudendal arteries.

Internal Organs   The internal male reproductive organs are the gonads or testes, a series of ducts (the epididymis, the vas deferens, and the urethra), and accessory glands (the seminal vesicles, the prostate, and the bulbourethral or Cowper's glands). The spermatic cords are internal supporting structures.

The *testes*, a pair of nearly symmetrical oval bodies situated in the scrotum, are the reproductive glands of the male that correspond to the ovaries in the female. They are covered by a dense, white, inelastic fibrous tissue called the *tunica albuginea*. Inside, fibrous septa extend into the testis and divide it into about 250 wedge-shaped lobes. Each lobe contains one to four narrow coiled tubes, the *seminiferous tubules,* which, if uncoiled, would measure about 60 centimeters (23 inches) in length. Male reproductive cells (spermatogonia) at different stages of development are found within these tubules. Smooth musclelike cells in the walls of the tubules cause tubular contraction. This contraction is thought to promote transport of spermatozoa and fluid within the tubules toward the *rete testis*, a network of larger straight ducts. About 20 small coiled ductules leave the upper end of the rete testis, perforate the tunica albuginea, and enter the head of the epididymis (Fig. 4-13).

In addition to reproductive cells, rather large *Sertoli's cells* are found within the testis. Spermatids (developing reproductive cells) attach themselves to the Sertoli's cells, which may provide the spermatids with nutrient material, hormones, or enzymes necessary for their maturation into spermatozoa. The *interstitial cells of Leydig* are also scattered among the tubules and are responsible for the production of male hormones.

The ductules leaving the testis open into the *epididymis*, a single convoluted duct that ends in the vas deferens. The epididymis is a tube nearly 5 meters (16

Figure 4-13. Male ductal system and developing reproductive cells. Enlargement on right shows cross section of seminiferous tubule and spermatogenesis.

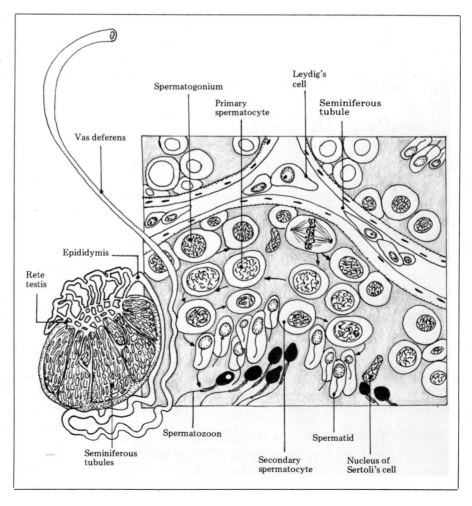

inches) long that is coiled into a space of about 4 centimeters (1½ inches) on the posterior aspects of the testis.

The *vas deferens (ductus deferens)*, the excretory duct of the testis, is a direct continuation of the duct of the epididymis. It ends, after a course of about 46 centimeters (18 inches), by joining with the duct of the seminal vesicle to form the ejaculatory duct. The peristaltic activity of its middle muscular layer is responsible for the passage of sperm along the duct. The vas deferens, nerves, lymphatics, and blood vessels form the *spermatic cord.*

The *ejaculatory duct* is approximately 2.5 centimeters (1 inch) long, penetrates the base of the prostate gland, and opens into the prostatic portion of the urethra. It ejects sperm and seminal vesicle fluid into the urethra.

The *urethra* is the last connecting link from the testis to the exterior. It is supplied with mucus derived from a large number of small glands located along its entire length, and also from the large bilateral bulbourethral glands, or Cowper's glands, located near its origin.

Accessory Glands of Reproduction

The *seminal vesicles* are two membranous pouchlike tubes lying behind the base of the bladder. The tube of each vesicle ends in a straight narrow duct, joining the vas deferens to form the ejaculatory duct.

The seminal vesicles are lined with secretory epithelium. The mucoid secretion contains much fructose, small amounts of ascorbic acid, inositol, ergothioneine, five of the amino acids, phosphoryl choline, and prostaglandins. During ejaculation, the seminal vesicle empties its contents into the ejaculatory duct while the vas deferens empties sperm. The seminal vesicle secretion adds bulk to the ejaculated semen. The fructose and other substances in the fluid probably provide nutrients and protection for the ejaculated sperm. Research suggests that prostaglandins may promote uterine contractions that help propel sperm toward the fallopian tubes [5].

The *prostate gland* is a chestnut-sized conical structure that surrounds the first several centimeters of the urethra. During ejaculation, the capsule of the prostate contracts simultaneously with contractions of the vas deferens and seminal vesicles, adding its thin, milky, alkaline fluid to the bulk of the semen. The alkalinity is important in fertilization, since the relatively acid fluid of the vas deferens may inhibit sperm fertility. It also helps to neutralize the acid vaginal secretions and enhance sperm motility.

The *bulbourethral glands (Cowper's glands)* are pea-sized structures found beneath the prostate on either side of the urethra. They contribute alkaline fluid to the semen.

FUNCTION OF THE MALE REPRODUCTIVE ORGANS

As in the female, puberty evokes a rapid growth spurt and many maturational changes in the male. At about age 10 a young man's testes, prostate, seminal vesicles, and penis begin to enlarge. By age 11 axillary sweating and odor appear, followed by pubic hair at 13 and enlarged larynx, axillary hair, and hair on the upper lip by 14. The average age at which boys acquire the ability to produce and ejaculate spermatozoa is 15, but it is not abnormal to find a range of 9 to 17 years. By age 18 the shoulders have broadened and the muscles have hypertrophied. At age 21 practically all skeletal growth has stopped.

During puberty the pituitary gland is stimulated to release FSH and LH

(interstitial cell stimulating hormone). FSH facilitates the production of spermatozoa, while LH acts on the Leydig cells of the testis to release androgens, namely
testosterone. The amount of testosterone serves as a feedback mechanism at the
level of the hypothalamus to regulate the amount of LH secreted from the
pituitary. The secretion of FSH is believed to be independently controlled by
inhibin, a nonsteroidal, water-soluble substance presumably secreted from the
seminiferous tubules [4].

Of the androgens, testosterone is the most significant male hormone. It is
formed by the interstitial cells of Leydig, which lie in spaces between the
seminiferous tubules. These cells are active in the fetus and the newborn, possibly
due to stimulation by a placental hormone, chorionic gonadotropin. They become
active again after puberty and at both of these times secrete large quantities of
testosterone. Some reports indicate that the testosterone level decreases rapidly
after the age of 40; other studies contradict these findings, reporting that levels of
testosterone remain remarkably stable after age 30 in healthy, vigorous men [6].
After secretion by the testes, testosterone circulates in the blood. Either it
becomes fixed to tissues where it performs intracellular functions, or it is
degraded into inactive products that are secreted in the urine as 17-ketosteroids.

The functions of testosterone are many. During fetal development it is
responsible for the development of the penis, scrotum, prostate gland, seminal
vesicles, and genital ducts. It provides the stimulus for descent of the testes and is
essential for the development of primary and secondary sex characteristics in the
male. After puberty, it stimulates enlargement of the penis, scrotum, and testes
until about the age of 20. Testosterone influences the distribution of body hair
and makes it more prolific. When there is a genetic predisposition for baldness,
testosterone may contribute to a decrease in the growth of hair on the top of the
head.

The effects of testosterone on the skin include an increase in thickness,
increased ruggedness of subcutaneous tissues, and increased pigmentation due to
elevated melanin production. Testosterone increases the rate of secretion of
sebaceous glands and is therefore believed to contribute to acne.

Under the influence of testosterone, the total quantity of bone matrix increases.
The bones become thicker and longer and the muscles increase in mass as a result
of the hormone's general protein anabolic function. This function is also thought
to be the cause of the higher hemoglobin and hematocrit levels in the male.

Testosterone may increase the basal metabolic rate. It also causes hypertrophy
of the laryngeal mucosa and enlargement of the larynx, which results in the
characteristically lower male voice.

Other androgens are produced by the male, but their masculinizing effects are
slight. Estrogen is also produced in small amounts, perhaps by the seminiferous
tubules or by the interstitial cells of the testes. Its function in the male is
unknown.

Spermatogenesis

Spermatogenesis occurs in the seminiferous tubules during active sexual life
beginning at puberty and continuing throughout the remainder of life. It is
stimulated by FSH in the presence of adequate testosterone. The tubules contain
two or three layers of *spermatogonia* (primitive germ cells) along the outer border
of the tubular epithelium. From puberty on, these cells continually proliferate

and differentiate to form mature spermatozoa. Each spermatogonium is capable of producing four descendant cells (Fig. 4-14).

At the time of sexual maturity, the spermatogonia become active and mature to form *primary spermatocytes*. Each primary spermatocyte undergoes an initial meiotic maturation division. The two resulting descendant cells, or *secondary spermatocytes*, contain the haploid number of chromosomes (23). These two cells divide mitotically during the second maturation division to form a total of four *spermatids*. Without further division the four spermatids, containing equal amounts of cytoplasm, are gradually transformed into four mature spermatozoa over a period of about 2 weeks. Each spermatozoon contains 22 autosomes and one sex chromosome, either an X or a Y.

During transformation each spermatid loses most of its cytoplasm and elongates into a spermatozoon with a head, neck, body, and tail. The head contains the nuclear material in a compact mass, and it is this part that fertilizes the egg. At the front of the head is a small structure called the *acrosome*, which is believed to play a role in the entry of the sperm into the ovum (Fig. 4-15).

The *centrioles* are found in the neck of the sperm and the *mitochondria* are found in the body. Attached to the body of the sperm is a long tail containing large amounts of adenosine triphosphate, which energizes its movement. When deposited in the vagina, the tail begins to move back and forth, driving the sperm forward at a maximum speed of 30 centimeters (12 inches) per hour.

Sperm mature in the epididymis; they develop their power of motility and become capable of fertilization within 1 to 14 days. Sperm are relatively dormant as long as they are stored (some are stored in the epididymis but most are stored in the vas deferens). As a result of their own metabolism, sperm secrete considerable CO_2 into the surrounding fluid, and the resulting acidity inhibits their activity. They are immotile at a pH greater than 12 or below 3. Sperm die rapidly in a strongly acidic environment, while a neutral or slightly alkaline medium greatly enhances their activity. Their activity is also increased with an increase in temperature, but this also causes an increase in their rate of metabolism and thus shortens their life span. The average life of sperm in ejaculated semen at normal body temperature is 1 to 7 days. Although sperm may be motile (alive), they may not be capable of fertilization. Their fertile life has been estimated at 24 to 48 hours [1].

Hyaluronidase, an enzyme found in the acrosomes of sperm heads, has the ability to break down intercellular cementing substances. When the ovum is expelled from the follicle, it is surrounded by the corona radiata, which must be removed before fertilization can occur. Hyaluronidase is thought to cause these cells to disperse, allowing the sperm to reach the ovum.

Seminal fluid consists of the ejaculum minus the sperm. Sixty percent of the seminal fluid comes from the prostate, 30 percent from the seminal vesicles, and the remainder from the epididymis and bulbourethral glands. It functions as a suspending medium, provides fructose and buffers, and contains substances that transform sperm into highly mobile cells.

Semen, a white viscous liquid with a pH of 7.35 to 7.50, consists of the seminal fluid plus the sperm. It normally forms a gel after leaving the male urethra but becomes more liquid within 10 to 15 minutes. The amount of semen per ejaculation is about 3 milliliters, with about 120 million sperm per milliliter. A

Figure 4-14. Maturation of male reproductive cells, resulting in formation of four mature sperm.

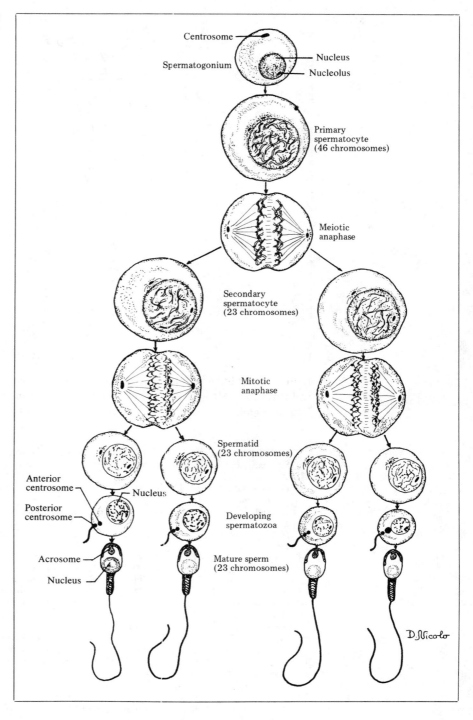

Figure 4-15. Mature sperm.

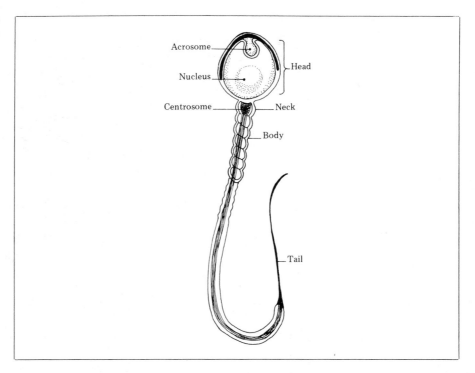

man is likely to be infertile when the number of sperm falls below 20 million per milliliter [3, 7]. It is possible that semen contains a mucolytic enzyme, similar to hyaluronidase, which can dissolve the mucous plug that frequently forms in the uterine cervix.

REFERENCES

1. Bedford, J. Developments in the Physiology of Conception. In R. Caplan and W. Sweeney (Eds.), *Advances in Obstetrics and Gynecology*. Baltimore: Williams & Wilkins, 1978.
2. Chiazze, L., Jr., et al. The length and variability of the human menstrual cycle. *Journal of the American Medical Association* 203:377, 1968.
3. Derrick, F. C., and Johnson, J. Reexamination of "normal" sperm count. *Urologie* 3.99, 1974.
4. Ganog, W. *Review of Medical Physiology*. Los Altos, Cal.: Lange Medical Publications, 1979.
5. Guyton, A. C. *Textbook of Medical Physiology* (5th ed.). Philadelphia: Saunders, 1976.
6. Harmon, S. M., and Tsitouras, P. Reproductive hormones in aging men. I. Measurement of sex steroids. *Journal of Clinical Endocrinology and Metabolism* 51:35, 1980.
7. Nelson, C. M. K., and Beinge, R. G. Semen analysis: Evidence for changing parameters of male fertility potential. *Fertility and Sterility* 25:503, 1974.
8. Reid, D. E., Ryan, K. J., and Benirschke, K. *Principles and Management of Human Reproduction*. Philadelphia: Saunders, 1972.
9. Schwartz, U., and Abraham, G. Corticosterone and aldosterone levels during the menstrual cycle. *Obstetrics and Gynecology* 45:339, 1975.
10. Shepard, R. S. *Human Physiology*. Philadelphia: Lippincott, 1971.
11. Speroff, L., Glass, R., and Kase, N. *Clinical Gynecologic Endocrinology and Infertility* (2nd ed.). Baltimore: Williams & Wilkins, 1979.
12. Zacharias, L., Rand, W., and Wurtman, R. A prospective study of sexual development and growth in American girls: The statistics of menarche. *Obstetrical and Gynecological Survey* 31:325, 1976.
13. Zacharias, L., Wurtman, R. J., and Schatzoff, M. Sexual maturation in contemporary American girls. *American Journal of Obstetrics and Gynecology* 108:833, 1970.

FURTHER
READING
Greenhill, J. P., and Friedman, E. A. *Biological Principles and Modern Practice of Obstetrics*. Philadelphia: Saunders, 1974.

Jacob, S. W. *Structure and Function in Man*. Philadelphia: Saunders, 1970.

Masters, W. H., and Johnson, V. E. *Human Sexual Response*. Boston: Little, Brown, 1966.

Pritchard, J. A., and MacDonald, P. C. *Williams Obstetrics* (16th ed.). New York: Appleton-Century-Crofts, 1980.

Romanes, G. J. (Ed.). *Cunningham's Textbook of Anatomy*. London: Oxford University Press, 1972.

Speroff, L., Glass, R., and Kase, N. *Clinical Gynecologic Endocrinology and Infertility* (2nd ed.). Baltimore: Williams & Wilkins, 1979.

Woods, N. *Human Sexuality in Health and Illness*. St. Louis: Mosby, 1975.

Chapter 5 Contraception, Infertility, and Therapeutic Abortion

The birth rate in the United States has been declining steadily during the past several years. One underlying factor has been the development of the nuclear family constellation, which promotes a couple's independence; it no longer seems desirable or valuable to many people to have a large number of children, which may have been an asset in the extended family group. What used to be sole functions of the family (i.e., socialization, education, food production) have been taken over by larger specialized institutions. The large middle class of today's society sees upward mobility as a goal within reach, so that a large number of children becomes a liability rather than an asset. In addition, the changing status of women, which involves the recognition of their individual goals and aspirations beyond that of motherhood, has been influential in decreasing family size. Although Catholicism discourages artificial methods of contraception, the majority of Catholic women report that they have used or will use them. Most other religious affiliations encourage parents to have only the number of children for whom they can adequately provide.

Because of these factors and because of the increased availability of contraceptive information and methods, it seems obvious that couples are planning their families; they are making choices about whether to have children, how many children to have, and when to have them. Contraception is the means by which family planning becomes a reality. It should be noted here that family planning, in its broad application, is also concerned with assisting infertile couples to become pregnant.

Most couples face decisions about contraception and often therapeutic abortion or infertility prior to coping with a pregnancy that proceeds to term. The traditional approach of nurses in counseling only the woman, and mainly after a pregnancy, is outmoded. Health education that includes sexuality, family planning, and preparation for parenthood should be imparted to both the woman and the man before choices actually have to be made.

CONTRACEPTION   Contraception is hardly a new practice but rather one that has been used through the ages. Wives of North African desert tribesmen mixed gunpowder solution to prevent pregnancy. Egyptian women inserted pessaries made from crocodile dung into their vaginas or used tampons made from lint soaked in citrus juice. They also partially hollowed out lemon halves and fitted them over the cervix. The Chinese swallowed 14 live tadpoles 3 days after menstruation.

During the second century, Greek women made vaginal plugs of wool soaked in sour oil, honey, cedar gum, and fig pulp, while others ate the uterus of a female mule. During the sixth century, Byzantine women attached a tube containing cat liver to their left foot. In the Middle Ages potions were prepared from willow leaves, iron rust or slag, clay, and the kidney of a mule. European brides in the seventeenth century were taught to sit on their fingers while riding in their coaches, or, in a figure-flattering move, to place roasted walnuts in the bosom, one for every barren year desired [22].

In the early 1900s, Margaret Sanger, a nurse in New York City's Lower East

Side, became incensed at the high incidence of illegal abortions and the high maternal death rate that followed. Accordingly, in 1916 in New York, she organized the first birth control clinic in the United States, only to be sent to jail as a result. Because of her initial persistence, birth control programs eventually became internationally funded by the Planned Parenthood Federation. Today you, as a nurse in the hospital or community, have broad opportunities to introduce the topic of family planning. This may be done initially during routine examinations, at the time of premarital examination, or in the prenatal period, as a part of the many kinds of planning being done at this time. The mother is usually very receptive immediately post partum in the hospital; also, when she is seen in the pediatrician's office during the period when coping with the baby occupies much of her energy, she is highly motivated to allow sufficient time before having another baby.

One of the most important factors in your ability to discuss family planning is your understanding and acceptance of your own attitudes and feelings regarding sex, sexuality, and the role of women in society. You are then more likely to be able to accept, without being judgmental, a variety of standards and modes of sexual behavior.

Since sharing contraceptive information involves very intimate areas of an individual's life, it is necessary that first contacts with couples be warm and meaningful. If you have the couple's respect and confidence, it is easier for you to perceive the couple's needs and to facilitate their choice, understanding, and use of a particular method. Because you are in a key position, it is imperative that you know the facts about various contraceptives; you should also know about the couple's attitudes, customs, mores, and vocabulary. You should be aware of the contraceptive methods used most frequently in the local community; this knowledge may be influential in helping couples make their choices. In many health centers, workers from the community are being trained and supervised by nurses to disseminate information about available services and to participate in activities within the center. These paraprofessionals can speak very effectively to couples as peers and as personal users of various contraceptive methods.

Follow-up appointments or perhaps a home visit by the family planning nurse should be scheduled to give the couple a chance to have their additional questions answered. In their expanded roles, nurses are doing counseling as well as performing routine vaginal examinations, taking Papanicolaou (Pap) smears, and fitting contraceptive devices. Although maternal-child health services are the traditional vehicles for sharing contraceptive information, you need to remember that patients in other health situations might like these resources to be made available to them. Postponement of pregnancy can be as important as medical treatment for a woman who has heart disease, cancer, tuberculosis, venereal disease, mental illness, or another disabling condition.

While some of the older methods of contraception were fairly successful, obviously today's methods enjoy far greater success rates. However, even today, methods that should be technically very reliable can have high failure rates. This may be due to misinformation regarding the method or may be caused by ambivalence or a negative attitude toward the method on the part of either the user or health personnel. Some methods require more motivation on the part of the user than others, which can contribute to increased failure rates. People also may be inadequately informed about the variety of methods available. In addition, people may not have adequate access to facilities where they may obtain today's methods of contraception. They may be unaware the service exists, or there may be a problem of distance to a health facility, inconvenient hours for service, or inordinate expense.

Tanis [39] points out a variety of reasons for failure or lack of use of birth control. These can be related to cultural, social, or educational influences such as poverty, ignorance, fear and anxiety, shame and embarrassment, or the feeling that an end result of birth control might be racial genocide. Inconsistent attitudes may involve denial, guilt, excitement due to risk, spontaneity, loneliness, hostility. Subconscious influences may be related to uncertainty in a relationship, coital gamesmanship, a sense of loss or grief, ambivalence, and attitudes of health care personnel toward the poor or toward sexuality in general.

The couple's attitude toward contraception is influenced by their feelings about infertility, sexuality, pregnancy, childbirth and parenthood, their cultural backgrounds, and the pressures they feel from their families and peers. Many people hesitate to interfere with the process of procreation on traditional or religious grounds. Effective prevention of pregnancy by contraception requires that the individual be extremely well motivated and, ideally, have a partner who is similarly committed.

The ideal contraceptive is recognized as one that is 100 percent effective, safe, simple to use, inexpensive, removed from the sex act itself, completely reversible, and easily accessible. No current method comes close to fulfilling all of these conditions. See Tables 5-1 and 5-2 for summaries of current contraceptive methods.

Condoms   Condoms were originally developed during the Renaissance to protect against venereal disease. During the eighteenth century their value as a contraceptive was recognized, and their use for this purpose became widespread during the nineteenth century after the discovery of vulcanization. Condoms have accumulated a number of synonyms, such as rubbers, skins, coats, softies, covers, protectors, shoes, bags, and prophylactics.

The earliest condoms were made from fabric impregnated with drugs or from the intestinal membranes of animals, usually sheep. Today there are numerous brands on the market, most made from latex, in a variety of colors, plain or reservoir ended, ribbed or pagoda shaped, structured or contoured. Some are made without a lubricant; others are lubricated with a dry lubricant such as a silicone compound or packaged with a wet lubricant, either a water gelatin colloid or a solution of glycerine in water. The lubricants often contain a preservative that acts as an antibacterial agent and also enables these condoms to be stored intact in a foil or plastic package at normal temperatures for approximately 5 years [19]. Lubricated types appear to be more popular, and since there is less friction when they are used, they also reduce the risk of tearing during intercourse. The two most common condom shapes are those with a dome-shaped end and those with a nipple or reservoir end. It is estimated that 20 to 30 million couples in the world use condoms as their only contraceptive method or in combination with another method.

When used consistently, condoms are a highly effective method of contraception

Table 5-1. Oral
Contraceptives and
Intrauterine Devices

Side Effects or Complications	Cause	Comments	Management
Oral Contraceptives			
Menstrual cycle alteration Reduced flow Missed period	Suppression of ovulation leads to incomplete development of endometrial glands or incomplete development of endometrium	Oligomenorrhea occurs in 50–70% of women. Amenorrhea is more common with products with low estrogen, occurs in 2–10% of cycles (mostly in first 3 cycles)	Counsel women regarding possible changes. Advise them to inform health care practitioner if amenorrhea in 2 consecutive cycles
Breakthrough bleeding in first half of cycle	Reduced absorption of oral contraceptive; lack of estrogen; pathology	Common during first 3 cycles, especially with low estrogen pills	Counsel women regarding possible irregularities. Advise them to inform their health care practitioner if bleeding persists after 3 cycles so that cause may be determined. May need pill with more estrogen
Breakthrough bleeding in second half of cycle	Reduced absorption of pill; lack of progestogen; pathology		May need new medication with more progesterone. Advise women to see their health care practitioner for her evaluation
Weight gain	Progesterone has anabolic effect, increases appetite. Estrogen may increase subcutaneous fat	Gain of 5–7 pounds common. Subcutaneous fat increases in breasts, hips, and thighs	Pill may be changed to one with different dosages of estrogen and progesterone
Nausea and vomiting, chloasma, headache, migraine	Due to estrogen	Unilateral and throbbing; usually not due to the pill	Another type of contraceptive is indicated
Fluid retention	Due to estrogen and/or progesterone	Associated with other signs of fluid retention	Pill may be changed to one with different dosages of estrogen and progesterone
Vaginal infections	May be due to changes in vaginal flora and pH	Increased discharge, itching	Treatment with appropriate medication is indicated
Nausea and vomiting	Due to estrogen	More common in first 3 cycles, with high doses of estrogen. May occur in 3% of users	Advise women to take pill with evening meal. May need different pill and/or antiemetic
Chloasma	Due to estrogen and progesterone	Will probably disappear slowly, but may never completely disappear. May occur in 30% of women	Advise women to avoid excessive exposure to sunlight, especially if they have a dark complexion and developed chloasma during pregnancy. May need a different pill
Edema	Due to estrogen and synthetic progestins	Usually disappears after third cycle. Less likely with low estrogen pill	If edema continues women may need new prescription, particularly if they have cardiac problems or wear contact lenses
Breast changes	No evidence of increase in incidence of breast cancer. Estrogen may increase growth of existing cancer	Increase in breast size is common. Some degree of tenderness may be present	Advise women to perform regular breast self-examination. Any breast changes should be evaluated by health care practitioner

Table 5-1 (continued)

Side Effects or Complications	Cause	Comments	Management
Hypertension	May be due to estrogen or progesterone	Blood pressure remains normal in 95% of women. If hypertension develops, it usually returns to pre-pill levels within 3 months after pill discontinued	Advise women to keep regular appointments for 6-month check-ups with health care practitioner
Increased incidence of myocardial infarction	May be due to effect of estrogen	Risk increases with age, duration of pill use, and smoking. Up to 5% of pill users may be at risk	If over 35, women should probably consider other types of contraception. They should stop smoking if they continue pill use. Low estrogen pill may be indicated
Increased incidence of thromboembolism	May be due to effect of estrogen	Risk increases in women over 35, who smoke heavily, or who have used the pill continuously for 5 years or more	Older women should stop smoking or discontinue pill use. Low estrogen pill may be indicated
Intrauterine Devices Cramps, bleeding	Due to foreign body in uterus	Effects usually diminish over time. In 2–20% of women may necessitate removal of IUD. IUD is inserted during menstrual period since cervix slightly softened and dilated and existing pregnancy is ruled out	IUD contraindicated in cases of uterine anomaly, uterine myomata, undiagnosed irregular bleeding. Advise women that they may experience discomfort and faintness immediately after IUD insertion. Menstrual blood loss may increase as well as dysmenorrhea but will gradually diminish in most women. Advise women to use supplemental vaginal foam for first 2 months and return for check-ups as indicated
Expulsion	Improper placement; natural effort of uterus to expel foreign body	Rates vary from 1–15%; higher in nulligravidas and with small devices	Advise women to check IUD string weekly at first and then after each period. If IUD cannot be located, notify health care practitioner
Infection	Introduction of microorganisms	Uterine or pelvic pain; uterine bleeding; abnormal vaginal discharge; fever; chills	Advise women to report signs of pelvic infection to health care practitioner

Sources: Adapted from R. Dickey. *Managing Contraceptive Pill Patients.* Aspen, Colo.: Creative Informatics, 1977; M. Gray and D. Grimes. Birth Control, Abortion, and Sterilization. In S. Romney, M. Gray, A. Little, J. Merrill, E. Quilligan, and R. Stander, *Gynecology and Obstetrics.* New York: McGraw-Hill, 1981; and J. McDonald and M. Currin. Management of Patients on Oral Contraceptives. In E. S. E. Hafez (Ed.), *Human Reproduction* (2nd ed.). New York: Harper & Row, 1980.

[17]. Breaks or tears have been cited as causes of failure, but the most common cause of failure is irregular use. It has been estimated that over 99 percent of the condoms sold in the United States are free of defects. Pregnancy rates when using condoms have been reported as low as 2.6 per 100 women using the method for a year, and as high as 18 percent [19]. Since the method requires motivation and some technical skill on the user's part, as well as the expense of purchasing the

Table 5-2. Other
Common Methods of
Contraception

Method	Advantages	Disadvantages	Effectiveness
Diaphragm (with cream, jelly, or foam)	No systemic side effects No routine schedule to be kept, as with the pill Used only when needed Can be used during menstruation or breastfeeding	Prescription required Rare local allergic side effects Must be inserted before intercourse and remain in place for at least 6 hours afterwards Requires yearly check-up Requires instruction on insertion technique Cannot be used by some women because of uterine variation Involves handling of genitals	Effectiveness depends on how correctly the method is used Failure rate may be 2–29%
Spermicidal agents (alone)	No prescription required Easy to obtain and use Can be used during lactation Can be used as adjunct to condom Provides lubrication	Requires motivation May be "messy" Rare local allergic side effects Not conducive to orogenital sex Must be used 1 hour or less before intercourse Must wait at least 6 hours to douche	Effectiveness depends on how correctly the method is used Failure rate may be 2–29% for foams alone, 4–36% for jellies and creams alone
Cervical cap	No systemic side effects Convenient for intercourse Oral sex may be more enjoyable than with other barrier methods	Not manufactured in the U.S. and may be expensive Many health care providers may not be knowledgeable about its use Requires instruction on insertion technique Effectiveness depends on female's anatomy	May be highly effective if used correctly
Condom	No systemic side effects No prescription necessary Gives partner some responsibility for contraception May afford some protection against venereal disease Inexpensive and easy to use	Requires motivation since foreplay must be interrupted to fit condom in place May occasionally slip or tear while in the woman's vagina May be some loss of sensation for the male	Effectiveness depends on how correctly the method is used Failure rate may be 3–36%
Natural family planning: Rhythm, ovulation, sympto-thermal	No systemic effects No prescription needed Sanctioned by Roman Catholic Church	Requires high motivation, education, and meticulous daily record keeping Health professional's guidance may be needed, especially in the beginning. May be difficult to use if menstrual cycles are irregular Often requires long periods of abstinence	Effectiveness depends on how correctly the method is used Failure rate may be from 1–47% depending on type used

Table 5-2 *(continued)*

Method	Advantages	Disadvantages	Effectiveness
Coitus interruptus (withdrawal)	Can be used in unexpected intercourse or when nothing else is available No medical risk No expense	Decreased sexual satisfaction Requires self-control and timing on male's part Danger of premature ejaculation	Effectiveness is low to fair if practiced with much self-control Generally considered ineffective
Postcoital douche			Completely ineffective for preventing pregnancy

Sources: Adapted from C. Garcia and D. Rosenfeld. *Human Fertility: The Regulation of Reproduction.* Philadelphia: Davis, 1977; and *Contraception: Comparing the Options.* HEW Publication No. (FDA) 78-3069. Rockville, Md.: U.S. Dept. of Health, Education, and Welfare, 1978.

condoms, the failure rates vary according to a group's education and socioeconomic level.

Condoms are unrolled onto the erect penis before any leakage of semen has occurred. In uncircumcised males, the foreskin is retracted prior to application. When the condoms with dome-shaped ends are used, approximately 1 centimeter (½ inch) of the condom should be allowed to protrude beyond the end of the penis. This acts as a reservoir and decreases the pressure of the semen against the tip of the condom during ejaculation. Air should be expelled from this reservoir before the condom is completely unrolled onto the penis. (This should also be done with the condom with the nipple end.) If this step is omitted, the trapped air may be released during the thrusting motions, escaping through the open end of the condom and carrying drops of semen with it.

After ejaculation the penis should be withdrawn from the vagina, with the condom held firmly at the base of the penis. If this is not done, the condom may slip off easily as detumescence occurs.

Overall, this method has many advantages. The condom has proven reliability, is inexpensive, requires no physician visit or prescription, has a long storage life, is portable, and can be purchased over the counter or in relative secrecy from vending machines. For this reason it is particularly popular among teenagers. The condom may also help protect against venereal disease and *Candida* and *Trichomonas* infections (this protection also depends on other health measures such as a good handwashing and proper condom disposal).

Although the condom has been used for many years, its use has decreased as other methods have become available. This is probably due to such disadvantages as fear of breakage, difficulty or discomfort encountered when insertion is attempted (with nonlubricated types of condoms), and the need to interrupt lovemaking to apply the condom. This may only add to the anxiety of a man who is already uncertain about his ability to maintain an erection.

Men often complain of impaired sensation during intercourse, but this may be an advantage in men who ejaculate prematurely. Women occasionally complain of being unable to feel the ejaculation. Some women who value "cleanliness" prefer their partners to use condoms, since then the semen does not touch them. For some individuals the condom is unacceptable because of its association with prostitution and protection against venereal disease.

Condoms are ideal for couples who have irregular and unplanned intercourse and for couples for whom other contraceptives are contraindicated. Many couples use them for intercourse during menstruation, during the early postpartum period, and during lactation if hormonal contraceptives are contraindicated.

Diaphragms   The original diaphragm was invented in the nineteenth century by a German physician who used the pseudonym Mensinga. Diaphragms did not appear in the United States then because of laws prohibiting the importation of contraceptives. It was not until the 1920s that United States companies began manufacturing them. Use of the diaphragm declined with the introduction of the intrauterine device and oral contraceptives. With the recent publicity given to the risks associated with these methods, however, there has been renewed interest in the use of the diaphragm as a desirable method of contraception. In general this increased interest has been expressed by educated women of a high socioeconomic level [4].

A diaphragm resembles a cup, with a circular rim and a dome made of thin rubber; its size ranges from 45 to 105 millimeters (1.8 to 4.1 inches) in diameter. The purpose of the diaphragm is to block access to the cervical canal by covering the external os and thus act as a barrier between sperm and egg.

For the diaphragm to be effective, however, it is essential that it be used with a vaginal spermicidal cream or jelly. About a teaspoon of cream or jelly is placed inside the dome of the diaphragm, and more is spread around the rim. Some women find it facilitates insertion if they spread some jelly or cream on the other side of the dome also. It is important that the diaphragm be inserted before vaginal penetration by the penis, since preejaculate fluid may contain viable sperm.

For insertion, the diaphragm is squeezed together so that the rim sides touch, with the dome side down. When the diaphragm is properly inserted, the dome covers the cervix and the woman then tucks the anterior rim under her pubic bone. She must check to see that the dome has covered her cervix by feeling for the cervix with her index finger.

A woman may squat to insert her diaphragm, or she may stand placing her foot on a chair or the toilet, or lie on her back with her knees bent. The diaphragm and spermicide may be inserted 1 hour prior to intercourse and should not be removed for a minimum of 6 hours following intercourse. Should intercourse take place a second time within the 6-hour period, an applicator of spermicide should be injected into the vagina (without removing the diaphragm) prior to intercourse.

The diaphragm is removed by hooking an index finger under the front rim and pulling downward and outward. Removal may be facilitated by bearing down as though having a bowel movement. An introducer (or inserter or director) may also be used to insert or remove the diaphragm. For insertion, the diaphragm is stretched over the introducer, spermicide is applied as already described, and the diaphragm is directed into the vagina, with the front end placed in the posterior fornix. When it is in place, the diaphragm can be unhooked with sideward motion of the introducer. The woman then tucks the anterior rim under her pelvic bone. By using the hook end of the introducer the diaphragm may be removed (Fig. 5-1).

After use, the diaphragm should be washed with warm soapy water, dried, and dusted with cornstarch or talcum. Cared for in this way it should last between 2

Figure 5-1. Diaphragm
and inserter. Diaphragm
attached to hooked end of
inserter (top). Diaphragm
hooked and ready for in-
sertion (bottom).

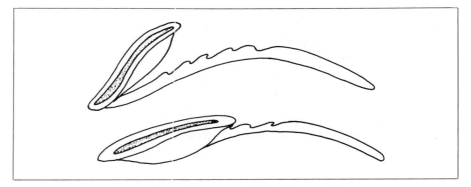

and 4 years; however, it must be inspected for holes or thinning prior to each insertion.

Diaphragms must be fitted to the individual by a physician, nurse, or health care worker prepared in this area, since a good fit is essential for its success. A virgin may be fitted with the diaphragm; however, after several months of sexual activity she should have the size rechecked, since she may now require a larger one. Diaphragm fit should also be checked following pregnancy or abortion, pelvic surgery, or a loss or gain of 10 or more pounds. Gara [15] emphasizes the importance of the relationship between effectiveness rate and adequate time devoted to diaphragm fitting, instruction in its use, and subsequent follow-up by the health care practitioner.

There are no side effects associated with the use of a diaphragm except in those rare people who are allergic to spermicides or rubber. However, the method does require high motivation, planning, patience, intelligence, some degree of mechanical aptitude, visits to a physician for fitting, and a prescription. There may also be associated psychologic problems for the woman who is uncomfortable touching her genitalia.

The diaphragm is contraindicated in women with moderate to severe pelvic floor damage, cystocele or rectocele, or a very long vagina or short fingers which would make insertion of the diaphragm difficult. The overall failure rates vary from 2 to 30 percent.

Cervical Caps   Widely used in Europe since the nineteenth century, the cervical cap has recently been the subject of renewed interest in the United States as an alternative contraceptive device. The function of a cervical cap is much like that of a diaphragm; it fits over the cervix and imposes a barrier between the sperm and egg. Cervical caps are made of rubber or plastic and are smaller, thicker, and less flexible than diaphragms. Rubber caps may be left in place for 24 hours at a time, while plastic ones may be left in place between menstrual periods, which separates their insertion from the sex act. Because of the incidence of infection, some practitioners are recommending that neither type of cervical cap be left in place for more than 24 hours.

Some of the difficulties associated with the use of the cervical cap are that it must be fitted by a well-trained practitioner and the wearer must learn and practice the techniques of its insertion and removal. The cervical cap is usually used with spermicidal cream or jelly and should remain in place after intercourse for 6 to 8 hours. The woman should not douche during this time period. The cervical cap has a failure rate of 2 to 15 percent [4, 8].

Spermicidal Agents   A variety of spermicidal agents have been developed since the early 1960s. Some of them are effective when used alone; some are used with diaphragms or other vaginal contraceptives. They are used by many women for whom the intrauterine device or oral contraceptives are inappropriate. Their failure rate may be due to inconsistent use, low motivation on the part of the user, or the necessity to use immediately before intercourse and to reapply when intercourse is repeated.

These agents contain two main ingredients: an inert base substance, such as soft soap or an oil in water emulsion, which acts as a barrier to sperm movement, and an active spermicidal agent which immobilizes or destroys sperm [4].

PASTES, JELLIES, AND CREAMS
Pastes and jellies are made of a water-soluble base that liquefies at body temperature and evenly covers the vaginal wall. They are applied with an applicator and plunger inserted as far as possible into the vagina. They can be used up to an hour before intercourse but must be repeated if more than an hour passes before actual intercourse occurs.

Many investigators feel that when used alone the jellies are inferior to vaginal creams since they do not disperse and adhere as well to tissue surfaces. Both creams and jellies are less effective when used alone than when used with a condom or diaphragm. Their failure rate averages 30 percent.

Some lubricating jellies that are often sold alongside contraceptive jellies in stores are intended for vaginal lubrication rather than for contraceptive purposes. When purchasing a jelly for contraceptive purposes one should check to see that it states on the label either that it contains a spermicide or that it is for contraceptive purposes.

Creams are made of water-insoluble substances such as stearates or glycerin and tend to remain wherever they are placed in the vagina. Many people feel that vaginal creams are the best substances to be used when a condom or diaphragm will not be used, since the creams adhere well to tissue surfaces. This is viewed by some as a disadvantage, since the creams coat the penis during intercourse and tend to cling to the labia and vulva as the penis is withdrawn. With jellies, pastes, and creams, the woman should not douche for at least 6 hours after intercourse.

SUPPOSITORIES
Contraceptive suppositories contain spermicide in a base of cocoa butter, glycerin, or other substance that melts at body temperature. Suppositories are cone-shaped and are usually inserted high in the woman's vagina either by hand or by an inserter about 15 minutes before intercourse. Their spermicidal effect usually lasts for 1 to 2 hours, but the woman or her partner should insert another suppository if intercourse is to be repeated. The woman should not douche for at least 6 hours after intercourse [4].

FOAMS—AEROSOLS AND TABLETS
Aerosol foams consist of an oil and water emulsion under gas pressure. When released, the gas propellant produces a foam which the woman can discharge into her vagina either directly or by means of an applicator. Foams should be inserted

30 minutes to 1 hour prior to intercourse and repeated with each intercourse. The woman should not douche for at least 6 hours after intercourse. Vaginal foams have become the most popular of all the chemical vaginal agents. They may be more effective than other agents since they cover the vagina and cervix more evenly [4].

Foaming tablets are also available. The foam-producing ingredients, tartaric acid and sodium bicarbonate, are mixed with other substances, including a spermicide. The mixture is pressed into a tablet and wrapped in foil. When the tablet is moistened (either by the secretions in the vagina or by wetting with saliva or water prior to insertion), the result is a foam plug that acts as a barrier and also as a releasing agent for the spermicide.

It takes approximately 5 minutes for the tablet to react completely. The failure rate is high, and a common side effect is an unpleasant burning sensation within the vagina. The tablets also need to be placed as far into the vagina as possible. As with the diaphragm, foams, creams, and jellies, douching should not take place for at least 6 hours after intercourse (douching is not really necessary at all).

With all chemical methods it is necessary to understand the method and the mechanics involved. Some women are repelled by the manipulation involved, while others incorporate it into their foreplay. Fastidious women may have a difficult time tolerating jellies, creams, and foams because of their "messy" nature and because they do not like to postpone douching following intercourse. Recent data show a positive association between vaginal spermicide use and a variety of congenital disorders in babies [44]. However, a well-defined syndrome among the infants whose mothers used spermicides is not present; therefore, the results are considered to be tentative. It is likely that more definitive research in this area will be reported in the future.

Postcoital Douche   The theory behind douching as a contraceptive measure is that semen can be flushed from the vagina before sperm have had a chance to enter the cervix. However, it is known that immediately after the ejaculation of semen into the vagina, the sperm penetrate the cervical mucus; some are passively carried to the place of fertilization in as short a time as 2 to 10 minutes; and some reach the internal os in 1.5 to 3 minutes. Since the woman must have extraordinary speed if her postcoital douche is to reach the sperm, its efficacy as a contraceptive measure is extremely doubtful. The pregnancy rate associated with it is at least 36 percent.

Occasionally women have used high concentrations of household disinfectants, vinegar, lemon juice, and carbonated soft drinks as douching agents. Not only are they ineffective but their caustic quality may irritate the lining of the female reproductive tract.

Coitus Interruptus   Coitus interruptus (withdrawal) requires the man to withdraw his penis immediately before he begins to ejaculate, a moment when the closest possible physical union is desired. It is also a time when the typical male impulse is to penetrate the vagina as deeply as possible. Consequently many couples find the use of coitus interruptus very frustrating, although some have relied on it for years with both success and satisfaction. Coitus interruptus is the oldest known form of contraception and, in some parts of the world, is still used more often than the condom and the pill. Depending on the care and timing of the man, the pregnancy rate is 8 to

40 percent. Effectiveness of this method may be compromised by the presence of viable sperm in preejaculate fluid.

Since even one drop of semen may contain 10,000 to 100,000 sperm, the effectiveness of coitus interruptus depends largely on psychologic factors. Withdrawal is best practiced by a conscientious man with a thorough knowledge of his own body, extremely good self-control, and a very strong desire to protect his partner. The woman has to be content to restrain her activity during intercourse so that she does not threaten her partner's control over his own sexual excitement. Coitus interruptus reduces the time for the woman to reach orgasm and may produce anxiety over whether her partner will withdraw in time.

Postcoital Contraceptives

Postcoital contraception involves the prevention of implantation after unprotected intercourse. Currently unavailable, the ideal method would be a contraceptive agent that would be given every month after ovulation. This might take the form of an agent to induce menstruation administered in the second half of the menstrual cycle.

Today the postcoital administration of estrogen appears to be an effective means of preventing pregnancy if enough is taken soon after unprotected intercourse. In 1975 the U.S. Food and Drug Administration approved diethylstilbestrol (25 mg) for such postcoital use, but only in cases of emergency such as rape. Such estrogen therapy begun as soon as possible (within 72 hours) after unprotected midcycle intercourse and continued for 3 to 6 days will probably be effective if implantation has not occurred. It is thought that the blastocyst is prevented from implanting in the woman's endometrium, perhaps by a disturbance in the estrogen-progesterone ratio or an alteration in the transport of the ovum through the fallopian tube [3].

High doses of diethylstilbestrol frequently cause nausea and vomiting within 6 to 8 hours after their ingestion. This may be severe during the first 1 to 2 days of treatment, but it can be minimized if the pills are enteric-coated or if the woman takes them at mealtime or with an antiemetic. It may be that intravenous injection may eliminate the nausea completely, but more testing of this method needs to be done. The woman may also experience breast tenderness, headache, dizziness, spotting, or ectopic pregnancy following the administration of this medication. There is no direct evidence that diethylstilbestrol or other estrogens administered after intercourse will result in genital cancer in offspring conceived if the treatment fails. (The timing of its administration does not coincide with vaginal organogenesis at 5 to 12 weeks of pregnancy [3, 18].)

Postcoital Prostaglandin

Little is known about the use of prostaglandins for contraception in women. Prostaglandins $E_2\alpha$ and $F_2\alpha$ are absorbed in the vaginal wall and successfully induce menstruation within a few days after the first missed menstrual period. In the future prostaglandins may be administered vaginally once a month at the time of the expected menstruation. They may achieve their effect by causing contractions which damage the embryonic endocrine function or deprive the corpus luteum of its luteotropic support. More research is required to fully evaluate available and future postcoital contraceptives [3].

Natural Family Planning

RHYTHM

The rhythm method of contraception is based on the facts that the egg is fertilizable for about 12 hours (not more than 24 hours) and that sperm usually maintain their total ability to fertilize for not more than 48 hours after ejaculation (although some have been found to survive in the female reproductive tract for as long as 7 days). Thus, theoretically a woman is potentially fertile for 2 days before ovulation and 1 day after—a total of 4 "unsafe" days per cycle. Even though it is known that ovulation occurs 14 ± 2 days before the onset of the next menstrual period, unfortunately it is impossible to make an accurate prediction of when ovulation will occur in each cycle, particularly if the cycles vary in length. There are two methods of rhythm birth control, which may be used singly or in combination to determine when ovulation occurs and to compute the number of infertile and fertile days per cycle.

With the *calendar method*, the accuracy of determining infertile days is greatly improved if the dates of the twelve previous cycles are known. If all the cycles were 28 days long, for example, the fertile phase would begin on day 10: 28 days minus 16 (14 plus 2 days for a long progestational phase or early ovulation) minus 2 more days for sperm life span. The fertile phase would end on day 17: 28 days minus 12 (14 minus 2 days for a short progestational phase or late ovulation) plus 1 day for ovum life span.

Since most cycles vary in length, the shortest cycle as well as the longest must be considered. The day on which menstruation begins is considered to be *day 1* of the cycle. In the general formula for the calendar method, the fertile phase extends from and includes the 18th day before the end of the shortest cycle through the 11th day before the end of the longest cycle. If, for example, a record of menstrual dates during the preceding twelve cycles shows that a woman has cycles as short as 23 days and as long as 33 days, her projected fertile phase for the current month would begin on day 5 (23 minus 18) and end on day 22 (33 minus 11).

It is fortunate that not very many women in their prime childbearing years (age 20–30) have such a wide range of cycle lengths, since if the woman in the example has an active flow of 4 days and her next menstrual period on day 24, she will have only two safe days. This would hardly be acceptable to most sexually active couples; this emphasizes the extremely strong motivation a couple must have if rhythm is to be successful. With *conscientious* use of this calendar rhythm method, the pregnancy rate is in the vicinity of 15 percent.

A woman may actually fail to ovulate once or twice a year. In these cases her menstrual flow, if there is any, will be slightly different in quality, amount, and duration, and it may occur earlier in the cycle. To safely use the rhythm method, she must not have intercourse until she has had at least two periods of normal flow, since ovulation may recur at any time after failure to ovulate.

It is possible to shorten the unsafe phase (as determined by the calendar method) with the use of the *basal body temperature method*. The basal body temperature is taken with a special thermometer that records 35.5° to 37.8°C in 0.05° rather than 0.1° units (96°–100°F in 0.1° rather than 0.2° units), so that minute temperature shifts may be read easily. The temperature is taken for 5 minutes, preferably rectally, at the same time each morning immediately upon wakening after at least 5 to 6 hours sleep. It is important that the temperature be taken before any kind of physical or emotional activity (e.g., eating, drinking, smoking, getting out of bed) and recorded at the time so that it is not forgotten.

The daily charting of the basal body temperature will reveal a characteristic pattern or curve, so that it is possible to determine the time of ovulation when there is a sudden and maintained shift of at least 0.3°C (0.5°F) (Fig. 5-2). This temperature shift reflects the thermogenic action of progesterone produced by the corpus luteum following ovulation, although the time relationship between the temperature rise and ovulation is still controversial. At the time of ovulation there may be a slight transient drop in temperature but this is not a constant finding [33].

Pinpointing ovulation is important for infertile couples as well as those hoping to avoid pregnancy, since infertile couples will want to take maximum advantage of their opportunities for fertilization. For the couple seeking contraception, the woman's safe period has begun when her temperature has been elevated by at least 0.3°C (0.5°F) for 3 consecutive days. This method is successful when intercourse is limited to the postovulatory period.

The basal body temperature method can be combined with the calendar method to determine a primary safe phase prior to ovulation, since the temperature rise

Figure 5-2. Basal body temperature during two menstrual cycles. Ovulation probably occurred on day 14 of each of these cycles.

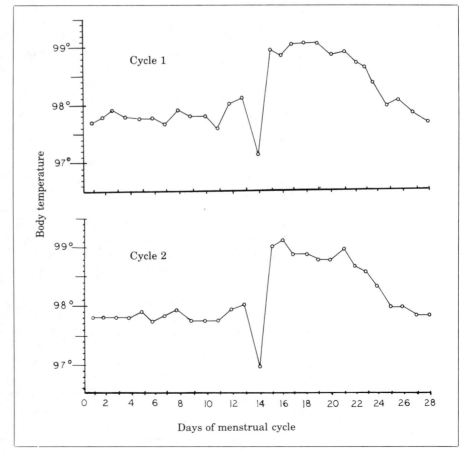

only determines the *end* of the abstinence period. Failures are more probable in this primary phase, however.

Although rhythm is effective when used correctly, necessity of a prolonged period of abstinence makes the method unacceptable to many couples. According to the National Fertility Survey, the use of all types of rhythm contraception fell significantly in the United States between 1965 and 1970. In 1965, 15 percent of couples using contraception used the rhythm method; in 1970 only 7 percent used it. Since the woman bears the responsibility of determining safe periods, she must be capable of accurate perception, faithful adherence to schedule, and simple calculations. In addition, her partner must be content to let her determine when intercourse is permissible; if he fears being dominated, he will not be able to tolerate this. By dictating periods of abstinence, the rhythm method makes the need for spontaneous sex impossible to meet. For those women in whom the sex drive is highest at ovulation, rhythm is extremely difficult to practice at the time when it is most necessary.

OVULATION METHOD

The ovulation method of natural family planning, based on the premise that fertilization cannot occur without the presence of a favorable cervical mucus, was introduced to the United States in 1952 by two Australian physicians, John and Lyn Billings [6]. The woman who uses this method of natural family planning must assess the consistency of her cervical mucus every day to determine when she is ovulating. She is taught to be aware of wetness or dryness around her vagina or vulva and to keep a careful record of her findings. Wet days represent the beginning of her ovulatory or fertile period when she should avoid intercourse. Observing mucus secretion as a method of family planning can be used in both ovulatory and anovulatory cycles, in menopausal and lactating women. Although its effectiveness can be reduced by infections such as cervicitis or vaginitis, the woman who is very familiar with the method will probably still be able to notice changes in the continuing vaginal discharge. Billings feels that the ovulation method is best used alone, not in combination with the basal body temperature method which may add confusing information. Advocates of the ovulation method proclaim that its effectiveness rate may be as high as 98 percent [9].

SYMPTO-THERMAL METHOD

Another method of natural family planning, the sympto-thermal method, was introduced in 1975 by the Kippleys [7]. This method involves both partners in identifying relevant signs and symptoms, keeping accurate records, and interpreting results. The method combines observations of cervical mucus, condition of the cervix (as ovulation approaches it dilates slightly, becomes softer, and feels more slippery), the basal body temperature, and secondary signs (increased sex drive, abdominal bloating, mittleschmerz, vulvar swelling, and slight bloody discharge).

All the methods of natural family planning require a high level of motivation on the part of the couple. One important advantage is that the woman learns more about her own body rhythms and how they are involved in the control of her own fertility. Natural family planning methods are becoming more popular as women become more concerned about the side effects that may accompany other methods of contraception.

Intrauterine Devices

Medical literature during the 1880s reported the use of intrauterine devices (IUDs) or intracervical devices for both contraception and treatment of gynecologic disorders. These devices were unpopular because it was believed that they initiated abortions and that they were associated with pelvic inflammations. In the early 1900s, opposition again developed shortly after two new models, silkworm gut rolled into rings and a coil of silver wire (Gräfenberg ring), were introduced. The IUD as a contraceptive was revived in 1959 by two physicians (one in Israel and one in Japan), with resulting low pregnancy rates and no serious side effects.

Since the early 1960s several types of polyethylene IUDs have become available, including the spiral, loop, and copper (Cu)-7. (Fig. 5-3). Their flexibility allows them to be inserted rather simply: The IUD is straightened full length in a narrow plastic tube and is inserted under sterile conditions into the uterus through the cervix; it then resumes its original shape as it is pushed from the inserter into the uterine cavity. The plastic devices are kept completely in the inserter for no more than 1 or 2 minutes to keep them from losing their shape "memory." Those with strings that project from the cervix can usually be removed

Figure 5-3. Types of IUDs. 1. Double coil. 2. Lippes Loop. 3. Multiload Copper, Cu-250. 4. Cu-7. 5. Spiral. 6. Copper T.

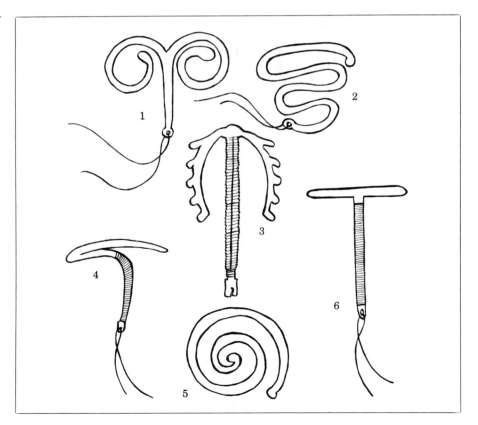

by gentle traction. Pregnancy rates with IUDs in place are 2 to 3 percent, depending on the device used.

Among women in the United States the rate of increase in use of intrauterine devices has been more rapid than that of any other reported method of contraception. They are used by over 3 million women in the United States and by over 15 million women worldwide with an effectiveness rate of 95 to 99 percent when they are inserted properly.

Rapid population growth, especially in underdeveloped countries, has created a need for more methods of population control. New inert materials have made it possible for IUDs to remain in the uterus for indefinite periods, and new treatments for pelvic inflammatory disease have made that a less serious complication. With more research into IUD development, new and improved models continually appear for clinical use, some with only small changes and others based on entirely new principles.

Intrauterine devices may be nonmedicated or medicated. All types are biologically active, however, since they create a change in the endometrium and in the endometrial environment. The IUD meets several criteria for ideal contraception: a high rate of effectiveness, reversibility, and low cost. The Lippes Loop remains the most widely used IUD in this country, followed by the Cu-7. The coil is the second most popular device among black women; among nulliparous women the Cu-7 ranks first in popularity.

MODE OF ACTION

The specific mechanism by which IUDs achieve their effect is not known. It is known that after IUD insertion a temporary intrauterine reaction occurs in response to microorganisms from cervical mucus on the surface of the IUD. The inflammatory reaction is usually self-limited as the woman's defense mechanisms neutralize the microorganisms. Another intrauterine reaction which is more lasting involves the IUD itself, a foreign body. An inflammatory response develops that depends on the chemical composition and size of the device. The reaction continues for as long as the IUD remains in the uterus and results from injury to the superficial endometrium and endometrial blood vessels, release of histamine, and inflammatory cell reactions. As a result blastocystic DNA synthesis decreases, and the cytotoxic effects are such that the blastocyst is lysed before implantation or is unable to implant normally [29]. The IUD may also exert its contraceptive effect by increasing the endometrial production or prostaglandins. Those IUDs that are medicated with copper or progesterone exert additional effects. It is thought that copper may produce an antifertility effect by modifying carbonic anhydrase, among other chemicals, believed to be essential for adhesion of the blastocyst to the superficial endometrium. Progesterone-medicated IUDs may alter the metabolism of the blastocyst or atrophy uterine glands [29].

EFFECTIVENESS AND RETENTION

Pregnancy rates and expulsion rates vary with the type and size of the IUD, the duration of its use, and the age and parity of the woman. The larger sizes are associated with higher pregnancy rates; the smaller sizes are associated with lower rates. Highest pregnancy rates exist for loops, then spirals. With a large loop, the pregnancy rates are highest for the first year and decrease with each subsequent year.

The actual effectiveness of the IUD approaches the theoretical effectiveness since it does not depend on daily or periodic medication or on insertion before, during, or after intercourse. About 30 percent of pregnancies with IUDs have occurred following unnoticed expulsion of the device. To lessen the chance of unnoticed expulsion, the woman should be taught to examine herself about once a week for the presence of the strings protruding from her cervix. Since a large proportion of expulsions occur at the time of the menstrual flow, especially during the first few periods following insertion, she should examine tampons or perineal pads to see if the device has been expelled. She should report expulsions immediately so that a new device can be inserted; she should be reminded to use other contraceptive measures in the interim.

IUDs of smaller sizes are associated with higher expulsion rates. The highest expulsion rates occur with spirals, then loops. Expulsion rates decrease with the age of the woman and, in most age groups, with parity.

The new Multiload Copper 250 is especially designed for nulliparous women with a small uterine cavity and uterine musculature with increased tone. In general the copper IUDs have fewer side effects and expulsions associated with their use than the larger nonmedicated IUDs sometimes used in nulliparas [30].

INDICATIONS AND CONTRAINDICATIONS

The IUD is most appropriate for women who prefer a method that requires no precoital preparation, who wish to dissociate intercourse from contraceptive measures, who are not successful in the use of other birth control methods, or who have contraindications to the use of other methods. The IUD should not be used by women who have pelvic inflammatory disease, known or suspected pregnancy, cervical or uterine cancer, uterine malformations or fibroids, or a history of abnormal uterine bleeding.

TIME OF INSERTION

A convenient time for insertion is during the woman's postabortion or postpartum check-up, which is a time when the cervix is still somewhat dilated, the risk of pregnancy is low, and her motivation for a method of contraception is high. Another time of choice is during the menstrual flow, when the cervix is again somewhat relaxed, the chance of pregnancy is minimal, and any bleeding after insertion (which could alarm the woman) is hidden in the menstrual flow.

If she has no difficulties, the woman can wear the plastic or stainless steel IUD indefinitely until menopause, although she is instructed to have an annual check-up. Copper-bearing IUDs are replaced from time to time, usually at 2-year intervals.

In clinics in the United States the IUD is the method of second choice, behind the pill and only slightly ahead of the diaphragm. In some of the developing countries, however, it forms the backbone of national family planning programs. IUDs are still most suitable for populations not accustomed to continued use of any form of preventive medicine.

SIDE EFFECTS AND COMPLICATIONS

The ideal IUD has not been developed at this time. Bleeding, pain, expulsion, uterine perforation, and an increased risk of pelvic inflammatory disease continue to be the chief complications associated with this contraceptive method. Uterine perforation occurs in one to seven women out of 10,000, usually when the IUD is being inserted (see Table 5-1).

The most common side effect (along with pain and discomfort) is bleeding, i.e., menorrhagia, metrorrhagia, or both. Women should be informed that they may normally expect some bleeding and some cramping after IUD insertion. The first few menstrual periods after insertion tend to be heavier and last longer than previously, and they are sometimes followed by postmenstrual staining or spotting. These symptoms tend to disappear within 3 months, but sometimes they are severe enough to cause the woman to have the IUD removed. (About 20–30 percent of women either have the device removed for these reasons or expel it involuntarily.) Associated cramping is usually eased by application of heat and by analgesics.

The most important complication associated with IUDs is that of pelvic infection which occurs in 2 to 3 percent of women, usually during the first or second year following insertion. Most of the pelvic inflammatory disease associated with IUDs is diagnosed as preexisting chronic or subchronic infection exacerbated by the insertion procedure rather than a new infection. IUD insertion may cause infection, although the bacteria in the cervical mucus carried along on the device are generally of low virulence. The host defenses of the endometrium are usually adequate to combat these organisms within a very short period of time. Most of these cases are mild and are treated with antibiotics, with or without removal of the device.

Users of IUDs are three to five times more likely to develop pelvic infections than nonusers. This is especially true of the nullipara who is under 25, has a history of pelvic inflammatory disease, and/or has multiple sex partners. The signs and symptoms that may herald the onset of such an infection are development of new menstrual disorders, abnormal vaginal discharge, fever, chills, abdominal or pelvic pain, and dyspareunia [21, 30]. There is no evidence at this time that the IUD has any carcinogenic effect.

EFFECTS ON FERTILITY AND REPRODUCTION
Fertility after removal of an IUD appears to be unimpaired. There is an increased incidence of ectopic pregnancy in women wearing an IUD compared to women in general. The incidence appears to be greater with IUDs containing progesterone [35], in cases where the IUD has been used for over 4 years, or where pelvic inflammatory disease has been a problem.

If a pregnancy occurs when an IUD is in place, a spontaneous abortion will usually occur about 50 percent of the time. If the IUD is removed, the risk of spontaneous abortion is reduced to 25 to 30 percent. Its presence has not been correlated with fetal malformation or injury.

OTHER EFFECTS
Infrequently some men have complained of pain during intercourse. This complaint was particularly associated with the Margulies spiral, which had a stiff, beaded projection from the cervix into the vagina. A few men complain about the nylon strings that protrude from the cervix; in these cases the strings are usually

clipped shorter. Ordinarily the IUD does not interfere with intercourse, douching, or use of tampons.

PSYCHOLOGIC IMPLICATIONS
Peaceful, secure, trusting women adapt well to the IUD. They do not have to be highly motivated or well organized. Some women may feel uncomfortable with the idea of a foreign body inside them or may fear that it will cause cancer.

The use of the IUD is contraindicated in women who have an unusually strong need to feel control over themselves. Sometimes such women become anxious when they are not permitted spur of the moment changes of mind regarding their fertility. However, since this method of contraception is dissociated from intercourse, women with guilt feelings about birth control may have fewer conflicts about using the IUD rather than the pill. On the other hand, the IUD is not usually an acceptable contraceptive measure for women who have strong feelings against abortion.

Other Contraceptive Methods

Some other contraceptive methods are currently being evaluated for long-term safety and effectiveness. They include rubber vaginal devices containing sustained-release progestational agents that abolish the midcycle LH surge. These are easily inserted and removed by the user and can be worn continuously for as long as 2 years or removed periodically in association with menstrual periods. Their placement in the woman's vagina is much like that of the diaphragm and does not interfere with intercourse [11].

Also being tested is a spermicide-impregnated sponge which the woman places in her vagina before intercourse and does not remove until 8 hours after intercourse. Currently not available for routine use are intracervical devices designed to release medication, especially progesterone, in the endocervix; in clinical trials to date they have remained in place for as long as 60 days without undesirable effects [11].

Subdermal silicone-rubber implants that release progestin have been shown to inhibit ovulation for as long as 1 year with a calculated lifetime as long as 5 years. (They are placed in the ventral aspect of the forearm.) Low pregnancy rates and no serious local or systemic side effects other than unpredictable bleeding have been noted. It is hoped that implants containing both estrogen and progesterone will be effective in improving the unpredictable bleeding pattern [11].

Injectable Contraceptives

Several types of injectable contraceptives are being tested, some containing estrogen-progestogen combinations and others containing progestogen only. Of these Depo-Provera has been the monthly injectable most widely tested; Cyclo-Provera and Deladroxate are two others. Tests have produced excellent results with very few contraceptive failures reported.

To date tests involving 2-month injectables have not been as favorable; however, one 3-month injectable has produced a pregnancy rate that compares favorably with that of oral contraceptives and exceeds that of intrauterine devices. One drug has been tested as a biannual contraceptive injection with good results. Side effects of the injectable contraceptives have involved irregular bleeding and a possible delay in fertility once the drug is discontinued. Increased risk of hypertension and thromboembolic disorders does not appear to be associated with this type of contraceptive [41].

Experimental Male Contraception

Many methods of male contraception are currently being investigated. They include efforts to isolate testicular inhibin, a hormone that selectively inhibits FSH secretion; the use of compounds to inhibit spermatogenesis; drugs that act directly on the cells of the seminiferous tubules to influence the metabolic activity of Sertoli cells; drugs that interfere with epididymal maturation of sperm; plugs and valves that interfere with sperm transport; drugs such as hyaluronidase inhibitors that inactivate sperm acrosome enzymes; and immunization with some form of LH to disrupt spermatogenesis. Problems with developing these types of male contraceptives involve the difficulty in separating the suppression of spermatogenesis and androgen production, the need for reversibility and restoration of fertility, and the lack of motivation in some men to use contraception [17].

Oral Contraceptives

Oral contraceptives (OCs) are currently the most popular and common method of birth control. Used by about 50 million women in the world, OCs consist of different combinations of synthetic estrogens and progesterone; OCs containing only progesterone are available in the United States but their use is somewhat limited [5].

OCs achieve their effect primarily by inhibiting ovulation though suppression of the hypothalamic-releasing hormones for FSH and LH. Under their influence the usual cyclic changes in the woman's endometrium occur earlier and with greater intensity than in nonmedicated cycles. This endometrium does not easily support implantation. The pills are also responsible for other secondary contraceptive mechanisms such as the production of cervical mucus that is scanty, thick, and generally unpenetrable by sperm [20]. Combination OCs, almost 100 percent effective in preventing pregnancy, have also been shown to reduce dysmenorrhea, premenstrual tension, endometriosis, and menorrhagia.

Combination OCs, pills that contain the same dosage of estrogen and progesterone, are taken each day for 20 to 21 days, followed by no more than 7 days without medication. During the nonmedicated period, the woman will experience a monthly blood flow—not true menstruation but rather withdrawal bleeding [5].

The pills are supplied in a number of ways. Some preparations have 28 pills per packet, the last seven being placebos. In the first month that a woman takes these, she takes the first pill on the fifth day of her period and then takes a pill each day until the packet is empty. When this happens she simply begins another packet.

A woman taking 21-day pills beings her first packet on the fifth day of her period. One pill is taken daily for 21 days, then the pills are discontinued for 7 days; a new packet of pills is begun on the eighth day.

Combination OCs are sold under the names Enovid, Norinyl, Norlestrin, Ortho-Novum, Ovral, and Ovulen, among others. Since synthetic estrogens and progesterones are much more potent than natural forms, they are given in much smaller doses than the amounts of estrogen and progesterone produced by the body. OCs are sold in varying hormone doses, since the correct dose depends on individual body chemistry: A particular woman may have undesirable side effects from one preparation and none from another.

The progestogen-only OC (mini-pill) does not always suppress ovulation because of its low dosage and for this reason is usually about 97 percent effective. It produces the same secondary effects of the combination pills. A distinct disadvantage of this type of OC is the unpredictable bleeding pattern that often accompanies its use. On the other hand, its use is not associated with increased risk of thrombosis or suppression of lactation [5].

The woman should take her pill at the same time each day; this helps her to form the habit of daily pill-taking and also helps to keep her blood level of medication constant. If she misses one pill, she should take it as soon as she remembers and the next one at her regular time. If she misses two pills, she should take two tablets as soon as she remembers and two tablets the following day. To be on the safe side, she should use an additional method of birth control for the rest of that cycle. If she misses three or more pills, she should use another method of birth control while she discards the remainder of that packet of pills, waits 4 days, and then begins a new packet of pills [26]. Many physicians advise women to use another contraceptive during their first packet of pills, since new pill users make more mistakes at this time than later.

The pill containing the lowest available dose of estrogen combined with the lowest available dose of progesterone is usually prescribed for women desiring oral contraception. Only if side effects persist after the third cycle is the medication changed, depending on whether the need is for a greater estrogenic or a greater progestational effect [26]. Because of a variety of the following complications and side effects, it is recommended that all OC users over 35 years of age reconsider their use of contraception.

SIDE EFFECTS AND COMPLICATIONS

Hypercoagulability.   A rather extensive body of literature links OCs to the development of a hypercoagulable state in users. It has been shown that these women have an increase in the number of platelets and in factor XII; 50 percent have an increase in fibrinogen activity; 25 percent have an increase in Factor VIII; and 75 percent have an increase in Factors II and IX. These changes are present even after short-term use, although the changes are reversed after OCs are discontinued. Related to these changes in clotting factors in OC users is the increased risk of developing thromboembolism or thrombophlebitis [5].

In a variety of prospective as well as retrospective studies, this increased risk (up to 11 times that of nonusers) has been linked to the estrogen dosage in the pill, with lower levels producing a decreased risk factor. Faulty research methods, however, leave this conclusion open to question. There also appears to be an increased risk of cerebral vascular disease in OC users, which is compounded if the woman smokes and/or is hypertensive. In addition, there appears to be an increased risk of myocardial infarction, compounded if the woman smokes, is over 40 years of age, and has used the pill continuously for 5 years or more [5].

Because of the risk of thromboembolic disease, the American Medical Association advises that any woman using the pill who has severe leg or chest pains, coughs up blood, has difficulty breathing, or has sudden severe headache or vomiting, dizziness, or fainting, disturbances in vision or speech, or weakness or numbness of an arm or leg should discontinue the pill and contact her doctor immediately (see Table 5-1).

Hypertension.   Research has confirmed the relationship between OC use and increased blood pressure, generally occurring after the first 2 years of use and becoming severe in about 5 percent of OC users. The mechanism of action appears to be related to changes in the renin-angiotensin-aldosterone system, with a consistent increase in plasma renin substrate associated with an increase in plasma renin activity and aldosterone excretion [5].

Hepatic Changes.   Oral contraceptives appear to have a stimulating effect on liver production of many proteins, including thyroxine-binding globulin, corticosteroid-binding globulin, copper-binding protein, iron-binding protein, and vitamin B_{12} binding capacity. The incidence of liver adenomas associated with OC use remains very low [31]. These tumors are usually benign [5].

Other Side Effects.   Women who use OCs usually have some increase in the cholesterol concentration contained in gallbladder bile and are therefore predisposed to cholesterol cholelithiasis. This effect of OCs on gallbladder disease does not become apparent until after 2 years of use, with the greatest incidence occurring after 5 years of use.

No definite relationship has been demonstrated between OCs and the development of breast cancer, although the estrogen they contain may increase the growth of *existing* breast cancer. Present evidence suggests that the pill may actually have a protective effect on the development or progression of benign fibrocystic disease of the breast, but data in human subjects are not conclusive [28]. There had been a link demonstrated between endometrial cancer and the use of sequential OCs (estrogen and progesterone in separate pills taken at different times in the cycle) but these have since been withdrawn from the market in the United States [25, 28, 37].

Through their effect on tryptophan metabolism, OCs may contribute to a decrease in vitamin B_6, an impairment of glucose metabolism, or emotional lability or depression. Several reports have indicated that for insulin-dependent diabetics using OCs, an adjustment of their insulin dosage is usually necessary [42].

The OCs can also produce temporary symptoms that are common during actual pregnancy. A woman may experience nausea, breast tenderness, weight gain or occasionally weight loss, and chloasma. The nausea, breast tenderness, and weight gain usually clear up during the first to third cycles as the woman's body adjusts to the synthetic hormone levels. The chloasma may remain even after the woman is no longer taking the pill.

Other side effects that have been attributed to OC use include amenorrhea, lighter periods, headache, hair thinning, regression of gum tissue, eye complaints (such as blurred vision and eyes tiring more easily), and changes in sex drive and appetite. Occasionally women develop corneal edema and are unable to wear their contact lenses. Women who are long-term OC users may also have changes in their vaginal pH from acidic to alkaline and thus an increased incidence of vaginal infections.

Breakthrough bleeding is an annoying side effect for many women. Often the estrogen dose is inadequate to maintain the integrity of the endometrium and it begins to slough. Some physicians will advise a woman to take two pills daily rather than one for the remainder of that packet, thus shortening that cycle; she then resumes taking the normal one pill per day starting on day 5 of the following cycle. A woman may also be asked to stop taking her pills at the first sign of breakthrough bleeding. This allows menstruation to begin; pill-taking is then resumed on day 5 following the beginning of the menstrual flow. If a definite flow does not begin, pill-taking resumes 7 days after the last pill was taken.

Some women have expressed concern that the ability to become pregnant will be decreased after using OCs for a few years. However, clinical studies indicate that this is not the case and that in fact 90 percent of the women attempting to become pregnant after discontinuing the pill do so within a year. There is also no evidence to indicate that pill use causes any abnormalities in the offspring of former pill users.

Nursing mothers should generally avoid OCs. The pill may cause a decrease in the mother's milk supply, and the hormones do pass through the milk. The long-range effects of these hormones on the infant are not known at this time.

CONTRAINDICATIONS

Absolute contraindications to a woman's use of OCs are pregnancy, vascular disorders, hepatic disease, blood dyscrasias where the risk of increased thrombosis may be aggravated, hyperthyroidism, epilepsy when anticonvulsants may make contraceptive action less effective, and breast or reproductive system cancer, which may be exacerbated. Relative contraindications include menstrual disorders when the cause has not been determined, lactation during the first 6 weeks (suppressive effect is minimized if OCs are started after that time), varicose veins (predisposition to thromboembolism), uterine fibroids (may increase in size), hypertension, and diabetes. Mortality for OC users is low when compared with the risk of death from pregnancy and childbirth except in women over the age of 40 [26].

Many times a client will be taking multiple medications, some of which interact to reduce or enhance the desired total effect. This is true in the case of OCs as well. The woman who takes laxatives or mineral oil may have impaired absorption of her OC. Antibiotics that change the bacterial content of the intestinal tract may have the same effect. Ampicillin, penicillin V, and neomycin appear to interfere with the hepatic circulation of estrogens and in this way may affect OC effectiveness. Because of the tendency of estrogen to increase clotting factors, if the woman is also taking an oral anticoagulant its effect will be lessened. Drugs that increase the metabolism of OCs, such as some barbiturates and the antituberculous drug rifampicin, will result in a decreased level of estrogen with the possibility of breakthrough bleeding or pregnancy. The woman who uses OCs should not take antimigraine agents containing ergotamine, since the resulting vasoconstriction may increase her risk of thrombosis. If she anticipates major surgery, she should discontinue OC use about 4 to 6 weeks before so that clotting factor changes will be reversed by the time the surgery is performed [26].

Sterilization   FEMALE STERILIZATION

History has always recorded a much greater interest in the sterilization of women than of men—from the use of chastity belts to various experimental surgical procedures. In ancient times closure of the vaginal entrance was achieved by sewing up the vulva and passing a ring through the labia majora, with the aim of preserving the purity of women by preventing adultery and illegitimate pregnancy. Sterilization itself was first proposed by Hippocrates as a means of reducing hereditary insanity. Oophorectomies were performed by the ancient Egyptians; the first tubal sterilizations were done in 1880.

By 1921, 42 different procedures had been proposed, and at the present time there are over 100 surgical techniques for sterilizing women. Generally these are variations on the following approaches: simple tubal ligation, tubal ligation with partial resection, cornual resection, bilateral salpingectomy, burial of the tubal stump in the broad ligament or in the uterus, transuterine cauterization of cornu, injection of sclerosing solutions into tubes, burying the ovary in the broad ligament, fimbriectomy, hysterectomy, and, more recently, electrocoagulation and transection via celioscopy or laparoscopy.

The choice of the specific procedure depends on many factors, among which are the patient's age, weight, history of previous pelvic surgery, presence of systemic or pelvic disease, risk of future pregnancies, failure rate and complexity of procedure, and the timing of the operation (whether or not post partum). Other factors to be considered include the safer alternative of vasectomy in the partner, psychologic factors, type of anesthesia, and availability of hospital or outpatient facilities.

Because of the expense and lack of trained personnel, surgical sterilization has not had much effect on the world population. Costs of sterilization should decrease as outpatient procedures are developed and refined, older techniques and their failures are evaluated, and culdoscopic and laparoscopic techniques are introduced.

In recent years elective voluntary sterilization has come to be increasingly accepted as a preferred method of contraception. Evans [13] postulates that in many areas close to 20 percent of women between the ages of 18 and 39 have had a sterilizing procedure performed. Vasectomy is requested by men despite the unconfirmed speculation that it may be related to isoimmune disease. The cost of sterilization procedures may be a deterrent for some couples, since many third-party medical insurance policies do not cover sterilization procedures, even though the end result would be reduction in the ultimate cost of health care.

Couples should not consider sterilization unless they regard it as irreversible. The more likely a procedure is to be reversible, the more likely it is to carry an increased risk of failure [13]. Fewer than 5 percent of individuals who are sterilized later express regret. However, sterilization is still difficult for many clients as well as physicians to accept and is a step that should not be taken without serious consideration of its consequences.

Informed consent following a discussion of risks and options involved is of the utmost importance. The best results are anticipated in the woman, man, or couple who have made an informed decision, who have had time for reflection, who are over 25 years of age, and who undergo the procedure during a nonstressful period in their lives.

Current Methods. In 1919 Madlener developed a more or less dependable method for female tubal ligation (at about the same time satisfactory techniques for vasectomy were developed). Today the tubal ligation techniques of Pomeroy (1930) and Irving (1950) are still widely used (Fig. 5-4).

Following the introduction of fiberoptics in 1964, endoscopic techniques began to be developed; laparoscopic sterilization (first developed in 1966) has become increasingly popular. During this procedure, which requires a very small abdomi-

Figure 5-4. A. Pomeroy tubal sterilization. Tubes are tied with plain catgut and a portion is resected. B. Irving tubal sterilization. Portions of the tubes are resected and the uterine stumps are buried in the uterine musculature. 1. Ligation and resection of the tube. 2. Securing opening in uterine musculature. 3. Tube being buried in the uterine musculature.

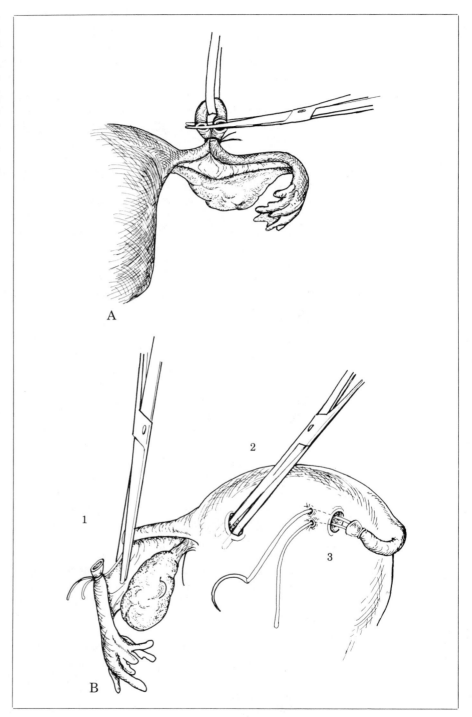

nal incision, a pneumoperitoneum is produced with carbon dioxide, the tubes are visualized, grasped with forceps, and electrocoagulated, and a portion of each is excised. This may be done on an outpatient basis.

Hysterectomy, of course, is another method of sterilization, one which is sometimes more easily accepted by Roman Catholics than procedures specifically designed to prevent conception. However, hysterectomy has a higher mortality associated with it.

On an experimental basis, intrauterine instillations of chemical cytotoxic agents for sterilization have been suggested, e.g., ethanol (100%) or ethanol and formalin (2 to 5%), which results in tubal obstruction. The endometrium does not seem to be affected. Studies are being made of tissue glues, for injection directly into either the fallopian tubes or the vas deferens, possibly producing closure of the tubal passageway.

Time of Procedure.   Although tubal ligations are performed at varying times, the first 48 hours post partum is a convenient period, since the patient is already in the hospital and her tubes are readily accessible. After 48 hours, tubal edema may make surgery more difficult, increase the risk of hemorrhage and infection, and contribute to a higher failure rate. Some increase of gynecologic disorders is associated with tubal ligations, but this is attributed to preexisting disease rather than to any interference with ovarian or uterine function.

MALE STERILIZATION

Vasectomy, the leading surgical procedure used for male sterilization, is also the leading method of contraceptive sterilization requested today. Compared to female sterilization, it is less expensive, less time-consuming, easier to perform, and more widely available and involves no risk to life. It does not affect sex drive, ability to enjoy intercourse, amount of ejaculate, or the quality, duration, or frequency of erection. The procedure is being performed in public health departments, hospital clinics, and doctors' offices.

The annual vasectomy rate in the United States has stabilized at about 500,000. It is a procedure increasingly being chosen by more highly educated men in higher income groups. It is rejected by men who regard it as a form of castration or for whom the ability to father children is a sign of their masculinity. The most common cause of vasectomy failure is ligation of some cord structure other than the vas. The majority of men who have a vasectomy are satisfied with the procedure and report no harmful effect on their potency, sexual performance, or level of pleasure [24].

The purpose of vasectomy is to sever the vas deferens in each testicle, thus making it impossible for sperm to pass from the testes into the urethra. The vas is severed and ligated in the straight portion, which is relatively close to the ejaculatory duct (Fig. 5-5). This portion of the vas is contained in the spermatic cord, along with blood vessels, lymph vessels, and nerves. The parts of the spermatic cord that lie within the scrotum can be located by feeling the posterior portion of the sac on either side. Once located, the skin and spermatic cord are injected with a local anesthetic, a small incision is made, and the vas deferens is isolated. The vas is then ligated and resected, or the ends may be electrocoagulated; then they are buried in surrounding structures, and the skin is closed. The procedure is then repeated on the other testis. The skin incisions in each testicle

Figure 5-5. Vasectomy. Vas deferens has been ligated and cut. Sperm are now blocked from entering ejaculatory fluid.

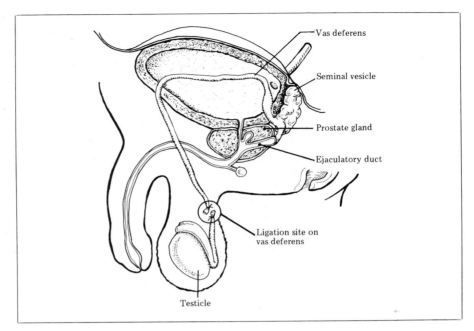

are covered with sterile gauze pads, which are held in place by some type of scrotal supporter. Both the pads and supporter may be removed after a day.

Following the procedure the man is asked to go home, rest, and apply an ice bag to the incisional area. Two aspirin tablets every 4 hours are recommended if he has pain. He is asked to keep the incisions dry and, while he may shower after a day, he should avoid swimming and baths. For 2 to 3 days following the procedure, he should avoid heavy physical activity, and some physicians recommend abstinence from intercourse. Vasectomies usually are performed Friday afternoon or evening, so that a minimum of time is lost from work. A man whose work does not require heavy physical activity may return to work when he feels comfortable.

Men must be told that they may not be sterile for 2 months or more following the procedure; therefore, they should bring a semen specimen less than 5 hours old to the clinic or doctor's office 2 to 3 months following surgery. Many physicians request two samples several weeks apart. The semen is examined for sperm content; a man is considered sterile when two samples of semen have been aspermatic.

Reported failure rates vary, but in general the method is more reliable than oral contraceptives. Failure may result from recanalization of the vas, ligation of a structure other than the vas, or failure to use another method of contraception during the unsafe period immediately following the procedure.

Postoperatively, the man may suffer from epididymitis, scrotal abscess, infection, or hematoma. Once thought to be rare, sperm granuloma of the vas is known now to be the most common postoperative complication of a vasectomy. The granuloma is painful and may contribute to vasectomy failure by initiating a spontaneous reanastomosis. This occurs when leaking sperm bridge the gap between the cut ends of the vas with subsequent recanalization. Although there are no permanent testicular changes or changes in LH, FSH, or testosterone levels following vasectomy, there does appear to be an increase in the number of sperm antibodies. To date there has been no well-controlled study to support the theory of an increased autoimmune phenomenon, but it is thought that if this is the case, it might be related to subsequent infertility following reanastomosis of the vas [24].

The severed vas can be rejoined through an operation called vasovasostomy, but fertility rates following the procedure remain low. Many intravasal devices and valves directed toward producing a reversible vasectomy have been tested. They are still being evaluated regarding their potential for inducing infection.

Some men have been encouraged to have vasectomies by the existence of banks to store frozen sperm. It has been reported that sperm may be preserved 2½ to 10 years or more in cold storage and be used for artificial insemination, resulting in normal offspring [12, 43]; however, these reports are controversial. The first individual born through the use of frozen sperm was 21 years old in 1974. As of the mid-1970s 300 to 400 healthy newborns conceived through the use of frozen sperm had been reported, and this group had a lower incidence of birth defects than that usually quoted for the normal population. The sperm banks have also been used to store semen of infertile men. The stored semen can be spun down and concentrated prior to artificial insemination.

PSYCHOLOGIC IMPLICATIONS OF STERILIZATION

Since many couples in the United States have their desired families at an early age, sterilization has become an inviting alternative to long-term use of temporary contraceptive measures for both men and women. The choice of this option should be made only after very serious consideration, since the reversal of male and female sterilizing procedures has not yet had a high rate of success. This leaves little room for a change of mind following circumstances such as death of existing children or remarriage. You can play a vital role as a listener and as a counselor when couples are contemplating such a step, helping them to make their decision based on knowledge of all the implications of the procedure.

As a rule, fewer than 5 percent of those men and women who are sterilized express regret over the decision. On the contrary, most report unchanged or improved health. When the fear of pregnancy has been removed, the couple's sex drive increases, as does the frequency of intercourse; many marriage bonds have become stronger. However, if the sterilization has been performed against the wishes of one partner, the result can be devastating to the relationship.

The emotional and psychologic impact of the loss of reproductive capacity can be very great, although more men than women tend to equate sterilization with castration. Roman Catholics may have more conflicts to resolve and may express guilt following the procedure. An individual who has had previous psychiatric problems is likely to be more disturbed while coping with the ramifications of being sterilized.

LEGAL ASPECTS

Accepted legal opinion supports the position that purely voluntary sterilization is permissible provided both partners have been informed of the implications of the procedure, including the chance of failure, and that permission in writing has been given. In most states the consent of the patient alone is all that is needed, provided he or she is legally competent, although it is highly desirable that both partners sign the permit. Lawfully married minors or "emancipated" minors (15 years or older and living apart from parent or guardian) may legally give consent; otherwise they need the consent of a parent or guardian.

INFERTILITY
Fertility is greatest in men and women around the age of 24. A woman's fertility gradually diminishes around the age of 30 and declines rapidly thereafter. Without using a method of contraception, 25 percent of all sexually active women will become pregnant in the first month, 63 percent in 6 months, 75 percent in 9 months, 80 percent in a year, and 90 percent in 18 months. According to the American Fertility Society, a couple who has had unprotected intercourse for a period of a year and who has not conceived may be considered infertile and is entitled to an infertility examination [8]. The infertility can be said to be primary if the couple has produced no children; it is secondary when a viable offspring has been born previously. Infertility affects approximately 10 percent of all couples.

Prior to more elaborate testing procedures, the couple should have thorough histories taken and thorough physical examinations performed. The woman's history would include her age at puberty, her menstrual, gynecologic, and obstetric history, and past and present illnesses. The couple should be interviewed separately and together regarding frequency of coitus and sexual technique. Attitudes toward intercourse may also be determined in these interviews.

Laboratory tests should be performed for urinary sugar and protein, complete blood count, serology, and semen analysis. Chest x-rays and thyroid function should be evaluated. The woman's pelvic examination could show an unduly tight hymenal ring, cervical or vaginal abnormalities, or deviations in the position and outline of the uterus, tubes, or ovaries. When nothing can be found to demonstrate infertility by means of these procedures, other factors must be investigated more thoroughly.

Infertility is reportedly due to cervical problems in 20 percent of couples, tubal problems in 30 percent, hormonal problems in 15 percent, and sperm deficiencies in 30 percent; these percentages vary according to the population studied. Low socioeconomic groups are reported to have higher tubal factors, often as a result of gonococcal or enterococcal pelvic inflammatory disease or postabortion sepsis. Despite all the progress in fertility management, no cause for infertility can be established in 5 to 10 percent of infertile couples.

Female Infertility
CERVICAL AND UTERINE FACTORS
An incompetent cervix can be a factor in infertility if the woman's history indicates two or more second-trimester abortions. The pregnancies usually terminate suddenly and painlessly after spontaneous rupture of the membranes, usually with no primary bleeding. Treatment can be performed surgically by placing plastic tubules or Dacron mesh around the circumference of the internal os.

The quality of cervical mucus can be a problem; it may be improved by low doses of estrogen, making it more favorable to penetration of sperm. The estrogen may also enhance ovarian response to pituitary gonadotropins. Progesterone and estrogen given during the luteal phase may also enhance endometrial quality, which aids in implantation.

Submucous uterine fibroids may disturb endometrial function or be large or numerous enough to prevent or interfere with implantation or fetal growth. These fibroids are diagnosed by palpation, curettage, or hysterography and are treated by surgical removal (Table 5-3). Third-degree retroversion of the uterus has also been considered to be a predisposing factor in infertility and may be treated with an intravaginal pessary.

Congenital anomalies, including bicornuate, septate, and double uteri, may also be contributing factors. Diagnosis of these anomalies is made by curettage or hysterography. Surgical treatment consists of removing the septum, joining the cornua, or uniting the horns of a double uterus (after the medial halves have been excised). Surgery should be delayed, however, until it has been established that a pregnancy cannot be maintained without intervention. If surgery is necessary, the woman should be advised to wait from 8 to 12 months after the operation before attempting to become pregnant. Delivery is usually by cesarean operation in order to minimize possibilities of uterine rupture and fetal loss.

TUBAL FACTORS

Occluded tubes may be diagnosed by tubal insufflation or hysterosalpingography. Occluded tubes may be opened by time, a period of sexual abstinence, antispasmodics, and weight loss. Some investigators believe that repeated tubal insufflations with carbon dioxide at pressures as high as 300 milligrams of mercury, along with pelvic heat and sexual abstinence, are superior to tubal surgery.

Surgical treatment (tuboplasty) for a closed oviduct is advisable when the male partner is normal and female reproductive function seems otherwise normal. The tuboplasty may take the form of a salpingolysis (separation of peritubal adhesions) or a salpingoplasty (opening of the totally occluded distal end of the tube). Reconstruction of the midsegment, cornual segment, or interstitial segment may also be performed.

Following surgery there is an increased incidence of tubal pregnancies. Smoldering pelvic inflammatory disease may also be reactivated at the time of tuboplasty. Formation or reformation of adhesions following tubal surgery is a major reason for failure to become pregnant. To reduce the incidence of adhesions, anti-inflammatory agents such as dexamethasone sodium phosphate (Decadron) and antihistamines such as promethazine hydrochloride (Phenergan) may be

Table 5-3. Diagnostic Tests Used for Infertility

Test	Procedure	Finding
Hysterosalpingogram	Cervix is injected with radiopaque dye, which flows into the uterus and fallopian tubes; radiologic examination follows	Determination of malformations, patency, or tumors
Laparoscopy	Small abdominal incision is made; laparoscope is passed into pelvic cavity	Visualization of ovaries, fallopian tubes, and uterus
Tubal insufflation (Rubin's test)	Carbon dioxide is introduced through the cervix into the uterus and fallopian tubes	Normally, pressure readings show a rise and fall. Shoulder pain signifies tubal patency

given preoperatively, intraperitoneally during surgery, and postoperatively for 2 days. Hydrocortisone may also be injected into the uterus and lavaged through the tubes postoperatively four to five times during the first 2 weeks after surgery to decrease the incidence of postoperative tubal adhesions [23].

OVARIAN FACTORS

The major ovarian abnormalities involved in infertility are irregular ovulation or anovulation and the anatomic and functional changes caused by endometriosis. It is essential in treating infertile couples to determine whether or not ovulation occurs; the methods most commonly used are endometrial biopsy, records of basal body temperature, and examination of vaginal cells and cervical mucus. Anovulation or oligo-ovulation may be due to pituitary, thyroid, adrenal, or ovarian dysfunction.

The ovarian cortex in Stein-Leventhal syndrome shows fibrosis and follicular cysts and is associated with anovulation. Following treatment with ovarian wedge resection, menstrual irregularity is corrected in many women, and ovulation and pregnancy following the procedure have been reported to occur in 13 to 89 percent of the women (depending on the population studied). Young women with irregular bleeding or endometrial hyperplasia are also believed to benefit from wedge resection, but it is recommended that they first be treated with administration of estrogen-progestin combinations.

Treatment. Two pharmacologic agents commonly used in treating anovulation are clomiphene citrate and human menopausal gonadotropins (HMG). Clomiphene is used in anovulatory women who have follicular function and adequate endogenous estrogen but lack adequate and cyclic stimulation by pituitary gonadotropic function. These women usually have normal or slightly decreased total pituitary gonadotropins but do not cycle with a burst of LH which causes release of the mature follicle. Clomiphene is believed to have an antiestrogenic effect that stimulates the hypothalamic-pituitary pathway to secrete increased FSH and LH.

Ovulation may be expected to occur in approximately 70 percent of women with secondary amenorrhea following clomiphene therapy; of this group, 40 percent will become pregnant. If pregnancy does not occur, it may be due to accelerated tubal transport or inadequate treatment time with the drug. Some resulting pregnancies are aborted before the fourth week. Women are advised not to attempt to become pregnant during the first treatment cycle, since the incidence of abortion is increased at this time, particularly if prolonged amenorrhea existed previously. Spontaneous abortion is not increased in pregnancies occurring after the first treatment cycle.

The incidence of multiple pregnancy in women who conceive following clomiphene therapy is increased to approximately one in every 16 pregnancies. The increase is undoubtedly due to fraternal twinning and superovulation after taking the drug. The most striking side effect during therapy is ovarian enlargement due to the enlargement of cystic follicles, cystic corpora lutea, or other physiologic cystic structures. These physiologic cysts regress spontaneously within 7 to 28 days following cessation of therapy, and the drug is administered again only after the ovaries have returned to pretreatment size. The drug should never be given to a woman who has an ovarian cyst.

Ovulation may also be induced by administration of the gonadotropic substances FSH and LH extracted from the urine of postmenopausal women, followed by doses of human chorionic gonadotropin (HCG). One preparation of menopausal gonadotropin, Pergonal, is in general use. In the course of the development of the drug, its FSH content has varied; currently each ampule contains 75 IU of FSH, 75 IU of LH, and 10 milligrams of lactose. Women with persistently low or absent gonadotropins may be treated with Pergonal if pituitary or hypothalamic tumors and cysts have been ruled out. Women with primary gonadotropin insufficiency and hypothalamic amenorrhea usually respond promptly to HMG and HCG therapy.

Women with normal gonadotropin levels are usually given at least six courses of clomiphene therapy before resorting to gonadotropin administration. Women who fail to ovulate with clomiphene alone may ovulate after clomiphene and HCG sequential therapy, e.g., 10 days of clomiphene followed 4 days later by a dose of HCG. Women who fail to respond to this therapy will usually respond to HMG if the ovaries have not been depleted of follicles.

Pergonal does not appear to influence the incidence of abortion in subfertile women the way clomiphene does. Following treatment with Pergonal, multiple births occur in approximately 20 percent of pregnancies, the majority of which are twin births. If no other cause for infertility exists, the pregnancy rate within the first two treatment cycles is 50 percent.

The recommended initial dose of Pergonal is one ampule given intramuscularly for 9 to 12 days followed by 10,000 IU of HCG given one day after the last dose of Pergonal. If the woman's ovaries become unusually enlarged, the dose of HCG may be omitted for that treatment cycle. Daily intercourse is encouraged, beginning on the day prior to administration of HCG and continuing until ovulation becomes apparent by the various indicators.

Couples attempting to conceive without the aid of drugs but by following the woman's basal body temperature are advised to have intercourse during days 11, 13, and 15, or 12, 14, and 16, of a 28-day cycle. It is not necessary to abstain before these days to increase sperm count, since evidence indicates that the motility decreases even though the count may increase. Men who have intercourse four or more times weekly have lower counts, but their partners have a higher rate of conception. Following intercourse the woman should remain supine for approximately an hour to facilitate upward sperm migration.

Much experimentation is now occurring with hypothalamic gonadotropic-releasing factors. They offer the advantages of being inexpensive and safer than gonadotropins and clomiphene [38].

OTHER FACTORS

Endometriosis has been identified as a factor in infertility about 10 to 15 percent of the time. In women with endometriosis the expectation of pregnancy is about one-half that of the general population; the incidence of sterility in these women approaches 30 to 40 percent.

Endometriosis may be treated with analgesics and patience, surgery, hormones, or a combination of the above. Pregnancy is considered the best treatment by some; they administer increasing doses of estrogen and progestins for 6 to 9 months to initiate a pseudopregnancy. This produces a decidual reaction in the areas of the endometriosis, and these areas undergo degeneration and necrosis and hopefully are absorbed, thus improving fertility. This treatment is successful 50 percent of the time if there is no other cause of infertility and if the endometriosis involves only the ovaries.

In Vitro Fertilization   In vitro fertilization has been successfully accomplished by aspirating ripe ovarian follicles during laparoscopy, fertilizing the egg with the male partner's semen, and then replacing the fertilized egg in the women's uterus. Couples for whom there is no other hope of having a child may find this method well worth whatever risks are involved [38].

In in vitro fertilization the woman is usually given an HCG injection to prepare the ovarian follicles. About 36 hours later preovulatory oocytes are obtained surgically from her ovaries. Other hormones may be given to her to prepare her uterus for implantation. A sample of sperm is diluted and placed in a saline solution to facilitate capacitation. Droplets of the sperm solution are placed in a petri dish and each preovulatory oocyte is propelled into one of the droplets. Within a few hours fertilization occurs and 12 hours later the growing organism is transferred to a solution designed for embryonic growth. When the developing blastocyst is 2 to 4 days old, it is inserted into the woman's uterus through a plastic cannula [46]. It may implant if all conditions are favorable.

Ethical and religious problems surrounding in vitro fertilization have been discussed widely in the popular media. These include whether conception via separation between procreation and intercourse is artificial and the potential loss of zygotes since several eggs usually become fertilized. Other issues that have received some attention are the risk of anomalies and the allocation of resources in competition with other priorities for funding. Since in vitro fertilization is unlikely to become a mass technology, Hellegers [17a] postulates that the ethical problems associated with it will not generate a major controversy.

Male Infertility   A man's fertility depends on his production of an adequate number of normal mature sperm (at least 20–40 million per milliliter of semen, with at least 60 percent normal forms). His fertility also depends on his being able to ejaculate and on his ability to produce an ejaculum that undergoes spontaneous enzymatic liquification within 30 minutes [38].

As the sperm move through the epididymis, they mature and become increasingly capable of motility and fertility. Mature sperm are stored in the end of the epididymis and the vas deferens, where they can survive for a much longer time than in the female reproductive tract. Their survival in the epididymis depends upon the endocrine activity of the testicular Leydig cells; this endocrine activity is responsible for the condition of the epididymal and ductal epithelium. Leydig cell failure leads to poor sperm motility, as a result of the absence of the hormonal support necessary for sperm maturation as well as their passage through the duct system.

Sperm are inactive in the epididymis and are transported through the duct via peristalsis and the spastic contractions at ejaculation. Sperm take about 3 weeks to pass through the duct system, a time that is influenced by the frequency of ejaculation. After a prolonged period of abstinence from ejaculation, there are often a high proportion of dead and aging sperm in the semen. After ejaculation the average man requires 30 to 40 hours to regain his normal sperm count. A man with a sperm count per ejaculation (2–4 cubic milliliters) of below 100 to 200 million is probably infertile. Specimens for semen analysis are obtained by masturbation; they should be collected in a clean, dry glass jar (not a condom), protected from cold temperatures, and transported to the doctor's office within 2 hours after collection.

Normally during ejaculation a sympathetic reflex action causes the sphincter of the urethra to close, while a parasympathetic reflex causes the external sphincter to open and the ejaculate is forced out through the urethral meatus. The contraction of the internal sphincter prevents retrograde passage of the semen into the bladder (retrograde ejaculation), which would result in a lack of seminal fluid upon ejaculation. This lack may occur following disruption of the internal sphincter as a result of surgery, the use of some antihypertensive blocking agents, or diabetic neuropathy.

At ejaculation, sperm respond to their changed environment by an increase in motility and metabolic activity; they rapidly become exhausted and die, probably as a result of the increased availability of oxygen. The life span of sperm at room and body temperature is relatively short, but their life may be prolonged by refrigeration, in some cases by increasing carbon dioxide tension and by freezing after treatment with a protective substance such as glycerol. Since sperm lose some motility in the process of freezing and thawing, sperm that already have poor motility are not the best specimens to be frozen.

Artificial Insemination Stored semen may be used to artificially inseminate the woman, a procedure timed to coincide with her ovulation, at which time the semen will be introduced into the vagina near the cervix with a syringe. Artificial insemination may be accomplished with the husband's sperm (AIH) or, if he is azoospermic, with a donor's sperm (AID). AID, while medically sound, may have legal, religious, and social implications that should be discussed with the couple. Only a minority of states have laws protecting the legitimacy of the babies that result from AID. Couples are usually referred to other practitioners for care during pregnancy. This eliminates legal problems such as perjury with respect to parenthood when the baby's birth certificate is signed. It may also avoid conflict of interest [46].

The combined problems of male infertility and the small numbers of adoptable babies have spurred interest in and demand for AID. Thousands of infants are born each year in the United States as a result, with a success rate for AID of about 70 percent (50% if frozen semen is used). Donors, while they remain anonymous to the couple, are usually chosen because their physical characteristics match those of the couple. Often the husband's semen is mixed with the donor's with the advantage that the husband's semen may be responsible for the pregnancy that results. The woman uses the basal body temperature chart to determine the approximate time of her ovulation, and one to three inseminations are done around that time in either the uterus, cervix, or vagina. About half of successful inseminations will occur within the first 2 months and 90 percent within 6 months.

FACTORS AFFECTING MALE FERTILITY

A common cause of male infertility (25%) is a *varicocele* which consists of dilated left scrotal veins due to incompetent valves in the left internal spermatic venous system with retrograde flow of blood from the renal vein into the scrotal circulation. In addition to increasing heat in the area, this blood from the renal vein may also carry a relatively high concentration of toxic metabolic substances such as steroids, which are potential inhibitors of spermatogenesis. This condition is surgically corrected, not with removal of the dilated veins but with the ligation of the left internal spermatic vein to prevent the retrograde flow of blood. This procedure usually results in an increase in sperm motility, a decrease in immature sperm forms, and a 40 to 50 percent pregnancy rate [1].

If the *semen volume* is less than 1 milliliter but is otherwise of normal quality, infertility may result from failure of the seminal fluid to make contact with the cervix. Artificial insemination is sometimes used in this case. Semen volume is occasionally increased by the administration of gonadotropins in high doses [1].

In most men the greatest concentration of motile normal sperm is in the first portion of the ejaculate. Insemination with this portion of the ejaculate often solves fertility problems, particularly when the man has a semen volume of 3 milliliters or more, with low sperm density or increased semen viscosity. Pregnancy also sometimes occurs in this case if the male withdraws his penis after the release of the first portion of the ejaculate [1].

Endocrine imbalances (i.e., decreased levels of pituitary gonadotropin, Leydig cell failure, thyroid dysfunction) may have an uncommon but devastating effect on male fertility.

Impotence, a factor in about 5 percent of male infertility problems, may have many causes, including diabetes, anticholinergic drugs, tranquilizers, certain antihypertensives, and surgery [1].

Sexual frequency may be related to infertility. If intercourse is too infrequent (abstinence for 5–7 days or more), not enough sperm will be deposited during the fertile period; however, if intercourse is too frequent, the semen may be of poor quality. Intercourse every other day during the fertile period is sometimes recommended. The woman should avoid immediate ambulation and/or douching. Sometimes couples have reported the use of spermicidal jellies as lubricants—an easily remedied cause of infertility [1].

Epididymal obstruction (congenital or secondary to infection from gonorrhea or tuberculosis), *testicular failure* (due to mumps, trauma, or tumor), or *cryptorchidism* may result in azoospermia. It is now thought that if the testes have not descended by the time a child is 5 years old, irreversible changes begin to occur. If the testes remain outside the scrotum until puberty, the male will be unable to produce sperm, since the testes have been subjected to the higher intra-abdominal temperature. Since Leydig cells are heat resistant, androgen function and secretion will continue. However, if the testes remain undescended by 30 to 35 years of age, hormone secretion will decrease as well. Active therapy with gonadotropins, followed by orchiopexy, is indicated between 5 and 9 years of age [1].

Sometimes, in association with epididymitis, the sperm penetrate the walls of the epididymis and invade surrounding tissue. In some infertile men this may result in the phenomenon of autoimmunization against their own sperm; the sperm appear to be ejaculated in an *agglutinated* condition. Other cases of sperm agglutination are sometimes remedied by ascorbic acid therapy, which increases the activity of antiagglutinin in the semen [1].

It is also possible that vaginally deposited sperm can provide an antigenic stimulus in susceptible women, who respond by developing antispermatozoal antibodies. These may be individual specific (only one partner's sperm) or species specific (any human sperm). It has been reported that if a condom is used during intercourse or if a couple abstains for periods ranging from 2 to 6 months, antibody titers will decrease, and pregnancy is likely to follow unprotected intercourse [1].

While *age* is not an important factor in sperm production, fertility is reduced with aging. *Allergic reactions* or *anxiety* or *emotional tension* can also have temporary adverse effects on sperm production [1].

Of the systemic diseases *diabetes* has a specific effect on fertility, since the accompanying vascular changes may accelerate aging. Diabetes may result in calcification of the vas deferens along with impotence and retrograde ejaculation [1].

With *chronic renal failure* there is often endocrine dysfunction, low levels of testosterone, oligospermia with poor motility, and germinal cell arrest. Although libido sometimes improves with continued dialysis, spermatogenesis often does not. Libido, potency, and ability to ejaculate may greatly improve after kidney transplant, but most patients on immunosuppressive therapy remain oligospermic. Return of ovulation and subsequent pregnancy have been reported in female patients. In most cases of *paraplegia* and *quadriplegia*, testicular atrophy is slow and progressive [1].

Infertility may also result from nutritional deficiencies in vitamin A (which causes germinal cell hypoplasia), vitamin B complex (which affects pituitary function), vitamin C (which affects sperm antiagglutinin), or certain trace elements such as zinc (which affects spermatogenic epithelium) [1].

Acute febrile or viral illnesses may result in temporary depression of sperm production and poor semen specimens. Too much *heat* affects the seminiferous tubules, arresting spermatogenic maturation. Frequent hot baths, sauna baths, close-fitting or thermal underwear, or occupations that require long hours of sitting may be contributing factors. Usually the semen returns to normal within 3 months after the extra heat is removed [1].

Damaged chromatin in *irradiated spermatozoa* may be incapable of fertilizing or of contributing to the normal development of the fertilized ovum. If a man receives 225 rads to his testes prior to puberty, it is predicted that three of every five of his children will have detrimental mutations. Therefore diagnostic x-rays and therapeutic radiation in boys should not be done without truly valid indications. Recovery of fertility in the adult male after accidental sterilization by nuclear radiation has been reported within 41 months [1].

Certain *drugs* adversely affect spermatogenesis. Colchicine arrests cell division at metaphase. Methotrexate interferes with folic acid metabolism in nucleic acid synthesis. Testosterone inhibits spermatogenesis by inhibiting pituitary FSH secretion. Nitrofurantoin (Furadantin) depresses spermatogenesis by interfering with carbohydrate metabolism in the germinal epithelium, producing primary spermatocyte arrest. Monoamine oxidase inhibitors are reported to produce an increase in the sperm count followed by a profound drop. Medroxyprogesterone (Depo-Provera) causes depression of sperm count and motility after a single injection; the use of such injections to induce periods of male sterility is currently under investigation [1].

It is known that alcohol can depress the level of serum testosterone. Working hours and alcohol intake are probably of importance in infertility as causes of impotence or decreased libido. There is also some question as to whether nicotine (smoking) can decrease semen quality. To date there is little sound evidence to confirm or deny the speculation. The effect of marijuana on spermatogenesis is still uncertain, but there is some evidence that it can depress androgen levels and thus decrease spermatogenesis.

Fertile males have higher levels of prostaglandin E (PGE) in their semen than males in couples with unexplained infertility. PGEs are known to relax the uterus and fallopian tubes, effects that may promote the union of sperm and ovum and prevent excessive motility from interfering with implantation. Theoretically a potential means of contraception would involve interference with the male prostaglandin physiology. It is known that this occurs after aspirin (600 mg, 4 times a day) has been taken for 1 week. It is possible, therefore, that medications, such as nonsteroidal anti-inflammatory agents, could be significant factors in previously unexplained male infertility [10].

MEDICAL THERAPY

Androgens may be used if there is a normal sperm count but decreased motility; they help to create an environment in the epididymis conducive to the development of motility. Clomiphene has been used to stimulate endogenous gonadotropin production in males with low sperm counts and normal or low FSH and interstitial cell-stimulating hormone levels. Semen responses have generally been unpredictable. Exogenous gonadotropins have been used in the past to stimulate testicular, germinal, and hormonal activity. Large doses of chorionic gonadotropin have shown good results in some instances.

Psychologic Implications

Infertility causes feelings of frustration, guilt, and depression; tests and treatment for it often bring about anxiety and fear [45]. A third party inquiring into private sexual activity is not without serious implications. The resulting tensions add their inhibiting effect to whatever organic factors are present via the hypothalamic pituitary pathways, autonomic smooth muscle systems, or pathways not fully delineated.

The tension involved in attempting to overcome infertility can cause a man to become impotent. It can also cause uterine or possibly tubal spasm, decreasing the chances of rapid passage of sperm.

The temptation to blame one another, particularly when one partner has been diagnosed as infertile, may lead to marital conflict. Couples need to share solutions to their problem; they may need to communicate more directly about their sexual relationship. Because the anxiety raised by this stressful time may block their understanding of what they are told about collecting specimens, timing ovulation, and so forth, you may have to repeat instructions several times [46].

Mocarski [27] points out that many infertile couples have health education needs regarding their reproductive functions and that you are in a position to dispel some of their myths and fallacies. By spending some time with the infertile couple you can elicit their concerns, answer their questions, and provide confirmation that their feelings are normal. At the same time you will be helping them to work through the tasks before them [36]: Recognizing and expressing their feelings about their infertility and how it has affected their lives; mourning the loss of their fertility (a normal and appropriate response); evaluating their reasons for wanting a child (Whose needs would a child meet? Theirs? Relatives? Are they concerned because they cannot bear a child or because they want children in their future?); making decisions about their future (Will they pursue adoption? Remain childless?).

THERAPEUTIC ABORTION
Historical and Legal Aspects

Laws and attitudes toward abortion have vacillated throughout history and may continue to do so. Catholic doctrine for 300 years, from 1450 to 1750, made specific distinctions about the status of the fetus in the mother's womb. The distinction, based on the concepts of "ensoulment" and "unensoulment," permitted abortion in the period up to 40 days of gestation. For the last century the Catholic Church has been opposed to any form of abortion; however, opinion polls carried out in the United States show that the majority of Catholics polled believe that the decision about abortion should be made by a woman and her doctor [14].

Orthodox Jews have been opposed to abortion in the past and remain so, while those less orthodox are not. Likewise some Protestant denominations have opposed abortion in the past and remain opposed today, while many no longer take an antiabortion stand.

There was a time in the early history of the United States when there was no legal prohibition against termination of pregnancy before quickening. Abortion reform began in the 1820s as a response to the high mortality of surgical procedures in general, particularly those carried out by back alley abortionists, and as a result of a movement by some to impose an ascetic morality on all. Laws passed by the states during this period outlawed abortion except when necessary to preserve the life of the woman.

On January 22, 1973, the United States Supreme Court, recognizing a woman's right to privacy and the current adequacy of medical practice, ruled in effect that in the first trimester of pregnancy the abortion decision is to be left to the woman and her doctor. The state of residence may not prohibit abortion in the second trimester but may regulate its procedures in the interest of protecting the woman's health; these regulations could include where abortions can be performed and who can perform them. During the final weeks of pregnancy the state may choose to protect the potential life of the fetus by prohibiting abortion except when necessary to preserve the life or health of the woman.

Since the Supreme Court decision, follow-up studies in the states that liberalized their abortion laws show a decrease in maternal mortality, a decrease in hospital admissions for women with complications of illegal abortion, a decrease in spontaneous abortion, and a decrease in out-of-wedlock births. Maternal mortality in New York City during the period October 1969 to March 1970 was 5.63 deaths per 10,000 live births, while during the comparable period of October 1970 to March 1971 (after a law had been passed permitting abortion on request) maternal mortality dropped to 2.6 deaths per 10,000 live births [19].

Statistics from San Francisco General Hospital reflect the California experience. In 1967 the hospital's rate of septic abortion was 68 women per 1,000 live births; after California's liberalized abortion law took effect, the rate of septic abortion dropped to 36 per 1,000 live births in 1968 and to 22 per 1,000 live births in 1969. The spontaneous abortion rate also dropped since, as one report notes, many abortions listed as spontaneous were not spontaneous but induced. The rate in 1967 was 125 per 1,000 live births and dropped to 49 per 1,000 live births in 1969. Maternal deaths from abortion fell in California from 8 per 100,000 live births in 1967 to 3 per 100,000 in 1969 [34]. Comparable changes can now be seen in many states with new, more liberal abortion laws. Currently between 30 and 55 million abortions are induced worldwide each year, making abortion one of the most common means of birth control.

Whether a state has a restrictive or liberalized law on abortion probably will not significantly change the number of abortions performed; abortions have been with us throughout history. In the past, abortion has been attempted by taking various drugs, starving, placing hot coals on the abdomen, jumping from high places, lifting heavy objects, diving into the sea from cliffs, sitting on a bucket of hot ammonia water, or inserting bent twigs or wires into the uterus as curettes. Substances such as lye, pine oil, alcohol, lysol, or other liquids were (and sometimes still are) also used to perform abortions. The complications from these various methods include hypotension and renal failure, infection, liver abnormalities, infarction, and necrosis of portions of the uterus.

The horrors of these methods and their subsequent complications dramatically underline the fact that decisions on abortion are made individually in response to social, economic, moral, religious, and psychologic factors, regardless of the status of the law. Liberalized laws should place more of the actual procedures under medical supervision.

Psychologic Aspects   Many nurses, especially those who have worked in maternity for some years, have difficulty caring for women who choose to terminate their pregnancies. Their orientation toward preserving life, as well as their own religious and moral philosophy, runs counter to abortion. Groups of nurses who work with women choosing abortions find it helpful to attend in-service education programs or to have counseling sessions among themselves in which they can explore their own thoughts and feelings about the procedure. In no instance should nurses be forced to care for patients having abortions when they themselves are opposed to the procedure. The experience is detrimental both to the nurses and to the women seeking abortions, who are already under stress and in need of care. Inevitably there is a decrease in the quality of care the nurses are able to provide, and their feelings about abortion are communicated to the woman, often leaving her with residual feelings of guilt [32].

A woman under the stress of carrying an unwanted pregnancy is in need of help. She has a right to expect counseling from nurses or other health professionals that will enable her to mobilize her inner strengths and outer resources. She needs an environment where she can openly examine her thoughts, wishes, and uncertainties without fear of judgment or coercion. The experience should help her toward a greater self-understanding and a feeling that she has some control over her life.

Counseling sessions should explore past psychologic and medical history, including past pregnancies, abortions, and living children, and the woman's experiences during pregnancy, labor, and delivery. It is important to know if the present pregnancy was planned or the result of contraceptive failure or failure to use a contraceptive. It is also vital to ask how she feels about this pregnancy, if she has made any decision about what to do, if she has felt life, and if she is now thinking in terms of a baby as opposed to an abstract pregnancy. All alternatives must be explored: having the baby and keeping it, adoption, foster care, or termination of the pregnancy.

Her religious feelings and convictions are important. Her current life situation should be explored, including her economic resources, current stresses, and availability of emotional support. What is the relationship with the man involved? How will other significant people in her life react? Will she receive support from them whatever her decision? How does she see this pregnancy affecting her future career or marriage goals? How does she feel about herself, about men, and about her own sexuality?

Help her focus on these important factors; correct misinformation and supply any information the woman might wish. Throughout the sessions you must be objective, refraining from judgment and intense emotional involvement. The woman must make her own decision; when she has made that decision, you should assist her in getting care through referral services.

If the woman chooses an abortion, refer her to an appropriate agency as soon as possible, because the complications of therapeutic abortion are lowest during the first trimester. The risk of complications is three to five times greater when the abortion is performed in the second trimester. Reports indicate that the majority of therapeutic abortions are now being performed during the first trimester, and the trend is toward a greater percentage being done during this period. Late abortions have been reported as being most frequent in young women under 18, black women, nonprivate patients, and women with six or more children [40].

Having an abortion does involve a certain degree of stress in women (and in some cases also their partner or support person). If the abortion occurs in the first trimester, the amount of stress may be less than in the second trimester when the woman is much more aware of the pregnancy and usually goes through labor during the termination procedure. Although many women may feel sad and somewhat guilty during the first weeks following the abortion, in most cases these feelings pass with time.

Methods of Therapeutic Abortion: First Trimester

The methods of abortion used during the first trimester (sometimes up to as late as 14 weeks) are varieties of curettage. These procedures are usually performed in an outpatient facility.

CURETTAGE

Curettage, a safe and efficient technique, probably accounts for the majority of legal abortions. There are three types of curettage procedures used in the first trimester [16].

Menstrual Regulation (endometrial aspiration or menstrual extraction). Menstrual regulation is a relatively new means of suction curettage used within a few weeks after the first missed menstrual period. A small flexible cannula is used to minimize the risk of uterine perforation. Under paracervical block anesthesia it is introduced into the woman's uterus, and after its position is checked the uterine contents are removed by suction. Occasionally this method fails to evacuate the pregnancy. Since anesthesia is used, the woman is asked to avoid eating for 3 to 4 hours prior to the procedure to avoid vomiting and aspiration.

Suction Curettage (vacuum aspiration).   Developed in China in 1958, suction curettage is the principal type of abortion technique in many countries. In fact, it may account for up to 90 percent of all legal abortions in the United States. Preparation is the same as for menstrual aspiration. Suction curettage involves dilation of the woman's cervix and then suction aspiration of the uterine contents with a rigid cannula. It is performed under paracervical block or general anesthesia. Dilation of the cervix is achieved over a period of several minutes by the gradual introduction of a series of progressively larger tapered cylinders (dilators). Cervical dilation can be achieved more slowly (over 4–6 hours or overnight) by means of laminaria (hygroscopic sticks of dried seaweed which when exposed to moisture in the cervix expand to several times their original diameters). With this technique, there may be less blood loss, less chance of uterine perforation, and a lower rate of complications than with sharp curettage.

Sharp Curettage.   Until recently the predominant method of abortion, sharp curettage now constitutes only about 4 percent of all legal abortions. The preparation and cervical dilation are similar to that for suction curettage, but instead of using suction the uterine contents are evacuated by using sponge or ovum forceps combined with sharp curettage.

Methods of Therapeutic Abortion: Second Trimester

Methods of abortion used during the second trimester include hysterotomy and intrauterine injection of saline or prostaglandins; hospitalization is required for each of these procedures. Because of the duration of the pregnancy, actual labor is involved in second-trimester abortions induced by saline or prostaglandins. Unlike most women in labor (who are about to have full-term infants that have been expected for some time), most women undergoing abortions have had the additional stress of deciding to terminate an unwanted pregnancy, finding health personnel and a facility to have the abortion performed, and having a procedure done to initiate labor prematurely. These women can use all the support you can provide—remaining with the woman during the procedure, helping her breathe and push properly, encouraging her by telling her that she is doing well and that labor is progressing, giving frequent back rubs in the lumbar area, and administering properly timed analgesics.

Ethical and legal issues surrounding abortion in the second trimester include the status of the liveborn abortus and the question of whether abortion methodology should maximize the possibility of fetal survival provided it does not increase maternal risk. Active treatment of liveborn viable fetuses usually continues for long periods of time at greatly increased costs for care and with the chance that the infant will be brain damaged. Debatable issues involve the quality of life versus physical existence [17a].

HYSTEROTOMY
Hysterotomy consists of incising the uterine wall, removing the products of conception, curetting the endometrium, and closing the incision. General or spinal anesthesia is used for the abdominal surgery. The method is not used often.

INTRAUTERINE INSTILLATION OF ABORTIFACIENT AGENTS
The infusion of hypertonic solutions (saline, urea) or of uterotonic agents (such as prostaglandin $F_2\alpha$) induces uterine contractions, usually resulting in the expulsion of the uterine contents. This is the most common method of second-trimester

pregnancy termination in the United States [16]. The agent is introduced into the amniotic sac or the extraovular space (outside the fetal membranes). Prostaglandins stimulate uterine contractions directly and usually produce a faster abortion than a hypertonic solution which acts indirectly. It is thought that the hypertonic solution causes fetal death, which is followed by uterine contractions, although the mechanism responsible for initiating uterine activity is actually unknown. In order to instill the abortifacient agent an amniocentesis is done. If prostaglandins are being used, an indwelling catheter may be placed since more than one injection of prostaglandins may be required [16].

Saline Injection.   After the fourteenth to sixteenth week of pregnancy, the amniotic sac is large enough and contains enough fluid for the saline injection procedure to be possible. A solution of 20 to 50 percent sodium is exchanged for an equal amount of amniotic fluid via amniocentesis (passing a catheter through the abdominal wall and into the amniotic cavity). A total of 50 to 200 milliliters of sodium solution is exchanged for amniotic fluid. It is believed that fetal destruction is caused by the increased osmotic pressure of the amniotic fluid.

Labor begins in 24 to 72 hours; the products of conception are usually completely expelled, making curettage unnecessary. The most serious complication of saline induction is intravascular absorption of the injected saline, leading to hypernatremia. The saline may be absorbed through torn blood vessels, through injection into myometrial or placental vessels, or by abnormally rapid transfer to the maternal circulation from fetal membranes. If this occurs, the woman will experience severe headache and thirst; if not treated, she will show signs of hypotension, bradycardia, apnea, and alterations in consciousness. Women who have kidney or cardiac problems should not have saline abortions.

Prostaglandins.   Of all the prostaglandins the actions of prostaglandins E_2 and $F_2\alpha$ are the most important in reproductive physiology. Prostaglandins are rapidly synthesized from fatty-acid precursors and have their effect almost immediately, binding to specific target cell receptor sites. Myometrial cells have specific receptor sites for PGE_2 and $PGF_2\alpha$. It is thought that activation of these sites produces the abortifacient and labor-stimulating effects of these prostaglandins, which are capable of causing sustained uterine contractions at all stages of pregnancy. When prostaglandins were first used intravenously, they had a high incidence of gastrointestinal side effects, such as nausea, vomiting, diarrhea, and chemical phlebitis at the infusion site. Vaginal administration proved to be no better. Currently intra-amniotic instillation of $PGF_2\alpha$ at around 14 to 16 weeks' gestation provides for a continuous release of the prostaglandin over several hours and has become a standard method of pregnancy termination. The incidence of side effects using this route is not that high and can be lessened by antiemetics and antidiarrheal medications. Occasionally a dilute intravenous infusion of oxytocin is used to augment the uterine contractions. It is also possible that laminaria tents may be placed in the woman's cervix to promote more rapid cervical dilation, especially if she is a nulligravida [10]. Intramuscular and vaginal forms of prostaglandin preparations are being investigated since these have the potential of self-administration or administration by personnel not skilled in amniocentesis.

Prostaglandins induce abortions by three possible mechanisms: stimulation of the myometrium, a decrease in estradiol and progesterone levels, and/or cervical relaxation. With the prostaglandin method there is little change in the woman's clotting factors in contrast to the hypertonic saline method which has been shown to alter Factor VIII and fibrinogen levels [2, 10].

Complications of Abortion

Complications of abortion include hemorrhage, uterine perforation, and cervical trauma (during dilation). Some blood coagulation defects have been reported with hypertonic saline and urea instillation abortions with late dilation and curettage procedures. Relevant pathophysiology is unclear, although hypernatremia, thrombus, or air or amniotic fluid emboli may be involved. Delayed complications include the possibility of retained products of conception and infection related to the retained tissue. Late complications involve infertility, cervical incompetence, ectopic pregnancy related to postabortion infection, and Rh sensitization. In the United States the risk of death from abortion is seven times less than the risk of death from term birth [16].

Follow-up Care

Following an abortion a woman should avoid douching and using vaginal sprays and tampons and should avoid intercourse, according to some physicians, for 2 weeks to prevent infection. If she has heavy bleeding (approximately twice that of her normal period), a temperature over 38°C (100.5°F), foul-smelling discharge, nausea and vomiting, or pain, she should see her physician at once. She can expect to have a menstrual period again in 4 to 8 weeks following the procedure.

All women should be seen for follow-up care after a therapeutic abortion to check for complications, including psychologic problems. Reports show, however, that severe psychologic aftereffects are uncommon and that the predominant reaction appears to be relief. Many women report moderate depression several days after the procedure. During the counseling session after the abortion or on follow-up visits, contraceptive information should be offered; the woman should be provided with a method of her choice.

CONTRACEPTIVE COUNSELING

Jean Michaels, 25, and her boyfriend, Carl Freed, 30, have recently decided to live together. Because they anticipate sexual activity on a regular basis, they have made an appointment at Family Planning Clinic. As you begin to talk with them, you discover that they feel very strongly about responsible parenthood and want to use the most effective means of birth control that would be acceptable to both of them. What are some of the parameters that you should explore with them to help them determine the type of contraception they should use?

REFERENCES

1. Amelar, R. D., and Dubin, L. Stimulation of Fertility in Men. In E. S. E. Hafez and T. N. Evans (Eds.), *Human Reproduction*. New York: Harper & Row, 1973.
2. Anderson, G. Prostaglandin versus saline for midtrimester abortion. *Contemporary Ob/Gyn* 4:91, 1974.
3. Aref, I., and Hafez, E. S. E. Postcoital Contraceptives. In E. S. E. Hafez (Ed.), *Human Reproduction* (2nd ed.). New York: Harper & Row, 1980.
4. Arrata, W. Vaginal Barrier Contraceptives. In E. S. E. Hafez (Ed.), *Human Reproduction* (2nd ed.). New York: Harper & Row, 1980.
5. Arrata, W., Tsai, A., and Ismail, M. Oral Contraceptives: General Considerations. In E. S. E. Hafez (Ed.), *Human Reproduction* (2nd ed.). New York: Harper & Row, 1980.
6. Billings, J. *Natural Family Planning: The Ovulation Method*. Collegeville, Minn.: Liturgical Press, 1975.
7. Britt, S. Fertility awareness: Four methods of natural family planning. *Journal of Obstetric, Gynecologic and Neonatal Nursing* 6(2):9, 1977.
8. Canavan, P., and Lewis, C. The cervical cap: An alternative contraceptive. *Journal of Obstetric, Gynecologic and Neonatal Nursing* 10:271, 1981.

9. Deibel, P. Natural family planning: Different methods. *American Journal of Maternal-Child Nursing* 3:171, 1978.
10. Dingfelder, J. Prostaglandins. In E. S. E. Hafez (Ed.), *Human Reproduction* (2nd ed.). New York: Harper & Row, 1980.
11. Duncan, G., Burton, F., and Skiens, W. Vaginal, Cervical, and Subdermal Delivery Systems. In E. S. E. Hafez (Ed.), *Human Reproduction* (2nd ed.). New York: Harper & Row, 1980.
12. Ersek, R. A. Frozen sperm banks. *Journal of the American Medical Association* 220:1365, 1972.
13. Evans, T. Female Sterilization. In E. S. E. Hafez (Ed.), *Human Reproduction* (2nd ed.). New York: Harper & Row, 1980.
14. Gallup, G. H. Abortion? Let doctor and patient decide, majority says. *Philadelphia Inquirer*, August 25, 1972.
15. Gara, E. Nursing protocol to improve the effectiveness of the contraceptive diaphragm. *American Journal of Maternal-Child Nursing* 6:41, 1981.
16. Grimes, D., and Cates, W. Abortion: Methods and Complications. In E. S. E. Hafez (Ed.), *Human Reproduction* (2nd ed.). New York: Harper & Row, 1980.
17. Hafez, E. Male Contraception. In E. S. E. Hafez (Ed.), *Human Reproduction* (2nd ed.). New York: Harper & Row, 1980.
17a. Hellegers, A. Ethical Issues in Obstetrics. In S. Aladjem (Ed.), *Obstetrical Practice*. St. Louis: Mosby, 1980.
18. Herbst, A. L., Robboy, S. J., and Scully, R. E. Clear cell adenocarcinoma of the vagina and cervix in girls: An analysis of 170 registry cases. *American Journal of Obstetrics and Gynecology* 119:713, 1974.
19. Hubbard, C. W. *Family Planning Education*. St. Louis: Mosby, 1973.
20. Huxall, L. Today's pill and the individual woman. *American Journal of Maternal-Child Nursing* 2:359, 1977.
21. Huxall, L. Update on IUD's. *American Journal of Maternal-Child Nursing* 5:186, 1980.
22. Kistner, R. W. *The Pill*. New York: Delacorte, 1968.
23. Kistner, R. W. The infertile woman. *American Journal of Nursing* 73:1937, 1973.
24. Lipshultz, L., and Benson, G. Vasectomy. In E. S. E. Hafez (Ed.), *Human Reproduction* (2nd ed.). New York: Harper & Row, 1980.
25. Lyon, F. The development of adenocarcinoma of the endometrium in young women receiving long-term sequential oral contraception. *American Journal of Obstetrics and Gynecology* 123:299, 1975.
26. McDonald, J., and Currin, M. Management of Patients on Oral Contraceptives. In E. S. E. Hafez (Ed.), *Human Reproduction* (2nd ed.). New York: Harper & Row, 1980.
27. Mocarski, V. The nurse's role in helping infertile couples. *American Journal of Maternal-Child Nursing* 2:264, 1977.
28. Moghissi, K. Oral Contraceptives and Endometrial, Cervical, and Breast Cancers. In E. S. E. Hafez (Ed.), *Human Reproduction* (2nd ed.). New York: Harper & Row, 1980.
29. Moyer, D., and Shaw, S. Mode of Action of Intrauterine Devices. In E. S. E. Hafez (Ed.), *Human Reproduction* (2nd ed.). New York: Harper & Row, 1980.
30. Moyer, D., Shaw, S., and Fu, J. Clinical Aspects of Inert and Medicated Intrauterine Devices. In E. S. E. Hafez (Ed.), *Human Reproduction* (2nd ed.). New York: Harper & Row, 1980.
31. Nissen, E., and Kent, D. Liver tumors and oral contraceptives. *Obstetrics and Gynecology* 46:460, 1975.
32. Olson, M. Helping staff nurses care for women seeking saline abortions. *Journal of Obstetric, Gynecologic and Neonatal Nursing* 9:170, 1980.
33. Pisani, B. Rhythm-Thermal Application. In M. S. Calderone (Ed.), *Manual of Family Planning and Contraceptive Practice*. Baltimore: Williams & Wilkins, 1970.
34. Profile of a typical patient seeking legal abortion given. (Editorial.) *Medical Tribune*, November 10, 1979.
35. Progestasert IUD and ectopic pregnancy. *FDA Drug Bulletin* 8:37, December, 1978–January, 1979.
36. Sawatsky, M. Tasks of infertile couples. *Journal of Obstetric, Gynecologic and Neonatal Nursing* 10:132, 1981.
37. Silverberg, S., and Makowski, E. Endometrial carcinoma in young women taking oral contraceptive agents. *Obstetrics and Gynecology* 46:503, 1975.
38. Speroff, L., Glass, R., and Kase, N. *Clinical Gynecologic Endocrinology and Infertility* (2nd ed.). Baltimore: Williams & Wilkins, 1978.
39. Tanis, J. Recognizing the reasons for contraceptive non-use and abuse. *American Journal of Maternal-Child Nursing* 2:364, 1977.

40. Tietze, C. Joint program for the study: Early medical complications of legal abortion. *Studies in Family Planning* 3:97, 1972.

41. Toppozada, M., and Hafez, E. S. E. Injectable Contraceptives. In E. S. E. Hafez (Ed.), *Human Reproduction* (2nd ed.). New York: Harper & Row, 1980.

42. Tpai, A., and Arrata, W. Effects of Steroid Contraceptives on Protein, Carbohydrate, and Lipid Metabolism. In E. S. E. Hafez (Ed.), *Human Reproduction* (2nd ed.). New York: Harper & Row, 1980.

43. Tyler, E. T. Frozen semen banks. *Medical Tribune*, March 22, 1972.

44. Walker, A., Jick, H., Rothman, K., Hunter, J., Holmes, L., Watkins, R., D'Ewart, D., Danford, A., and Madsen, S. Vaginal spermicides and congenital disorders. *Journal of American Medical Association* 245:1329, 1981.

45. Wiehe, V. Psychological reactions to infertility: Implications for nursing in resolving feelings of disappointment and inadequacy. *Journal of Obstetric, Gynecologic and Neonatal Nursing* 5(4):28, 1976.

46. Woods, N. Infertility. In C. Fogel and N. Woods, *Health Care of Women: A Nursing Perspective*. St. Louis: Mosby, 1981.

FURTHER READING

Ayvazian, A. Contraception choices of female university students. *Journal of Obstetric, Gynecologic and Neonatal Nursing* 10:426, 1981.

Bradbury, B. Preventing the "diaphragm baby syndrome": A matter of technique, teaching, and time. *Journal of Obstetric, Gynecologic and Neonatal Nursing* 4(2):24, 1975.

Calderone, M. S. (Ed.). *Manual of Family Planning and Contraceptive Practice*. Baltimore: Williams & Wilkins, 1970.

Contraception: Science, Technology, and Application. Washington, D.C.: National Academy of Sciences, 1979.

Dodds, D. J. Reanastomosis of the vas deferens. *Journal of the American Medical Association* 220:1498, 1972.

Fromer, M. *Ethical Issues in Health Care*. St. Louis: Mosby, 1981.

Gilbert, S. Artificial insemination. *American Journal of Nursing* 76:259, 1976.

Granberg, D. The abortion activists. *Family Planning Perspectives* 13:157, 1981.

Hale, R. W., and Pion, R. J. Laminaria: An underutilized clinical adjunct. *Clinical Obstetrics and Gynecology* 15:829, 1972.

Hatcher, R. A., Stewart, G. K., Stewart, F., Guest, F., Schwartz, D. W., and Jones, S. A. *Contraceptive Technology* 1980–81 (10th rev. ed.). New York: Irvington, 1980.

Kilby-Kelberg, S. Why some won't try the diaphragm method—why others try and fail. *Journal of Obstetric, Gynecologic and Neonatal Nursing.* 4(2):24, 1975.

McCusker, M. The subfertile couple. *Journal of Obstetric, Gynecologic and Neonatal Nursing* 11:157, 1982.

Manisoff, M. T. *Family Planning: A Teaching Guide for Nurses*. New York: Planned Parenthood–World Population, 1969.

Martin, M. Natural family planning and instructor training. *Nursing and Health Care* 11:554, 1981.

Menning, B. Resolve—A support group for infertile couples. *American Journal of Nursing* 76:258, 1976.

Menning, B. *Infertility: A Guide for the Childless Couple*. Englewood Cliffs, N.J.: Prentice-Hall, 1977.

Menning, B. The psychosocial impact of infertility. *Nursing Clinics of North America* 17:155, 1982.

Osegbe, D., Akinyanju, O., and Amaku, E. Fertility in males with sickle cell disease. *Lancet* 11:275, 1981.

Shinzo, I., Tien, S. L., and Yoshio, A. Immunologic analysis of sperm-immobilizing factor found in sera of women with unexplained sterility. *American Journal of Obstetrics and Gynecology* 101:677, 1968.

Swenson, I. Psychologic considerations in vasectomy: A review of the literature. *Journal of Obstetric, Gynecologic and Neonatal Nursing* 4(6):29, 1975.

T-mycoplasmas and male infertility. (Editorial.) *Science News* 109:37, 1976.

Zeitz, A. Oral contraceptives: Women's rights, nurses' responsibilities. *Journal of Obstetric, Gynecologic and Neonatal Nursing* 5(3):54, 1976.

Zipper, J. Metals as intrauterine contraceptives. *Contemporary Ob/Gyn* 4:85, 1974.

PART 2 PREGNANCY

Chapter 6 The Development of the Placenta and Fetus

FERTILIZATION   The process of fertilization involves the penetration of the ovum by a spermatozoon and the mingling of the nuclear material of each, resulting in a one-celled *zygote,* a term that is also loosely applied to later stages of cell division. This initiates cellular division, leading to the formation of a new individual. In the union of egg and sperm, which usually takes place in the ampulla of the tube, there are several significant biologic implications: (1) The diploid number of chromosomes (46) is restored; (2) the sex of the zygote is determined by the spermatozoon through its contribution of an X or a Y chromosome; and (3) a series of mitotic divisions begins that result in cleavage and further development of the zygote.

Although only one of the many millions of spermatozoa deposited in the female genital tract actually fertilizes the ovum, the others may aid the fertilizing sperm in penetrating the ovum. This occurs in the following manner. Sperm undergo a physiologic change called capacitation and a structural change called the acrosome reaction. During capacitation, a protective covering is removed from the head of the sperm. Following this, small perforations appear in the acrosome wall. This acrosome reaction allows enzymes to escape, helping sperm to penetrate the corona radiata and the zona pellucida. Movement of the sperm tail probably aids the penetration process. Although several sperm become embedded in the zona pellucida, only one sperm will enter the ovum and fertilize it (Fig. 6-1).

Soon after the spermatozoon enters the ovum, two reactions take place. First, a change in the zona pellucida prevents the entry of additional sperm; presumably this occurs in response to a substance released from the cytoplasm of the ovum. Additionally, the ovum finishes its second maturational division and its chromosomes arrange themselves in a vesicular nucleus known as the female pronucleus. Meanwhile, the head of the spermatozoon swells, forming the male pronucleus. The fusion of the two pronuclei provides the diploid number of chromosomes to the new individual (Fig. 6-2). A series of mitotic divisions now begins.

Following the two-celled stage, the zygote continues its division into an increasingly larger number of cells, but these cells become smaller with each cleavage division. Therefore, while the number of cells increases rapidly, the total mass increases little. The dividing cells in this stage are known as *blastomeres.*

During this cell division, the zygote passes down the tube. Transport of the cleaving egg along the tube is brought about by ciliary activity and tubal peristalsis, which probably act on the fluid in the tube rather than directly on the egg. During this phase, the egg lives mainly on the meager nutritional store of the blastomeres themselves. It is also possible that it derives some nutritional elements, such as amino acids and monosaccharides, from the breakdown products of tubal secretions [2].

On the third or fourth day after ovulation, the zygote, containing 12 to 16 cells and called the *morula* at this stage, enters the uterus. The morula consists of an *inner cell mass,* which develops into the embryo, and a surrounding *outer cell mass,* which forms the *trophoblast* and later develops into the placenta. During the next 2 or 3 days, as the morula continues to divide, fluid from the uterine cavity passes into the intercellular spaces of the inner cell mass. As the fluid

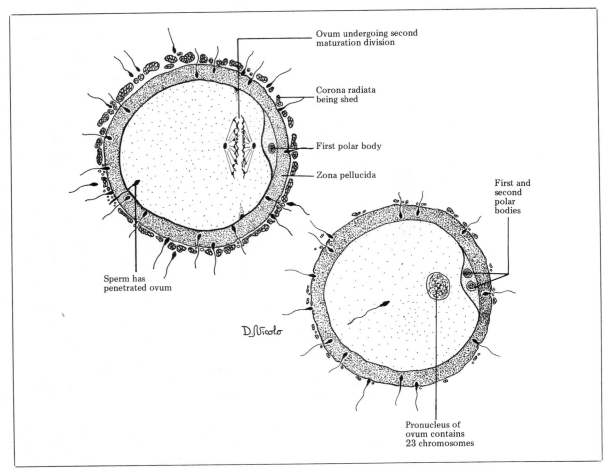

Figure 6-1.   Ovum being fertilized.

continues to increase, these spaces form a single cavity, the *blastocele*. The zygote is now known as the *blastocyst, blastula,* or *blastodermic vesicle.* The inner cell mass, now known as the embryoblast, is located on one pole, while the outer cell mass (trophoblast) forms the wall of the blastocyst. The blastocyst, now floating free in the uterine cavity, derives its nutrition from the uterine glands, which secrete a mixture of mucopolysaccharides, glycogen, and lipids [2]. During this period the zona pellucida is lost, and the trophoblast is then able to become attached directly to the surface of the endometrium.

Around the eighth day, a second cavity, the primitive yolk sac, forms in the area of the blastocyst cavity. Although it does not store yolk, it is important for several reasons [8]. Apparently the yolk sac has some role in the early transport of nutrients to the embryo while uteroplacental circulation is being established. Blood forms on the walls of the yolk sac in the third week and continues to form there until hematopoiesis begins in the liver. Primitive germ cells appearing in the wall of the yolk sac in the third week subsequently migrate to the developing gonads, where they become germ cells. During the fourth week, the dorsal part of the yolk sac becomes the primitive gut of the embryo.

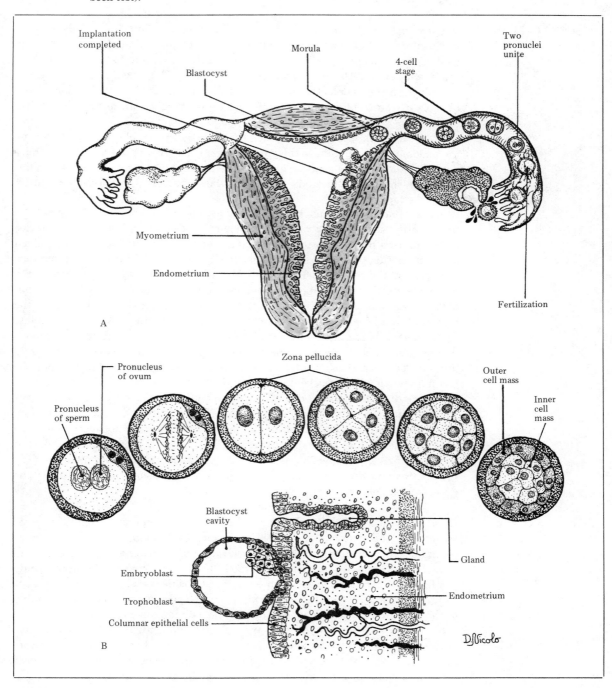

Figure 6-2. Implantation of the blastocyst. A. Serial representation of ovum from ovulation to implantation. B. Blastocyst beginning implantation (zona pellucida has been lost).

After the twelfth week, the yolk sac is located in the chorionic cavity between the amnion and the chorionic sac; it begins to shrink and solidify as pregnancy advances. It may sometimes be seen on the fetal surface of the placenta at the time of delivery.

OUTER CELL MASS
Implantation

The trophoblast begins implanting in the endometrium 6 to 7 days after fertilization. This occurs most often on the upper part of the posterior uterine wall. The trophoblastic cells burrow between the columnar epithelial cells, and these epithelial cells soon begin to degenerate. The blastocyst is partially embedded in the endometrium by the eighth day. At the embryonic pole of the blastocyst, the trophoblast, also referred to as the chorion, forms a solid disc composed of an inner layer, the *cytotrophoblast,* and an outer layer, the *syncytiotrophoblast* or *syncytium,* which is derived from the cytotrophoblast. At this time the endometrium adjacent to the implantation site is edematous and increasingly vascular, and its large tortuous glands secrete glycogen and mucus. The syncytial layer has the ability to erode maternal tissues, and once the process begins it advances rapidly.

Spaces known as trophoblastic lacunae appear by the ninth day in the proliferating syncytium. Soon the syncytium invades small, irregular capillaries in the uterine mucosa, forming maternal sinusoids. By the eleventh day blood oozes from the sinusoids into the lacunae, thus establishing a rudimentary uteroplacental circulation. This allows hormones already being produced by the trophoblastic tissue to enter the maternal circulation providing for maternal changes that maintain the pregnancy. (Detection of one of these hormones in the maternal circulation provides the basis for pregnancy testing.) As the trophoblast continues to invade more sinusoids, the lacunae eventually become continuous with maternal arterial and venous capillaries. Because of the difference in pressure between these capillaries, maternal blood begins to flow through the lacunar complex by the seventeenth day (Fig. 6-3) [16].

By this time (the twelfth day) the uterine epithelium has usually healed over the area through which the trophoblast eroded its way into the mucosa. Occasionally, bleeding may occur at the implantation site as a result of increased blood flow into the lacunar spaces in this area. (The pregnant woman may think that the resulting vaginal bleeding is her menstrual period, since it occurs around the thirteenth day after ovulation; this may cause confusion in determining the expected date of delivery.)

Placental Formation

By the twelfth day cells of the trophoblast have begun to form organized structures, the *chorionic villi.* These structures sequentially form primary, secondary, and tertiary villi (Fig. 6-4). *Primary villi* begin to form when syncytial strands, which previously surrounded the lacunae in an irregular fashion, radiate out from the cytotrophoblast. Cytotrophoblastic cells project into the organized syncytial strands, completing the formation of the primary villi. By the beginning of the third week, the trophoblast has developed many primary villi.

Secondary villi form when primary villi develop central cores of connective tissue. *Tertiary villi* form when small capillaries begin to arise in the villous core and branch out into the villus. During the fourth week of development these capillaries make contact with the intraembryonic circulatory system.

Figure 6-3. Blastocyst embedded in the endometrium approximately 12 days after fertilization. Syncytium invades maternal sinusoids.

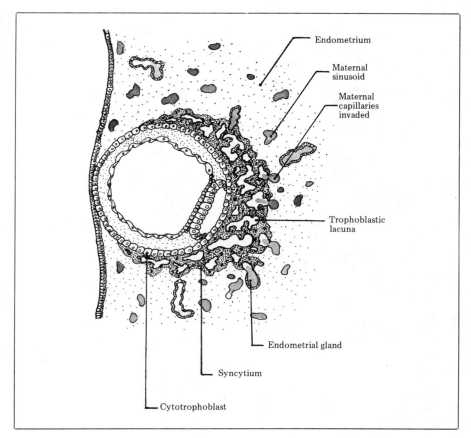

Primary villi become anchored deep in the uterine endometrium, and soon numerous small fingerlike projections branch from existing villous stems into surrounding *lacunar,* or *intervillous, spaces.* These villi are known as *free,* or *terminal, villi.* Some researchers have stated that the fetus relies on these villi for exchange between fetal capillaries and maternal blood in the intervillous space [2]. By the fourth month, these terminal villi have only the syncytium and the endothelial wall of the capillaries to separate maternal and fetal circulations.

Villi cover the entire surface of the chorion early in pregnancy. Those villi beneath the embryo that are in contact with a succulent uterine endometrium will continue to grow and form the *chorion frondosum,* or bushy chorion. Having little or no contact with the endometrium, the villi on the side opposite the embryo degenerate, leaving that side smooth by the third month. This portion of the chorion is known as the *chorion laeve,* or bald chorion (Fig. 6-5).

During pregnancy the thickened uterine endometrium is known as the *decidua.* The layer in contact with the chorion frondosum is called the *decidua basalis.* It is composed of a compact layer tightly connected to the chorion and a spongy layer with dilated glands and spiral arteries. The placenta is formed from the decidua basalis and the chorion frondosum (the only functional part of the chorion). The decidual layer covering the chorion laeve is known as the *decidua capsularis.*

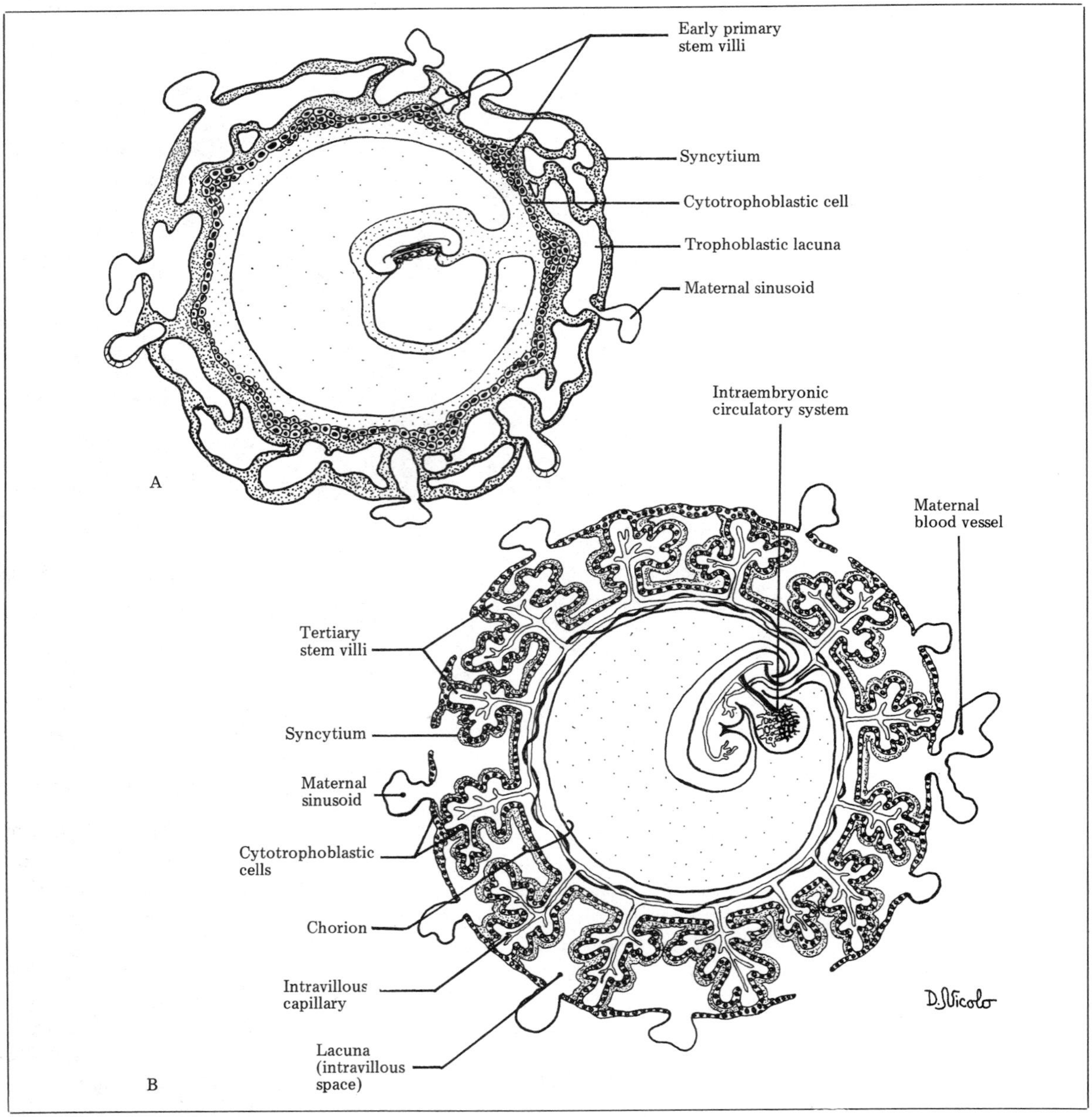

Figure 6-4. A. During the second week of embryonic development cytotrophoblastic cells begin to form primary stem villi. B. At 4 weeks of development there are many villi. Capillaries have formed within them and have made contact with the intraembryonic circulatory system.

Early in its development the decidua capsularis has a structure similar to that of the decidua basalis. Later, the growing conceptus causes it to project into the uterine cavity; the decidua capsularis becomes stretched and degenerates by the third month. The chorion laeve then comes in contact with the epithelium of the *decidua vera* on the opposite side of the uterus. By the fourth month the two fuse, obliterating the uterine cavity (Fig. 6-6).

Another important membrane, the amnion, begins to develop by about the seventh to eighth day after ovulation. It begins as a small vesicle and grows into a small sac that eventually surrounds the embryo between the fourth and fifth

Figure 6-5. Uterine decidua and developing chorion.

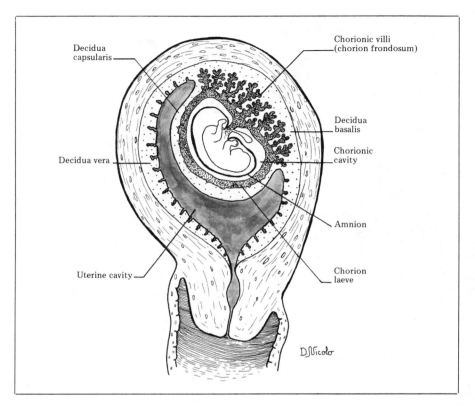

months. Further growth of the sac brings the amnion into contact with the chorion, and the two, although slightly adherent, can be separated at term.

In early pregnancy the normally clear alkaline fluid that collects within the amniotic cavity is a product of the amnion and the maternal blood. Its functions are to cushion the fetus against injury, provide a medium in which it can move, and maintain a relatively constant temperature. The amount and constituents of the fluid change as pregnancy progresses. Many tests to assess fetal maturity and well-being are based on the measurement of these constituents.

During the first half of pregnancy, the amniotic fluid is similar in composition to maternal plasma but has less protein and little solid material. In the latter half of pregnancy it contains varying amounts of desquamated fetal cells, lanugo, scalp hair, and vernix caseosa, as well as other solutes. Also in the latter half of pregnancy the fetus contributes to amniotic fluid composition and volume by both urinating and swallowing large amounts of fluid. The fetal urine raises the concentration of urea, creatinine, and uric acid. Although the total volume may vary, there is an average of about 1,000 milliliters of amniotic fluid at term [9].

Maturing Placenta   The placenta continues to increase in both size and weight throughout pregnancy. At term it weighs approximately 450–680 grams (1–1½ pounds), or about one-sixth of the weight of the baby. It has a discoid shape, and the appearance of its two surfaces is markedly different. The fetal surface is covered by the shiny amnion. The rough, red maternal surface is divided into an average of 22 lobes, or

Figure 6-6. Fusing of the decidua vera and the chorion laeve occurs by the fourth month of embryonic development. The uterine cavity is now obliterated.

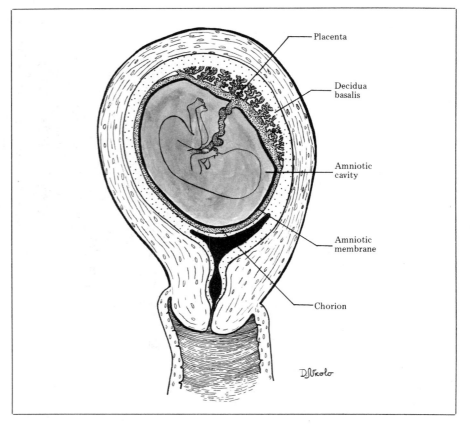

cotyledons, which develop between the fourth and fifth months as a result of septum formation by the decidua basalis (Fig. 6-7).

Overly large placentas may be a sign of fetal infections such as syphilis, tuberculosis, toxoplasmosis, and cytomegalovirus. Hemolytic disease of the newborn is another disorder related to extra large placental size. Small placental size is often associated with growth-retarded or immature infants.

The placenta's functions, many of which begin soon after implantation, include fetal respiration, nutrition, excretion, and hormone exchange. It also synthesizes hormones and probably has an immunologic and protective role [7]. As the placenta grows and fetal demands increase, certain necessary changes alter placental efficiency. The syncytium thins and the number of blood vessels close to its surface increase, facilitating transport of materials to and from the fetus. Later in pregnancy its efficiency is decreased by other changes, including the obliteration of certain vessels and deposits of fibrin and calcium in the placenta.

PLACENTAL EXCHANGE

Placental exchange of substances between mother and fetus occurs across the *placental barrier,* or *membrane,* which is composed of a layer of syncytium and fetal capillary endothelium. The exchange is dependent on adequate maternal blood flow in the intervillous space and fetal blood in the chorionic villi. Transfer

Figure 6-7. Full-term placentas. A. Maternal surface, showing cotyledons and grooves. B. Fetal surface, showing blood vessels running under the amnion and meeting at the umbilical cord. C. Inner amnion and outer smooth chorion. D. Marginal attachment of cord, often called battledore placenta. (From K. L. Moore. *Before We Are Born.* Philadelphia: Saunders, 1974.)

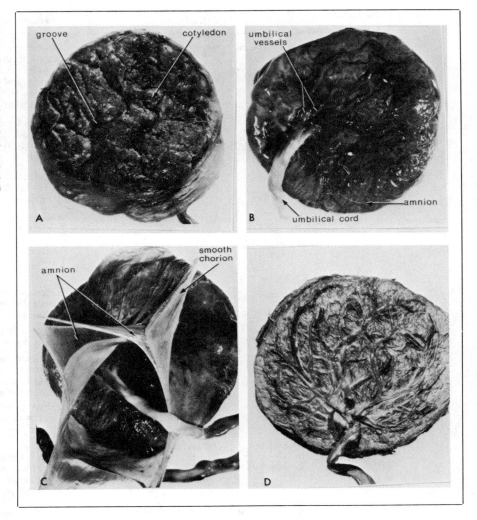

of substances across the placental membrane has been shown to occur via four mechanisms: simple diffusion, facilitated diffusion, active transport, and pinocytosis (Table 6-1) [2,8,9].

Substances crossing the placental membrane have been classified into four general groups. *Substances concerned with the maintenance of biochemical homeostasis or protection against sudden fetal death* transfer at a rate of milligrams per second. The predominant mechanism of transfer is rapid diffusion. This group of substances includes electrolytes, water, and respiratory gases. *Substances concerned primarily with fetal nutrition,* whose transfer is measured in milligrams per minute, are moved by carrier systems in addition to diffusion and include amino acids, sugars, and most of the water-soluble vitamins. *Substances concerned primarily with the modification of fetal growth and the maintenance of pregnancy* transfer by slow diffusion at a rate of milligrams per hour. Most of the hormones are in this group. *Substances of immunologic*

Table 6-1. Placental Transport

Substance	Mechanism	Characteristics
Oxygen, carbon dioxide, carbon monoxide	Simple diffusion	Efficiency of gas exchange approaches that of lung. Dependent on rate of maternal blood flow in intervillous space and flow of fetal blood in chorionic villi and on thickness and surface area of placental barrier
Water	Diffusion	Peak in transfer at 36th week, when it is 3½ liters/hour to and from fetus—70 times as great as at the 9th week
Sodium and potassium	Diffusion and active transfer	Less than 0.1% of sodium that reaches fetus is retained. Equal amounts in mother and fetus
Calcium	Active transfer	Fetus obtains calcium at expense of maternal reserves. Maternal calcium metabolism increased in pregnancy. Placental barrier offers little resistance. Higher in fetus than in mother
Iron	Active transfer	Fetus obtains iron at expense of maternal reserves. Higher in fetus than in mother
Phosphates	Active transfer	Inorganic phosphates twice as high in fetal blood as in maternal blood
Fluoride	Unknown	Readily crosses placental barrier. Appears to be concentrated in the placenta and this perhaps regularizes its transfer
Iodide	Similar to that of iodide concentration by thyroid gland	Taken up by fetal thyroid gland as early as 14th week of gestation. Readily crosses placental barrier
Carbohydrates	Diffusion and active transport	Principal source of energy for the fetus. Concentration of glucose in fetal blood is 20–30% lower than that of mother, perhaps due to utilization by placenta itself
Lipids, fats, and fatty acids	Not resolved. May be diffusion, active transport, pinocytosis	Concentration greater in maternal blood than in fetal blood. Absorption of fat, fatty acids, and glycerol in placenta may be similar to absorption in intestinal canal
Amino acids, polypeptides, and proteins	Probably active transport; pinocytosis	Amino acids used in fetal circulation for synthesis of plasma and tissue proteins. Higher in fetus than in mother. Significant levels of gamma globulin antibodies reached between 22nd–30th week. Increased to equal maternal level at 9th month
Vitamins	Very complex; probably active transport	Most known vitamins present in the placenta although precise localization indefinite. Water-soluble vitamins cross more readily than fat-soluble vitamins. Levels of vitamin A and E lower in fetus than in mother; B complex, C, and D higher in fetus; B, C, D, E stored in placenta

Table 6-1 (continued)

Substance	Mechanism	Characteristics
Bilirubin	Diffusion	Quickly cleared
Protein hormones	Slow transfer	Do not reach fetus in significant amounts (exception: thyroxine)
Steroid hormones	Diffusion	Pass placental membrane freely
Antibodies	Active transport, pinocytosis	Some passive immunity for fetus by transfer of maternal antibodies for diphtheria, smallpox, measles. None for pertussis or chicken pox
Drugs and antibiotics	Diffusion; some active transport	Placenta is permeable to most drugs; the higher the molecular weight, the slower the passage. Passage of insulin controversial. Drugs taken by the mother may affect the fetus directly or indirectly by altering maternal or placental metabolism
Infectious agents	Unknown	Some bacteria, protozoa, viruses, rickettsiae. Permeability of placenta to *Treponema pallidum* greatly increased after the 5th month

importance, including plasma proteins, probably transfer primarily by pinocytosis; transfer is measured in milligrams per day [4].

HORMONE PRODUCTION

Presently only five hormones are known to be produced by the placenta: the protein hormones, namely human chorionic gonadotropin (HCG), human chorionic somatomammotropin or human placental lactogen (HPL), and thyrotropin; and the steroid hormones, namely estrogen and progesterone. There is some evidence for the production of adrenocorticotropic hormone [13]. Evidence for the synthesis of hormones such as melanocyte-stimulating hormone, relaxin, corticosteroids, and aldosterone is not conclusive. It is generally believed that the syncytium is the site of hormone production (Tables 6-2 and 6-3) [10].

Since the placenta must be considered a homograft, one wonders why the products of conception do not habitually provoke an immune response in the mother; the reason (or reasons) that they do not remains a mystery. The most acceptable explanation for the survival of this homograft is that the placental membrane results in fairly complete anatomic separation of maternal and fetal circulations [5]. The apparent immunologic inertness of the trophoblast may reflect either the presence of few antigenic sites, their masking by a barrier, or both. It is possible that HCG may block an attack on the trophoblast by maternal lymphocytes [6].

INNER CELL MASS
Embryonic Period (2 to 8 Weeks)

From the beginning of the second week until the eighth week, the embryo undergoes morphogenesis (i.e., all major features of the external body take recognizable form) and organogenesis (i.e., the main organ systems are established). During the long fetal period that follows, the organs undergo little more than maturation.

Table 6-2. Placental Hormones	Hormone	Source	Characteristics, Values, Functions
	Human chorionic gonadotropin (HCG)	Syncytium	Chemical and biologic properties similar to pituitary luteinizing hormone. Has thyroid-stimulating properties. Appearance in urine is used as test for pregnancy. Detected in blood and urine soon after implantation (10 days after conception). Peak between 50–70 days of gestation (500,000–1,000,000 IU/24 hours). Low level maintained thereafter (80,000–120,000 IU/24 hours). Disappears within 1 week postpartum. Stimulates and prolongs existence of corpus luteum, thereby maintaining local environment favorable for implantation and growth of embryo. Probably helps to regulate estrogen production and to suppress maternal immunologic reactions against the fetus
	Human placental lactogen (HPL), chorionic somatomammotropin	Syncytium	Composition similar to that of human pituitary growth hormone. Present in urine. Detected between 4th and 8th weeks after conception. Concentration rises rapidly throughout pregnancy, reaching peak (serum level) in last trimester—10–20 mcg/ml at term. Rapidly disappears from maternal circulation within 1 day after delivery. Plays possible role in mammary development. Might be synergistic with HCG in maintenance or corpus luteum. May potentiate activity of growth hormone but has no growth-producing activity itself. May be "diabetogenic" factor in pregnancy. Significant physiologic antagonist of insulin. Mobilizes free fatty acids from maternal stores. Glucose then available for fetal use
	Progesterone ("hormone of pregnancy")	Syncytium	Necessary for maintenance of pregnancy. Transition from dependence on ovarian production to dependence on placental production at 6–8 weeks of gestation. Daily production in late pregnancy is about 250 mg. Reduces smooth muscle excitability. Effect greatest in myometrium. (Additional effects in Chap. 4.) Principal metabolite is pregnanediol (found in urine). Fetus contributes little to production directly or by provision of precursors. Precursor is maternal cholesterol. Small amount of progesterone enters fetal circulation for adrenal production of steroids
	Estrogen	Syncytium	By 7th week of gestation, more than 50% of estrogens in maternal circulation produced by the placenta. Increased amount of estriol excreted in urine during pregnancy; 24–28 mg/24 hours is the average excretion at term. Significant fetal contribution to placental production of estrogen. Maintenance of fetal circulation essential to adequate placental function. Fetus provides estrogen precursors (19 carbon androgens) from adrenal gland and liver. Therefore, determination of urinary estriol during pregnancy can be a test of placental function and fetal well-being. (Additional effects of estrogen in Chap. 4.)
	Human chorionic thyrotropin (HCT)	Syncytium	Small amount in human placenta. Similar in action to pituitary TSH. Responsible for raised levels of thyrotropin in mother's plasma
	Human chorionic adrenocorticotropin hormone (HCACTH)	Syncytium	Some evidence that rise in free cortisol during pregnancy may be due to placental ACTH. Content of ACTH higher than can be accounted for by maternal production. Cortisol levels in mother resistant to suppression by dexamethasone, suggesting a maternal ACTH supply not from maternal pituitary gland. Placental ACTH may increase maternal adrenal activity to provide basic building blocks (cholesterol and pregnenolone) for steroidogenesis by placenta

Table 6-3. Dynamics of Steroid Production During Pregnancy

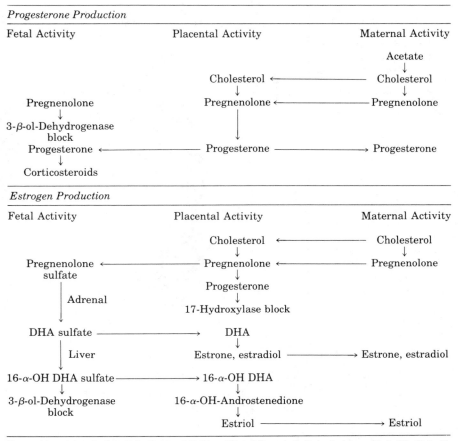

Progesterone Production

Fetal Activity	Placental Activity	Maternal Activity
		Acetate ↓
	Cholesterol ←	Cholesterol ↓
Pregnenolone ↓	Pregnenolone ← ↓	Pregnenolone
3-β-ol-Dehydrogenase block		
Progesterone ←	Progesterone	→ Progesterone
↓ Corticosteroids		

Estrogen Production

Fetal Activity	Placental Activity	Maternal Activity
	Cholesterol ← ↓	Cholesterol ↓
Pregnenolone ← sulfate	Pregnenolone ← ↓	Pregnenolone
	Progesterone ↓	
Adrenal	17-Hydroxylase block	
↓		
DHA sulfate ——→	DHA ↓	
Liver	Estrone, estradiol ——→	Estrone, estradiol
↓		
16-α-OH DHA sulfate ——→	16-α-OH DHA ↓	
↓	16-α-OH-Androstenedione ↓	
3-β-ol-Dehydrogenase block	Estriol ——————→	Estriol

Source: Adapted from L. Speroff, R. Glass, and N. Kase. *Clinical Gynecologic Endocrinology and Infertility* (2nd ed.). Baltimore: Williams & Wilkins, 1979.

SECOND WEEK

By the eighth day of development, the cells of the growing embryo (embryoblast) differentiate into two distinct cell layers. The layer of small flattened polyhedral cells is known as the entodermal germ layer, and the layer of high columnar cells is known as the ectodermal germ layer. The ectodermal and entodermal cells form the *bilaminar germ disc.* The ectodermal cells are initially attached to the growing cytotrophoblast. With further development, spaces that have appeared between the two layers form the amniotic cavity. The entodermal disc shows a slight thickening by the end of the second week. This thickening is located in the midcephalic region of the embryonic disc and is called the *prechordal plate;* it is this structure that establishes a cephalocaudal axis (Fig. 6-8).

THIRD WEEK

Approximately at the beginning of the third week, ectodermal cells in the caudal region of the germ disc multiply and move toward the midline, forming a narrow groove with small bulges on either side. This structure is known as the *primitive streak.* It appears to mark the main axis of the embryo, along which the spinal cord will later develop. Research indicates that modified ectodermal cells travel to the region of the primitive streak and eventually pass between the ectodermal

Figure 6-8. During the second week of embryonic development the ectoderm and entoderm are formed. The prechordal plate develops, establishing a cephalocaudal axis in the embryo.

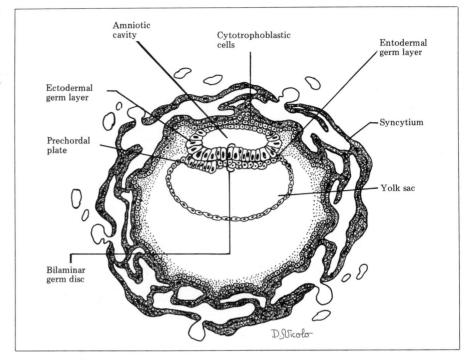

and entodermal layers. There they form a new germ layer, the mesoderm, which is the last embryonic layer to develop (Fig. 6-9).

By the middle of the third week, the embryonic disc has become elongated and pear-shaped, with a broad cephalic end and a narrow caudal end. Most rapid growth takes place in the cephalic region, where the three germ layers begin further specific development. Such development in the caudal region will not occur for approximately another week. Thus, a maturational developmental pattern (i.e., one of cephalic priority) for all later growth is set. By the end of the third week the three basic layers of the embryo proper, entoderm, ectoderm, and mesoderm, have been formed (Fig. 6-10).

During this period, a midline thickening of the embryonic ectoderm appears. This is known as the neural plate, in which a longitudinal groove develops. Neural folds form along the neural groove. By the end of the third week these folds have begun to meet and fuse, forming the neural tube.

Also at this time isolated spaces form in the mesoderm. These spaces subsequently coalesce to form a single horseshoe-shaped cavity (intraembryonic coelom) that in turn becomes the pericardial, pleural, and peritoneal cavities. During this same period, the developing heart appears as paired tubes that are joined to blood vessels in the embryo and in the extraembryonic membranes.

By the end of the third week, mesodermal blocks known as somites appear on each side of the midline. They appear in a craniocaudal sequence and by the end of the first month approximately 40 pairs have formed. Their formation shapes the contours of the embryo, and during this time the size of the embryo is usually expressed in terms of the number of somites. The 33 pairs of vertebrae that form the spinal column develop from these somites (Fig. 6-11).

Figure 6-9. Developing mesoderm at the beginning of the third week of embryonic development.

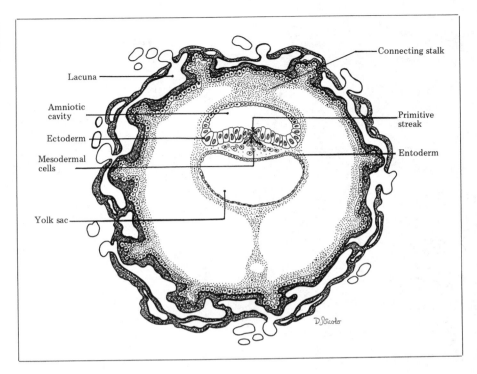

FOURTH WEEK

By the end of the first month, the embryo is 6 millimeters (¼ inch) long and slightly curved, and its head comprises one-third of its total length. Externally there is no distinguishable face; however, outlines of the eyes can be seen on the side of the face just above a large opening, the primitive mouth cavity. The foundations for the brain, spinal cord, and entire nervous system have been established. The neural tube is now closed at the center. Most organs are just beginning to form. The heart, an S-shaped bulb, is now pulsating rhythmically. The liver, stomach, intestines, pancreas, arm buds, lung buds, and primordia of the thyroid gland are definable.

During the second month, the external appearance of the embryo becomes more human. Even though somites are still visible, the age of the embryo at this stage is expressed as crown-rump (C.R.) length (the measurement from the vertex of the skull to the midpoint of the buttocks).

FIFTH WEEK

In the fifth week growth of the head is extensive, mainly due to rapid brain development. The ear pits appear on the side of the head and the jaws begin to form, giving the face a more humanlike appearance. The pituitary gland is forming, as are the pharyngeal branches that will later give rise to the bronchi. The neural mechanisms for vestibular function and hearing are developing. Leg buds become visible, and the umbilical cord is now a distinct structure that connects the embryo to the placenta (Fig. 6-11C).

The umbilical cord develops from the attaching body stalk that is readily distinguishable in the 21-day embryo; the body stalk usually grows from the

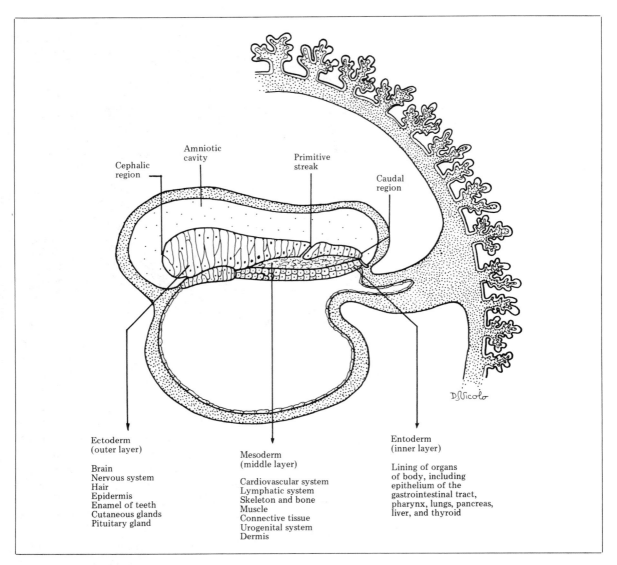

Cephalic region

Amniotic cavity

Primitive streak

Caudal region

Ectoderm
(outer layer)

Brain
Nervous system
Hair
Epidermis
Enamel of teeth
Cutaneous glands
Pituitary gland

Mesoderm
(middle layer)

Cardiovascular system
Lymphatic system
Skeleton and bone
Muscle
Connective tissue
Urogenital system
Dermis

Entoderm
(inner layer)

Lining of organs
of body, including
epithelium of the
gastrointestinal tract,
pharynx, lungs, pancreas,
liver, and thyroid

Figure 6-10.   By the end of the third week of embryonic development, three germ layers have evolved that later form various body systems.

center of the implantation site. Since an equal amount of trophoblastic proliferation occurs on either side of the implantation site, the umbilical cord is most often centrally located on the placenta [14]. In the early somite stage a chain of vessels in the body stalk provides circulation between the developing embryo and the chorionic villi. These vessels are soon reduced to four main stems, two on the right and two on the left. The right vein degenerates early, thus leaving the cord with one large vein and two smaller arteries. The vessels of the cord are supported by a specialized connective tissue known as Wharton's jelly, and both the vessels and Wharton's jelly are surrounded by a membrane of amniotic tissue. Cords vary in size; at term the umbilical cord averages 2 cm (1 inch) in diameter and 55 cm (22 inches) long. Because the vessels are longer than the cord itself they must coil and twist, which frequently results in false knots. With fetal movement, a long cord is

Figure 6-11.   Four- and 5-week-old embryos with formed somites (size is now expressed by the number of somites). A. Embryo at 4 weeks. B. Internal structures of embryo at 4 weeks. C. Embryo at 5 weeks.

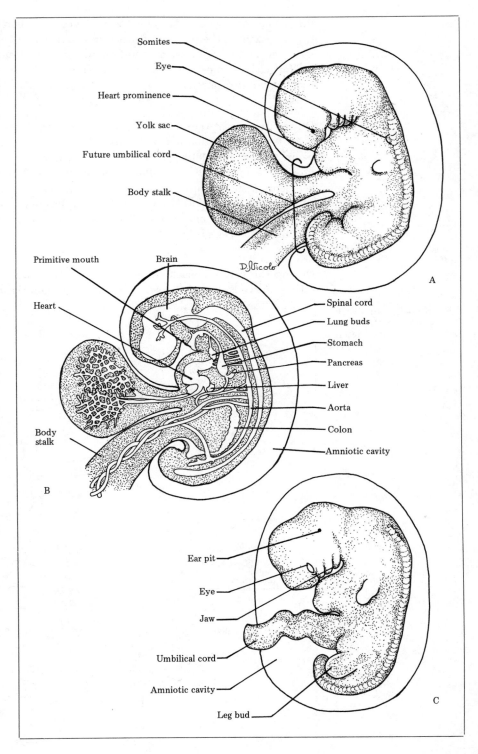

likely to become wrapped around the baby's neck. A short cord may be instrumental in detaching the placenta if traction is put upon it. About 1 percent of cords lack one of the arteries, a condition that is associated with congenital fetal malformations, most frequently cardiovascular defects, genitourinary defects, esophageal atresia, and imperforate anus [1,3,8].

SIXTH WEEK

During the sixth week the eye muscles form, the eyes become pigmented, the basis for the sensation of smell is established, and the teeth and facial muscles begin to form. Paddlelike rudiments of hands develop, while cartilage centers for later bone formation take shape. The embryonic kidney is in the process of developing, and the urethra becomes patent at this time, establishing a communication with the amniotic cavity. The penis is forming in the male, and testes can be distinguished from ovaries. The liver is beginning to take over the job of forming blood cells (Fig. 6-12).

SEVENTH WEEK

During the seventh week the eyes and ears continue rapid development. The retinal nerve cells and the semicircular ear canals become established, and the

Figure 6-12. Six-week-old embryo with paddle-like hands.

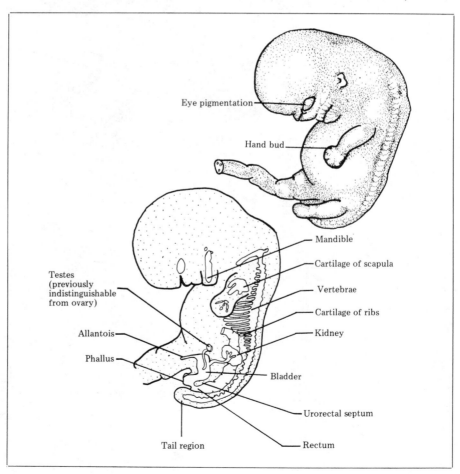

palate and tongue take form in the mouth. The eyelids are forming, and nipples are visible. The neck now becomes distinct, connecting the head with the body. The cartilage of the jaws, ribs, and vertebrae begins to be replaced by bone, and most muscles become well organized. The urogenital and rectal passages become completely separate (Fig. 6-13).

EIGHTH WEEK

By 8 weeks, the embryo weighs 1 gram (0.04 ounce) and is 3 centimeters (1.2 inches) long (C.R.). The hands and feet are well formed. The eyes have moved to the front of the head, giving a more human look to the face. By the end of the eighth week the eyelids begin to fuse. The auricles, although low set, begin to

Figure 6-13. Seven-week-old embryo. Palate and tongue have now formed.

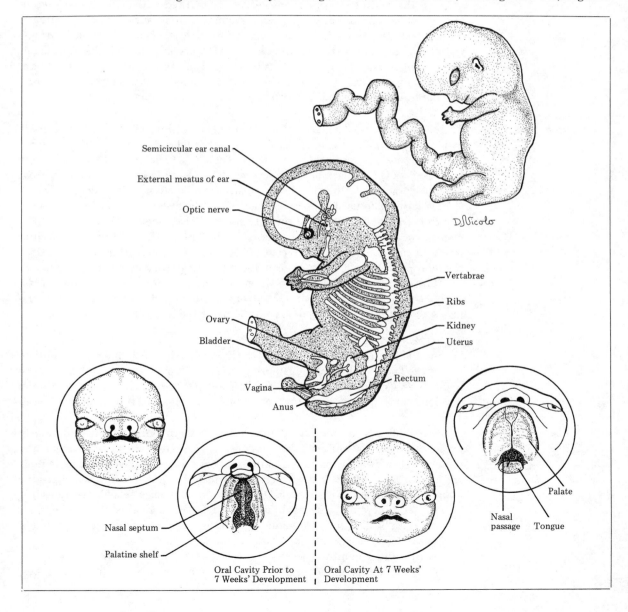

Semicircular ear canal

External meatus of ear

Optic nerve

Vertabrae

Ribs

Ovary

Kidney

Bladder

Uterus

Rectum

Vagina

Anus

Nasal septum

Palate

Palatine shelf

Nasal passage   Tongue

Oral Cavity Prior to 7 Weeks' Development

Oral Cavity At 7 Weeks' Development

assume their final shape. Bone is now rapidly replacing cartilage, and the major blood vessels are forming their final pattern. The heart, which is now functionally complete, has attained the form it will have during fetal life. The thyroid, thymus, and adrenal glands are developing, and the taste buds are forming. Intestinal villi are beginning to develop. The clitoris appears in the female fetus, and the ovaries or testes begin their descent toward their final location. While differences in the appearance of the external genitalia exist, they are not distinct enough to identify the sex of the embryo. The gasp reflex, a primitive breathing movement, is now present, and somatic movements can be seen although they are not felt by the mother at this time.

Thus, the end of the embryonic period is marked with a certain degree of completeness. Because all major organ systems have been started, if not already established, the fetus is not so susceptible to the effects of disease, drugs, radiation, and other external threats as it was earlier. Although the fetus is not out of danger, the above factor plus its larger body size increases its resistance. Figure 6-14 indicates those critical periods of development when the embryo and fetus are most susceptible to developmental malformations.

Fetal Period (9–40 Weeks)

The developmental phase from the beginning of the third month until delivery is called the *fetal period*. It is primarily a time of rapid body growth, although some further tissue differentiation does occur (Table 6-4). The age of the fetus is now expressed as C.R. length or as crown-heel (C.H.) length, the measurement from the vertex of the skull to the heel. (Haase's rule is often used to determine the C.H. length of a fetus of known gestation: Up to the fifth month, the number of the month is squared, thus giving the C.H. length in centimeters; following the fifth month, the number of the month is multiplied by 5. Thus a 4-month-old fetus would have a C.H. length of 16 centimeters, or 6 inches.) During the first half of the fetal period, the fetus grows rapidly in length, particularly during the fourth and fifth months. The weight of the fetus, however, increases relatively little during this time. During the latter half of the fetal period, particularly during the last 2½ months, the fetus gains about 50 percent of its full-term weight.

THIRD MONTH

During the third month the limbs reach their relative length in proportion to the rest of the body, with the lower limbs a little shorter and less developed than the upper ones. Fingernails, toenails, and hair follicles begin to form, and the thumb develops opposition. The eyelids seal and remain closed for three months (Fig. 6-15).

Tooth buds appear for all 20 temporary teeth, making this a particularly important time for the fetus to receive an adequate amount of calcium and minerals. The swallowing and sucking reflexes are better developed, taste buds are numerous, and salivary glands begin to form. The thyroid and digestive glands are complete. The pancreas forms insulin and the gallbladder secretes bile into the fetal intestine, where villi are more definable and peristalsis of the small intestine can be observed. The kidneys begin to form urine, which passes into the bladder and from there into the amniotic fluid.

The ill-defined genital structures of both sexes begin to take recognizable shape. The prostate gland is forming in the male, as are the fallopian tubes,

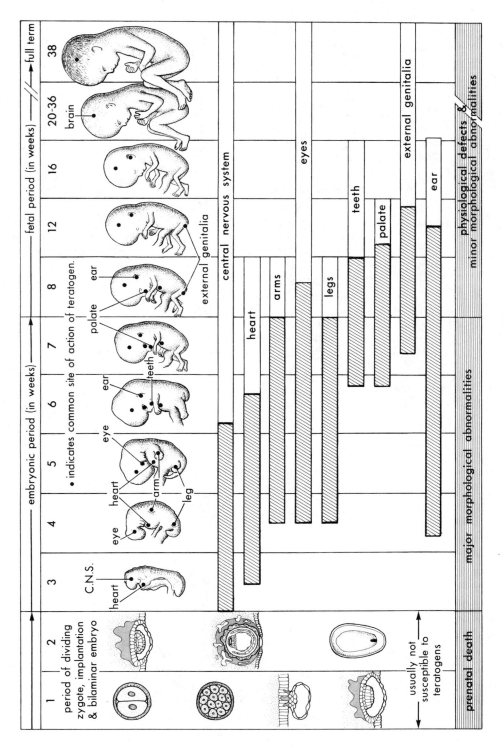

Figure 6-14. Schematic illustration of the sensitive or critical periods in human development. During the first 2 weeks of development, the embryo is usually not susceptible to teratogens. During these predifferentiation stages, a substance either damages all or most of the cells of the embryo, resulting in its death, or damages only a few cells, allowing the embryo to recover without developing defects. The left (shaded) sides of the bars denote highly sensitive periods; the right sides indicate stages that are less sensitive to teratogens. (From K. L. Moore. *The Developing Human: Clinically Oriented Embryology* [3rd ed.]. Philadelphia: Saunders, 1982.)

Table 6-4. Average Fetal
Length and Weight

Age (weeks)	Length	Weight
8	4 cm (1.6 in)	1–4 gm (0.04–0.1 oz)
12	9 cm (3.5 in)	30–40 gm (1.1–1.4 oz)
16	16 cm (6.3 in)	120–130 gm (4.2–4.6 oz)
20	25 cm (10 in)	300–400 gm (10–14 oz)
24	30 cm (12 in)	600–700 gm (1.3–1.5 lb)
28	35 cm (14 in)	1,000–1,200 gm (2.2–2.6 lb)
32	43 cm (17 in)	1,800–2,000 gm (4.0–4.4 lb)
36	46 cm (18 in)	2,500–2,700 gm (5.5–6.0 lb)
40	50 cm (20 in)	3,100–3,400 gm (6.8–7.5 lb)

uterus, and vagina in the female. The lungs have taken shape, and respiratory movements can be observed. The vocal cords are beginning to form, and bone marrow is a site for blood production. Numerous connections develop between muscles and nerves, and the fetus at this time becomes responsive to a touching stimulus. During the third and fourth months, specialized sensory endings begin to develop in the skin. It is questionable, however, if distinct senses of pain, touch, or temperature exist in prenatal life. Similarly, there is no evidence that the fetus has a sense of position [15].

FOURTH MONTH

The fetus is more erect in the fourth month, since its back has become more muscular and its bony skeleton more developed. It stretches and exercises its

Figure 6-15.   Three-month-old fetus.

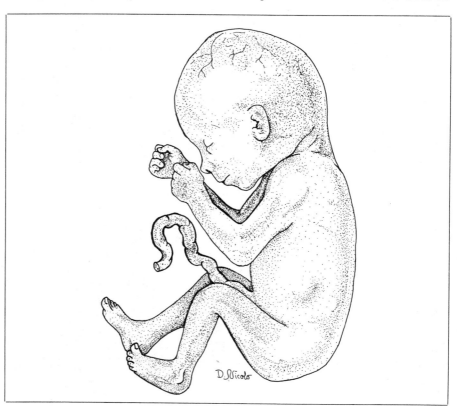

arms and legs. Its skin is pink or red, thin, loose, and wrinkled; lips have formed on the mouth, and fingerprints have developed (Fig. 6-16).

The basal metabolic rate begins to show a progressive increase. The surface of the fetal brain has many convolutions. The sealed eyes are sensitive to light, but sound evokes little reaction from a 4-month-old fetus. If the maternal abdominal wall is thin enough, the heartbeat of the fetus can be heard with a fetoscope. With the use of various sound amplification techniques, fetal heart sounds may be heard weeks earlier. Oocytes are developing in the ovaries of the female fetus.

Meconium, a sterile, viscid, odorless, dark green substance, is present in the fetal intestinal tract. At term, meconium contains desquamated epithelial cells, hair, and vernix from the amniotic fluid swallowed by the fetus, and mucus, bile, and other secretions of the intestinal glands. This comprises the first stool of the newborn.

During the fourth month the fetus makes sucking motions and swallows some amniotic fluid. (Some babies are born with calluses on their thumbs from sucking them in utero.) It has been suggested that the sugars and proteins swallowed may contribute nutritionally to the fetus, and that amniotic fluid provides the fetus with some gamma globulin and antibodies [15]. There is some evidence that fetal

Figure 6-16. Four-month-old fetus with intact chorion and amnion and attached placenta. (From E. Page, C. Villee, and D. Villee. *Human Reproduction* [2nd ed.]. Philadelphia: Saunders, 1976. By permission.)

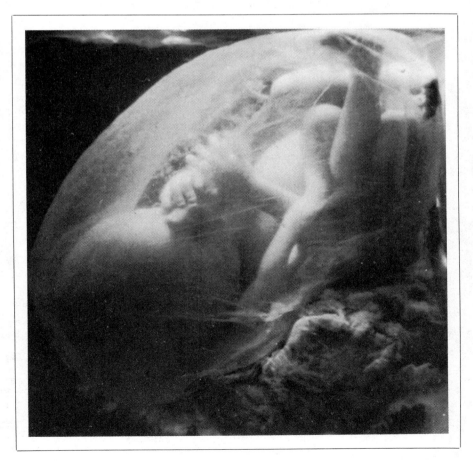

taste buds may be activated in utero by sweetening the amniotic fluid. One study seemed to indicate that sweetening the amniotic fluid enticed the fetus to swallow greater quantities [15]. There have also been attempts to feed the fetus in utero by injecting assimilable proteins into the amniotic fluid. The injection of dye into the amniotic fluid is sometimes used as a diagnostic tool, since the fetus swallows it and it lodges in the stomach and intestines, where it can be viewed on x-ray. Partial ossification of the fetal skeleton may also be seen on x-ray by the beginning of the sixteenth week.

FIFTH MONTH

By the fifth month the fetus has settled into a favorite lie or resting position. Fetal movements can now be recognized by the mother as kicking or turning (quickening). Sleeping habits begin to appear, and the fetus responds to loud noises or music. The fetus's hand grip (grasp reflex) denotes muscular strength, coordination, and reflex action.

Sweat glands are forming, and the sebaceous glands are secreting a fatty substance that forms a protective, cheeselike paste known as *vernix caseosa*. This substance protects the fetus's delicate skin from chapping, abrasions, and hardening as a result of being in amniotic fluid. At this stage, the fetus is covered with fine hair, or *lanugo,* and has baby hair on its head and eyebrows and a faint fringe of eyelashes. Nipples are more apparent over the mammary glands. Brown fat begins to form; this is the major site of heat production, particularly in the newborn infant.

During the fifth month adult hemoglobin can be identified in fetal blood. In the early months of gestation, fetal blood contains fetal hemoglobin, which is progressively replaced by adult hemoglobin as term approaches. Fetal hemoglobin has a greater affinity for oxygen and a constant, high oxygen-carrying capacity. Gamma globulin, identified in fetal blood as early as 20 weeks, reaches a concentration at term that either equals or exceeds that found in maternal blood.

SIXTH MONTH

During the sixth month the skin begins to thicken on the hands and feet; the body skin appears reddish and wrinkled, with little or no subcutaneous fat. The hair on the head is growing long, and the fetus is covered with abundant vernix. The grasp reflex has strengthened; the startle reflex is present at the end of the sixth month. The eyes are structurally complete, and the lung alveoli are beginning to develop.

Ossification is advancing; the first true bone formation has occurred in the breastbone. At 6 months the fetal bones contain as little as 12 percent calcium, compared to a calcium content of 90 percent in adult bone [15]. At this time the bony fetal skeleton can be seen on x-ray.

SEVENTH MONTH

The 7-month fetus has a chance for survival if born prematurely but mortality is high, usually because of respiratory distress. During this time, the brain makes tremendous strides in its development, and the localization of functional areas occurs. The nervous system has developed enough to make rhythmic breathing movements possible if air is available. The fetus is able to swallow if food is put in the mouth, and body temperature can be regulated. By the seventh month, the lanugo has begun to fade, appearing primarily on the back and shoulders, and the eyes reopen during this period. Much subcutaneous fat has formed, smoothing out many of the skin wrinkles. The testes begin to descend into the scrotal sac of the male fetus.

The lungs have reached the stage of development at which the expansion of air passages will permit them to function in oxygenating the blood. Pulmonary surfactant, a phospholipid-rich substance with very low surface tension, now coats much of the alveolar epithelium [11]; this helps to prepare the alveoli for expansion by air at birth.

EIGHTH MONTH

If born during the eighth month, the fetus will have a much better chance of survival. Its weight gain at this time results from an increase in subcutaneous fat, the insulating properties of which help to control the body temperature of the fetus. The skin, which is now pink (or pale in dark-skinned babies), has lost its wrinkled appearance.

NINTH MONTH

During the ninth and last calendar month of gestation, the fetus is less active than previously, perhaps because it is so large and there is so little space left in the uterus. The remaining vernix caseosa appears mostly on the back. The fetus has firm breasts. The eyes are blue since the eye pigmentation needs a period of exposure to light before it is fully developed. The gums are ridged. Considerable meconium is in the large intestine. The fetus has acquired maternal antibodies that will protect it for approximately the first 6 months after birth, until the immune system begins functioning. The immunities include measles, rubella, mumps, whooping cough, and scarlet fever.

Development of Body
Systems

Although all body organ systems begin their development in the embryonic period, it is during the fetal period that further differentiation takes place. The following material highlights the development of the major body systems and indicates the predominant anomalies that result when development does not proceed normally [8].

THE CARDIOVASCULAR SYSTEM

The cardiovascular system begins to develop during the third week from the mesodermal germ layer. Two heart tubes fuse to form one. As the heart tube grows, it twists to the right and soon assumes the external appearance of the adult heart. During the fourth to seventh weeks, the heart is partitioned into four chambers. The critical period of cardiac development occurs between days 20 and 50. Many critical and complex events are occurring during this time, and deviation from any one of them may result in cardiac defects.

Problems in partitioning of the heart may result in septal defects, especially ventricular septal defects. Some malformations result from abnormal transformation of the aortic arches into the adult arterial pattern. Failure of the usual changes in the circulatory system at birth results in two of the most common abnormalities of the heart and cardiac vessels: patent foramen ovale and patent ductus arteriosus.

Figure 6-17. Developing respiratory system. Abnormal development with esophageal atresia and tracheoesophageal fistula is shown.

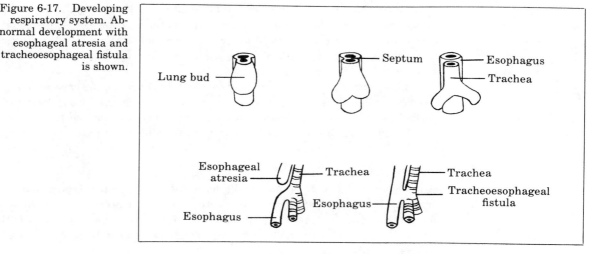

THE RESPIRATORY SYSTEM

The respiratory system begins to develop early in the fourth week from a groove in the primitive pharynx. The groove deepens to produce a diverticulum or pouch which soon becomes separated from the foregut by a septum, thus forming the esophagus and the laryngotracheal tube. Should this septum fail to form or form incompletely during the fourth and fifth weeks, the infant is left with a communicating passage between his esophagus and trachea known as a tracheo-esophageal fistula (Fig. 6-17).

The laryngotracheal tube subsequently divides to form two lung buds: a left bud, which later divides into two branches or main bronchi, and a right bud, which divides into three bronchi. Thus the primordia of the adult lobes of the lung are established.

Subsequent lung development may be divided into the following four stages [8]:

1. Pseudoglandular (5–17 weeks): The bronchi and terminal bronchioles form.
2. Canalicular (13–25 weeks): Bronchi and terminal bronchioles enlarge, the respiratory bronchioles and alveolar ducts develop, and lung tissue becomes highly vascular.
3. Terminal sac (24 weeks to birth): Alveolar ducts give rise to terminal air sacs. By 28 weeks the capillary network has proliferated close to the alveolar epithelium, and the lungs may be sufficiently developed to permit survival if the fetus is born.
4. Alveolar (late fetal period to 8 years of age): The development of pulmonary alveoli is completed.

THE NERVOUS SYSTEM

The central nervous system develops from the neural plate, which appears around the middle of the third week of development. The neural plate invaginates, forming folds on both sides which develop into the neural tube. The cranial end of the neural tube forms the brain, while the remaining, longer part becomes the spinal cord. The lumen of the tube forms the ventricles of the brain and the central canal of the spinal cord.

Congenital malformations of the central nervous system may be caused by genetic abnormalities or environmental factors, such as infectious agents, drugs, or toxic pollutants. Most abnormalities result from failure of the neural tube to close completely, resulting in openings in the vertebral column or in portions of the spinal meninges and/or spinal cord protruding through such openings. Defective openings in the vertebral column (spina bifida) occur most commonly in the lower thoracic, lumbar, and sacral regions. Failure of the neural folds in the cranial end of the neural plate to fuse and form the forebrain is known as anencephaly. Congenital abnormalities of the ventricular system result in hydrocephalus.

THE DIGESTIVE SYSTEM

A primitive gut (foregut, midgut, and hindgut) forms during the fourth week when the roof of the yolk sac is incorporated into the embryo (Fig. 6-18). The embryonic foregut gives rise to the pharynx, lower respiratory tract, esophagus, stomach, duodenum, liver, pancreas, and biliary apparatus. Because the esophagus and trachea have a common origin in the foregut, abnormal partitioning by the tracheoesophageal septum results in fistulas between them.

The midgut gives rise to the duodenum beyond the common bile duct, the jejunum, the ileum, the cecum, the appendix, the ascending colon, and the right half or more of the transverse colon. During the fifth week of development, the midgut herniates into the umbilical cord because of inadequate room in the abdomen. During the tenth week the intestines return to the abdomen; failure to do so results in an omphalocele. Additionally, the gut is closed at one stage of development; if the gut fails to reopen normally, stenosis (narrowing), atresia, or

Figure 6-18. Developing digestive system. Note rotation and growth of ventral pancreatic bud. In development of the hindgut, note progression of urorectal septum dividing the rectum and developing urinary bladder.

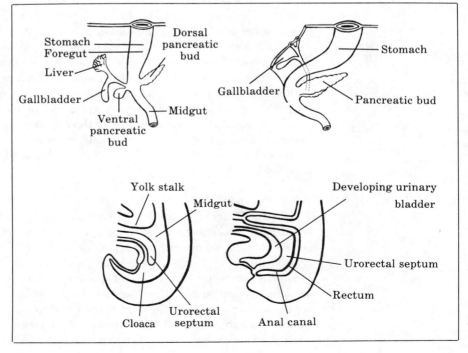

obstruction may occur. If remnants of the yolk sac persist, abnormalities such as Meckel's diverticulum may occur.

The hindgut gives rise to the distal third or more of the transverse colon, the descending colon, the sigmoid colon, the rectum, and the upper portion of the anal canal. The caudal portion of the hindgut forms the cloaca, which is divided by the urorectal septum into the urogenital sinus and the rectum. The urogenital sinus gives rise to the bladder and the urethra. Initially the rectum is separated from the exterior by an anal membrane, which breaks down at the end of the eighth week of development. Abnormal development of the hindgut may result in anal atresia, persistent anal membrane, or fistulas between the bladder or urethra and the rectum.

THE UROGENITAL SYSTEM

During development three successive sets of kidneys develop. The first are the pronephros, a nonfunctional set. They are followed by the mesonephros, which may function as a temporary excretory organ. The third and permanent kidneys are the functional metanephros. Initially the kidneys are located in the pelvis, but they gradually rise into the abdomen. Abnormalities of the kidney may result from failure to rise out of the pelvis or from early division of the ureteric bud, resulting in a double ureter and supernumerary kidney.

The reproductive system develops in association with the urinary tract. The germ cells, first seen on the yolk sac, migrate to the developing gonads. Gonadal sex is controlled by the Y chromosome's exerting its action on the indifferent gonad which, prior to this effect, could develop into a male or female. Under the influence of a Y chromosome, testes develop and produce male hormones, which stimulate development of the mesonephric ducts into male genital ducts and the indifferent external genitalia into the penis and scrotum. The male hormones suppress development of the paramesonephric ducts.

If two X chromosomes are present but no Y chromosome, ovaries develop and the paramesonephric ducts develop into the uterus and uterine tubes. The indifferent genitalia develop into the clitoris and labia, while the vagina develops from the urogenital sinus. The mesonephric ducts regress.

Developmental abnormalities may occur in the male if fetal testes fail to produce adequate male hormones, or in the female if the adrenal glands produce too much androgen. In both of these instances a pseudohermaphroditism occurs. Structural abnormalities may also occur in the developing organs when growth is impeded.

THE SPECIAL SENSES

The eyes and ears begin to develop during the fourth week. Most serious defects result from disturbances in development during the fourth to sixth weeks, but defects of sight and hearing may occur during the fetal period as well. The sense organs, especially the eyes, are sensitive to teratogens. Congenital cataracts and glaucoma may result from intrauterine infections, while low-set malformed ears are often associated with chromosomal abnormalities. Congenital deafness may result from abnormal development of the membranous and/or bony labyrinth as well as from abnormalities of the ossicles, from recessive inheritance, and from environmental factors, such as prenatal rubella virus infection.

THE MUSCULOSKELETAL SYSTEM AND LIMBS

The skeletal system is derived from mesoderm; the vertebral column and ribs develop from the sclerotome regions of the somites while most skeletal muscle is formed from the myotome regions of the somites. Ossification begins in the long bones by the end of the embryonic period. By 12 weeks primary ossification centers have appeared in nearly all bones of the extremities. Secondary centers of ossification appear after birth.

The limbs begin to appear toward the end of the fourth week, with the arm buds developing slightly before the leg buds. By the end of the eighth week, both the fingers and the toes are no longer webbed but have separated into distinct digits. Most limb malformations seem to be caused by genetic factors, but many probably result from an interaction of genetic and environmental influences.

FETAL CIRCULATION

Since the fetal lungs are not called upon to function independently while in utero, oxygenation of the fetus depends on a specialized circulatory flow. Aspects of the fetal circulation, which become altered after birth, include the umbilical vessels, and the ductus venosus, foramen ovale, and ductus arteriosus (Fig. 6-19).

The umbilical vein carries oxygenated blood from the placenta to the fetus, and the umbilical arteries carry blood with a low oxygen content from the fetus to the placenta. The umbilical vein divides into two branches just below the liver; the larger branch becomes the ductus venosus and empties directly into the inferior vena cava, while the smaller branch unites with the portal vein to empty blood into the liver. After the blood from the smaller branch circulates through the liver, it enters the inferior vena cava through the hepatic vein. Thus the inferior vena cava above the hepatic vein contains oxygenated blood from the placenta and unoxygenated blood returning from the lower portion of the fetus. The superior vena cava contains unoxygenated blood returning from the fetal head, neck, and arms.

Blood coming into the heart from the inferior vena cava is for the most part immediately deflected by a fold of endocardial tissue from the right atrium into the left atrium; it flows through the foramen ovale, an opening between the two chambers. From the left atrium, blood flows into the left ventricle. Eighty percent of this blood comes from the inferior vena cava and 20 percent from the fetal lungs via the pulmonary veins. The heart, brain, and upper portion of the fetus are supplied by 25 percent of the left ventricular output into the aorta, while the other 75 percent goes directly to the descending aorta [12].

Little or none of the less oxygenated blood from the superior vena cava normally passes through the foramen ovale; rather it passes into the right ventricle and from there into the pulmonary artery. This blood, for the most part, is shunted to the descending aorta through the ductus arteriosus, a wide channel connecting the two vessels. Only a small volume of blood, enough for tissue oxygenation, goes through the lungs before the onset of respiration, thereby making the pressure in the left atrium low. From the descending aorta, most of the deoxygenated blood flows through the hypogastric arteries to the umbilical arteries and back to the placenta. The remainder flows into the inferior vena cava, where it mixes with blood returning from the placenta via the umbilical vein.

Figure 6-19. Fetal circulation.

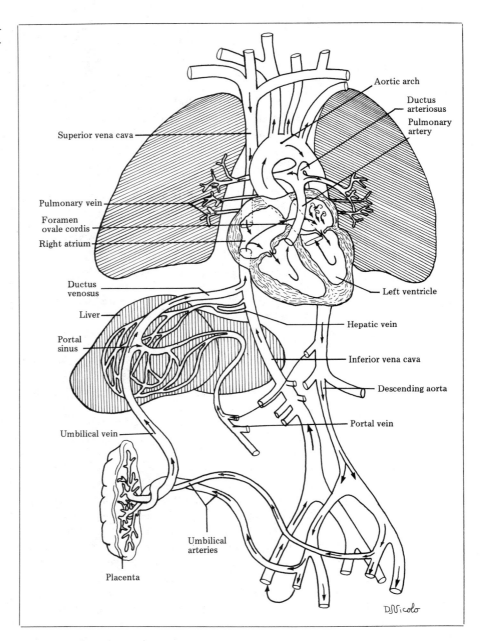

Aortic arch
Ductus arteriosus
Pulmonary artery
Superior vena cava
Pulmonary vein
Foramen ovale cordis
Right atrium
Ductus venosus
Left ventricle
Liver
Hepatic vein
Portal sinus
Inferior vena cava
Descending aorta
Portal vein
Umbilical vein
Umbilical arteries
Placenta

REFERENCES

1. Ainsworth, P., and Davies, P. A. The single umbilical artery: A five-year survey. *Developmental Medicine and Child Neurology* 11:297, 1969.
2. Boyd, J. D., and Hamilton, W. J. *The Human Placenta*. Cambridge, England: Heffer and Sons, 1970.
3. Feingold, M., Fine, R. N., and Ingall, D. Intravenous pyelography in infants with single umbilical artery. *New England Journal of Medicine* 270:1178, 1964.
4. Kaiser, I. Fertilization and the Physiology and Development of Fetus and Placenta. In D. Danforth (Ed.), *Obstetrics and Gynecology*. New York: Harper & Row, 1977.
5. Langman, J. *Medical Embryology*. Baltimore: Williams & Wilkins, 1963.

6. Lanman, J. Immunological Functions of the Placenta. In P. Gruenwald (Ed.), *The Placenta and Its Maternal Supply Line*. Baltimore: University Park Press, 1975.
7. Marrs, R., and Mishell, D. Placental trophic hormones. *Clinical Obstetrics and Gynecology* 23:721, 1980.
8. Moore, K. L. *The Developing Human: Clinically Oriented Embryology*. Philadelphia: Saunders, 1977.
9. Pritchard, J., and MacDonald, P. *Williams Obstetrics* (16th ed.). New York: Appleton-Century-Crofts, 1980.
10. Reid, D., Ryan, K., and Benirschke. K. *Principles and Management of Human Reproduction*. Philadelphia: Saunders, 1972.
11. Reynolds, E. O., and Strang, L. B. Alveolar surface properties of the lung in the newborn. *British Medical Bulletin* 22:79, 1966.
12. Rugh, R., and Shettles, L. B. *From Conception to Birth: The Drama of Life's Beginnings*. New York: Harper & Row, 1971.
13. Speroff, L., Glass, R., and Kase, N. *Clinical Gynecologic Endocrinology and Infertility* (2nd ed.). Baltimore: Williams & Wilkins, 1979.
14. Thomsen, K., and Hiersche, H. The Functional Morphology of the Placenta. In A. Klopper and E. Diczfalusy (Eds.), *Foetus and Placenta*. Oxford, Engl.: Blackwell, 1969.
15. Windle, W. F. *Physiology of the Fetus*. Springfield, Ill.: Thomas, 1971.
16. Wynn, R. Principles of Placentation and Early Human Placental Development. In P. Gruenwald (Ed.), *The Placenta and Its Maternal Supply Line*. Baltimore: University Park Press, 1975.

FURTHER READING   Abdul-Karim, D. Human fetal medicine—a symposium. *Clinical Obstetrics and Gynecology* 17:37, 1974.

Babson, S., Pernoll, M., Benda, G., and Simpson, K. *Diagnosis and Management of the Fetus and Neonate at Risk*. St. Louis: Mosby, 1980.

Beaconsfield, P., Birdwood, G., and Beaconsfield, R. The placenta. *Scientific American* 243:95, 1980.

Chez, R. Fetal and placental endocrinology. *Clinical Obstetrics and Gynecology* 23:719, 1980.

Cook, C. Intrauterine and extrauterine recognition and management of deviant fetal growth. *Pediatric Clinics of North America* 24:431, 1977.

Fetus's vulnerability to foreign chemicals. *Science News* 109:72, 1976.

Fuchs, F. Genetic amniocentesis. *Scientific American* 242:47, 1980.

Jones, J. Fetal metabolism and fetal growth. *Journal of Reproduction and Fertility* 47:189, 1976.

Kulovich, M., Hallman, M, and Gluck, L. The lung profile. *American Journal of Obstetrics and Gynecology* 135:57, 1979.

Levine, A., and Imai, P. Intrauterine treatment of fetal hydronephrosis. *Association of Operating Room Nurses Journal* 35:655, 1982.

Martin, C., and Gingerich, B. Uteroplacental physiology. *Journal of Obstetric, Gynecologic, and Neonatal Nursing* 5(5):16s, 1976.

Miller, C., et al. Uterine malformation and fetal deformation. *Journal of Pediatrics* 94:387, 1979.

Muir, H. Concept of the fetus as a transplant. *Nursing Mirror* 146(3):25, 1978.

Niswander, K. *Obstetrics*. Boston: Little, Brown, 1981.

Patterson, P. Fetal therapy: Issues we face. *Association of Operating Room Nurses Journal* 35:663, 1982.

Schuster, C. S., and Ashburn, S. S. *The Process of Human Development*. Boston: Little, Brown, 1980.

Speroff, L., Glass, R., and Kase, N. *Clinical Gynecologic Endocrinology and Infertility* (2nd ed.). Baltimore: Williams & Wilkins, 1979.

Chapter 7 Normal Pregnancy

The primary aim of health care during pregnancy is to ensure a healthy and happy outcome for families experiencing pregnancy and birth. The goal encompasses more than simply preventing or minimizing physical complications for mother and infant. Since childbearing is such a significant and personal experience, health care must include the teaching and support necessary to make this event as positive and rewarding as possible. The experiences a man and a woman encounter during the period of pregnancy, labor, delivery, and the early days after birth have far-reaching effects, not only on their own self-images but also on their relationships with each other and with their newborn. Their ability to cope, their resources and support systems, and the teaching, guidance, and support they receive from health care personnel will do much to make this a period that will either foster or inhibit their personal growth.

Nurses as members of a health care team must initially determine the health care needs and expectations of the woman and her family if the pregnancy is to be an experience that supports the personal growth of the family unit. The development of scientific nursing practice requires research and the use of the nursing process (assessment, planning, intervention, evaluation). A first step in the process, the nursing history, is the systematic collection of data as a basis for planning and implementing quality care for the woman and her family. A thorough health history and physical assessment enable the health care provider to determine whether the woman can be expected to have an uncomplicated pregnancy and delivery or whether she will be at risk for the development of complications. The earlier any possible risk factors can be identified, the earlier the woman can begin to receive special attention to ensure the best possible outcome for her, her baby, and her family. A variety of scoring systems have been developed to give weight to known high-risk categories (see Table 7-1 and Fig. 7-1).

When the initial assessment process is completed during the first meeting with the woman, a plan of care is formulated based on the data collected. This plan will be continually evaluated and modified as the woman progresses through her pregnancy, labor, delivery, and postdelivery periods. To provide for continuity of care, the format of the care plan should be constructed so that it will accompany the woman's record throughout her pregnancy, delivery, and postpartal period, whether she is seen initially in the practitioner's office or in the outpatient facility. As nurses, it is our responsibility to carefully document and update such items on the plan of care as the continued assessment of the expectations held by the woman and her family regarding the care they are to receive; their adjustments to the pregnancy; special problems of this family that need continued assessment; teaching that has been done; and evaluation of the learning that has occurred.

HEALTH HISTORY   While a variety of formats can be used in the data collection process (Fig. 7-2), it is essential to address the following items early in the woman's pregnancy. Concentrate initially on the starred categories; the remaining information can be

Table 7-1. Obstetric Scoring

Obstetric Patients—High-Risk Score Sheet	
Assign High Risk if Score Is +5 or Greater:	
I. Socioeconomic (+1 for each factor)	
Age—less than 18 or greater than 34	———
Parity—0 or greater than 4	———
Marital status—unwed	———
Educational status—less than 12 years	———
II. Nutritional (+2 for each factor)	
HB—less than 10 gm	———
Un/Tn ratio—less than 60	———
Height—less than 60 in	———
Weight—less than 100 lb or greater than 200 lb	———
III. Past Pregnancy Performance (+3 for each factor)	
Difficult labor—prolonged labor	———
Damaged infant	———
Congenital major anomaly	———
Previous cesarean section	———
IV. Past Pregnancy Outcome (+4 for each factor)	
Fetal death	———
Neonatal death	———
Low birth weight (less than $5\frac{1}{2}$ lb)	———
V. Medical or obstetric complication, present pregnancy (+5 for this factor)	———
High-Risk Score	Total: ———

Source: Adapted from H. C. Heins. Identification of the high risk obstetrical patient: The use of an objective scoring method. *Journal of the South Carolina Medical Association* 46:213, 1976.

more easily elicited in subsequent visits when the woman will be more familiar with you and the clinical setting.

*Age

There is an increased risk of complications in the very young woman, including anemia, preeclampsia, and prematurity. In the older woman, hemorrhage and hypertension are two examples of risk factors.

*Family History

Elicit information on important health problems of family members, such as diabetes, renal or hematologic disorders, hypertension (especially during pregnancy), heart disease, multiple pregnancy, congenital defects, or mental retardation.

*Woman's Past Medical and Gynecologic History

Include a history of urinary or venereal infections, bacterial or viral infections during pregnancy, diabetes, hypertension, heart disease, endocrine disorders, anemia, genital tract history (anomalies, vaginal infections, surgery), rubella screening, Pap test results, use of oral contraceptives or other contraception, menstrual history (menarche, type of menstrual periods, length, regularity), medication history, use of alcohol, tobacco, caffeine, mood-altering drugs.

*Woman's Past Obstetric History

Note dates of deliveries, duration of gestation, abortions (spontaneous or induced), significant problems during pregnancy, woman's perception of the process of the pregnancy for self and her family, description of labor (spontaneous, induced, length, complications), description of delivery (type—vaginal or cesarean; anesthesia), presentation of infant at delivery (vertex, breech), condition and weight of infant, woman's perception of labor and delivery process and outcome

Score	Factor	Score	Factor	Score	Factor
	Biological/Genetic I		Specify _____	3	Syphilis, untreated after 20 wk
1	Age ≥ 35/<18	2	Hx of pelvic operations (uterus, tube, etc.)	2	Gonorrhea, untreated
2	Age ≥ 40	2	Hx of neoplasm/tumor	1	Venereal disease, adeq. Rx
2	Elderly primigravida (>35 yr)	1	Neurological disease	2	Maternal fever (cause unknown)
2	Adverse hereditary disorder _____ state		Other (specify) _____	3	Maternal fever (FHS > 160)
2	Hemoglobinopathy		*Fertility VI*		Other _____
2	Rh negative (with increase titer this pregnancy)	1	Para 0		*Social VIII*
3	Rh negative (with zone III)	2	Para ≥ 6/problem getting pregnant		SCORING FOR FACTORS
	Other _____	1	Interval of pregnancy 2 yr (end to EDC)	0	Factor present, no effect on ability to function
	Habits this Pregnancy II		FOR EACH OCCURRENCE:	1	Factor present, can cope reasonably well
1	Heavy smoker (≥ 20 cigarettes/day)	1	Abortion (< 20 wk)	2	Factor present, can cope marginally
3	Drug use (heroin, etc.)	1	Stillbirth	3	Factor present, can't cope, intervention necessary
2	Alcohol use (mod. to heavy)	1	Neonatal death (4 wk old)		FACTORS (CIRCLE, UNDERLINE, AND SCORE)
1	Previous drug use	1	Low birth weight (full-term)	a.	Need for basic services (transportation, day care, foster care)
	Other _____	1	Surviving premature (2,500 gm)	b.	Public assistance—Medicaid
	Nutritional III	1	Antepartum hemorrhage (previous preg.)	c.	Finances (no PA, MA, medical care payments, etc.)
1	Overweight: 20# above ideal weight/≥ 200#	1	Toxemia (previous preg.)	d.	Housing hazardous to health (no heat, peeling paint, overcrowded, etc.)
2	Underweight: 15# below ideal weight	1	Difficult mid-forceps/operative vaginal delivery	e.	Need for housing (no place to live; unsatisfactory living arrangement)
1	Inadequate diet (this pregnancy)	1	C-section for prolonged labor/dystocia	f.	Out of wedlock
2	Weight loss/failure to gain weight (this pregnancy <10# by 30 wk)	1	Major congenital abnormality (life threatening)	g.	Emotional adjustment to pregnancy (accepting, rejecting, ambivalent, requests delivery before 37 wk, fear of harm by baby)
	Excessive weight gain (>35#)	2	Rh incompatibility, cohort homozygous	h.	Distracts clinical personnel—fear of hospitalization
	Other (specify) _____	3	Erythroblastosis	i.	Preoccupation with physical complaints
	Endocrine IV		Hx of affected isoimmunization	j.	Mental health problems: hx/ staff impression
1	Abnormal GTT/class A diabetes		*This Pregnancy/Complications VII*	k.	Delinquency/adult crime
1	Family hx of diabetes/hx of large babies 10# (>4.5 kg)	1	Bleeding, early (<20 wk)	l.	Alcoholism/drugs (in any significant person to patient)
2	Diabetes class B, C, D	2	Bleeding, with pain	m.	Stressful life event (death/ separation of significant person, broken home, unemployment, etc.)
3	Diabetes class E, F, G, R		Bleeding, late (>20 wk)		
3	Diabetes any class with decreasing insulin requirement	1	Bleeding, ceased	n.	Interpersonal relationship difficulties (social isolation, rebellions, antisocial behavior, disturbed relationship, poor adult relationships)
2	Thyroid disease (needs therapy)	2	Bleeding, continues		
	Other (specify) _____	3	Bleeding, pain		
	Medical/Surgical V	3	Bleeding, hypertension	o.	Legal problems other than delinquency or adult crime
2 (3)	Heart disease class I, II (III, IV)	3	Bleeding, coagulopathy	p.	Education (good reading and comprehension, unable to read or follow oral instruction, etc.)
	Preexisting hypertension	2	Placental insufficiency/fetal growth retardation (>3 wk)		
1 (2)	≥ 140/90 mm Hg			q.	Other
	≥ 160/110 mm Hg	3	Possible/probable fetal death		
2	Debilitating pulmonary disease (asthma, etc.)	2	Multiple pregnancy		
1	Chronic renal dis/recurrent UTI	2	Spontaneous rupture of membranes (< 37 wk)		
3	Chronic renal dis/with decreased function	2	Hydramnios (singleton), chronic		
3	Chronic renal dis/with increased creatinine/BUN	3	Hydramnios (singleton), acute		
1	Nondebilitating acquired disease, e.g., collagen disease, etc.	2	Suspected dystocia/serious pelvic deformity		
		3	Suspected uterine rupture		
		1 (2)	Anemia, Hgb < 11 gm (Hgb > 8 gm)		
		1 (3)	Toxemia, mild (severe)		
		3	Toxemia eclampsia		
		3	First rubella infection/exposure (<8 wk pregnant)		
		(2) [1]	First rubella infection/exposure (8–12 wk) [>12 wk]		

Total Score (add scores in all categories):

Class	0–1 = Low risk	2 = Medium risk	≥3 = High risk
Management	Routine	Close watch; consultations as needed	Ancillary tests; very close supervision by physician and others

Figure 7-1. Maternal and Infant Risk Index (MIRI) developed by the staff of the Maternal and Infant Care Project of Erie County, New York. The number to the left of each applicable item is circled and that item is underlined. Then the circled scores are totaled and averaged. An average score of 0–1 is classed as low risk and receives routine management. A score of 2 indicates a medium risk and is observed closely, with consultations as needed. A score of 3 or higher indicates a high-risk patient in need of ancillary tests and very close observation by physician and others. (Social factors [VIII], are scored by writing the score, as determined by the guide, beside the applicable factor.) (From A. S. Ademowore and E. Myers. Use of the problem-oriented medical record by nurses caring for high-risk antepartum patients. *Journal of Obstetric, Gynecologic and Neonatal Nursing* 6(1):17, 1977. By permission.)

PRENATAL RECORD

Hospital	Doctor		Date
Hosp. No.	Office No.	Insurance	
Pts. Name	Age	Race	Relig.	Country of Birth	Occupation
Address	Phone	Marital Status S M W D Sep.	Years Married	Education
Name of Father of Child	Age	Ht.	Wt.	Significant disease
Business Address	Business Phone	Occupation	Education

FAMILY HISTORY: (Tbc, Hypertension, Heart D., Diabetes, Neuro-Psych., Epilepsy, Allergies, Mult. Births, Congenital Anom.)

MENSTRUAL HISTORY: Onset at ___ Yrs. | Interval ___ Days | Duration ___ Days | Amt. ___

Months Preg. Attempted ___ L.M.P. ___ Normal? ___ E.D.C. ___

PRIOR MEDICAL HISTORY	✓ Pos.	Remarks (Include date and time of Rx)	HISTORY SINCE LAST MENSTRUAL PERIOD	✓ Pos.	Remarks (Include date and time of Rx)
Kidney Disease			Nausea		
Heart Disease			Vomiting		
Hypertension			Indigestion		
Rheumatic Fever			Constipation		
Tuberculosis			Headache		
Venereal Disease			Bleeding (Specify)		
Gyn. Disorder			Vaginal Discharge		
German Measles			Edema		
Nervous & Mental			Abdominal Pain		
Diabetes			Urinary Complaints		
Thyroid Dysfunction			German Measles		
Phlebitis, Varicosities			Other Virus		
Epilepsy			Radiation (Specify)		
Drug Sensitivity			Accidents		
Allergies			Medications		
Blood Dyscrasia					
Blood Transfusions					
Rh, ABO Sensitivity					
Operations, Accidents					

SUMMARY OF PREVIOUS PREGNANCIES	Full Term	Premature	Abortions	Now Alive	Mult. Births

No.	Year	Place of Confinement	Dur. of Gestation	Dur. of Labor	Type of Delivery	Born A or D	Weight	Complications Maternal	Child

Figure 7-2. Form for antepartal history and physical examination. (Form developed jointly by the Committee on Maternal and Child Care of the American Medical Association and the American College of Obstetricians and Gynecologists.)

Patient's Name: Date of Birth:

PHYSICAL EXAMINATON:

T.   P.   R.   B.P.   Hgt.   Pres. Wt.   Wt. at L.M.P.

Eyes   Teeth   Thyroid   Throat   Skin

Heart

Lungs

Breasts   Nipples   Tumors

Abdomen   Height of Fundus

Fetal Heart   Presentation and Position

Extremities   Varicosities   Edema

General Body Type

PELVIC EXAMINATION (bi-manual and speculum):

Vulva

Vagina

Perineum

Cervix

Uterus

Adnexae

Rectal Exam.

Diag. Conj.   cm. Trans. Diam. Outlet   cm. Shape Sacrum

Arch   Coccyx   S.-S. notch

Ischial Spines

Inlet:	Mid Pelvis:	Outlet:	Prognosis for Delivery:
☐ Adequate	☐ Adequate	☐ Adequate	
☐ Borderline	☐ Borderline	☐ Borderline	
☐ Contracted	☐ Contracted	☐ Contracted	

LABORATORY EXAMINATIONS: For Syphilis   Type   Date   Result

Blood Type and Rh: Patient   Father of Child

Hemoglobin   Hematocrit or RBC

Urinalysis: Albumin   Sugar   Microscopic

Exam. for Tbc: Type   Date   Result
(Cytology, Chemistry, etc.)

FACTS OF SPECIAL IMPORTANCE:
Initial Over-all Evaluation of Patient:

Sensitivities   Nutritional Status

Type of Del. planned   Anesthesia planned

Physician to call if attending M.D. not available

M.D. who will attend infant   Is breast feeding planned?

Date   Signed

(Original to be submitted to hospital upon completion.)

Figure 7-2 (continued)

American Medical Association 1968
Printed in the U.S.A.

Price: Single copy, 25¢ each; 50-99, 23¢ each;
100-499, 21¢ each; 500-999, 19¢ each;
1000 or more, 17¢ each.
Prices are subject to change.

0138-366 H; 671-150 M

(OP-65)

SUBSEQUENT PRENATAL VISITS

Name	Hosp.	Hosp. No.	Office No.

Date	SYMPTOMS						Blood Pressure	Weight	Ht. of Fundus	Position & Presentation	Fetal Heart	Urine		Hemoglobin	Nutrition		Rx and Remarks	Initials
	Headache	Dizziness	Edema	Nausea & Vomiting	Bleeding							Albumin	Sugar					

Date	Progress Notes & Consultation	Date	Progress Notes & Consultation

Rh antibody titer followup: date: result:

date: result: ; date: result:

Speculum examination in third trimester, including cytologic examination, if made:

Date	Signed

(Original to hospital at approximately 38 weeks.)

Figure 7-2 (continued)

for herself and her family, description of postdelivery period (problems—infection, hemorrhage), description of infant after birth (problems—jaundice, infection, respiratory distress, anomalies), type of feeding, infant's current health, woman's perception of postdelivery process and outcome for herself and her family, woman's perception of infant's temperament (irritable, pleasant, placid).

Woman's Present Obstetric History

Include the number of pregnancies the woman has had (gravidity), and the number of living children she has. A 4-digit code is often used: first digit—number of full-term births; second digit—number of preterm births; third digit—number of abortions; fourth digit—number of living children. Thus, 3-2-1-5 would mean 3 full-term births, 2 preterm births, 1 abortion, and 5 living children. See Table 7-2 for complete definitions of terms applied to pregnancy.

Date and Description of Last Normal Menstrual Period (LNMP)

Include the date, length, and amount and type of bleeding of her last normal menstrual period. This information is important in determining the expected date of delivery or expected date of confinement (EDC). A last menstrual period much lighter than normal may be a sign of developing trophoblastic circulatory activity, thus causing confusion in determining the EDC. The average duration of pregnancy from conception to birth is 266 days. If counted from the first day of the last menstrual period, as it often is, the average duration of pregnancy is approximately 280 days or 40 weeks. Fifty percent of all live births occur within 40 to 41 weeks; however, pregnancies extending a week beyond the expected date of delivery are fairly common and are generally regarded as within acceptable limits, as are pregnancies of 38 weeks' gestation (Table 7-3).

Nagele's rule, based on a 28-day menstrual cycle, is generally used to estimate the EDC. This is done by counting back 3 months from the first day of the last menstrual period and adding 7 days. For example, if the woman's menstrual period began December 2 (12/2), subtract three months and add 7 days, and the EDC would be September 9 (9/9). Although this method is only an approximation, it has been found to be highly dependable.

Pregnancy is sometimes divided into 10 lunar months. A lunar month consists of 28 days, a period coinciding with the average menstrual cycle. The first lunar month of pregnancy is calculated from the first day of the last menstrual period. Pregnancy is also divided into trimesters, or periods of approximately 3 calendar months. The first trimester begins from the time of conception; pregnancy then consists of a total of three trimesters, approximately 8¾ calendar months.

Table 7-2. Definition of Terms Applied to Pregnancy

Term	Definition
Gravidity	Number of pregnancies regardless of duration
Gravida	A woman who is or has been pregnant
Primigravida	A woman who is pregnant for the first time
Multigravida	A woman who has been pregnant more than once
Nulligravida	A woman who has never been pregnant
Para	Number of pregnancies that have continued to the period of viability
Primipara	A woman who has had one pregnancy that reached the period of viability
Multipara	A woman who has had more than one pregnancy that reached the period of viability
Nullipara	A woman, either primigravida or multigravida, who has not yet delivered a viable infant

Table 7-3. Number and Percentage of Births Related to Gestational Interval (Weeks 26–52)

Week	Number of Births	Percentage of Total Births	Week	Number of Births	Percentage of Total Births
26	1	0.03	40	745	25.18
27	0	0	41	818	27.64
28	4	0.14	42	397	13.42
29	3	0.10	43	152	5.14
30	4	0.14	44	41	1.39
31	7	0.24	45	16	0.54
32	6	0.20	46	12	0.41
33	13	0.44	47	3	0.10
34	22	0.74	48	1	0.03
35	21	0.71	49	2	0.07
36	49	1.66	50	0	0
37	92	3.10	51	2	0.07
38	160	5.40	52	2	0.07
39	386	13.04			
			Total	2,959	100

Source: Modified from A. Treloar, B. Behn, and D. Cowan. Analysis of gestational interval. *American Journal of Obstetrics and Gynecology* 99:36, 1967.

Signs and Symptoms of Pregnancy

Signs and symptoms of pregnancy include amenorrhea, breast changes, nausea and vomiting, fetal movement, skin pigmentary changes, urinary frequency, and fatigue (Table 7-4). Include a history of bleeding or other unusual signs (Table 7-5) and any exposure to infections or x-rays. Investigate the woman's current medications and current and past immunizations. A pregnant woman should take as few medications during her pregnancy as possible, since it is not known what effect many drugs have on fetal growth and development. Before any drug is given, its advantages must outweigh the factor of such unknown risks as well as any known fetal effect (Table 7-6). Vaccinations with live viruses that can cross the placental barrier and be hazardous to the fetus are generally to be avoided during pregnancy. Therefore, it is important that a woman receive her immunizations prior to pregnancy (or have a pregnancy test done before being immunized if there is the possibility that she may be pregnant). In addition, women who are vaccinated with live viruses should be advised to use a contraceptive during the subsequent 2 or 3 months.

Diet History

Assess and evaluate weight gain, nutritional patterns, and eating habits. Optimal weight gain during pregnancy based upon the lowest rate of complications is 24 to 28 pounds. Recommended weight gain is 2 to 4 pounds during the first trimester and from 0.5 to 1 pound per week during the second and third trimesters. (See Chapter 8 for further information on total weight gain and a detailed methodology of nutritional assessment.)

Alcohol Consumption

Assess and evaluate the woman's alcohol consumption and counsel her accordingly. Excessive use has been shown to produce abnormal changes in the fetus, which result in a common pattern of craniofacial, limb, and cardiovascular defects associated with prenatal and postnatal growth retardation [16,25]. There is no agreement on what a safe level of alcohol consumption is. The best advice to give a woman is that offered by the March of Dimes: "If you are pregnant don't drink; if you drink heavily don't get pregnant" [6,25,26]. For a more complete description of the fetal alcohol syndrome see Chapter 21.

*Table 7-4. Signs and
Symptoms of Pregnancy*

Signs or Symptoms	Time of Appearance	Other Possible Causes
Presumptive signs or symptoms		
Amenorrhea	Usually reliable 14 or more days after date period expected	Emotional disturbance, chronic disease, hormone imbalance
Breast changes		
Enlargement	Usually after 10 weeks	Hormonal therapy or imbalance, various tranquilizers, intracranial tumors
Tenderness	After 4 weeks	
Nausea and vomiting	Usually after 4–6 weeks	Emotional disturbance, drugs, infections, gastrointestinal irritations
Fetal movement (quickening)	Usually 14–17 weeks	Intestinal gas
Blueness of vagina, vulva, and cervix (Chadwick's sign)	Usually 6–12 weeks	Pelvic tumors, obesity, heart disease
Skin pigmentary changes	8 weeks until term	Hormonal imbalance, drugs
Urinary frequency	Usually 8–12 weeks	Infection, drugs
Fatigue	First trimester	Increased activity, infection, anemia, drugs
Probable signs or symptoms		
Enlarged abdomen	Usually after 4th month	Weight gain, abdominal tumor
Soft uterine isthmus (Hegar's sign)	After 6 weeks in multigravida; 8 weeks in primigravida	Uterine tumors
Soft cervix (Goodell's sign)	4–6 weeks	Pelvic infection
Braxton Hicks' contractions	May begin as early as 6–8 weeks	
Fetal outline	After 6th month	Uterine tumors
Ballottement	4th to 5th months	
Pregnancy tests	Reliable by 4 weeks	Endocrine imbalance
Positive signs		
Fetal heart sounds	By Doppler, 10 weeks; by stethoscope, 20–22 weeks	Funic souffle, uterine souffle, maternal pulse, intestinal gas
Fetal movements felt by an examiner	Usually after the 5th month	
Fetal outline by:		
X-ray	Usually 4 months or later	
Sonography	6 weeks or later	

Smoking Habits   Assess and evaluate the woman's smoking habits and counsel her accordingly. The clearest finding of research to date is that smoking mothers are more likely than nonsmoking mothers to have low birth weight babies, particularly if they smoke more than one-half pack per day [19,23]. The risk of spontaneous abortion, of fetal death, and of neonatal death increases directly with increasing levels of maternal smoking during pregnancy [7]. The observation is consistent over national, racial, socioeconomic, and geographic lines. Although the mechanisms by which tobacco decreases birth weight have not been precisely identified, it seems that the most likely explanation is oxygen deprivation caused by carbon monoxide. However, the placentas of these babies are not smaller, indicating an attempt to increase oxygen transport to the fetus. In addition to carbon monoxide, nicotine may contribute to the smaller size of smokers' babies by its vasoconstricting action. Vitamin depletion (B_{12}) due to detoxification of cyanide, a smoke by-

Table 7-5. Unusual Signs to Report During Pregnancy

1. Swelling or puffiness of the face and/or hands and fingers
2. Persistent headaches
3. Blurred vision, double vision, or spots before the eyes
4. Fainting or dizziness
5. Abdominal pain or cramps
6. Persistent vomiting
7. Pain on urination
8. Chills or fever
9. Bleeding or loss of fluid from the vagina
10. Epigastric pain

product, may also contribute to lower weights of the infants [25]. A few researchers have suggested that cigarette smoking depresses a woman's appetite during pregnancy and that decreased caloric intake accounts for lesser fetal growth, an opinion mirrored in the popular notion that a pregnant woman can compensate for the effect of smoking by eating more. Other research contradicts the nutrition hypothesis [27].

*Caffeine Consumption

Assess and evaluate the woman's caffeine consumption and counsel her accordingly. Caffeine is the most popular drug in North America and many other parts of the world. The caffeine content of beverages as reported in the literature varies considerably. When the caffeine content of coffee and tea consumed in the home was examined, considerable variation was found [4]. In some instances the caffeine content of tea exceeded that of coffee. Significant amounts of caffeine are also found in cola beverages, the average bar of chocolate, cocoa, and a number of over-the-counter headache and cold medications (Table 7-7).

The teratogenic significance of caffeine has not been confirmed, although some retrospective research has indicated that in women with a high daily intake of caffeine (600 mg or 8–9 cups of coffee) the chances of a poor pregnancy outcome are high [5,9,13,29,31,32,33]. Caffeine apparently is not metabolized by the fetus in utero. Alcohol and caffeine both possess the ability to affect fetal levels of cyclic AMP and potentially alter the course of fetal development. Until the evidence is more conclusive, pregnant women should be counseled that it would be wise to avoid caffeine during pregnancy [5].

Activities

Assess the woman's activities including her exercise, rest, sleep, sexual activity, employment, and plans for travel.

EXERCISE, REST, AND SLEEP
A woman's prepregnancy exercise pattern forms the basis for her level of activity during pregnancy. In general, it is not necessary to limit exercise, provided the woman does not become excessively fatigued. However, she should remember that it will take her longer to become rested following exercise and that her balance and coordination may be impaired. For these reasons, if a woman is not used to exercising or active sports, now is not the time for her to begin. A woman who is an enthusiastic jogger may be reluctant to give up running during pregnancy. If her health is good, there does not seem to be any compelling reason for her to limit this form of exercise. There is some evidence that maternal physical fitness during pregnancy is positively correlated with higher maternal and fetal pH at the time of delivery; this may result from a more efficient

*Table 7-6. Maternal Drug
Ingestion and Fetal Effect*

Maternal Drug	Effect(s) Seen in Fetus and/or Newborns
Analgesics	
Narcotics (especially if abused)	Decreased responsiveness of neonate (fetal level = 70% of maternal level), death (4–10% mortality), apnea, depression, bradycardia, hypothermia, withdrawal symptoms, feeding problems, decreased incidence of hyaline membrane disease (heroin), enhanced glucuronyl transferase activity
Salicylates (excessive)	Fetal death, hemorrhage, decreased albumin binding capacity (increased bilirubinemia), platelet dysfunction, prolonged gestation (prostaglandin inhibition)
Acetaminophen (excessive)	Nephrotoxic effect
Anesthetics	
General	Apnea, depression (ether has direct narcotic effect on infant)
Conduction or local	Indirect effect of maternal hypotension; direct effects: acidosis, bradycardia, neurologic depression, decreased muscle tone
Anti-infectives	
Ampicillin	Decreased maternal urinary and plasma estriol levels, interfering with monitoring of fetal well-being
Chloramphenicol	May be dangerous to neonate if mother takes drug late in pregnancy; neonatal enzyme too immature to metabolize and eliminate drug
Quinine, quinidine	Possible ototoxicity, thrombocytopenia, congenital anomalies of central nervous system
Streptomycin	Nerve deafness if mother treated for prolonged period
Sulfonamides	Icterus (competes with bilirubin for albumin-binding sites), hemolytic anemia (should not be prescribed in last trimester of pregnancy)
Tetracycline	Placental transfer after 4 months' gestation, inhibition of bone growth, discolored deciduous teeth, defective enamel development after 4th month of pregnancy
Isoniazid	No reported fetal effect; mother should be on pyridoxine supplement to prevent pyridoxine deficiency in infant
Metronidazole (Flagyl)	Not recommended during first trimester
Anticoagulants	
Dicumarol	Death in utero, hemorrhage, coanal atresia, ocular malformations, mental retardation (contraindicated throughout pregnancy)
Heparin	No neonatal effect; high molecular weight does not permit it to cross placenta
Anticonvulsants	
Phenytoin and barbiturate	Congenital malformations, cleft lip and palate, hernias, congenital heart disease, central nervous system, genital, and skeletal anomalies, withdrawal symptoms
Antidiabetic drugs	
Chlorpropamide (Diabinese) Tolbutamide (Orinase)	Respiratory distress and neonatal hypoglycemia; teratogenic effects suggested but never proved
Anti-inflammatory drugs	
Indomethacin	May prolong onset of labor (prostaglandin inhibitor); respiratory distress in infant due to pulmonary hypertension
Steroids	
Cortisone	Possible cleft palate
Dexamethasone	May be placental insufficiency
Progestin	Masculinization of female fetus
Diethylstilbestrol	Adenocarcinoma of lower genital tract in female offspring years later; abnormalities of genital tract in males; potential for malignancy not known

Table 7-6 (continued)

Maternal Drug	Effect(s) Seen in Fetus and/or Newborns
Antithyroids	
Propylthiouracil	Fetal goiter, hypothyroidism
Potassium iodide (compound commonly found in asthmatic medications, expectorants)	Fetal nontoxic goiter
I^{131}	Uptake by fetal thyroid, exophthalmos, arrest of brain development
Ataractics	All tranquilizers may cause changes in postnatal behavior (withdrawal), which may last for months
Librium, Valium	Loss of beat-to-beat variation in fetal heart rate pattern; some evidence of congenital anomalies
Reserpine	Nasal congestion with respiratory distress, lethargy, bradycardia, hypothermia
Thorazine	Chromosomal abnormalities, jaundice
Cancer chemotherapeutic agents	
A-methopterin (Methotrexate)	Contraindicated. Fetal death, multiple malformations
Aminopterin	
Cytoxan	
Cardiovascular drugs	
Propranolol (Inderal)	Hypoglycemia and postnatal bradycardia, decreased platelets, respiratory depression
Cigarette smoking	Effect equal to number of cigarettes smoked
Over one pack/day	Increased incidence of stillbirths, mortality
Under one pack/day	Decreased birth weight by 400 gm, decreased length, cardiac anomalies, decreased fetal breathing
Diuretics	
Ammonium chloride, chlorothiazide, thiazide	Maternal and fetal acidosis, thrombocytopenia, hemorrhage, respiratory distress
Sedatives	
Alcohol	Infant blood level = maternal level; convulsions, withdrawal syndome, fetal alcohol syndrome
Barbiturates	Withdrawal symptoms early or late, lasting 4–6 months; possible congenital anomalies
Bromides	Growth failure, lethargy, feeding difficulty, high-pitched cry
Magnesium sulfate	Respiratory depression, hypotonia
Toxins	
Carbon monoxide (air pollution, smoking)	Stillbirth, fetal brain damage
Lead, mercury	Abortion, growth retardation, congenital anomalies, cerebral palsy
Naphthalene	Hemolysis, jaundice
Polychlorinated biphenyls (PCBs) (environmental contaminant)	May cause dark brown staining of skin and mucous membranes; growth retardation
Vaccines	In general, pregnant patients should not receive vaccines containing live viruses
BCG	Attenuated bacteria. Contraindicated
Cholera	Inactivated bacteria. Only to meet travel requirements
DPT toxoid	No effect
Influenza	May be recommended to prevent influenza
Measles	Live virus. Contraindicated
Mumps	Live virus. Contraindicated
Polio	Not routinely indicated but not contraindicated when protection necessary. Sabin vaccine–live virus. Salk vaccine–inactivated virus.
Rabies	Killed virus. Not contraindicated. Each case considered individually
Rubella	Live virus. Contraindicated. Isolated in fetus when mother immunized 7 weeks before conception
Smallpox	Live virus. Contraindicated

Table 7-6 (continued)

Maternal Drug	Effect(s) Seen in Fetus and/or Newborns
Typhoid	Inactivated bacteria. Not recommended; only with continued exposure
Yellow fever	Live attenuated virus. Contraindicated
	If necessary defer as long as possible
Vitamins	
K	Icterus, hemolysis, anemia
Other	
LSD	Possible chromosomal damage, limb and skeletal anomalies
Methadone	Found in amniotic fluid by 16th week; no chromosomal abnormalities but some rearrangement may occur; withdrawal symptoms

Sources: From R. Hill and L. Halbouty. *Perinatal Pharmacology: Maternal Drug Ingestion and Fetal Effect*. Evansville, Ind.: Mead Johnson & Company, 1979; M. Klaus and A. Farnaroff. *Care of the High-risk Neonate* (2nd ed.). Philadelphia: Saunders, 1979; and T. O'Brien and C. McManus. Drugs and the fetus: A consumers' guide by generic and brand name. *Birth and the Family Journal* 5:58, 1978.

oxygenation system with greater elimination of CO_2 [34, 35]. It has been reported that several women, even in the last trimester of pregnancy, have run in marathons without apparent fetal or maternal ill effects [20]. In general, however, it appears that in pregnancy endurance during exercise may be decreased. Activities or sports that have a risk of bodily injury (such as skiing and snowmobiling) should be considered very carefully with each woman, in terms of her individual history and the length of her pregnancy.

An adequate amount of rest is very important, especially during the last 6 weeks. Sometimes several short periods of rest are more convenient than longer ones; take each woman's daily activities into consideration when making suggestions. Encourage half-hour rest periods in the morning and afternoon. Counsel a woman who works to use her break periods to best advantage by sitting with her legs elevated, if possible, and perhaps closing her eyes for a few minutes. Encourage women to sit rather than stand whenever possible.

The sleep center is probably a central site of action for progesterone so that it is common for pregnant women to be listless, tired, and sleepy [8,15]. Counsel pregnant women to try to get at least 8 hours of sleep a night.

The most comfortable relaxation position for some pregnant women is lying on the side with a pillow under the flexed upper knee or with a pillow under the abdomen. If she is on her back, she might be more comfortable with a small pillow under her head and feet, a cushion or pillow under her knees, and a folded towel under her lumbar spine; this tends to lessen the strain on her back (Fig. 7-3).

Resting is sometimes difficult for a mother who has several small children.

Figure 7-3. A comfortable position for relaxing during pregnancy.

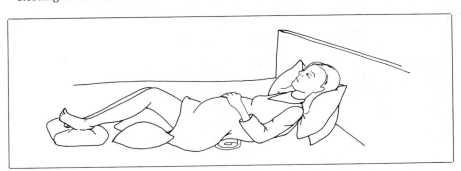

Table 7-7. Caffeine Content of Selected Products

Product	Caffeine Content (mg)
Coffee (5 oz cup)	
Instant, decaffeinated	2
Instant, regular	66
Freeze-dried	66
Percolated	110
Dripolated	146
Soft Drinks (12 oz can)	
Diet Mr. Pibb	52
Mountain Dew	52
Mellow Yello	51
Tab	44
Sunkist Orange	42
Shasta Cola	42
Dr. Pepper	38 (60 mg Bunker)
Diet Dr. Pepper	37
Pepsi Cola	37
Royal Crown Cola	36
Diet Rite Cola	34
Coca Cola	34 (64.7 mg Bunker)
Cragmont Cola	Trace
7-Up	0
Sprite	0
Diet 7-Up	0
RC-100	0
Diet Sunkist Orange	0
Patio Orange	0
Fanta Orange	0
Fresca	0
Hires Root Beer	0

Tea (5 oz cup)

	Brewing Time		
	1 min	3 min	5 min
Bagged Tea			
Black	21–33	35–46	39–50
Green	9–19	20–33	26–36
Oolong	13	30	40
Leaf Tea			
Black	31	38	40
Darjeeling	19	25	28
Green (American)	28	33	35
Japanese green	15	—	20
Iced tea (12 oz can)		22–36	

Product	Caffeine Content (mg)
Cocoa and Chocolate	
Cocoa beverage (water mix, 6 oz)	10
Milk chocolate (1 oz)	6
Sweet or dark chocolate	20
Baking chocolate (1 oz)	35
Chocolate syrup (2 tbsp)	13
Nonprescription Drugs	
Stimulants (standard dose)	
Caffedrine capsules	200
No Doz tablets	200
Vivarin tablets	200
Pain Relievers (standard dose)	
Anacin	64
Excedrin	130

Table 7-7 (continued)

Product	Caffeine Content (mg)
Midol	65
Plain aspirin, any brand	0
Diuretics (standard dose)	
Aqua-Ban	200
Pre-Mens Forte	100
Cold Remedies (standard dose)	
Coryban-D	30
Dristan	32
Coricidin	30
Sinarest	30
Weight-control Aids (daily dose)	
Dexatrim	200
Dietac	200
Spantrol capsule	150
Appedrine tablet	100

Sources: From M. Bunker and M. McWilliams. Caffeine content of common beverages. *Journal of the American Dietetic Association* 74:28, 1979; Caffeine: How to consume less. *Consumer Reports* 597, October 1981; C. Lecos. Caution on caffeine. *FDA Consumer* 6, October 1981; and M. Tull and A. Brown. Effects of caffeine on pregnancy and lactation. *Pediatric Nursing* 6:51, 1981.

Encourage her to coordinate her rest periods with their nap times or to plan for several periods of quiet activity during the day. During this time, she might sit with her feet elevated and read stories to them. They might spend time together in a room where the children can play safely, occupied with toys or television, while the mother rests. Encourage women in a clinic or practitioner's office to help each other by sharing their methods for providing for periods of rest.

SEXUAL ACTIVITY

There is no evidence to indicate that a pregnant woman with no unusual complications should not engage in intercourse or masturbation to orgasm until late in the third trimester or even until the time of labor, depending on the woman's or couple's needs (and assuming that the woman's membranes are intact). Masters and Johnson [18] have detailed some of the physiologic changes that relate to the pregnant woman's response for which she can be prepared. Breast tenderness during advanced sexual tension, which may be severe in the first trimester, tends to decrease in the second and third trimesters. Increased pelvic vascularity and chronic engorgement contribute to high levels of sexual tension in the last half of pregnancy; the woman's sexual drives may become more intense at this time. Vaginal lubrication is greatly increased, and orgasms may be very strong.

Patterns of sexual activity are likely to change throughout pregnancy, due to physical discomfort, loss of interest, fatigue, fear of injury to the baby, or (toward term) difficulty in finding a compatible position. Mutual masturbation or oral-genital techniques may be used more frequently, and alternative positions for intercourse may be attempted. The side-by-side position (either with the couple face to face or with the man facing the woman's back) is less exhausting, avoids deep penetration, and puts less pressure on the woman than other positions do. She may find the female superior position uncomfortable, and this disadvantage may outweigh the advantage of being able to control the depth of penetration. The sitting position often results in deep penetration, which may also be uncomfortable or harmful for the woman.

Whatever position or technique the couple chooses, they should take sensible precautions against excessive abdominal pressure, deep penile penetration, and infection. Vaginal intercourse during pregnancy may be contraindicated if the woman has a history of spontaneous abortion or premature labor, a ripe cervix, ruptured membranes, pain, spotting, or bleeding. Strong uterine contractions occur with orgasmic response, both from intercourse and masturbation; caution couples that orgasm may initiate labor contractions if the woman is within 3 weeks of term. Whether or not premature labor can be attributed to orgasmic response remains controversial [18].

EMPLOYMENT

At least one-third of all women of childbearing age in the United States are now actively employed, for reasons of both self-satisfaction and economics. Generally there is no reason for them to stop working during pregnancy, provided that they have no complications and provided that the nature of their work does not pose a threat to them or their babies. Certain safeguards are recommended: The pregnant woman should avoid severe physical strain; she should have adequate periods of rest; she should use good body mechanics; and she should avoid toxic substances, such as benzene and toluene, carbon monoxide, chlorinated hydrocarbons, lead and its compounds, mercury and its compounds, phosphorus, potent pesticides, x-rays and radioactive substances, and turpentine.

Traveling   Generally travel has no bad effect on pregnancy. During the last trimester, however, the woman should be cautious about traveling long distances from home; if she should go into labor it would be best for her to be delivered by the practitioner who has been caring for her and in whom she has confidence. Airlines may refuse to transport a woman expecting delivery within 7 days unless she has her doctor's certification that she is physically fit for travel. The pregnant woman should not go through x-ray security but should ask for a hand check instead. No matter what form of transportation she uses, she should walk about at least every 2 hours to enhance her circulation.

When driving, the woman should use a seat belt. The lap belt should be worn low so that much of the impact of a collision will be absorbed by the stronger pelvic bones. Whenever possible, the shoulder belt should be used in conjunction with the lap belt, since if the lap belt is used alone, the collision forces could cause the mother's body to jackknife over the belt. In cold weather, pregnant women should be advised not to fasten their safety belts over several layers of clothing, since they might create slippery surfaces under the force of impact and the belt could creep up and cause injury. The American Automobile Association advises pregnant women to warm the car, unbutton outer clothing, and pull the belt snugly over as few layers of clothing as possible.

PSYCHOSOCIAL ASSESSMENT AND EVALUATION   It is important to assess and evaluate any emotional changes the woman may be experiencing, her reactions to the pregnancy, her family support system, ethnic practices that may be influential in her care, and her learning style. Provide the woman with information and suggestions where appropriate based upon your assessment and evaluation.

Emotional Changes   Inadequate sleep and rest may contribute to a woman's susceptibility to mood swings. Furthermore, a physiologic basis for the emotional lability of pregnancy has been hypothesized by a number of researchers. Some reports note that a decrease in vitamin B_6 (pyridoxine) occurs as a result of increased levels of estrogen and progesterone. Adequate supplies of B_6 are necessary in the formation of catecholamines [3].

For some time researchers [24] have postulated a link between affective disorders (depressions and elations) and changes in central nervous system catecholamine metabolism, particularly those leading to a decrease in norepinephrine. Treadway and his colleagues [28] hypothesize that the decrease in norepinephrine levels in pregnancy and in the postpartum period may predispose the mother to affective disorders during these times. Help the woman to understand that these mood swings, which can be very disturbing to her and her family, are a common occurrence during pregnancy and may be relieved by adequate rest and sleep.

Reactions to Pregnancy   When the woman describes her reactions to her pregnancy, listen carefully and try to evaluate the woman in relation to the following questions:

What is the woman's level of maturity and self-esteem?
Does she perceive pregnancy as an illness or state of wellness?
How strong is her need to have a sense of control?
What was her motivation for becoming pregnant?
How does she usually react to stressful situations?
Was the pregnancy planned?
What is the baby's father's reaction to the pregnancy? The family's reaction?
How does she describe the fetus (as an object, a person)?
Preferred sex? Preferred name?
When appropriate, are preparations being made for the baby?
Does she wear maternity clothes (how early)?
What changes in her life situation will this pregnancy initiate?
Will her career plans be interrupted or altered?
What are her perceived physical discomforts?
How will she react to a change in body image?
What are her expectations of pregnancy, delivery, and parenting?
How did her mother view pregnancy and labor?
What has been her past experience in caring for children?
What was the quality of her parents' parenting?

Remember to elicit the answers to these questions over a period of *several visits*.

Family Support System   Assessment of the woman's family support requires the following information:

What is her marital status?
Who lives with her?
Who are her most significant others?
Who are the members of her immediate family?

What are the relationships within the family that will provide support or conflict during the pregnancy?

Is the family aware of what she considers to be important about this pregnancy?

What is her perception of the major effect of the pregnancy on her family?

What is the predominant family style (autocratic, democratic)?

Will there be changes in economic status relative to the family's life style because of the pregnancy?

Will family members be able to support her economically and emotionally?

Is there someone who can help with the work at home?

Is there someone nearby with whom she can talk?

How is the baby's father coping with the pregnancy?

Who is answering his questions and giving him support?

Is he involved in planning for the new family member?

Ethnic Background   It is important to have an understanding of ethnic practices specific to childbearing and of the pregnancy complications specific to ethnic groups (e.g., sickle cell anemia for blacks, Tay-Sachs disease for Jews). Also, the woman may have cultural values that are different from your own. Consider whether they will influence your ability to provide care (Table 7-8).

Learning Style   As you work with the woman over the next few months, you will want to evaluate many of the following points:

How does she learn best? With written material, audiovisual material, discussion, demonstration and return?

Can she read and comprehend the material commonly distributed to pregnant women?

Is she comfortable asking questions?

Is she likely to believe everything she hears?

Is she skeptical or resistant to information shared?

Is it difficult for her to ask for help?

What does she do when her progress is unsatisfactory?

Once she understands something, to what extent does she apply it to her situation?

Does she usually follow directions as given or does she modify them?

Is she reluctant to change old habits?

Remember to complete this information over a number of visits. Do not try to obtain it all or even most of it during a single visit.

PREGNANCY TESTING   Following the health history you may want to have the woman change her clothing and void before the physical examination. She will be more comfortable during the examination when her bladder is empty and you may test the voided specimen for glucose, acetone, and protein. You may also use this time, while the woman changes her clothes, to perform a pregnancy test.

Pregnancy is most often tested for by seeking evidence of the presence of human chorionic gonadotropin (HCG) in the woman's urine. In the past, many of these tests required the sacrificing of laboratory animals, and results were not

Table 7-8. Cultural
Practices During
Pregnancy

American Indian	Pregnancy is considered a normal event. Tribal practices differ. Many prenatal women visit clinics and the medicine man for his blessings and help
Crow	Pregnant woman avoids looking at anything deformed to prevent it from occurring in the child
Pueblo	Pregnant woman is encouraged to be happy and to speak only of things that will bring joy to the baby. She walks slowly while pregnant and does not use sewing needles which might have an unkind effect on the infant
Navajo	Pregnant woman concentrates on good thoughts and is cheerful. Mental stimulation is minimized. The woman is supposed to avoid exposure to illness and death and tying or braiding rope. The latter is believed to cause difficult labor. Pregnant woman is supposed to limit salt and fat intake and drink much goat's milk. Raisins are avoided since they are believed to result in brown skin spots on mother and infant
	In general during pregnancy many tribes believe that the woman should refrain from stepping over a gun, a snake's tail, or a deep ravine, and from tying knots and using sharp instruments such as knives, needles, and nails
Mexican-American	Pregnant women are to avoid cool air in motion. Moonlight is to be avoided; a moon in eclipse is perilous. *Antojos* or cravings must be satisfied or the fetus will be marked. Milk is often avoided since it may make the baby large and difficult to deliver. Pregnant women are supposed to work and move about so the baby will not grow large. Massage treatments monthly are believed to fix the fetus in a favorable position for delivery. Sexual activity is continued through pregnancy to lubricate the birth canal for delivery
Filipino	Pregnancy is viewed as a normal, happy time. Diet should be rich in vitamins and proteins but cravings are to be satisfied to avoid birthmarks on the infant. Squid is avoided since it may make the baby's cord wrap around his neck; crab may result in clubbed fingers; dark foods such as prunes will result in a dark skinned infant
Indochinese	Pregnancy is viewed as a normal life event. The taking of blood (for tests) weakens the body. Tonics and medicines (even vitamins) are avoided during pregnancy since they may make the baby large and difficult to deliver. A preference for sweet foods means the baby will be male; a sour food preference will yield a female child. The woman is supposed to avoid unclean foods such as dog, mouse, rat, and snake so the child will be born intelligent. She is supposed to avoid carrying heavy loads, reaching for high places, and attending weddings and funerals. The latter will result in unconsolable crying in the newborn. She is also supposed to avoid the spirits that are found in places of worship and on the streets at noon and at 5 o'clock

Sources: From A. Clark. *Culture Childbearing Health Professionals*. Philadelphia: Davis, 1978; A. Hollingsworth, L. Brown, and D. Brooten. The refugees and childbearing: What to expect. *RN* 43:44, 1980; P. Stern. Solving problems of cross-cultural health teaching: The Filipino childbearing family. *Image* 13:47, 1981; and L. Todd. Indochinese refugees bring rich heritages to childbearing. *International Childbirth Education Association News* 21:2, 1982.

available for several days and sometimes up to a week or more. Currently these methods have been replaced by the use of immunologic tests using either red blood cells or latex particles coated with HCG, which agglutinate when exposed to antiserum containing antibodies against HCG. When the antiserum is mixed with a pregnant woman's urine, the HCG in her urine and the antibodies in the antiserum are bound together. The subsequent addition of red blood cells or latex particles results in no agglutination; they precipitate out, yielding a positive pregnancy test (Fig. 7-4). If the woman is not pregnant, the antibodies against HCG remain unbound and are agglutinated when red blood cells or latex particles are added.

The method using red blood cells takes approximately 2 hours and has been reported to be 98 percent accurate, while the method using latex particles takes about 2 minutes and its accuracy is reported to be about 92 percent [14]. The more sensitive immunologic tests can detect pregnancy from as early as 6 to 8 days after conception [22] to 3 to 4 days after the first missed period [10], but they may yield false positive results because the same reaction may occur with urinary follicle-stimulating hormone (FSH), luteinizing hormone (LH), or both. Thus, the tests will give the same results with LH during ovulation and with the high levels of FSH during menopause.

False negative reactions may occur early in pregnancy (first 20 days after the first missed menstrual period) with the less sensitive tests or with dilute urine specimens. For this reason, women are asked to bring the first voided morning urine to be tested, since HCG levels should be high. Specimens allowed to stand 8 hours or longer at room temperature may lose HCG activity and also produce false negative reactions. While few false negatives are seen after 14 days following the first missed menstrual period, the less sensitive tests may yield negative reactions during the second and third trimesters when HCG levels are low [10,22].

The use of these pregnancy tests provides just one indication of pregnancy; a positive result from such a test is a probable but not positive sign of pregnancy. Other signs and symptoms indicative of pregnancy are elicited during the history and physical examination (see Table 7-4).

PHYSICAL ASSESSMENT

The physical assessment described below is not a comprehensive approach but rather one that combines a general assessment applicable to all women with an emphasis on the major physical changes that may be found in women due to pregnancy. This approach is necessary since the initial physical findings will vary depending upon when the woman seeks care. The assessment may be performed very early in pregnancy before many bodily changes have occurred, or it may take place later when changes due to pregnancy are well underway.

Initial physical evaluation of a pregnant woman is comprehensive. This initial

Figure 7-4. Positive pregnancy test shows no agglutination. Negative reaction shows agglutination, which appears as solid dots.

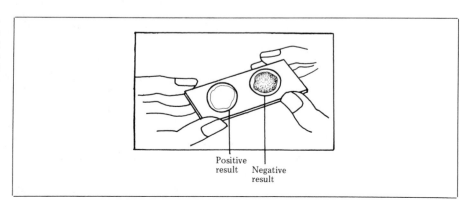

Positive result   Negative result

examination begins with a general assessment of the woman's body build, weight, apparent age, posture and body movements, personal hygiene, mental status, and vital signs. This general assessment is followed by a comprehensive examination of her body systems and evaluation of changes due to pregnancy; physical examinations performed during her return visits are focused primarily on the latter (Table 7-9).

Table 7-9. Physical Assessment on Return Antenatal Visits

Assessment	Significant Findings
Vital signs	
Blood pressure	Elevation of 15 mm Hg or above diastolic may signify a hypertensive disorder of pregnancy; seek physician consultation
Temperature	Elevations above 99.6°F (37.6°C) may indicate infection, possibly respiratory or urinary tract; question the woman about signs and symptoms of infection and evaluate further; seek physician consultation
Pulse	Elevations above 90 bpm may indicate anxiety or cardiac or other disorders; evaluate and consult with physician as appropriate
Respirations	More than 24 respirations per minute may indicate cardiac, respiratory, or other disorders; evaluate and consult with physician as appropriate
Weight gain	Usual weight gain is 2–4 lb in first trimester, and approximately 11 lb in both the second and third trimester for a total weight gain of 24–28 lb. Usual weight gain per week during the second and third trimesters is 0.5–1.0 lb. Weight gain of 2 lb or more per week may indicate hypertensive disorders of pregnancy; consult physician
Edema	After the 8th month of pregnancy, dependent edema of the ankles and feet is common. Edema of the face, hands, and fingers may indicate a hypertensive disorder of pregnancy; consult physician
Urinalysis	Significant amounts of protein may indicate renal disorder or a hypertensive disorder of pregnancy; significant amounts of glucose may indicate diabetes mellitus; consult physician

Uterine size	Using McDonald's rule
	Height of fundus (in cm) $\times$ 2/7 (or $\div$ 3.5)
	    = Duration of pregnancy in lunar months
	Height of fundus (in cm) $\times$ 8/7
	    = Duration of pregnancy in weeks
	Usually the fundus is found halfway between the symphysis and umbilicus at 16 weeks; just below the umbilicus at 20 weeks; at xiphoid at 36 weeks. Uterine height ahead of that expected may indicate miscalculation of EDC, multiple gestation, or hydatidiform mole; below that expected may indicate miscalculation of EDC, growth-retarded fetus; consult physician if findings appear deviant

Fetal heart rate	Normal fetal heart rate is between 120 and 160 bpm and audible with a fetoscope after about 20 weeks' gestation; inability to hear fetal heart tone after this time with fetoscope or amplifier (Doppler) may be due to maternal obesity, polyhydramnios, miscalculated EDC, or fetal demise; consult physician where appropriate
Sleeping and eating patterns	The woman needs about 8 hours of sleep a night plus periodic rest periods during the day; inability to sleep may be due to excessive fatigue during the day, anxiety regarding

Table 7-9 (continued)

Assessment	Significant Findings
	employment or financial matters, or an uncomfortable position at night; nausea and vomiting usually subside after the first trimester and the woman is able to consume a nutritious diet; nausea and vomiting after the first trimester may indicate hyperemesis gravidarum; irregular non-nutritious meals may reflect prepregnant eating habits, cultural practices for pregnancy, a hurried lifestyle, or economic problems; evaluate and plan accordingly, using other members of the health team as appropriate
Common discomforts of pregnancy	The woman may experience fatigue, heartburn, hemorrhoids, backache; evaluate and counsel accordingly
Unusual reportable signs	Signs of hypertensive disorder: facial, hand, or finger edema, persistent headache, blurred or double vision, fainting, epigastic pain Signs of infection: chills, fever, pain on urination Signs of possible abortion or labor: abdominal pain or cramps, bleeding or fluid loss from vagina

General Assessment and Evaluation

The inspection of a woman's general state of health and outstanding characteristics begins with observations made during introductions, as the woman moves about the examining room, and as she follows instructions prior to and during the interview or health history. Often the initial impression provides direction for pursuing selected parts of the interview and physical examination in particular depth; for example, very short stature and obesity in a pregnant woman indicate a particular need to evaluate nutritional status and eating patterns, blood pressure, and adequacy of pelvic dimensions, and perhaps to ask about hemorrhoidal difficulties and the height of the fetus's father.

The survey generally proceeds in a cephalocaudal direction. Observe the woman's face for symmetry, contour, facial tics, and facial expression. Facial edema in a pregnant woman may indicate hypertension, particularly during the last trimester. Facial expression may reflect adaptation to the pregnancy as well as anxiety level [17].

Evaluate the woman's overall body build, amount of muscle mass, adipose tissue, height, and weight for clues to the woman's nutritional status, eating habits, and bony pelvic structure as well as for clues to metabolic or genetic disorders.

There is often a great deal of difference in the apparent age of women of the same chronologic age. As individuals grow older, the skin loses turgor, appears dull, moves less readily, sags, and wrinkles. While these changes usually occur in middle age and are first observable in the anterior neck and chin, they may also be seen in women who have experienced rapid weight loss. During pregnancy, women who experience hypertensive disorders of pregnancy may develop facial edema giving them the appearance of being much older than their stated age.

Evaluate the woman's posture and body movements for clues to her sense of balance, muscular coordination, mobility of joints, and self-image. Abnormal posture may result from pathology of the muscles, bones, joints, or neurologic system. Poor posture maintained over a long period of time may result in painful joints, ligaments, and muscles, especially during pregnancy when the woman's center of gravity is altered by her growing uterus. Improved posture, proper shoes, and certain exercises will prevent or relieve ligament and muscle pain. Continue the assessment by observing body movements for lack of coordination and tremor occurring at rest or stimulated by voluntary movement.

A woman's personal hygiene is an important indication of her self-esteem as well as of the availability of facilities and supplies to maintain good body care. The woman's nails may reflect the level of concern and care she has for her appearance, as may her manner of dress. The general cleanliness and press of clothing may provide clues to cultural and socioeconomic status and to the ego strength of the woman. Note the odor of her body and breath; the smell of alcohol or the fruity odor of acetone (diabetic acidosis) is indicative of conditions often incompatible with a favorable fetal outcome.

The woman's manner of speech provides clues to her emotional health and mental status. Note characteristics of speech such as pace, clarity, vocabulary, sentence structure, tone, and strength of voice. A focus on the woman's mental status helps to evaluate her problems in living and often the psychodynamics underlying them. Focus on her state of awareness, from alert to dull, her ability to comprehend what she is told, level of education, length of attention span, and level of cooperation from passive acceptance to rigid resistance. Information on the woman's mood, described in terms of behaviors she exhibits, is helpful.

The general inspection made during introductions and interview provides an overall impression of the woman's general state of health and outstanding characteristics. Having formed an initial impression, now proceed to a physical examination of the woman following up on clues provided by the initial survey. At the beginning of the physical examination measure the woman's height and weight, and obtain her vital signs.

Physical Examination   HEAD

Assessment and Evaluation.   Examination of the woman's head includes assessment of the size and shape of the skull and the condition of her scalp and hair. A large head may result from osteitis deformans in which body thickness increases or from excessive growth hormone secretion (acromegaly) in which the skull becomes enlarged and the facial features appear coarsened. Local deformities of the skull often result from trauma or surgery.

Inspect her scalp by parting her hair in several areas and assessing it for dandruff, parasites, and sebaceous cysts. The latter result from occlusion of sebaceous gland ducts and are palpable as smooth, rounded nodules attached to the scalp. Assess hair for texture, thickness, and pattern of distribution. Texture may reflect thyroid metabolism: The hair is coarse, dry, and brittle in hypothyroidism; fine, soft, and silky in hyperthyroidism [17]. Thinning or loss of hair accompanies stress and the taking of some drugs, and occurs hereditarily and in some disorders such as myxedema or malnutrition. The stress of pregnancy may cause thinning or loss of hair.

FACE

Assessment and Evaluation.   Examine the woman's face by observing her facial expression, the color and condition of her facial skin, and the shape and symmetry of her facial structures, including her eyebrows, eyes, nose, mouth, and ears. Normally the palpebral fissures (the distance between the eyelids) are equal, as are the nasolabial folds (the creases extending from the angle of the nose to the corner of the mouth). Within the range of normal, however, are many women with slightly asymmetrical expression. The muscles of facial expression are supplied by the seventh cranial nerve, the facial nerve. Test facial muscle function by asking the woman to elevate her eyebrows, frown, lower her eyebrows, close her eyes tightly, puff her cheeks, and smile. Asymmetry or abnormal movements or both may result from facial nerve disorders such as Bell's palsy. The major accessible artery on the face, the temporal artery, which passes anterior to the ear over the temporal muscle and into the forehead, should be palpated to assess any thickening, hardness, or tenderness.

Changes in facial shape can result from numerous situations, including thyroid disorders, adrenal dysfunction, prolonged illness and edema caused by cardiovascular or kidney disease, or hypertensive disorders of pregnancy. Hyperthyroidism may be associated with protrusion of the eyeballs (exophthalmos) and elevation of the upper lids, giving the woman an excited, startled, or staring expression. Hypothyroidism may be manifested by a dull and puffy face with a sleepy expression, dry skin, and coarse features. Increased adrenal hormone production may result in a round face ("moon face") with red cheeks and excessive facial hair. Edema of the face is often initially evident in the eyelids.

Note facial coloring and changes in coloring in areas such as the lips, nose, cheeks, ears, and oral mucosa. Cyanosis or bluish coloration may result from cardiac or pulmonary disease; pallor may indicate anemia. Pallor is particularly prominent in the face. Jaundice may be evident in the skin, sclera, mucous membranes of the mouth under the tongue, and on the palate. Changes in skin pigmentation may be due to changes in melanin production and deposition. During pregnancy a woman's forehead and cheeks may become more darkly pigmented resulting in chloasma, or the "butterfly mask" of pregnancy. This effect, which may be exaggerated by exposure to the sun, disappears or regresses after delivery.

EYES

Assessment and Evaluation.   Examination of the woman's eyes involves evaluation of visual acuity, ocular motility, ocular structures, and estimation of intraocular tension. While you will not perform a complete eye examination, you may want to test the woman's visual acuity and examine several structures of the eye. Assessing visual acuity is a simple test of ocular function. Findings in the normal range of visual acuity give an indication of the clarity of the transparent media (cornea, anterior body, lens, and vitreous body), the adequacy of macular, or central, vision, and the functioning of the nerve fibers from the macula to the occipital cortex. Traditionally, Snellen's chart, with various sizes of letters or with the letter E facing various ways, is used for this purpose.

Inspect the woman's eyelids for their ability to close completely, for position and color, and for any lesions, infection, or edema. When the lids do not close properly, drying of the cornea may result in serious damage.

Examine her conjunctivae by separating the eyelids and holding them against the ridges of the bony orbit surrounding the eye. Next, have the woman look up and down and to each side. Many small blood vessels are normally visible through the clear conjunctivae. The sclera is normally white, although some pigmented deposits are within the range of normal. Some darkly pigmented women may have a yellow coloring to their sclerae.

Examine the woman's pupils for size, shape, reaction to light, and accommodation. The pupils are normally round in shape and equal in size. The pupillary response to light consists of both a direct and a consensual reaction. The beam of a penlight is brought in from the side and directed on one eye at a time. The eye toward which the light is directed is observed for the direct response of constriction; simultaneously, the other eye is observed for a consensual response of constriction.

Evaluate pupillary accommodation by observing the change in pupillary size as the woman's gaze is switched from a distant to a near object. (Visualization of a distant object normally causes pupillary dilation.) Next, ask the woman to fix her gaze on your index finger, which is placed 5 to 6 inches from her nose. The normal response is pupillary constriction and convergence of the eyes. Record the evaluation of the pupils by using the notation PERRLA, which stands for pupils equal, round, react to light, and accommodate.

With an ophthalmoscope, examine the optic disc for size, shape, color, the distinctness of its margins, and the physiologic cup. The retinal vessels are examined for color and the ratio in size of arterioles to veins; arteriovenous crossings are examined for their light reflex. The retinal background is examined for color and regularity of appearance and for any areas of light or dark color alterations. Changes in caliber and alterations of the vessels can occur in areas of crossing. Changes in these vascular structures are often indicative of systemic diseases such as hypertension. Because caliber changes may or may not be evenly distributed along the course of the vessel, vessels should be observed from the disc to the periphery. Arterioles, normally about two-thirds to three-fourths of the diameter of the corresponding veins, are subject to a decrease in diameter as a result of constriction of the vessels or reduced blood flow to the eye; in hypertension, the arteriole-vein ratio may be 3:5, 2:4, or less [17].

Changes at arteriovenous crossings include an apparent narrowing or blocking of the vein where an arteriole crosses over it. This appearance is the result of some degree of concealment of the underlying veins by an abnormally opaque arteriole wall and occurs with longstanding hypertension; it is initially apparent as venous narrowing and later as a more complete interruption of the vessel. These changes are referred to as arteriovenous nicking. Emboli in a retinal vessel cause abrupt narrowing of arterioles and abrupt dilatation of a vein as it impedes return flow. Women with vascular changes indicative of hypertension are at risk during pregnancy for premature delivery, premature separation of the placenta, growth-retarded infants, and other complications.

EARS, NOSE, AND THROAT

Assessment, Evaluation, and Intervention.   Examination of the woman's ears, nose, and throat is an important part of every physical examination because it provides the opportunity to inspect directly or indirectly most parts of her upper respiratory system and the first portion of her digestive system. Examine the woman's external ear by inspecting both auricles for position, size, and symmetry. Examine the lateral and medial surfaces of each auricle and surrounding tissues to determine skin color and presence of deformities, lesions, or nodules. Palpate the auricles and mastoid areas for evidence of swelling, tenderness, or nodules. Occasionally, women have unusual yet quite normal auricles as a result of heredity; this should be noted on the woman's chart since the same auricles found in her newborn may otherwise be interpreted as outward signs of congenital defects by health care personnel.

Inspect the auditory canal for cerumen, redness, or swelling. Bulging of the tympanic membrane may occur when pus forms in the middle ear. Retraction of the membrane occurs when pressure is reduced due to obstruction of the eustachian tube, a condition usually associated with upper respiratory system infection. During pregnancy increased blood flow in the tympanic membranes and blockage of the eustachian tubes may cause the woman to experience a sense of fullness in her ears, decreased hearing, or earaches [14]. Explain these changes to her if she experiences them.

Inspect the external portion of the nose for deviations in size or color; the nares are inspected for flaring or discharge. The ridge and soft tissues of the nose are palpated for displacement of bone or cartilage and for tenderness or masses. The examination can also be carried out by pushing the tip of the woman's nose upward while shining a light into her naris.

Inspect the nasal septum for deviation, exudate, and perforation. The septum is seldom straight. Examine the lateral walls of the nasal cavities and the inferior and middle turbinates for polyps, swelling, exudate, and color changes. Nasal mucosa is usually redder than oral mucosa. Increased redness indicates infection while pale, boggy turbinates are typical of allergy. Drainage from the middle meatus, which drains several of the paranasal sinuses, is important and should be described and recorded. As a result of increased blood flow and peripheral vasodilatation during pregnancy, the woman may experience nasal congestion and nosebleeds, especially during the last trimester. As a result of this congestion some women may snore during sleep when they are pregnant and may experience voice changes due to capillary enlargement which affects the larynx and vocal cords. Explain these changes to her if she experiences them.

Examination of the woman's mouth proceeds from the anterior to the posterior areas and begins with the external components of the mouth and jaw. Inspect the woman's lips for symmetry, color, edema, or surface abnormalities. Ask her to open and close her mouth to demonstrate the mobility of her mandible and occlusion of her teeth. Examine her oral mucosal surfaces.

During pregnancy, increased progesterone production may cause the woman's gums to become hyperemic and softened. Mouth secretions may become acidic, and many women mention an increase in salivation. Occasionally, a vascular swelling of the gums known as an epulis of pregnancy may develop; it regresses after delivery. Because of these changes and the incidence of nausea and vomiting in early pregnancy, good oral hygiene is essential. If her gums bleed, suggest that brushing be done with a softer toothbrush and a mild toothpaste; an alkaline mouthwash may also be used.

Examine the woman's tongue by inspecting the dorsum for any swelling, variation in size or color, coating, or ulcerations. While an examination of the woman's teeth and gums is not a substitute for a dental examination, it will reveal gross problems such as caries, missing teeth, and malocclusions. Contrary to the popular notion that each pregnancy costs a tooth, there is no demineralization of teeth during pregnancy. What seems like an increased incidence of dental caries during pregnancy may actually be the discovery of preexisting conditions as a result of more thorough health examinations. However, the acid content of the mouth, a change in eating habits, and the increased blood supply to the teeth may contribute to tooth decay during pregnancy. Dental work is not contraindicated; however, if dental x-rays are necessary, they should be postponed until the latter half of pregnancy. In addition, a lead apron should be used to protect the woman's abdomen.

Following the examination of the woman's teeth and gums, inspect her palate and uvula; use a tongue depressor if necessary. Next, inspect the woman's oropharynx while her head is back and the base of her tongue is gently depressed with a tongue depressor. Inspect the anterior palatine arches and the posterior arches for inflammation or swelling. The size of her tonsils should be estimated, and any exudate noted. Examine the posterior wall of her oropharynx for any change in color.

NECK

Assessment and Evaluation. Examine the woman's neck by assessing her neck muscles and cervical vertebrae, her trachea, her thyroid gland, her carotid arteries, her jugular veins, and her cervical lymph nodes. Inspect her neck muscles for symmetry of the musculature and for any abnormal masses or inflammations. Assess the function of her neck muscles by evaluating the normal centered position and the range of motion of her head and by testing her muscle strength against the resistance of your hands.

Common abnormalities of the neck muscles include stiffness and pain. Some degree of muscle spasm may occur in tense individuals and tenderness on palpation may be found over the affected muscles. Stiffness of the neck may also result from vertebral disease or meningitis.

Examine her thyroid gland by observation and palpation. Since the effects of thyroid activity are widespread and may adversely affect fertility, observations of the woman's behavior, appearance, skin, eyes, hair, and cardiovascular status are important in evaluating the gland's level of activity.

In examining the thyroid, observe the lower half of her neck first in normal position, next in slight extension, and then while the woman swallows a sip of water. Movements of the cartilages are easily noted. Normally no unusual bulging of thyroid tissue in the midline of the lobes or behind the sternocleidomastoid muscle is observed. Gross enlargement (goiter) may be seen on inspection.

Next, palpate the woman's neck for the presence of an enlarged thyroid, for consistency of the gland, and for any nodules. The normal thyroid gland is not palpable; however, in very thin persons the isthmus is occasionally palpable. Palpation may be accomplished by either standing in front of or behind the woman. Although examination techniques vary, the principles of examining movement of the gland during swallowing, adequate exposure of the gland by relaxation and manual displacement of surrounding structures, and comparison of one side of the gland with the other remain the same. Since the thyroid gland is fixed to the trachea, it ascends during swallowing and is thus distinguished from other neck masses.

One satisfactory technique is to press gently on one side of the gland, displacing the larynx and trachea laterally. The opposite side is then exposed and palpated lightly. Next, keeping the fingers lightly in place, ask the woman to swallow; this motion will move the gland past the fingertips and will identify nodules if present.

Normal lymph nodes are not visible or palpable. Cervical nodes lie grouped in four major areas which should be examined: under the jaw, in the anterior triangle of the neck, in the posterior triangle, and above and below the clavicles. If palpable, lymph nodes should be described carefully.

SKIN

Assessment and Evaluation.   Begin the examination of the woman's skin with an observation of the skin that is exposed, followed by an inspection of the skin, mucous membranes, and epidermal appendage of each body part. Inspect the skin for color and vascularity and for evidence of perspiration, edema, injuries, or lesions. Note changes that are indicative of past injuries and habits, such as calluses, stains, scars, needle marks, and insect bites. Note the grooming of the woman's hair and nails.

Skin color varies from person to person and from one part of the body to another. The vascular flush areas include the cheeks, the bridge of the nose, the neck, the upper chest, the flexor surfaces of the extremities, and the genital area. Increased color in these areas may be caused by vascular disturbance, blushing, or an elevated temperature; they should be compared with areas of less vascularity. The areas that readily show pigmentary changes are the face, the backs of the hands, the flexors of the wrists, the axillae, the mammary areolae, the midline of the abdomen, and the genital area.

Other changes in skin color may indicate systemic disorders. Cyanosis, a dusky blue color, may be observed in the nailbeds or in the lips and mouth area, indicating decreased tissue oxygenation. When tissue bilirubin is increased, the tissues appear yellow; this may be observed first in the sclerae and then in the mucous membranes and skin. Pallor is most noticeable in the woman's face, conjunctiva, mouth, and nails. Generalized redness of the skin may be indicative of fever, while defined areas of redness may be the result of a localized infection or sunburn. Other localized changes in skin color may indicate a problem such as edema, which tends to blanch skin color. Changes in the normal pattern of pigmentation result from changes in the distribution of melanin or in the function of the melanocytes in the epidermis. Color changes in the skin of dark-skinned women can be observed in the sclerae, conjunctivae, buccal mucosa, tongue, lips, nailbeds, palms, and soles [17].

Describe any skin lesions in terms of location and distribution, configuration, and morphologic structure. Obtain a history of any eruption—i.e., how long it has been present, whether it itches, whether it appeared abruptly or seemed to start in a specific area and spread, and whether the lesions are primary or secondary. Primary lesions are those that appear initially in response to some change in the external or internal environment of the skin; secondary lesions result from modifications in the primary lesion.

Changes in Pregnancy. There are several skin changes that occur during pregnancy. From the second trimester there is increased pigmentation of the breast areolae. In addition, a line of increased pigmentation, the *linea nigra*, may appear over the lower abdomen from the umbilicus to the symphysis pubis. The woman's forehead and cheeks may become more darkly pigmented, resulting in chloasma, or the "butterfly mask" of pregnancy. Scars or moles may also darken.

Little is known about the etiology of these pigmentary changes. It is known, however, that the level of melanocyte-stimulating hormone (MSH) is increased from the end of the second month of pregnancy until term. In addition, estrogen and progesterone are reported to have a melanocyte-stimulating effect.

During pregnancy, many Caucasian women (though fewer black women) develop palmar erythema and/or spider angiomas (vascular spiders). These angiomas are dilated precapillary vessels radiating out from a central dilated arteriole, probably as a result of high estrogen concentrations.

In the last trimester, about 50 percent of all pregnant women develop slightly depressed red streaks over the abdomen and sometimes over the breasts (Fig. 7-5). These stretch marks (striae gravidarum) fade and become silvery two or three months after delivery, but the silvery markings persist indefinitely. Several theories have been advanced to explain the cause of striae, ranging from hyperactivity of the adrenal cortex to stretching of the skin with rupture of underlying elastic fibers. Occasionally such stretch marks are seen in women with abdominal distention or increased fat tissue. Although various ointments have been suggested to prevent striae, there is no known effective prevention.

The woman's umbilicus, which usually remains deeply indented during the first trimester, becomes steadily more shallow as pregnancy advances. At term it

Figure 7-5. Woman at term with marked abdominal striae. (From L. M. Hellman and J. R. Pritchard. *Williams Obstetrics* [14th ed.], 1971. Courtesy of Appleton-Century-Crofts, Publishing Division of Prentice-Hall, Inc.)

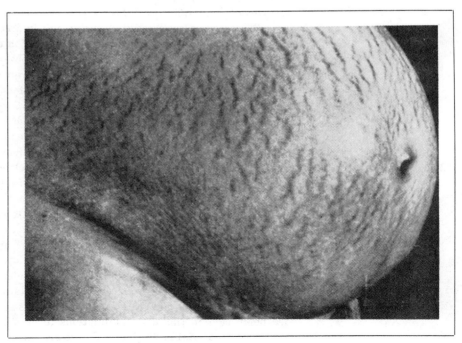

may be level with the surface or protrude somewhat. There is increased vascularity of the skin and muscles of the perineum as well as softening of the connective tissue.

Because perspiration is more profuse during pregnancy and activity of sebaceous glands may increase, advise the woman to bathe daily. In the last 2 months of pregnancy, when keeping her balance becomes more of a problem, the woman may have difficulty getting in and out of a bathtub. It is for this reason, rather than avoidance of vaginal contamination, that tub baths are discouraged at this time, since it is now generally accepted that tub water does not enter the vaginal canal as was once believed.

HAIR AND NAILS

Assessment and Evaluation. Examine the woman's body hair to determine the distribution, quantity, and quality. Deviations from the normal female hair pattern that evolves after puberty may indicate an endocrine problem. Hirsutism (increased body hair) is found in conditions such as Cushing's syndrome and acromegaly, while decreased hair growth or loss of hair may be associated with hypopituitarism or a pyogenic infection. Patchy gray hair may develop following nerve injuries. Dry and coarse hair is found in hypothyroidism, while in hyperthyroidism the hair is silky and fine.

Assess the woman's nails to determine not only their condition but also possible evidence of generalized disorders. Examine her nails for shape, normal dorsal curvature, adhesion to the nail bed, regularity of the nail surface, color, and thickness. Examine the skin folds around the nails for any color changes, swelling, increased temperature, or tenderness.

RESPIRATORY SYSTEM

Assessment, Evaluation, and Intervention. Assessment of the woman's respiratory efficiency is accomplished by direct and indirect appraisal of structures supporting alveolar function. For adequate inspection of the thorax, the woman should be sitting and uncovered to her waist. First observe the general shape and symmetry of her thorax. In adults the anteroposterior diameter of the thorax is less than the transverse diameter. In the normal infant, and in some adults with pulmonary disease, the thorax is almost round.

Normally, men and children breathe diaphragmatically, and women breathe thoracically or costally. If the woman appears to have labored respiration, observe her for the use of the accessory muscles of respiration—the sternocleidomastoid and trapezius muscles—and for supraclavicular retraction. Obstruction in air inflow is often accompanied by retraction of intercostal spaces during inspiration. Obstruction in the outflow of air results in an excessively long expiratory phase of respiration. Resting respiratory rate in adults is 16 to 20 breaths per minute and is regular. The ratio of respiratory rate to pulse rate normally is $1:4$ [17]. Observe the woman's lips and nail beds for color and observe her nails for clubbing.

Palpate the muscle mass and the thoracic skeleton, noting any areas of abnormality. If the woman has no respiratory complaints, a rapid general survey of the anterior, lateral, and posterior thoracic areas should be sufficient.

Use percussion in thoracic examinations to determine the amounts of air, liquid, or solid material in the lung and to determine the positions and boundaries of organs.

Auscultation of the lungs provides information about the functioning of the respiratory system and about the presence of any obstruction in the passages. First, instruct the woman to breathe through her mouth and to breathe more deeply and slowly than usual. Systematically auscultate the apices and the posterior, lateral, and anterior chest, evaluating breath sounds and the sounds produced by the spoken voice and listening for abnormal sounds (Fig. 7-6).

Note any abnormal breath sounds such as rales, rhonchi, or friction rubs. A *rale* is a short, discrete, interrupted, crackling or bubbling sound that is most commonly heard during inspiration. Rales are thought to be produced by air passing through moisture in the bronchi, bronchioles, and alveoli, or by air rushing through passages and alveoli that were closed during expiration and opened abruptly during inspiration. Low-pitched, coarse rales occurring early in inspiration are thought to have their origins in the bronchi, as in bronchitis. Medium-pitched rales in mid-inspiration occur in diseases of small bronchi, as in bronchiectasis. High-pitched, fine rales are found in diseases affecting the bronchioles and alveoli and occur late in inspiration.

Rhonchi are continuous sounds produced by the movement of air through narrowed passages in the tracheobronchial tree. Low-pitched rhonchi, sometimes called sonorous rhonchi and usually heard in early expiration, originate in the larger bronchi; high-pitched, sibilant rhonchi, sometimes called wheezes, originate in small bronchioles and often occur in late expiration.

A pleural *friction rub* is a loud, dry, creaking or grating sound indicative of pleural irritation. It is produced by the rubbing together of inflamed and roughened pleural surfaces during respiration and therefore is heard best during the latter part of inspiration and the beginning of expiration.

Normal vocal resonance is heard as muffled, nondistinct sounds; it is loudest

Figure 7-6. Location of breath sounds. (1) Tracheal sounds; (2) bronchial sounds; (3) bronchovesicular sounds; (4) vesicular sounds. Begin at the upper locations, listening first at one site and then at the corresponding site on the opposite side, using one lung field as a control for the other.

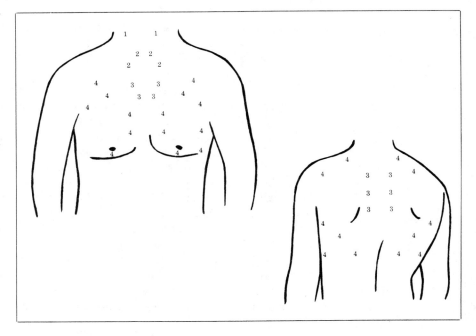

medially and is less intense at the periphery of the lung. Vocal resonance is assessed if there has been any respiratory abnormality detected on observation, palpation, percussion, or auscultation.

Changes in Pregnancy.   During pregnancy, deep respirations, a slight increase in respiratory rate, and sighing may be more prevalent. The woman's PCO_2 is lowered by the increase in progesterone production. It has been reported that the respiratory centers are far more sensitive to stimulation by CO_2 during pregnancy, causing the woman to hyperventilate. She breathes more deeply and has an increased tidal volume and alveolar ventilation. Her hyperventilation causes a respiratory alkalosis, which is compensated for by the kidney through an increase in bicarbonate excretion and a corresponding decrease in plasma sodium concentration. Because of this mechanism, there is little or no change in blood pH.

Later in pregnancy, the woman's enlarged uterus causes elevation of her diaphragm. For the same reason, her lower ribs flare out and may not recover their normal position after pregnancy. The transverse diameter of the rib cage increases, probably due to increased mobility of the rib attachments.

These changes in the respiratory system often interfere with the woman's sleep and comfort. Counsel her in good body mechanics and good erect posture (both standing and sitting) to alleviate discomfort. So she may obtain relief by increasing space within the rib cage, teach her to raise both arms above her head; encourage her to use two or more pillows under her head and shoulders when lying down.

HEART AND BLOOD VOLUME CHANGES

Assessment, Evaluation, and Interventions.   Examination of the woman's heart includes inspection, palpation, and auscultation. Examination of her peripheral pulses, including the radial, brachial, femoral, popliteal, dorsalis pedis, and posterior tibial, is an essential element in evaluation of the woman's cardiovascular system. Assessment of her abdominal aorta and assessment of her blood pressure in the upper and lower extremities in the sitting, standing, and lying positions are also very important.

Inspect the woman's chest wall and epigastrium while she is lying down. Standing to the woman's right side, observe her chest for size and symmetry, pulsations, lifts, heaves, or retractions. The normal apical impulse may be observed as a pulsation in the midclavicular line in the fifth left intercostal space; this impulse is caused by the contracting left ventricle and is seen in approximately 50 percent of normal adults. Since it occurs synchronously with the carotid impulse, simultaneous palpation of a carotid artery will help to identify it. Since the apical impulse helps to identify the location of the cardiac apex, it aids in assessing cardiac size. Slight retraction of the chest wall may normally be found just medial to the midclavicular line in the fifth interspace. A lift or heave may be noted when the work of the right ventricle is greatly increased; it appears as a diffuse lifting impulse along the left sternal border each time the heart beats.

Palpate the entire precordium, beginning at the apex, moving to the left sternal border, and then proceeding to the base of the heart. During palpation look for the apical impulse at or near the apex and for any abnormal heaves, thrills, or retractions elsewhere on the precordium, which may indicate cardiac hypertrophy, dilatation, or murmurs. The abnormal flow of blood resulting in an audible murmur may also result in a palpatory sensation known as a thrill.

To locate the apical impulse, stand to the woman's right side and palpate first over the apex, particularly in the area of the fifth interspace in the midclavicular line. Normally, the apical impulse is palpable in or just medial to the midclavicular line and is felt as a faint, short-duration, localized tap less than 2 centimeters in diameter. During pregnancy, when the woman's diaphragm is raised, the apical impulse may normally be located anterior to the midclavicular line. Evaluate and record the presence, location, size, and character of the apical impulse.

Continue palpation along the left sternal border where a diffuse, lifting systolic impulse along the lower sternal border may be found in women with right ventricular hypertrophy. Palpation at the base of the heart is normally "quiet" but evaluation of pulsations, thrills, or vibrations should be made.

The stethoscope you use for auscultation of the heart should have both a bell and a diaphragm. The diaphragm accentuates higher-frequency sounds while the bell accentuates those of lower frequency and filters out those of higher frequency. Most low-pitched sounds are diastolic filling sounds or murmurs and are often best heard with the woman lying down, since orthostatic pooling on standing may cause such sounds to diminish in intensity. Although heart sounds are referred to as being of "high" or "low" frequency, these terms are relative; all heart sounds are generally low pitched (low in frequency) and are in a range ordinarily difficult for the human ear to hear.

When auscultating the woman's heart, first note the rate and rhythm of the heartbeat. At each auscultatory area, concentrate initially on S_1, noting its intensity and variations, possible duplication, and the effects of respiration. Do the same with S_2. Next concentrate on the systole and then on diastole, listening first for any extra sounds and then for murmurs [17].

If the initial part of the examination was done with the woman lying on her back, ask her now to roll to her left side. Apply the bell lightly at the apex and listen for the presence or absence of low-frequency diastolic sounds, such as a filling sound or a mitral valve murmur. Next ask the woman to sit up and lean slightly forward. Pressing the diaphragm firmly against her chest, listen at both the second left and the second right intercostal spaces at the sternal border to detect the presence of high-pitched diastolic murmurs of aortic or pulmonic valve insufficiency. Listen during normal respiration and then with the woman holding her breath in deep expiration (Fig. 7-7).

Changes in Pregnancy.   During pregnancy, the heart is pushed upward by the diaphragm and is rotated forward. Heart sounds heard now, such as pulmonic and apical systolic murmurs, might be considered pathologic in the nonpregnant state. During pregnancy the mean cardiac output rises from 4.5 liters per minute to a maximum of about 6 liters per minute, an increase of about 33 percent. The heart rate increases from 70 to 85 beats per minute, an increase of only about 20 percent. To compensate for the difference, the stroke volume must increase also. It has been reported that the peripheral resistance of the vessels is reduced, possibly because of the effects of estrogen and progesterone. This results in venous dilatation in the woman's pulmonary vascular bed and in her legs.

Blood volume at term rises to about 45 to 50 percent above nonpregnant levels.

Figure 7-7. A. Precordial areas palpated to determine the presence of thrills, thrusts, heaves, retractions, bulges, and lifts. B. Cardiac auscultatory sites.

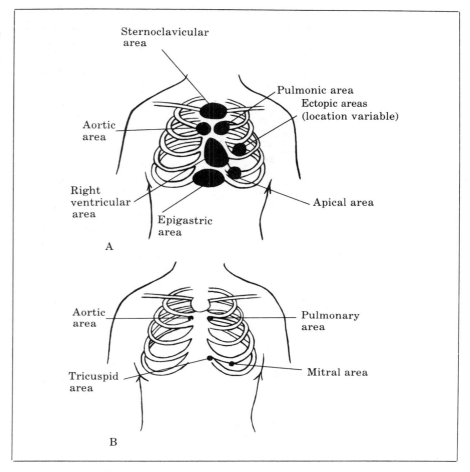

This increase begins in the first trimester, is most rapid during the second trimester, peaks at approximately 32 to 36 weeks, and then plateaus. Some studies [20, 30] report a drop in volume in the 36- to 40-week period, although this may be related to testing methods and the position of the woman. The increased volume serves to meet the demands of the enlarging uterus, helps to maintain adequate circulation when the woman is standing or lying down, and acts as a reserve for blood loss at delivery. The blood volume increase is several hundred milliliters higher in multigravidas than primigravidas; the reasons for this are unknown.

The woman's uterus receives the greatest proportion of the increased blood flow; early in pregnancy, her kidney receives a significant increase. Blood flow to the skin and mucous membranes increases by 70 percent by the thirty-sixth week, causing peripheral vasodilatation and complaints of "feeling the heat," sweating, and nasal congestion. The increased blood flow to the woman's hands may explain the increased rate of fingernail growth during pregnancy.

During pregnancy, the increase in plasma volume is followed by an increase of about 30 percent in the production of red blood cells. It should be noted that the increase in red cell volume is proportionately less than the increase in plasma volume. This results in a physiologic anemia, or pseudoanemia, most evident in the second trimester of pregnancy. The hemoglobin may fall to an average of 11 to 12 grams per 100 milliliters of blood, from an accepted norm of 13.7 to 14.0 grams per 100 milliliters. The hematocrit may drop to an average of about 34 percent from an accepted norm of 40 to 42 percent.

Because of the increased number of red blood cells, the woman's iron requirement also rises. Her increased need, though slight in the first half of pregnancy, is great during the second half of pregnancy, when she needs approximately 6 to 7 milligrams of iron per day to meet the demand of her own body and that of the growing fetus. If these demands are not satisfied, the fetus can receive iron from the placenta, but the woman suffers a drop in hemoglobin.

In addition to the increase in red blood cells, there is a rise in white blood cells, platelets, globulins, cholesterol, and sedimentation rate, while albumin and total proteins decrease. Some clotting factors show an increase during pregnancy. Fibrinogen levels may be increased by as much as 50 percent or more, and Factor VIII is also markedly increased. There are also significant rises in Factors VII, IX, and X, although the reasons for these increases are unknown. Controversy exists with regard to changes in the fibrinolytic system in late pregnancy, normal labor, and postpartum period, but it is generally believed this system is depressed in pregnancy and enhanced in the postpartum period [2, 8].

During the latter part of pregnancy, there is a decrease in the woman's venous return from her lower extremities, partly caused by pressure from her enlarged uterus on the pelvic veins and inferior vena cava. This commonly results in dependent edema, leg cramps, and the development or aggravation of varicosities in her legs, vulva, and anal area. If this occurs, encourage the woman to rest more during the day, with her legs elevated if possible. When she is in bed, a pillow under the mattress will maintain the elevation more consistently than a pillow placed under her legs. Teach her to avoid constricting clothing, such as garters or rolled stockings. Support stockings may be helpful but should be put on after her legs have been elevated for several minutes, or preferably before she gets out of bed in the morning. Encourage her to avoid activities that require prolonged standing.

Varicosities in the woman's anal area (hemorrhoids) may be painful and may itch and/or bleed. Instruct her to use her finger (lubricated with a substance such as petroleum jelly) to push protruding hemorrhoids back inside her rectum. In addition, cold or witch-hazel compresses may relieve the discomfort and itching. Also tell her that hemorrhoids may be aggravated by constipation, and that she will need to take measures to avoid constipation. Hemorrhoids usually regress after delivery; if surgical removal is necessary, it is usually delayed until that time.

Teach the woman that vulvar varicosities may be relieved by placing a pillow under the buttocks or by elevating the hips for frequent rest periods (Fig. 7-8). During delivery, vulvar varicosities may make it difficult to choose the site for an episiotomy if one is necessary.

In the latter months of pregnancy women will notice that their feet swell, especially around the ankles, after normal activity. This dependent edema is common, whereas edema of the hands and face is not and should be reported to the

Figure 7-8. Position for relief of vulvar varicosities.

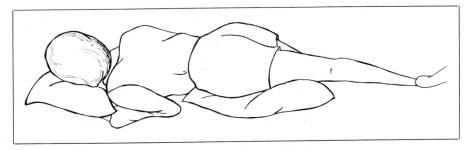

midwife or obstetrician. Dependent edema will be relieved somewhat when the woman goes to bed at night; as she assumes a horizontal position, venous return from her legs will increase. This often causes nocturia, since the woman's body now rids itself of the extra fluid that has collected in her legs during the day.

BREASTS

Assessment, Evaluation, and Interventions.   Using the techniques of inspection and palpation, examine the woman's breasts while she is seated with her arms at her sides, with her arms abducted over her head, and while she pushes her hands into her hips, in order to inspect contraction of the pectoral muscles and dimpling if a breast mass is present (Fig. 7-9). Next, examine her while she is bending forward. Inspect her breasts for symmetry, bulging, retraction, and fixation. Breast masses may prevent her breasts from moving upward or forward normally as well as produce dimpling. Her breasts also are inspected for color, size, lesions, moles, pigmentation, and distribution of hair. Inspect her areolar area for size, shape, symmetry, color, and lesions. Inspect her nipples for size, shape, color, erection, lesions, and discharge. If her breasts are symmetrical, both nipples should point laterally in the same direction.

Begin palpation with the axillary, subclavicular, and supraclavicular lymph nodes. Relaxation of the woman's muscles is important during palpation in order to detect enlarged nodes. This can be achieved partially by supporting the woman's wrist or forearm on the side being palpated.

Next, ask the woman to lie down in order to palpate her breasts. Unless the woman's breasts are small, a small pillow placed under her shoulder on the side to be palpated will help spread her breast more evenly across her chest and make it easier to locate masses. Palpate the woman's breasts while they are flattened against her rib cage. The examination may be carried out in one of two ways: The breast may be visualized as a wheel with six or eight spokes, with palpation occurring along each spoke until the breast has been thoroughly palpated; or the breast may be treated as a group of concentric circles with the nipple as the center, with palpation beginning at the outermost circle and continuing along the inner circumferences until the total breast has been examined. Ridges of breast tissue found underneath very large breasts may be confused with breast masses but are nonpathologic. Palpate the areolar areas to detect underlying masses. Compress each nipple to detect masses or discharge. If discharge is found, "milk" the breast with both index fingers along each "spoke" to identify the lobe from which the discharge is originating. Compression of this lobe will result in discharge from the nipple.

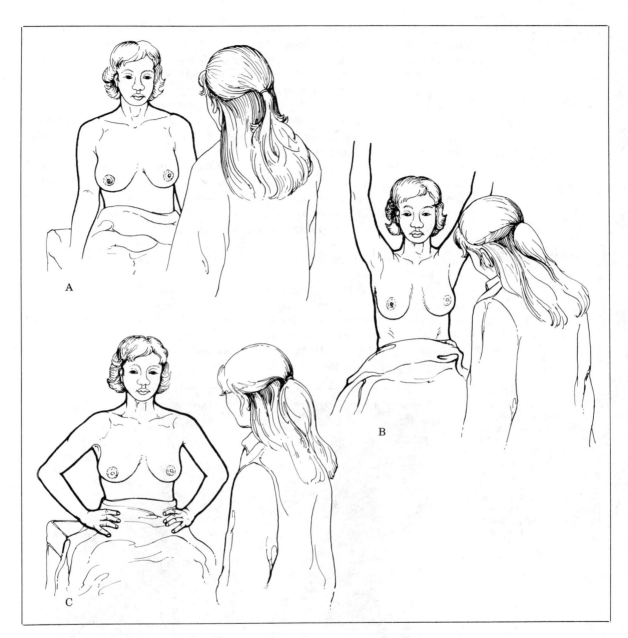

Figure 7-9. Positions for examination of the breast. A. Inspect the woman's breasts while her arms are at her sides; B. with arms abducted over her head; C. with hands pressed against her hips. (From R. D. Judge, G. D. Zuidema, and F. T. Fitzgerald [Eds.]. *Clinical Diagnosis: A Physiologic Approach* [4th ed.]. Boston: Little, Brown, 1982.)

Normally the breasts feel granular. Young women's breasts may feel very firm and elastic while older women's breasts may feel much more granular and stringy. The breasts may feel full, tender, and nodular premenstrually. If a mass is detected, describe it in relation to its location, size, consistency, mobility, tenderness, discreteness, dimpling, and erythema.

Changes in Pregnancy.   During pregnancy, mammary growth is stimulated by the continued presence of progesterone and estrogen and by the lactogenic properties of chorionic somatomammotropin. Estrogen enhances development of the breast ductal system, while progesterone stimulates the development of the alveolar system. Increased blood supply contributes to initial breast enlargement. After the second month, hypertrophy of mammary alveoli causes the breasts to continue to increase in size and become nodular. As the breasts enlarge further, veins become visible just below the skin (Fig. 7-10). With extensive enlargement, stretch marks (striae gravidarum) may develop.

Nipples become larger, more deeply pigmented, and more erectile. After the first few months, a thick yellowish fluid, colostrum, may be expressed from them with gentle massage.

At the same time the areolae become broader and more deeply pigmented. The depth of the pigmentation varies with the woman's complexion: the darker her complexion, the deeper the pigmentation (Fig. 7-11). Scattered throughout the areolae are a number of small elevations, hypertrophied sebaceous glands called Montgomery's glands (Montgomery's tubercles). Their secretions protect the surrounding skin and keep it pliable.

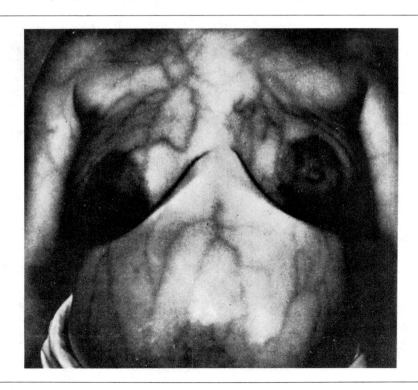

Figure 7-10. Infrared photograph of woman one month before term, showing accentuated venous pattern over breasts and abdomen. (From L. M. Hellman and J. A. Pritchard. *Williams Obstetrics* [14th ed.], 1971. Courtesy of Appleton-Century-Crofts, Publishing Division of Prentice-Hall, Inc.)

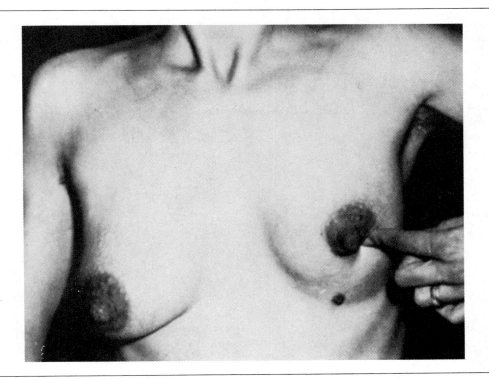

Figure 7-11. Breast changes of pregnancy. Note the deep pigmentation of the areolae and nipples and the prominence of Montgomery's glands. The accessory nipple beneath the left breast is also pigmented. (From J. R. Willson, and E. Carrington. *Obstetrics and Gynecology* [6th ed.]. St. Louis: Mosby, 1979.)

Special breast care, according to Atkinson's [1] research, is helpful in enhancing the ability to nurse, to toughen the nipples (and thereby decrease the incidence of cracking and nipple pain), and to enhance erectility and eversion of the nipples. Daily cleansing with warm water and a soft clean cloth, followed by careful drying, is important. Using soap may remove protective natural skin oils and leave the nipple more subject to damage. Since the skin on the surface of the nipples is thin, measures such as rubbing them gently with a washcloth are used to toughen them. When crusts form as a result of breast secretions, they may be softened by applying a suitable nipple cream or lanolin.

Occasionally inversion of the nipples occurs. If the woman plans to breast-feed, this inversion can be counteracted by placing the thumbs on opposite sides of the areola close to the nipple (Fig. 7-12). The woman then presses firmly but gently into the breast tissue, gradually pushing away from the areola; she then releases pressure but keeps her thumbs in position. This is done four or five times in succession in both the horizontal and vertical directions and is carried out daily.

Nipples can be made more erect by rolling them between the thumb and forefinger, applying even, gentle pressure for 15 to 30 seconds. Cream may be massaged into the tissue by using this method.

Any of the above conditions may be discovered as you examine the woman's breasts. This is usually a good time to teach the mother the technique of breast self-examination and to stress the importance of doing it monthly when she is no longer pregnant (Fig. 7-13). She should also be alerted to the nodular breast changes that occur during pregnancy and regress afterward.

Figure 7-12. Technique of correcting inverted nipples. The nipples may be everted by placing the thumbs on opposite sides of the areola close to the nipple and applying firm but gentle pressure into the tissue and then pushing away from the areola.

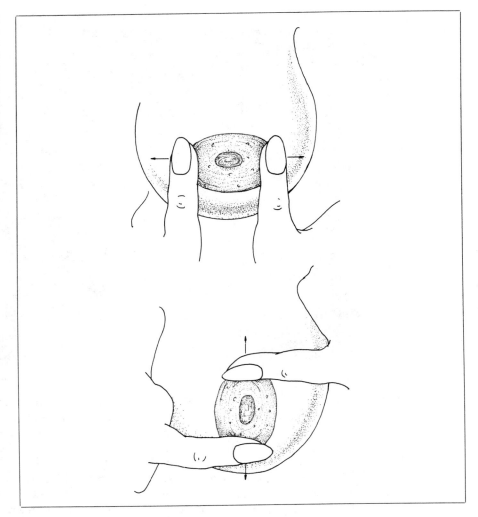

In addition check the fit of the woman's brassiere. Since the increasing size of the breasts may make them pendulous, a well-fitting supporting brassiere is very important. The brassiere should fit smoothly below the breasts, supporting and lifting them so that the nipples are on a line with the midpoint of the upper arm (Fig. 7-14). Wide adjustable shoulder straps will be more comfortable and should keep the brassiere from riding up in the back or slipping down in the front. Usually the cup size should be one size larger than before pregnancy.

ABDOMEN AND DIGESTIVE TRACT

Assessment, Evaluation, and Interventions.   Assess the woman's abdomen by using inspection, auscultation, percussion, and palpation. To inspect her abdomen, ask the woman to lie on her back with her hands at her sides in order to relax her abdominal muscles as much as possible. Next ask her to take a deep breath, forcing her diaphragm downward and decreasing the size of her abdominal cavity. In this way, masses such as an enlarged liver or spleen are more

Figure 7-13. Breast self-examination. A. Stand with hands on hips and observe for symmetry or changes, looking in a mirror. B. Follow same procedure with hands in air. C. Squeeze palms together to contract pectoral muscles. Breasts should project outward. Observe for bilateral motion and signs of dimpling. Tumors on the pectoral muscle may cause dimpling and uneven projection. Squeeze nipples to see if fluid may be expressed, which would indicate possible lesions in the ductal system. D. Palpate breast in a circular motion beginning from the outermost circle. E. While lying on side, palpate the breast and axilla area for lumps.

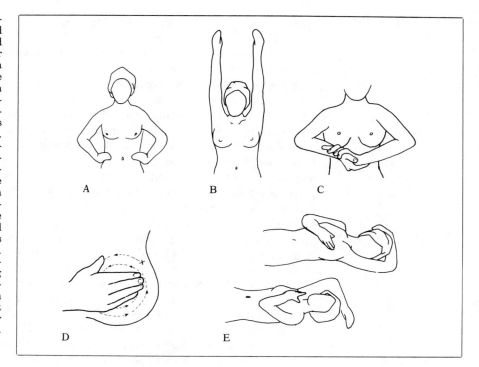

Figure 7-14. Maternity brassiere. A well-fitting maternity brassiere supports the breasts so that the nipples are on a line with the midpoint of the upper arm.

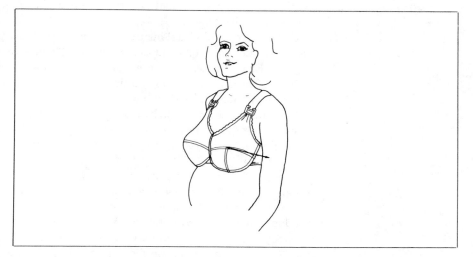

obvious. A separation of the rectus abdominis muscles (diastasis recti abdominis) may be observed or palpated as a ridge between these muscles when intra-abdominal pressure is increased by having the woman raise her head and shoulders. Diastasis recti generally occurs late in pregnancy or in marked obesity and does not interfere with functions of the abdominal structures.

For further inspection of the woman's abdomen, stand at the foot of the bed or examining table; asymmetry of the abdominal contour may be detected more readily from this position. Both sides of the abdomen are normally symmetrical in both contour and appearance.

Asymmetrical distention of the abdominal wall may be seen on inspection and may be due to a hernia, tumor, cysts, or bowel obstruction. In a thin woman you may see movement in the abdominal wall due to motility of her stomach and intestines. Observe the woman's abdominal skin for pigmentation, lesions, striae, scars, dehydration, general nutritional status, and venous patterns, all of which yield valuable information about her general state of health.

Auscultate the woman's abdomen before percussing, since bowel motility and thus bowel sounds will be increased by percussion. Use a stethoscope with a diaphragm to hear the sounds of air and fluid as they move through her gastrointestinal tract. Normal bowel sounds are high-pitched gurgling noises that occur approximately every 5 to 15 seconds. (Some clinicians suggest that the number is as high as 15 to 20 per minute, or roughly one bowel sound for each breath sound.) However, peristaltic sounds may be quite irregular. Normally, a hum originating from the inferior vena cava and its large tributaries is audible through the stethoscope. If a bruit is heard, and is detected with the woman in a variety of positions and with the bell of the stethoscope held lightly against her abdomen, it may indicate a dilated, tortuous, or constricted vessel [17].

Percuss the woman's abdomen in order to detect fluid, gaseous distention, masses, and solid structures within her abdomen. The woman's entire abdomen should be percussed lightly to identify areas of tympany and dullness. Tympany will predominate because of the presence of gas in the large and small bowel, while resonance will be heard in some areas. Solid masses will percuss as dull, as will a distended bladder.

Following careful visual inspection, auscultation, and percussion, use palpation to substantiate findings and to explore the abdomen further and evaluate major organs. Examine organs for shape, position, mobility, size, consistency, and tension. Thorough and systematic screening is performed to detect areas of tenderness, muscular spasm, masses, or fluid.

Examine all of the quadrants of the woman's abdomen systematically by palpation. Initially, use light palpation followed by deep palpation. Evaluate any abdominal mass for consistency, contour, movement with respiration, and mobility.

Changes in Pregnancy.   An essential part of the abdominal examination of a pregnant woman is an assessment of the height of her fundus. Prior to the twelfth week of pregnancy the uterus is contained in the pelvic cavity. At 16 weeks the fundus is found approximately halfway between the symphysis and umbilicus; at 20 weeks, just below the umbilicus; at 36 weeks, at the xiphoid. During the last month of pregnancy, as the fetal head drops into the bony pelvis, the fundal measurement may decrease (Fig. 7-15).

Palpate the woman's abdomen to find the top of her fundus. When it has been located, measure the distance between the top of her fundus and the top of her symphysis pubis with a tape measure, as in Figure 7-16. Using McDonald's rule, you can now calculate the woman's total weeks of gestation by multiplying the distance in centimeters between her symphysis and fundus by 8/7. To calculate the length of her pregnancy in lunar months, multiply the same measurement by 2/7 or divide that figure by 3.5. Discrepancies between fundal height and

Figure 7-15. By the end of the fourth month the uterus has risen out of the pelvic cavity.

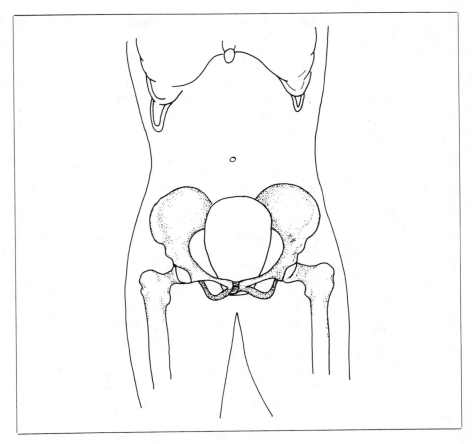

Figure 7-16. Measuring fundal height from the top of the symphysis pubis to the top of the fundus.

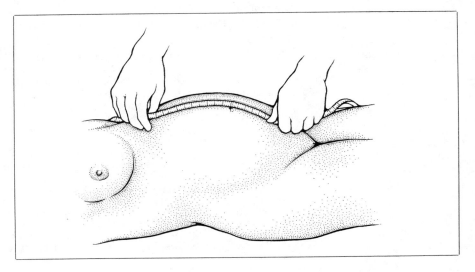

estimated gestational age should be explored for the possibility of twins or fetal growth retardation.

Next, palpate the woman's abdomen to determine fetal lie, presentation, and position (Table 7-10). This may be done by following the four maneuvers suggested by Leopold and Sporlin. These maneuvers are generally performed after 26 to 28 weeks' gestation when the fetus is large enough for its body parts to be differentiated through the abdominal and uterine walls (Fig. 7-17). With the woman on her back, stand to her side, facing her head for the first three maneuvers and facing her feet for the fourth.

The first maneuver is done by outlining the uterus with your fingertips, then gently palpating her fundus to determine if the fetal head or breech occupies that portion of the cavity. The head feels hard and round and is freely movable and ballottable, while the breech feels large and nodular.

For the second maneuver, outline the sides of the uterus while applying gentle but deep pressure. On one side the fetus's back will be palpated as a hard, continuous structure, while the other side will feel nodular, reflecting portions of the fetal extremities. If the woman is obese or has excessive amniotic fluid, apply deep pressure on one side of her abdomen while palpating the other side; then reverse the procedure.

In the third maneuver, grasp the woman's abdomen above the symphysis pubis with one hand. If the fetal part grasped is movable, engagement has not occurred; if engagement has occurred, the part feels fixed in the pelvis. As in the first maneuver, determine if the head or breech has been grasped. If the head is the presenting part and the cephalic prominence (brow) can be felt on the same side as the small parts, the head must be flexed and the vertex presenting. If the cephalic prominence is felt on the same side as the back, the head must be extended.

For the fourth maneuver, face the woman's feet and palpate the lower portion of her uterus, sliding your fingers toward the birth canal. If the head is presenting, your fingers on one side will meet an obstruction (the cephalic prominence), while those on the other side will descend more deeply into the pelvis (Fig. 7-18).

Once you have determined the position of the fetus, auscultate the fetal heart rate. Fetal heart sounds are best heard through the fetus's back. The fetal heart

Table 7-10. Fetal Lie, Presentation, and Position		
Fetal lie		The relationship of the long axis of the fetus to the long axis of the mother. A fetus may lie transversely in the mother's uterus (horizontally) or longitudinally (vertically)
Fetal presentation		The portion of the fetus that is deepest in the birth canal and is felt on vaginal examination is referred to as the presenting part. Presentations include cephalic (head), breech (buttocks or feet), face, shoulder, and several other unusual presentations
Fetal position		The relationship of the fetal presenting part to the right or left side and anterior or posterior portion of the mother's bony pelvis. For example, fetal position might be recorded as LSA (left, sacral, anterior). L represents the left side of the mother's pelvis; S signifies sacrum (identifying landmark in a breech presentation); A signifies the anterior portion of the maternal bony pelvis (see Chap. 12). This indicates that the fetus is presenting in the breech with his sacrum directed toward the left anterior portion of the mother's bony pelvis

Figure 7-17. Leopold's maneuvers. A. First maneuver. B. Second maneuver. C. Third maneuver. D. Fourth maneuver.

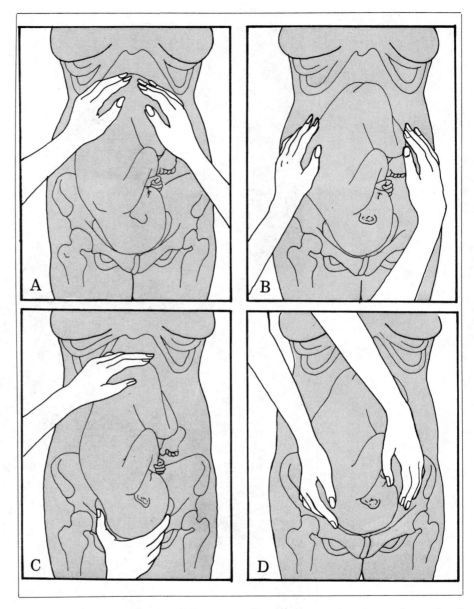

rate can often be heard with a fetoscope as early as the sixteenth week of gestation. By using a Doppler, which amplifies sound, the fetal heart rate can be heard after about 10 weeks' gestation. The heart sounds at this time are usually found at the woman's midline and slightly above her pubic hairline. Normally the fetal heart rate is between 120 and 160 beats per minute. You may also hear a uterine souffle, a soft blowing or swishing sound, as the blood rushes through the placenta. Locate both the uterine souffle and the fetal heart sounds to be sure that you can distinguish between them.

Following examination of the woman's abdomen, assess, evaluate, and counsel

Figure 7-18. Midwife teaches a father-to-be to palpate his growing baby.

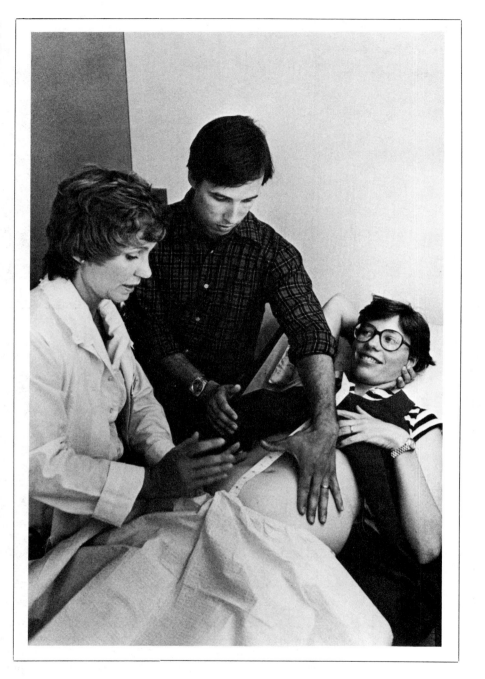

the woman regarding digestive changes she may be experiencing. Nausea and vomiting are common occurrences during pregnancy, appearing for the most part in the morning. These symptoms occur in about 50 percent of all pregnant women, beginning between the fourth and sixth weeks and generally easing by about the twelfth week. The cause is unknown. Negative feelings about pregnancy (e.g., ambivalence, uncertainty, and anxiety) may play a role. Hypoglycemia has also been suggested as a cause, as has the decreased gastric motility and the relaxation of the alimentary tract. It has also been noted that the period of nausea and vomiting coincides with the period of high levels of chorionic gonadotropin. If the woman is experiencing nausea and vomiting, suggest that she eat smaller meals or have a rapidly absorbed carbohydrate, such as orange juice, toast, or crackers, before arising or when nauseated. Dry high-carbohydrate foods seem to work better than liquids. Encourage her to avoid greasy foods and strong food odors. Antiemetics may be needed if these measures fail.

During the first two trimesters of pregnancy, there is a decrease in the production of gastric acid and pepsin. The large amounts of progesterone produced by the placenta contribute to a relaxation of the woman's alimentary tract, resulting in decreased tone and motility, delayed gastric emptying, and an increased absorption of nutrients. Constipation commonly occurs in pregnancy, as a result of decreased tone and motility of the intestines and displacement and pressure from the enlarging uterus. Lack of exercise and inadequate intake of fluids and roughage can be important contributing factors in constipation; these areas should be explored with the woman before other remedies are suggested. If a laxative is necessary, suggest prune juice, bulk-producing agents, stool softeners, or milk of magnesia. Discourage the use of mineral oil, since it tends to interfere with the absorption of the fat-soluble vitamins.

Heartburn may also be a problem for the pregnant woman. Her enlarging uterus puts pressure on her stomach and alters its position. This effect, in addition to decreased gastric motility, which can cause a reverse in peristaltic waves, results in a reflux of stomach contents into her lower esophagus. To relieve heartburn, suggest local antacids, such as aluminum hydroxide gels, to soothe the mucosa and neutralize the acid reflux. Advise the woman not to use sodium bicarbonate, a systemic antacid, since it results in absorption of excessive sodium. In addition to the use of antacids, suggest that she have smaller, more frequent meals.

Pregnancy has also been described as a period of cholestasis. The woman's gallbladder may become atonic and distended, with the bile quite thick, which predisposes her to gallstone formation.

Eating patterns may also change during pregnancy. The woman may notice an increase in appetite and thirst, particularly in early pregnancy, while later in pregnancy she may have a reduced capacity for large meals which leads to frequent snacking. Many women report a desire for highly flavored foods such as pickles, which is perhaps related to a dulling of the sense of taste. Some women may experience pica (a desire to eat bizarre substances), leading to the eating of such items as clay, coal, solid laundry starch, and refrigerator frost. Clay and laundry starch eaten in sufficient quantities cause anemia, weight loss, and other problems related to nutritional deficiencies.

Dirt-eating (geophagia) seems to be the result of a superstition handed down from the past. In Africa warriors carried earth from their homeland with them into distant battles, where the earth was eaten for strength. Other people believed that eating dirt stimulated sexual prowess. During pregnancy, eating clay was believed by some to benefit bowel evacuation, aid in proper positioning of the fetus, prevent syphilis, and help avoid nausea and dizziness. Starch ingestion supposedly aided blood clotting and made the delivery easy [21].

MUSCULOSKELETAL ASSESSMENT

Assessment, Evaluation, and Interventions.   Begin assessing the woman's neuromuscular coordination when you first meet and observe her. Continue the assessment as she enters the room, sits, rises from a sitting position, moves onto the examining table, lies down, and rolls over. Note her speed, coordination and strength of motion, and any clumsy, awkward, or involuntary movements.

A general inspection of her musculoskeletal system includes a visual scanning for symmetry, contour, size, and involuntary movement of the two sides of her body; gross deformities; areas of swelling or edema; and ecchymoses or other discoloration. Note her posture, stance, and body alignment; the structural relationships of her limbs to her trunk; and the shape of her spine and its structural apposition to her shoulder girdle, thorax, and pelvis. Use palpation to examine her musculoskeletal system to detect swelling, temperature changes, and changes in muscle shape.

Changes During Pregnancy.   During the last trimester of pregnancy, women sometimes experience aching, weakness, and numbness in the upper extremities. This may be a result of the traction placed on ulnar and median nerves by the anterior flexion of the neck and by the slumping of the shoulders characteristic of the pregnancy posture. Encourage the woman to stand tall, wear comfortable shoes, and rest frequently.

EXTERNAL GENITALIA AND PELVIC ORGANS

Assessment, Evaluation, and Interventions.   An examination of the woman's external genitalia and internal pelvis is an important part of the physical assessment. You will find that individual women need varying degrees of support during this exam. If the woman has not had a vaginal examination previously, provide a skillfully worded explanation, depending on her level of understanding, anxiety, and knowledge of her own body. When you are examining her, provide privacy and explain what you are doing and what you are about to do. Communicate to her the significance of relaxation. You may ask her to keep her buttocks on the examining table while letting her legs fall loosely apart or to breathe deeply through her mouth to help relax her abdominal muscles. If you are not the examiner, your role as support person and advocate is just as vital in these areas.

Begin inspection of the woman's external genitalia with observation of the skin surfaces and distribution of pubic hair. Pubic hair normally is shaped as an inverse triangle. Beginning with external skin surfaces and proceeding to the labia minora and clitoris, inspect skin surfaces for parasites, leukoplakia, varicosities, hyperpigmentation, erythema, swelling, and lesions. The clitoral region is a common site for chancres of syphilis in younger women and for cancerous lesions in older women. The visible portion of the clitoris usually does not exceed 2 centimeters in length and 1 centimeter in width. Inspect the slitlike urethral orifice for signs of infection. While the openings to Skene's glands are normally not visible, inspect for erythema, polyps, or discharge in this area. Examine the area of Bartholin's glands for abnormalities such as swelling, erythema, discharge, or ductal enlargement. Examine the woman's perineum for the presence of a previous episiotomy.

Follow inspection of the woman's external genitalia with palpation. Palpate any abnormal masses to determine size, shape, consistency, and tenderness. Upon palpation the labia feel soft with a consistent texture. Insert your gloved index and middle fingers into the woman's vagina to palpate the glands, perineum, and vaginal orifice and to check the adequacy of her vaginal wall. Gently milk the urethra and region of Skene's glands' openings toward her vaginal orifice in order to detect any pain or discharge. Palpate the area of Bartholin's glands for swelling and tenderness. With your index and middle fingers in the woman's vagina and your thumb on the external surface of her perineum, palpate her perineum. In the nullipara the perineum feels firm, while in a multipara who has had an episiotomy the structure is thinner and rigid due to scar tissue. Ask the woman to constrict her vaginal orifice around the two fingers in her vagina. The nullipara should demonstrate much muscle tone; the multipara, less tone. Spread your two fingers laterally in the vagina and instruct the woman to bear down against them in order to observe stress incontinence, cystocele, rectocele, enterocele, or uterine prolapse (Table 7-11).

Following the above inspection and palpation, perform speculum and bimanual examinations to assess internal pelvic organs (Fig. 7-19). With the speculum placed properly in the vagina, inspect the cervix for color, size, position, shape and symmetry, surface characteristics, shape and patency of the os, and discharge. After inspection of the cervix, obtain a Pap smear and culture for gonorrhea. Examine the vagina during insertion and withdrawal of the speculum. Inspect the vaginal mucosa for color and general condition and observe vaginal secretions for color, odor, and consistency. Normally vaginal secretions are odorless, thin or mucoid, and clear or somewhat cloudy; some white creamy material may also be present. Vaginal secretions tend to increase during pregnancy [17].

Table 7-11. Disorders Detectable on Vaginal Examination

Cystocele	A portion of the anterior vaginal wall and the bladder prolapse into the vagina. When the woman bears down, a bulge appears on the anterior vaginal wall
Rectocele	A portion of the posterior vaginal wall and the rectum protrude into the vagina. When the woman bears down, a bulge appears on the posterior vaginal wall
Enterocele	The pouch of Douglas protrudes into the vagina, appearing as a bulge in the posterior fornix
Uterine prolapse	Weakening of the uterine supports and classified as first, second, and third degree prolapse
First degree prolapse	When the woman bears down and her cervix appears at the introitus
Second degree prolapse	When the woman bears down and her cervix protrudes outside of the introitus
Third degree prolapse	When the woman bears down and her uterus is outside the introitus and her vagina is turned inside out

Figure 7-19. Insertion of the vaginal speculum. A. Blades held obliquely on entering the vagina. B. Blades rotated to the horizontal position as they pass the introitus. C. Blades separated by depressing thumbpiece and elevating handle. D. Normal parous cervix. (From R. D. Judge, G. D. Zuidema, and F. T. Fitzgerald [Eds.]. *Clinical Diagnosis: A Physiologic Approach* [4th ed.]. Boston: Little, Brown, 1982.)

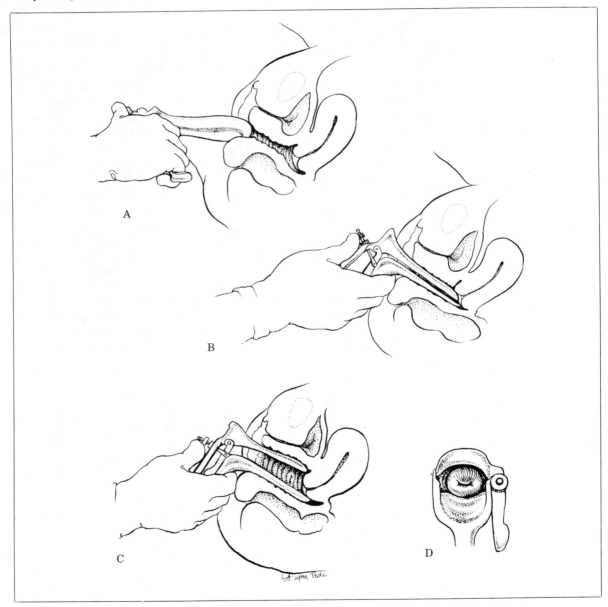

Follow the speculum examination with the bimanual examination in order to palpate the pelvic structures between your two hands. Insert your gloved index and middle fingers of one hand into the woman's vagina while your opposite hand is used to press her abdominal and pelvic contents toward your intravaginal hand. Assess her cervix for location, size, contour, surface characteristics, consistency, position, mobility, and patency of the os. The cervix and fornices should be completely palpated. Introduce one finger into the external os to assess its patency. With your fingers in the lateral fornices, move the cervix back and forth. The cervix and uterus should be freely moveable with no accompanying tenderness.

Normally the surface of the woman's cervix is smooth. However, Nabothian cysts, tumors, or lesions will make it feel nodular or irregular. The consistency of the cervix is firm and slightly resilient; it feels analogous to the tip of the nose in nonpregnant women, while it softens in pregnancy and hardens with tumors. The cervix normally is located midline on the anterior vaginal wall or on the posterior wall. If located laterally, it may indicate a tumor or adhesion. In the nonpregnant woman, the external cervical os should admit a finger for about a quarter-inch. A stenosed external os is abnormal.

Assess the size, shape, surface characteristics, consistency, position, mobility, and tenderness of the uterine body and fundus. First determine uterine position. The cervical position provides clues. Since most uteri are anteflexed, begin palpation anteriorly. With your fingers in the woman's anterior fornix, gently lift the tissues against your hand which is on her abdomen midway between her symphysis pubis and her umbilicus. If her uterus is in anteposition, it will be palpable between your hands. If her uterus is not palpated in this position, place your fingers in her posterior fornix and again lift forward toward your hand on her abdomen. If her uterus is in retroversion, you will feel only the isthmus between your hands, and you may feel the corpus with the back of your fingers.

If her uterus is in anteposition or midposition, attempt to palpate all its anterior and posterior surfaces by maneuvering its position and by "walking up" its surface with your fingers that are in her vagina. Following uterine palpation examine the adnexal areas. These structures may be difficult to locate due to their size and position [17].

With your fingers in one of the lateral fornices, place your other hand on her iliac crest on that same side. Next bring your hands together in a downward and medial direction, allowing the tissues lying between your hands to slip between them. While your hand on the woman's abdomen provides resistance, palpate the organs between your hands with your fingers in the fornix. Often no specific organ is palpated. If normal ovaries are palpated, they should feel smooth, firm, ovoid, slightly flattened, and very moveable. While sensitive to touch, ovaries should not be tender. Fallopian tubes normally are not palpable. The round ligaments may be located and feel cordlike.

Changes in Pregnancy. UTERUS AND CERVIX. There are marked uterine changes during pregnancy. From a small, almost solid organ, weighing between 30 and 60 grams (1–2 ounces), the uterus enlarges to a thin-walled muscular sac, weighing between 700 and 1,000 grams (1.5–2.2 pounds), increasing its capacity 500 to 1,000 times. During the first trimester the uterus becomes almost spherical in shape. During the second and third trimesters it changes from a globular to an ovoid shape.

Uterine enlargement is most marked in the fundus, with the greatest growth occurring in the first half of pregnancy. In the first trimester, uterine enlargement is due primarily to tissue hypertrophy, stimulated principally by increased levels of estrogen and perhaps progesterone. Even in those pregnancies that are extrauterine, the uterus itself may double in size during the first trimester due to this hormonal stimulation. During the second and third trimesters, further uterine enlargement is due to mechanical stretching and thinning of the uterine wall caused by the growing fetus.

The uterine musculature hypertrophies considerably; although the growth of new muscle fibers is quite limited, there is a great increase in the amount of fibrous and elastic tissue. All of these changes strengthen the uterine wall.

During the first half of pregnancy, uterine lymphatics and blood vessels, particularly veins, hypertrophy. Blood vessels become increasingly coiled and later uncoil as the uterus stretches, thus supplying the expanded surface area. Uterine oxygen consumption, as well as blood flow, is increased, and the nerve supply, like the blood vessels, hypertrophies.

The mechanism of uterine contractions is not fully understood. The general consensus is that progesterone reduces the excitability of the uterus, possibly by affecting the membrane potential of the myometrium, particularly over the placental site. This effect is antagonized somewhat by estrogen. The gradual increase in contractility has been attributed to increased concentrations of actomyosin in the uterine muscles.

During the first 30 weeks, uterine activity consists of slight contractions of low intensity occurring about every minute and localized to small areas in the uterus. At the same time, other contractions (Braxton Hicks' contractions) occur over a larger area approximately every hour with a greater intensity. It is thought that they aid placental function by enhancing circulation in intervillous spaces. As term approaches, Braxton Hicks' contractions become more frequent and intense. Because of this, they may be the cause of false labor, in which these contractions are mistaken for the contractions of true labor. At this time they also pull the muscle fibers that surround the internal cervical os and contribute to effacement (thinning of the cervix), particularly in the primigravida. If Braxton Hicks' contractions cause discomfort to the woman, abdominal breathing may help.

During the fourth month, the uterus rises out of the pelvic cavity and partially fills the abdominal cavity. As this happens, tension is placed on the broad ligaments, and the round ligaments begin to hypertrophy and elongate. The round ligaments now help to stabilize the upper part of the mobile uterus, while its lower portion remains anchored by cervical connections.

Because the upper portion of the uterus is free in the abdominal cavity, when the woman stands it falls forward and rests on her anterior abdominal wall, thus altering her center of gravity. To compensate for this, she walks with her head and shoulders thrust backward and chest protruding. The walking stride she now assumes is called "the pride of pregnancy."

This posture may cause a lordosis, resulting in backache. If the woman's backache is mild, you may suggest the use of a light maternity girdle, maintenance of good posture, pelvic rocking exercises, or possibly a bed board. It is important that she wear well-fitting, comfortable shoes with good arch supports. Her shoes need not be low-heeled unless she develops a backache or is unable to maintain good balance with high-heeled shoes.

When she is supine, her uterus falls backward and rests on her vertebral column and anterior large vessels. The compression of these vessels leads to a decrease in venous return to the heart, possible decrease in cardiac output, and hypotension, a condition sometimes referred to as the "inferior vena cava syndrome." When it occurs, a change to the left lateral position removes the pressure of the uterus from the vessels.

As the uterus fills the abdominal cavity, it gradually pushes the intestines to the sides and upward. It elevates the diaphragm, causing dyspnea and shifting the position of the heart. Because of the position of the sigmoid colon on the left, the uterus tends to turn toward the right.

The cervical portion of the uterus undergoes pronounced softening (Goodell's sign) and cyanosis as early as 1 month after conception (see Table 7-4). These changes are due to increased vascularity, hyperplasia of cervical glands (which increases their secretion), and edema. The glands of the cervical mucosa proliferate, and as a result a meshlike mucosal structure, the mucous plug, is formed. This helps to seal the uterine contents from contamination (Fig. 7-20).

Uterine changes cause a number of common complaints during pregnancy. The enlarged uterus causes pressure on the pelvic blood vessels, impairing circulation to the lower extremities, which may be responsible for muscle cramps in the legs. The actual cause of these cramps is not certain, however; they have also been attributed to inadequate or impaired absorption of calcium, parathyroid deficiency, hyperventilation, and excess loss of chloride from the body. Instruct the woman that she may get immediate relief from the cramps by standing with her feet flat on the floor, or by dorsiflexing her foot, while straightening her leg by downward pressure on her knee (Fig. 7-21, p. 223). Suggest preventive measures such as exercise and good body alignment in order to improve circulation.

Effective utilization of calcium depends on a proper ratio of calcium to phosphorus. When large quantities of milk are taken in, the calcium-phosphorus ratio is disturbed since more phosphorus is absorbed than calcium. Therefore, you will want to assess the milk intake of the pregnant woman who has muscle cramps and possibly suggest a decrease. A calcium preparation taken at bedtime will elevate ionizable calcium levels in her plasma. Another suggestion is that she take aluminum hydroxide with milk to remove some of the phosphorus.

The pregnant woman's enlarging uterus contributes to bladder irritability in the first trimester. Increased anteflexion displaces the cervix and stretches the base of her bladder. This feeling simulates that of a full bladder, resulting in urinary frequency. The frequency disappears as the uterus rises into the abdomen, only to reappear at or near the end of pregnancy when the fetal head descends into the pelvis. If a woman finds frequency a real problem in the first trimester, suggest that she limit her fluids in the evening so that her sleep will not be repeatedly disturbed by nocturia.

VAGINA. During pregnancy, under the influence of increased estrogen, the vaginal walls show a thickening of the mucosa, a loosening of connective tissue (to facilitate expansion), and a hypertrophy of smooth muscle cells. Increased vascularity gives the vagina its violet color (Chadwick's sign). Copious thick

Figure 7-20. The mucous plug during pregnancy helps to seal the uterine contents from contamination.

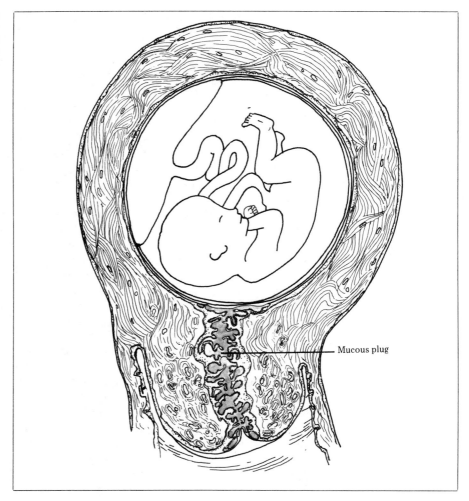

Mucous plug

white secretions result from increased production of lactic acid from the glycogen in the vaginal epithelium. The acid pH (3.5–6.0) helps to keep the vagina free from pathogenic organisms; however, all these changes contribute to an increased incidence of vulvovaginitis in pregnancy.

Two infections in particular, candidiasis and *Trichomonas vaginalis*, appear frequently. Candidiasis, a yeast infection caused by *Candida albicans*, may cause a profuse, cheesy, white irritating discharge. This organism has been cultured from the vagina in about 25 percent of women approaching term; this is not surprising since the vaginal mucosa has a high glycogen content, which serves as an excellent growth medium. The treatment of candidiasis in the past consisted of local applications of gentian violet; currently the fungicide nystatin (Mycostatin) is used without known fetal effects.

Trichomonas vaginalis, a protozoal infection, is characterized by a foamy white or yellow leukorrhea with irritation and pruritus. This infection is treated by the use of local medications such as Vagisec, Floraquin, and AVC cream. Flagyl, while very effective, has not been fully evaluated for use during pregnancy;

Figure 7-21. The woman can relieve leg cramps by dorsiflexing her foot while straightening her leg, with downward pressure on her knee.

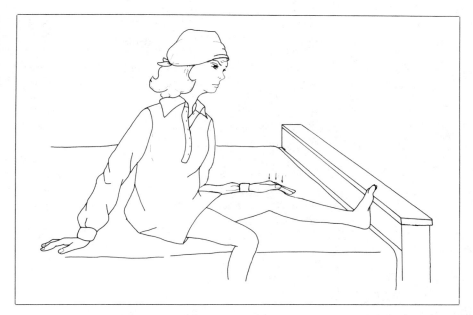

however, no adverse effects on the fetus have been reported following its use after the first trimester. A vinegar douche (3 tablespoons of white vinegar in 2 quarts of water) is sometimes used. Since men may also be infected with *Trichomonas* organisms, the woman's partner should be examined and treated; in this way reinfection of the woman is avoided.

Most cases of increased vaginal discharge during pregnancy have no pathologic cause. If the secretions are troublesome, a vinegar douche is often used. You should instruct the woman that douching during pregnancy should be kept to a minimum. It should never be done with a bulb syringe, to avoid a possible air embolism. If she uses a douche bag, it should not be placed more than 2 feet above her hip level to prevent high fluid pressure. She should not insert the nozzle more than 3 inches into her vagina. You might suggest to the woman that vulvar pruritus and discomfort may be relieved if she keeps the area as free from discharge as possible by washing frequently with water and a mild soap. In addition, she should avoid the combination of panty hose and nylon panties, since they can prevent the evaporation of normal perspiration and retain heat, thus providing a good environment for the incubation of organisms.

OVARIES AND FALLOPIAN TUBES. During pregnancy, ovulation ceases, maturation of new follicles is suspended, and ovarian veins hypertrophy. The corpus luteum of pregnancy probably functions maximally during the first month of pregnancy, primarily producing progesterone; this serves to maintain the uterine environment necessary for proper implantation and retention of the pregnancy. The tubal musculature probably undergoes little or no hypertrophy during pregnancy; under the influence of progesterone, its activity is at a low ebb.

PELVIC STRUCTURE

Evaluation of the woman's bony pelvis is a very important part of prenatal care, since its diameters must be large enough to accommodate the fetal head as it passes through the birth canal. The woman's pelvis is made up of four bones: The two innominate bones (or hip bones) form the sides and the front, and the sacrum and the coccyx form the back. The pelvic bones are held together by the fibrocartilage of the symphysis pubis and several ligaments.

The bony pelvis is divided into two parts, the false pelvis and the true pelvis, separated by a line referred to as the linea terminalis, or pelvic brim. The false pelvis lies above the line and is bounded by the lumbar vertebrae posteriorly, the iliac crests to the sides, and the lower portion of the abdominal wall anteriorly. The false pelvis provides support for the abdominal organs, including the pregnant uterus (Fig. 7-22).

The true pelvis lies below the linea terminalis; its walls are formed by the sacrum, coccyx, and lower portion of the hip bones. Because the true pelvis forms the passage through which the baby must travel during birth, it is of great obstetric significance. The true pelvis is divided into three parts: the inlet, the midpelvis, and the outlet.

The inlet is the uppermost boundary of the true pelvis and is bounded by the

Figure 7-22. Bony pelvis. The false pelvis lies above the linea terminalis, the true pelvis below.

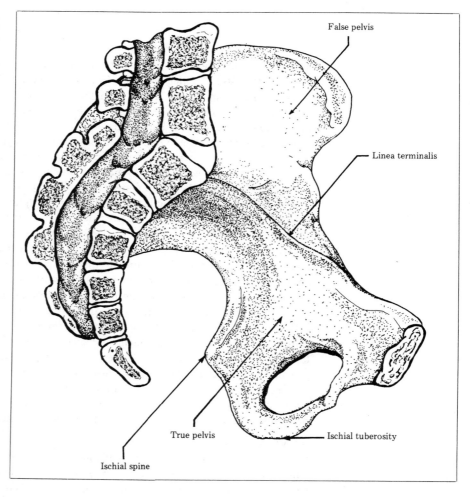

upper margin of the symphysis pubis in the front, the linea terminalis on the sides, and the first sacral vertebra or sacral promontory (an important obstetric landmark) in the back. The largest diameter of the inlet is the transverse diameter. Its smallest diameter (anterior-posterior) is the most important measurement and is measured three different ways, depending on the point on the symphysis from which the measurement is made. The *true conjugate* is the distance from the top of the symphysis to the middle of the sacral promontory. It usually measures 11 centimeters (4.3 inches) or more; the minimum acceptable measurement for most vaginal deliveries is 10 centimeters.

The *obstetrical conjugate*, the distance between the inner surface of the symphysis and the sacral promontory, is a few millimeters shorter than the true conjugate. Exact measurement of the obstetrical conjugate may only be obtained by x-ray, but it can be estimated by subtracting 1.5 to 2 centimeters (0.6–0.8 inch) from the third diameter, the *diagonal conjugate* (usually 12.5 centimeters, or 4.9 inches). The diagonal conjugate is the distance from the lower margin of the symphysis to the sacral promontory. You can usually measure this diameter by placing two fingers in the woman's vagina and touching the sacral promontory

Figure 7-23. Measuring the diagonal conjugate from the lower margin of the symphysis to the sacral promontory.

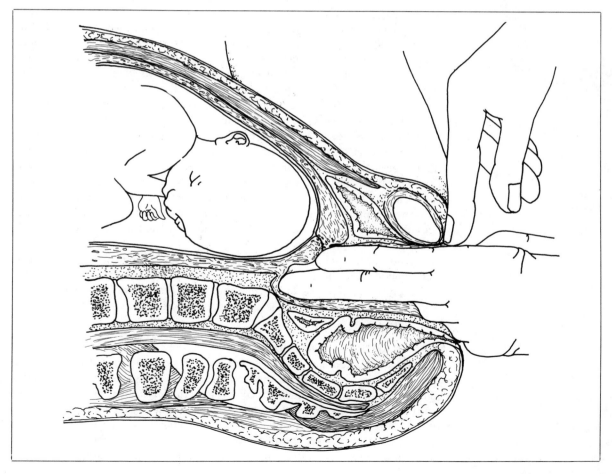

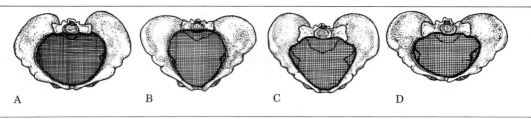

A   B   C   D

Figure 7-24. Four main types of pelvic shapes: A. Gynecoid. B. Anthropoid. C. Android. D. Platypelloid.

(Fig. 7-23). This process may be uncomfortable for the woman, so she will require preparation and support. You may prefer to defer this part of the pelvic examination until the second trimester, when vaginal and perineal tissues are more easily stretched.

The diameters of the midpelvis cannot be measured clinically. The smallest diameter of the midpelvis, the distance between the ischial spines, averages 10.5 centimeters (4.1 inches). The spines themselves are another obstetric landmark and can be palpated on pelvic examination to determine their prominence. Prominent ischial spines may indicate a contracted midpelvis.

The outlet is the lowest boundary of the true pelvis. It is bounded by the lower margin of the symphysis anteriorly, the ischial tuberosities to the side, and the tip of the sacrum posteriorly. Its most critical diameter is between the ischial tuberosities; ideally this diameter should be 9 centimeters (3.5 inches) or more. The minimum acceptable measurement that will allow vaginal delivery is 8 centimeters (3.1 inches). Since this diameter is shortened when the pubic arch is narrow, you should always check the arch during the pelvic examination.

In addition to these measurements, check the coccyx for mobility. If it is fixed, it may shorten the diameters of the outlet and may fracture during delivery.

The woman's pelvic size and shape can be influenced by a number of things: sex, racial characteristics, general body build, nutritional status (especially conditions such as rickets during childhood), congenital defects, and disease or injury of the spine, pelvic bones, or lower extremities. There are four main types of pelvic shapes. The gynecoid pelvis (the normal female pelvis) is found in about half of the obstetric population. Since important diameters may be smaller in the other pelvic shapes, they may be the source of difficulty at the time of delivery (Fig. 7-24).

As a result of hormonal increases (possibly estrogen, progesterone, and relaxin), the pelvic joints begin to relax in the first half of pregnancy and become increasingly mobile in the last 3 months. As a result, walking may become difficult and uncomfortable. These changes tend to regress within 3 to 5 months after delivery.

ANUS AND RECTOSIGMOID AREA

Assessment, Evaluation, and Interventions.   Following vaginal examination, while the woman is still in lithotomy position, place your gloved, lubricated index finger against her anal sphincter until it begins to yield. Then insert your finger upward. Ask the woman to tighten her sphincter around your finger so that you may evaluate the muscle strength of her sphincter. Examine her levator ani muscle by palpating laterally and posteriorly where it is attached to the rectal wall on both sides. Palpate the mucosa of her anal canal for tumors or polyps.

Palpate her coccyx to determine its mobility and sensitivity. You should be able to feel her cervix as a small round mass through the anterior wall of her rectum. Following the rectal examination, examine any feces that cling to your glove for blood and pus.

ENDOCRINE SYSTEM

The pituitary changes during pregnancy are not great. The pituitary gland enlarges somewhat, and there is increased activity of the posterior pituitary hormone, oxytocin. The anterior pituitary hormones FSH and LH are decreased. The reported low blood levels of pituitary somatomammotropin (growth hormone) may perhaps be due to increased levels of chorionic somatomammotropin. The blood level of MSH is also increased.

The thyroid, like the pituitary, enlarges during pregnancy. The basal metabolic rate rises progressively during pregnancy as a result of the increasing growth of the fetus. The increased amount of estrogen causes a rise in the concentration of thyroid hormone; since most thyroid hormone is protein bound, the amount of unbound active hormone does not rise appreciably.

During pregnancy there is some increase in the level of adrenal corticosteroid, which has been implicated as the cause of abdominal striae, glycosuria, hypertension, and heavier facial features. Early in the second trimester, significant amounts of aldosterone are secreted, and the level becomes even higher in the third trimester. Some studies [9,10] suggest that these elevated levels protect the women from the natriuretic effects of progesterone.

The level of ionized or active calcium is not significantly lower during pregnancy as compared to its level during the nonpregnant state.

URINARY SYSTEM

During pregnancy the glomerular filtration rate is increased from 50 to 60 percent without an increase in tubular reabsorption. This results in the excretion of many solutes, e.g., urea, uric acid, creatinine, amino acids, folic acid and other water-soluble vitamins, and glucose. Progesterone is believed to cause relaxation of the smooth muscle in the renal pelvis, ureters, and bladder, which contributes to dilatation of the pelvis and ureters and results in urinary stasis. The dilated ureters also elongate and in so doing tend to curve or coil (Fig. 7-25). Dilatation of the ureters is always greater on the right side above the pelvic brim, due to the dextrorotation of the pregnant uterus; the left ureter may be cushioned somewhat by the sigmoid colon. These changes regress following pregnancy.

Because of the increased collecting space of the urinary tract and the resulting urinary stasis, pregnant women are more likely to have large numbers of bacteria in their urine, even in the absence of symptoms. Cystitis and upper urinary tract infections are common.

Follow-up Evaluation   This initial health assessment is comprehensive. It is followed on subsequent visits by assessments that are briefer. Encourage the woman to make return visits every 4 weeks for the first 7 months of pregnancy, every 2 weeks for the next month, and every week during the last month. During these return visits her general health, including eating and sleeping habits and discomforts of the pregnancy, is explored. A history of the woman's normal daily diet forms the basis for assessment of her specific dietary needs. Usually she receives vitamins and supplementary iron. Her weight, blood pressure, fundal height, fetal heart tones,

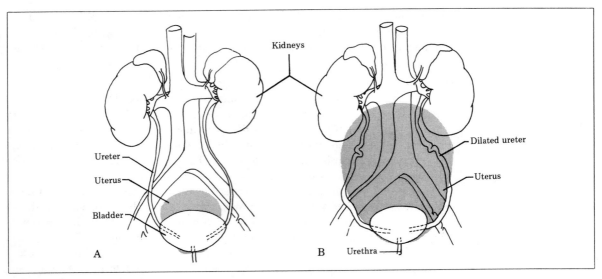

Kidneys

Ureter

Uterus

Bladder

A

Dilated ureter

Uterus

B   Urethra

Figure 7-25. A. Normal urinary system. B. Urinary system during pregnancy. The ureters dilate, elongate, and coil, increasing the collecting space of the urinary tract and adding to urinary statis. These changes increase the incidence of urinary tract infections during pregnancy.

and urinary sugar and protein are checked, and she is evaluated for signs of complications.

During the woman's initial visit answer her questions, begin health teaching according to her and her family's individual needs (Table 7-12), and develop an initial plan of care with her in keeping with her desires and expectations regarding health care. Each woman will have different expectations for the care she and her family are to receive, and her needs will vary according to those expectations and according to the trimester of her pregnancy.

Before she leaves, discuss with her the objectives for her next visit. Following the woman's initial visit, assess the information you have already gathered and identify that which you still need. The plan of care for the woman and its quality and implementation also depend upon what you bring to the situation. Your

Table 7-12. General Areas of Antepartum Teaching

Physiologic changes of pregnancy
General hygiene, discomforts of pregnancy, normal daily activities, common feelings about
 pregnancy
Nutrition
Fetal growth and development
Labor and delivery
Anesthesia and analgesia
Breathing techniques and other coping measures
Tour of labor and delivery area
Routines of the agency and available alternatives
  During labor
  On the postpartum unit
  Involvement of significant others
Child care
  Newborn care
    Breast or bottle feeding
    Bathing, dressing
    Needs and characteristics—physical, developmental, temperamental
Sibling rivalry
Normal responses while adjusting to new roles and responsibilities
Community groups and agencies offering supporting services

knowledge of current nursing practice, current nursing research, and local, state, and national resources available for aid to the family is essential for developing and providing comprehensive quality care.

At each subsequent visit, review and evaluate the plan of care with the woman and her family and modify it where appropriate. Whatever the personal goals of the woman, broad goals of care should include a healthy outcome for mother and baby and personal satisfaction and growth of the family members.

Case Study   The Thomases

You are in practice with Dr. Jean Thompson, a certified nurse midwife. You will be providing much of the care, teaching, and counseling to the Thomases in this busy nursing practice. Develop a plan of care for Janice and her husband including your interventions at each of her visits for the remainder of her pregnancy. You will develop your own approach and style in providing care to pregnant couples. Applying the nursing process to the outline following the case study will serve as one guide in organizing your approach to the couple during pregnancy.

INITIAL VISIT   The Thomases have been married 1 year. David, 22, is a printer; Janice, 19, works as a cashier in a local diner. On her first visit to Dr. Thompson, the nurse midwife, Mrs. Thomas appears tense. She believes she is pregnant. Dr. Thompson greets her and begins talking with her. Janice states that her last menstrual period began November 10 (the date of the visit is January 26). She has had no bleeding or spotting since. She is very tired, has been nauseated upon arising, and complains of having to void frequently. Dr. Thompson tests the urine specimen Janice has brought along for sugar and albumin. She also performs an immunologic pregnancy test and finds that it is positive.

Janice meanwhile is being examined by Dr. Thompson. She listens to Janice's heart and lungs, records her blood pressure, and performs a vaginal examination. Dr. Thompson then talks with Janice and tells her she believes she is pregnant. The pregnancy test is positive, her uterus is enlarged, and her other signs and symptoms point to the fact that she is pregnant. She notes in her folder positive Hegar's and Chadwick's signs. She now takes a history. She begins by recording gravida 1, para 0. Janice's answers are short and precise, but at times she needs questions repeated. After the history the midwife talks further with Janice and mentions some signs and symptoms to be reported immediately should they occur. Janice has difficulty concentrating on these and attempts to write them down.

Janice, somewhat overwhelmed at this point, wants to know her expected date of confinement. She also wants to know how a pregnancy test could be done so quickly and how accurate it is. She asks when she will begin to show, stating that her husband might be concerned about this. Not being able to think of another thing to ask at this point, she leaves Dr. Thompson's office with an appointment to return in 1 month.

THIRD VISIT   In her fourth month Janice returns for her third visit. She is no longer fatigued or complaining of nausea or frequency. You look over the results of her blood studies and find that she is blood type O, Rh+; her STS is negative, hemoglobin 13, hematocrit 39 percent. Janice is complaining of a fullness and tenderness in her breasts and sore nipples. While not enjoying these feelings, she is enjoying the fact that she is now a 36D: "I always had large breasts so I should have gallons of milk to feed the baby now." Janice is planning to continue working but would like to know when she should quit. The visit goes well until Janice steps on the scale; to everyone's amazement, Janice has gained 8 pounds since her last visit. Janice is 5 feet 2 inches tall. Her prepregnancy weight was 126 pounds. Thus far in her pregnancy, Janice has gained 12 pounds.

After much discussion Janice is about to leave but remembers another thing she wanted to ask. The hospital where she is to deliver is offering a series of classes for expectant parents. She wants to know whether these are worth her time and effort.

FOURTH VISIT   In her sixth month Janice brings her husband along with her. Her uterus is now at the level of her umbilicus. She has been feeling well, but complains of constipation and gas. Her varicose veins seem to be bothering her more now, and she has noticed some ankle swelling at the end of the day. She also says she notices a periodic tightening in her abdomen.

While Janice is preparing for her examination, you notice that David Thomas seems to be trying to start a conversation. After some time he states that Janice "sure has changed." Commenting that women do show changes during pregnancy, you wait for him to continue. With a great deal of hesitation he tells you that Janice doesn't seem to love him any longer and that she gets upset very easily. After Janice's examination, the Thomases talk with Dr. Thompson. They are planning a trip to Minnesota by car for a week and want to know if that will be okay.

FIFTH VISIT   In her seventh month Janice again is feeling fairly well but her back has begun to ache in the past month or two. She also is bothered by excess vaginal secretions and wants to know if she should douche. She tells you about one incident last week when she awoke from her sleep with a horrible cramp in her leg. Janice's weight gain is fine, and she comments, "It's fine because I started smoking again. When I don't smoke a lot I eat more. I'm going to stop working soon and I'm afraid I'll be eating more when I'm home. I've never had a lot of free time and I'm not sure how I will adjust to it."

SIXTH VISIT   In her eighth month Janice comes to the office and is very upset. "I think I've been pregnant for 2 years. I'm ugly—just look at me! I've got brown spots on my face, stretch marks, a black line on my stomach. I can't eat right because I can't breathe very well. I'm not even comfortable when I sleep. I can't wait until it's all over. I almost wish I could wish the whole thing away."

After talking with Janice and reassuring her, you are able to calm her down. She seems to have a lot of free time and doesn't appear to know what to do with it. Janice asks if tub bathing isn't allowed because the water and soap might get up the birth canal and hurt the baby. Having no more questions, Janice leaves and is to return the following week.

Assessment Form			
Assessment	Plan	Intervention	Evaluation

I. Health history
  A. Age
  B. Family history
    1. Significant health problems
    2. Chronic diseases
  C. Woman's past medical and gynecologic history
    1. Past medical problems
      a. Infections
      b. Chronic diseases
    2. Past gynecologic history
      a. Menstrual history (menarche, length, character, regularity of periods)
      b. Pap test results
  D. Woman's past obstetric history
    1. Abortions
    2. Deliveries (date, gestation, problems length of labor, type of delivery, presentation, condition of infant)
    3. Postpartum experience (perception, complications)
  E. Woman's present obstetric history
    1. Gravida, para
    2. EDC
    3. Signs and symptoms present
    4. Unusual signs
    5. Exposure to infections
    6. Current medications, past and current immunizations
  F. Diet history
    1. Weight gain
    2. Nutritional pattern
    3. Eating habits
    4. Alcohol consumption
    5. Caffeine consumption
    6. Smoking habits
  G. Activities
    1. Rest and sleep (amount, pattern)
    2. Exercise (type, appropriateness)
    3. Sexual (needs met, adjustments needed)
    4. Employment (outside home, possible hazards, plans to continue)

Assessment Form			
Assessment	Plan	Intervention	Evaluation

5. Travel plans
H. Psychosocial
  1. Emotional changes
  2. Reactions to pregnancy (woman's, father's, family's, adjustment required in life-style, planned, motivation for pregnancy, preparations for infant, wearing maternity clothes, preferred sex, preferred name, characteristics and features attributed to fetus)
  3. Family support system (marital status, who lives with her, significant others, type of support available—financial, emotional—from whom, predominant family style)
  4. Ethnic practices (specific to childbearing, complications common to ethnic group)
  5. Learning style (How does she learn best [method]? Can she read, understand, remember? Does she ask questions? Does she apply knowledge?)
II. Laboratory Results
  A. Pregnancy test
  B. Hb, Hct
  C. Urine (protein, glucose, acetone)
  D. STS, gonococcal culture
III. Physical Examination
  A. General survey
  B. Vital signs, height, weight
  C. Head
  D. Face (expression, color and condition of facial skin, symmetry of facial structures)
  E. Eye (visual acuity, lids, conjunctivae, sclerae, pupils, optic disc)
  F. Ear (external—size and location; auditory canal, tympanic membrane)
  G. Nose (deviation, discharge, congestion)
  H. Mouth (teeth, gums, mucosal surfaces, tongue)
  I. Throat (tonsils, oropharynx)
  J. Neck (muscles, cervical vertebrae, trachea, thyroid, carotid arteries, jugular veins, cervical lymph nodes)

Assessment Form

Assessment	Plan	Intervention	Evaluation

K. Skin (color, vascularity, edema, injuries, lesions)

L. Hair (distribution, quantity, quality)

M. Nails (shape, texture, curvature, adherence to nail beds)

N. Respiratory system (shape and symmetry of thorax, respiratory rate, abnormal breath sounds)

O. Heart and blood volume changes (heart sounds, rate, peripheral pulses, varicosities—legs, vulva, anus)

P. Breasts (symmetry, bulges, retraction, fixation, masses, nipples, color, size, tenderness, discharge)

Q. Abdomen and digestive tract (diastasis, stria, pigmentation, scars, masses, uterine height, lie, presentation and position of fetus, fetal heart rate, nausea, vomiting, heartburn, constipation)

R. Musculoskeletal (posture, deformities, swelling, involuntary movements, pain)

S. External genitalia and pelvis (color, distribution of hairs, signs of infection, position and condition of uterus, ovaries, cervix, vagina, measurements of pelvic inlet, midpelvis, outlet)

T. Anus and rectosigmoid area (adequacy of sphincter, polyps)

U. Urinary system (pain on urination, frequency)

IV. Specific Learning Needs (to cope with physical changes)

V. Needs Identified (by woman, husband or baby's father, significant others)

VI. Plans and Expectations of Childbirth Experience

   A. Idealized experience

   B. Childbirth education classes

   C. Labor support

   D. Anesthesia

   E. Idealized child

   F. Method of infant feeding

REFERENCES
1. Atkinson, L. Prenatal nipple conditioning for breast feeding. *Nursing Research* 28:267, 1979.
2. Basu, H. K., and Jeffcoate, N. Local fibrinolytic activity in the pregnant uterus. *American Journal of Obstetrics and Gynecology* 107:1188, 1970.
3. Butterworth, C., Jr. Interactions of nutrients with oral contraceptives and other drugs. *Journal of the American Dietetic Association* 62:510, 1973.
4. Caffeine: How to consume less. *Consumer Reports* 46:597, 1981.
5. Caffeine: What it does. *Consumer Reports* 46:595, 1981.
6. Davidson, S. Smoking and alcohol consumption: Advice given by health care professionals. *Journal of Obstetric, Gynecologic and Neonatal Nursing* 10:256, 1981.
7. Hasselmeyer, E., Meyer, M., Catz, C., and Longo, L. *Pregnancy and Infant Health.* Washington, D.C.: U.S. Department of Health, Education and Welfare (PHS) 79-50069, 1979.
8. Hytten, F., and Leitch, I. *The Physiology of Human Pregnancy.* Oxford, Eng.: Blackwell, 1971.
9. Jacobson, M., Goldman, A., and Syme, R. Coffee and birth defects. *Lancet* 2:1415, 1981.
10. Krieg, A., and Henry, J. Pregnancy tests. *Postgraduate Medicine* 42:48, 1967.
11. Laidlaw, I., Reese, J., and Garnall, A. The influence of estrogen and progesterone on aldosterone secretion. *Journal of Clinical Endocrinology* 22:161, 1962.
12. Landau, R., Platz, E., and Lugibihl, K. Effect of pregnancy on metabolic influence of administered progesterone. *Journal of Clinical Endocrinology* 20:1561, 1960.
13. Linn, S., Schoenbaum, S., Monson, R., Rosner, B., Stubbfield, R., and Ryan, K. No association between coffee consumption and adverse outcomes of pregnancy. *New England Journal of Medicine* 306:141, 1982.
14. Llewellyn-Jones, D. *Fundamentals of Obstetrics and Gynecology,* Vol. 1. London: Taber and Taber, 1971.
15. Luce, G., and Segal, J. *Sleep.* New York: Coward-McCann, 1966.
16. Luke, B. Maternal alcoholism and fetal alcohol syndrome. *American Journal of Nursing* 77:1924, 1977.
17. Malasanos, L., Barkauskas, V., Moss, M., and Stoltenberg-Allen, K. *Health Assessment.* St. Louis: Mosby, 1981.
18. Masters, W., and Johnson, V. *Human Sexual Response.* Boston: Little, Brown, 1966.
19. McKay, S. Smoking during the childbearing year. *American Journal of Maternal-Child Nursing* 5:46, 1980.
20. Physicians seek reason for clay eating. *Journal of the American Medical Association* 201:26, 1967.
21. Pritchard, J., and MacDonald, P. *Williams Obstetrics* (16th ed.). New York: Appleton-Century-Crofts, 1980.
22. Radioreceptor assay of human chorionicgonadotropin: Detection of early pregnancy. *Science* 184:793, 1974.
23. Rush, D. Effects of smoking on pregnancy and newborn infants. *American Journal of Obstetrics and Gynecology* 135:281, 1979.
24. Schildkraut, J. The catecholamine hypothesis of affective disorders: A review of supporting evidence. *American Journal of Psychiatry* 122:509, 1965.
25. Smith, D. *Mothering Your Unborn Baby.* Philadelphia: Saunders, 1979.
26. Stephens, C. The fetal alcohol syndrome: Cause for concern. *American Journal of Maternal-Child Nursing* 6:251, 1981.
27. Tobacco hazards to health and human reproduction. *Population Reports,* Series L, No. 1, March 1979.
28. Treadway, C., Kane, F., Jarrahi-Zadel, A., and Lipton, M. A psychoendocrine study of pregnancy and the puerperium. *American Journal of Psychiatry* 125:1380, 1969.
29. Tull, M., and Brown, A. Effects of caffeine on pregnancy and lactation. *Pediatric Nursing* 6:51, 1981.
30. Ueland, K., Novy, M.J., Peterson, E., and Metcalfe, J. Maternal cardiovascular dynamics. *American Journal of Obstetrics and Gynecology* 104:856, 1969.
31. Weathersbee, P., and Lodge, J. Alcohol, caffeine, and nicotine as factors in pregnancy. *Postgraduate Medicine* 66:165, 1979.
32. Weathersbee, P., and Lodge, J. Caffeine: Its direct and indirect influence on reproduction. *Journal of Reproductive Medicine* 19:55, 1977.
33. Weathersbee, P., Olsen, L., and Lodge, J. Caffeine and pregnancy. *Postgraduate Medicine* 62:64, 1977.
34. Woodward, S. How does strenuous maternal exercise affect the fetus? A review. *Birth and the Family Journal* 8:17, 1981.
35. Wright, V., Emmons, P., and Larson, D. Running through pregnancy. *Runner's World* 13:54, 1978.

FURTHER READING   Abril, I. Mexican-American folk beliefs: How they affect health care. *American Journal of Maternal-Child Nursing* 2:168, 1977.

Allgaier, A. Alternative birth centers offer family-centered care. *Hospitals* 16:97, 1978.

Barnard, K. The family and you. *American Journal of Maternal-Child Nursing* 3:83, 1978.

Bettoli, E. Herpes: Facts and fallacies. *American Journal of Nursing* 82:924, 1982.

Brink, P. (Ed.). *Transcultural Nursing: A Book of Readings.* Englewood Cliffs, N.J.: Prentice-Hall, 1976.

Brownlee, A. The family and health care: Explorations in cross-cultural settings. *Social Work in Health Care* 4:179, 1978.

Cameron, J. Year-long classes for couples becoming parents. *American Journal of Maternal-Child Nursing,* 4:358, 1979.

Candy, M. Birth of a comprehensive family-centered maternity program. *Journal of Obstetric, Gynecologic and Neonatal Nursing* 8:80, 1979.

Carter-Jessop, L. Promoting maternal attachment through prenatal intervention. *American Journal of Maternal-Child Nursing* 6:107, 1981.

Chung, H. Understanding the oriental maternity patient. *Nursing Clinics of North America* 12:67, 1977.

Cohn, S. Sexuality in pregnancy: A review of the literature. *Nursing Clinics of North America* 17:91, 1982.

Collins, E. Maternal and fetal effects of acetaminophen and salicylates in pregnancy. *Obstetrics and Gynecology* 58:57 (Suppl.), 1981.

Corby, D. Aspirin in pregnancy: Maternal and fetal effects. *Pediatrics* 62:930 (Suppl.), 1978.

Cranley, M. Development of a tool for the measurement of maternal attachment during pregnancy. *Nursing Research* 30:281, 1981.

Danaher, B. G., et al. A smoking cessation program for pregnant women: An exploratory study. *American Journal of Public Health* 68:896, 1978.

Fawcett, J. Body image and the pregnant couple. *American Journal of Maternal-Child Nursing* 3:227, 1978.

Gortmaker, S. The effects of prenatal care upon the health of the newborn. *American Journal of Public Health* 69:653, 1979.

Grudzinskas, J., et al. Does sexual intercourse cause fetal distress? *Lancet* 29:692, 1979.

Gullekso, D. J., et al. Maternal drug use during the perinatal period. *Family and Community Health* 11:31, 1978.

Harris, R., Dombro, M., and Ryan, C. Therapeutic uses of human figure drawings by the pregnant couple. *Journal of Obstetric, Gynecologic and Neonatal Nursing* 9:232, 1980.

Herbst, A. Coitus and the fetus. *New England Journal of Medicine* 301:1235, 1979.

Herpes can spread to endometrial cavity. *Sexually Transmitted Diseases Bulletin* 2:6, 1982.

Himell, K. Genital herpes: The need for counseling. *Journal of Obstetric, Gynecologic and Neonatal Nursing* 10:446, 1981.

Hogan, R. *Human Sexuality: A Nursing Perspective.* New York: Appleton-Century-Crofts, 1980.

Holey, E. S. Promoting adequate weight gain in pregnant women. *American Journal of Maternal-Child Nursing* 2:86, 1977.

Josten, L. Prenatal assessment guide for illuminating possible problems with parenting. *American Journal of Maternal-Child Nursing* 6:113, 1981.

Kindley, K. The sexuality of women in pregnancy and postpartum: A review. *Journal of Obstetric, Gynecologic and Neonatal Nursing* 7:28, 1978.

Leininger, M. Cultural diversities of health and nursing care. *Nursing Clinics of North America* 12:5, 1977.

Lion, E. *Human Sexuality in Nursing Process.* New York: Wiley, 1982.

Luakaran, V., and van den Berg, G. The relationship of maternal attitude to pregnancy outcomes and obstetric complications. *American Journal of Obstetrics and Gynecology* 136:374, 1980.

Mehl, L. Options in maternity care. *Nursing Dimensions* 7:26, 1979.

Mercer, R. She's a multip . . . she knows the ropes. *American Journal of Maternal-Child Nursing* 4:301, 1979.

Mercer, R. A theoretical framework for studying factors that impact on the maternal role. *Nursing Research* 30:73, 1981.

Moghissi, K. Risks and benefits of nutritional supplements during pregnancy. *Obstetrics and Gynecology* 58:68(Suppl.), 1981.

Moore, D. The body image in pregnancy. *Journal of Nurse Midwifery* 12:17, 1978.

Primeaux, M. American Indian health care practices—A cross-cultural perspective. *Nursing Clinics of North America* 12:55, 1977.

Sadowsky, E., Laufer, N., and Allen, J. The incidence of different types of fetal movements during pregnancy. *British Journal of Obstetrics and Gynaecology* 86:10, 1979.

Stichler, J., and Bouden, J. Pregnancy: A shared emotional experience. *American Journal of Maternal-Child Nursing* 3:153, 1978.

Tamez, E. Curanderismo: Folk Mexican-American health care system. *Journal of Psychiatric Nursing and Mental Health Services* 12:34, 1978.

The pregnant drinker. *American Journal of Public Health* 68:836, 1978.

The pregnant smoker. *American Journal of Public Health* 68:835, 1978.

Tripp-Reimer, T., and Friedl, M. Appalachians: A neglected minority. *Nursing Clinics of North America* 12:51, 1977.

Worthington, B. S. Nutrition during pregnancy, lactation and oral contraception. *Nursing Clinics of North America* 14:269, 1979.

Chapter 8 Nutritional Needs During Childbearing

Many hormonal, biochemical, and physiologic changes occur during pregnancy and influence both the woman's need for nutrients and the efficiency with which her body uses them. These changes are necessary for adequate fetal growth, maternal maintenance during pregnancy, and preparation of the mother for childbirth and lactation. We have knowledge of some of these changes. Decreased gastric motility and peristalsis during pregnancy, for example, slow the passage of food through the woman's gastrointestinal tract and possibly enhance the absorption of nutrients. The effect of human placental lactogen (HPL) in increasing maternal lipids for use as an energy source for the mother while maternal glucose is made more readily available to the fetus for energy use is another such change. Unfortunately, our knowledge and understanding of many of these changes are incomplete.

It is not known how the levels of most nutrients are controlled during pregnancy. Most of the nutrients that have been measured are found to exist at lower concentrations in pregnant women than in nonpregnant women. Dietary deficiency or failure of absorption is probably not responsible for most of the low levels, although many of them can be artificially raised by large dietary supplements [10]. Excretion by the kidney probably plays only a small role. The reduced level of many nutrients may be due to a resetting of different maternal homeostatic mechanisms. It may also be that the lowering of nutrient levels in maternal blood reflects a balance that favors transfer to the fetus rather than to maternal tissues.

Many of the adjustments in the pregnant woman's carbohydrate and insulin metabolism have been documented; for instance, fasting blood sugar values are lower in pregnancy. Insulin responds differently to a glucose load, a phenomenon that is observed throughout pregnancy but is more obvious in the later stages of pregnancy. These changes are exaggerated in pregnant women who are overweight, women with a family history of diabetes, and women who had diabetes in previous pregnancies [7]. While insulin seems to have a normal effect on blood glucose in early pregnancy, in late pregnancy the increased quantities of insulin that are released do not have a corresponding effect on blood glucose levels [10]. This same reaction has been noted in both men and nonpregnant women who have received large doses of progesterone [13]. During pregnancy there is also increased resistance to injected insulin; the fall in blood sugar it produces is not so great as that in the nonpregnant woman.

Several sources of insulin antagonism in pregnancy have been identified. It has been postulated that insulin, like thyroxin and many other hormones, might be more protein bound and thus less active. Progesterone, estrogen, and HPL are believed to play a part in promoting a state of insulin resistance. The elevated levels of serum corticosteroids in pregnancy might also be expected to antagonize insulin, probably by accelerating its destruction in the liver. Another contributing factor may be the increased levels of fatty acids; their high levels in late pregnancy may result from increased lipolysis due to HPL. It has been suggested that the mechanism of insulin antagonism by HPL and by growth hormone may be through higher levels of serum fatty acids. Insulin is also thought to be destroyed by a placental enzyme reaction.

Increased amounts of circulating insulin and low blood glucose may be responsible in part for the increased appetite and food intake during pregnancy, and increased insulin action might explain the amount of fat storage that takes place. It may also be that the fainting episodes that are common at the beginning of pregnancy are hypoglycemic rather than vasovagal in nature [10]. The increasing need for more insulin in later pregnancy to counteract increasing insulin metabolism puts additional stress on the woman's pancreas. It is not surprising that the woman whose pancreas has little natural reserve may not be able to produce enough insulin, resulting in the development of gestational diabetes.

Plasma lipids are generally high in pregnancy, and the level tends to rise throughout its course. This may be a reflection of increased fatty-acid synthesis, possibly by the liver. There is extensive storage of fat in adipose tissue. Progesterone may act to reset a lipostat in the hypothalamus during pregnancy. Following delivery this mechanism probably returns to its nonpregnant level and the woman loses much of her added fat.

In most normal pregnancies, there is a positive sodium balance. This results from the increased glomerular filtration rate as well as the presence of large amounts of progesterone secreted by the placenta. Progesterone slows absorption of filtered sodium through the renal tubules. Through the renin-angiotensin-aldosterone pathway, aldosterone is released as part of a compensatory mechanism to counterbalance the salt-losing tendency of progesterone. With the resulting sodium reabsorption that occurs in the kidneys, a positive sodium balance is achieved. To maintain fluid balance and proper osmosis, extra water is retained in maternal tissues and contributes to the woman's weight gain during pregnancy [23].

The basal metabolic rate is increased during pregnancy for many reasons: increase in muscle mass of the uterus, breast growth, fetal mass and placenta, and increased cardiac and respiratory loads. The total increase is about 20 to 25 percent over the nonpregnant state. The energy needed to meet these demands has been found to vary from 38 to 50 calories per kilogram per day [2] (300 calories more than the woman's nonpregnant caloric maintenance needs is often used as a rule-of-thumb figure). Since the exact energy expenditure of these metabolic changes is difficult to predict in any given pregnant woman, satisfactory weight gain is often assumed to reflect appropriate caloric consumption [40].

NUTRITIONAL NEEDS DURING PREGNANCY
Weight Gain

The average weight gain of the typical adult woman during pregnancy with an unrestricted balanced diet is 11 to 13 kilograms (24–28 lb) [12]. A range of 20 to 35 pounds more satisfactorily includes the majority of women in the United States. Most of the weight gained can be accounted for by the products of pregnancy and by maternal physiologic changes (Table 8-1). The weight gain is minimal in the first trimester (1–2 kg or 2–4 lb); over the second and third trimesters it occurs at a rate of about 0.2 to 0.5 kg (0.5–1.0 lb) per week (Fig. 8-1). During the second trimester about 60 percent of the weight gain is maternal, while during the third trimester 60 percent is fetal [29]. Pitkin has suggested that inadequate weight gain would be a gain of 1 kilogram or less per month in the second or third trimester while excessive weight gain would be a gain of 3 kilograms or more per month [28].

Table 8-1. Components of Maternal Weight Gain During Pregnancy

Tissue	Weight (gm)	Weight (lb)
Fetus	3,150	7
Placenta	675	1.5
Amniotic fluid	900	2
Subtotal	3,725	10.5
Mother		
Uterus	900	2
Breasts	450	1
Increase in blood volume	1,350	3
Tissue fluids	1,350	3
Fat	4,050	9
Subtotal	8,100	18.0
Total	11,825	28.5

Source: H.S. Guthrie. *Introductory Nutrition* (4 ed.). St. Louis: Mosby, 1979. Used by permission.

It has been reported that the mother's weight gain and prepregnancy weight are the two strongest influences (except gestational age) on birth weight [11,12,21,22,26,37]. In previous decades stringent restriction of maternal weight gain was advocated, presumably to produce a baby whose weight would ensure easy delivery and reduce the incidence of preeclampsia. Now it is recognized that maternal weight restriction and nutritional inadequacy may contribute to a high perinatal mortality in the United States through their association with fetal growth retardation, hypertensive disorders, abruptio placentae, and premature delivery [23,25]. Weight gain above the average during pregnancy results in no significant hazard to fetal development or delivery of the infant but maternal fat stores may remain following delivery. Shedding this additional weight will require a weight reduction program and effort on the mother's part (Tables 8-2 and 8-3).

While some women in the United States do suffer from severe malnutrition, many others will begin a pregnancy with inadequate nutritional reserves. The increased demands of pregnancy deplete their nutrient stores, and deficiencies soon become evident. Even with treatment it may take months for these mothers to feel recovered. The nutritional needs of the pregnant woman mainly depend on a well-balanced diet, with nutrients from each of the basic food groups (Table 8-4). It must be remembered that the woman's general health at the time of her infant's conception is a result of dietary habits that have been established throughout her lifetime; thus, her prepregnancy nutrition may be most important of all (Table 8-5).

Protein Needs

The woman's carbohydrate and fat intake will automatically increase as she consumes the recommended 300 additional calories per day during pregnancy. Those extra daily calories should include 30 grams of protein from the second month of pregnancy until term. This figure may be adjusted according to the size and age of the woman following guidelines suggested by King [15,16]:

Mature women—1.3 grams of protein per kilogram of pregnant weight
Adolescent girls (15–18 years)—1.5 grams of protein per kilogram of pregnant weight
Younger girls—1.7 grams of protein per kilogram of pregnant weight

Figure 8-1. Prenatal weight gain is low in the first trimester; it increases to up to 1 pound per week in the second and third trimesters. (From Committee on Maternal Nutrition, Food and Nutrition Board, National Research Council, National Academy of Sciences. Maternal nutrition and the course of pregnancy. Washington, D.C.: U.S. Government Printing Office, 1970.)

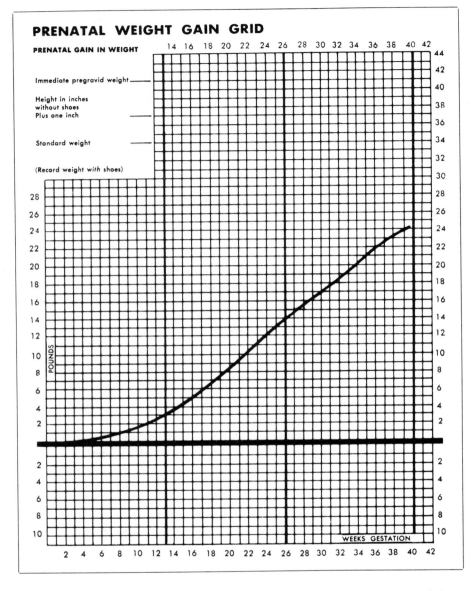

The higher recommended protein intake for adolescents and younger girls is to support continued maturation. Protein requirements for pregnant women are usually between 70 and 80 grams per day.

The protein consumed during pregnancy is used for a number of physiologic changes in pregnancy. The nitrogen composition of fetal tissue rises from 0.9 grams at conception to 55.9 grams at term. In addition, 17 grams of nitrogen is stored in the placenta, 1 gram in amniotic fluid, 17 grams in maternal breast tissue, and 40 grams in the uterus. The protein synthesis necessary for the developing fetus is dependent on the amino acids that preferentially pass from the maternal to the fetal circulation where the amino acid concentration is higher.

*Table 8-2. Percentiles for Weight and Height of Girls 12–18 Years of Age**

	Weight (kg)			Height (cm)		
Age	5	50	95	5	50	95
12	30.52	41.53	60.81	139.8	151.5	162.7
13	34.14	46.10	67.30	145.2	157.1	168.1
14	37.76	50.28	73.08	148.7	160.4	171.3
15	40.99	53.68	77.78	150.5	161.8	172.8
16	43.41	55.89	80.99	151.6	162.4	173.3
17	44.74	56.69	82.46	152.7	163.1	173.5
18	45.26	56.62	82.47	153.6	163.7	173.6

* Data have been used to derive reference points. It is not intended that they necessarily be considered standards of normal growth and development.
Source: Food and Nutrition Board. *Recommended Daily Allowances* (9th ed.). Washington, D.C.; National Academy of Sciences, 1980.

Maternal reserves of 200 to 350 grams of nitrogen are stored to protect the woman against losses during labor and delivery and to prepare her for lactation. Increased blood volume and blood constituents, especially hemoglobin and plasma protein, contribute to the woman's need for increased intake of protein. Complete protein foods include milk, eggs, cheese, fish, and meat; legumes, nuts, and whole grains are additional protein sources (Table 8-6).

Mineral Needs

CALCIUM AND PHOSPHORUS

The recommended daily requirements of calcium and phosphorus for pregnant women are between 1,200 and 1,600 milligrams of each, an increase of 400 milligrams over those recommended for nonpregnant women. Calcium and phosphorus are normally involved in energy and cell production as well as in acid-base buffering. While there is some increased need for these minerals early in pregnancy, most of the calcium is required in the last trimester. Calcium stores of the woman increase from 4 grams at the middle of pregnancy to 30 grams at term. Fetal stores increase from 1 gram at the middle of pregnancy to 23 to 28 grams at term. Calcium is necessary for rapid mineralization of fetal skeletal tissue as well as formation of fetal tooth buds [31]. Dairy products are an excellent source of

*Table 8-3. Desirable Weights for Women 25 Years and Older**

Height		Small Frame	Medium Frame	Large Frame
Feet	Inches			
4	10	92–98	96–107	104–119
4	11	94–101	98–110	106–122
5	0	96–104	101–113	109–125
5	1	99–107	104–116	112–128
5	2	102–110	107–119	115–131
5	3	105–113	110–122	118–134
5	4	108–116	113–126	121–138
5	5	111–119	116–130	125–142
5	6	114–123	120–135	129–146
5	7	118–127	124–139	133–150
5	8	122–131	128–143	137–154
5	9	126–135	132–147	141–158
5	10	130–140	136–151	145–163
5	11	134–144	140–155	149–168
6	0	138–148	144–159	153–173

*Weight in pounds in indoor clothing. For girls 18–25, subtract one pound for each year under 25.
Source: Metropolitan Life Insurance Company.

Table 8-4. Daily Food Guide

	Number of Servings		
Food Group	Nonpregnant Woman	Pregnant Woman	Lactating Woman
Protein foods (animal and vegetable)	3	4	4
Milk and milk products	3	4	5
Grain products	3	3	3
Vitamin C–rich fruits and vegetables	1	1	1
Leafy green vegetables	2	2	2
Other fruits and vegetables	1	1	1

Source: Adapted from *Nutrition during Pregnancy and Lactation*. Sacramento, Calif: Maternal and Child Health Branch, California Department of Health Services, 1975.

calcium; other sources are whole or enriched cereal grain and green or leafy vegetables (Table 8-7).

IRON

Only about 10 to 20 percent of the iron in food is normally absorbed. While the absorptive efficiency of most pregnant women may increase near term, this change is generally not adequate to meet the iron requirements optimally during pregnancy without the use of iron supplements [38].

The total iron requirement of pregnancy is approximately 1,000 milligrams— 300 milligrams for the increase in total red cell volume, 300 milligrams for the fetus, 70 milligrams for the placenta, and 500 milligrams or more in blood loss at delivery and post partum. Some iron is saved (about 150 milligrams), since during

Table 8-5. Recommended Dietary Allowances of Selected Nutrients for Pregnancy and Lactation

Nutrients	11–14 Years (101 lb–62 in)	15–18 Years (120 lb–64 in)	19–22 Years (120 lb–64 in)	23–50 Years (120 lb–64 in)	Added for Pregnancy	Added for Lactation
Protein (gm)	46	46	44	44	+30	+20
Fat-soluble vitamins						
Vitamin A (μg RE)	800	800	800	800	+200	+400
Vitamin D (μg)	10	10	7.5	5	+5	+5
Vitamin E (mg αTE)	8	8	8	8	+2	+3
Water-soluble vitamins						
Vitamin C (mg)	50	60	60	60	+20	+40
Thiamine (mg)	1.1	1.1	1.1	1.0	+0.4	+0.5
Riboflavin (mg)	1.3	1.3	1.3	1.2	+0.3	+0.5
Niacin mg NE	15	14	14	13	+2	+5
Vitamin B_6 (mg)	1.8	2.0	2.0	2.0	+0.6	+0.5
Folacin (μg)	400	400	400	400	+400	+100
Vitamin B_{12} (μg)	3.0	3.0	3.0	3.0	+1.0	+1.0
Minerals						
Calcium (mg)	1,200	1,200	800	800	+400	+400
Phosphorus (mg)	1,200	1,200	800	800	+400	+400
Magnesium (mg)	300	300	300	300	+150	+150
Iron (mg)	18	18	18	18	30 to 60 mg of supplemental iron is recommended	
Zinc (mg)	15	15	15	15	+5	+10
Iodine (μg)	150	150	150	150	+25	+50

Source: Food and Nutrition Board, National Academy of Sciences—National Research Council, 1980.

Table 8-6. Foods High in Protein

Food Source*	Protein Content (gm)
Milk, whole	9
American or cheddar cheese, grated	28
Cottage cheese	31
Swiss cheese (1 oz)	8
Eggs (one, 2 oz)	6
Meat, poultry, seafood	
Beef (4 oz)	31
Hamburger, lean (4 oz)	31
Chicken (4 oz)	26.6
Liver (4 oz)	20
Pork chop with bone (4 oz)	18.3
Bluefish, baked (4 oz)	29
Shrimp, cleaned (4 oz)	28
Legumes, whole grains, nuts	
Navy beans	15
Lima beans	16
Oatmeal	5
Long grain rice	4
Whole wheat flour	10
Cashews, roasted	23
Peanuts, roasted	37
Walnuts, shelled	26

*1 cup unless otherwise noted

pregnancy no iron is lost through menstruation. Most iron demands occur in the second half of pregnancy, during which time the fetus stores a 3- to 4-months' supply in its liver to meet iron demands and to avoid anemic conditions during pregnancy. In addition, it is recognized that 90 percent of anemia in pregnancy is caused by iron deficiency associated with limited iron intake (4–6 mg/1,000 cal) combined with limited iron stores [17]. The National Research Council of the

Table 8-7. Foods High in Calcium

Food Source*	Calcium Content
Milk or equivalent milk foods	
Whole milk	288
Nonfat (skim) milk	298
Evaporated, unsweetened, undiluted milk	635
Cheese	
Cheddar or American (1 oz)	219
Creamed cottage cheese	212
Ice cream (8 fl oz)	175
Yogurt	295
Whole or enriched cereal grains	
Self-rising enriched wheat flour	292
Long grain parboiled rice	33
Oatmeal	21
Green, leafy vegetables	
Broccoli	132
Cabbage	222
Collard greens	289
Spinach	167
Turnip greens	267
Seafood	
Clams (3 oz)	59
Oysters	226
Sardines (3 oz)	372

*1 cup unless otherwise noted

National Academy of Sciences has recommended that pregnant women receive 30 to 60 milligrams of ferrous iron as a daily supplement during the second and third trimesters [5]. Food sources rich in iron include liver, other meats, dried fruit and beans, green vegetables, eggs, and enriched cereals (Table 8-8).

MAGNESIUM, ZINC, IODINE, AND SODIUM

The recommended daily allowance (RDA) of magnesium for pregnant women is 450 milligrams, an increase of 150 milligrams above that for nonpregnant women. This mineral is important in cellular metabolism and structural growth. Foods containing magnesium include whole grains, milk, nuts, and legumes.

Zinc, a component of numerous enzymes, is important for overall growth. Zinc deficiency in pregnant rats is teratogenic [8,33]. The RDA of zinc during human pregnancy is 20 milligrams, an increase of 5 milligrams over that of the nonpregnant state. Foods high in zinc include milk, shellfish, and wheat bran.

Iodine, important in the functioning of the thyroid, is recommended to be increased by 25 milligrams during pregnancy to a total daily intake of 175 milligrams. This increase can be met by using iodized salt.

For decades many physicians restricted the sodium intake of pregnant women on the assumption that it prevented preeclampsia. Subsequent research indicates that normal sodium intake is essential in pregnancy. While particularly salty foods such as ham, potato chips, and sodium-based seasonings should be avoided,

Table 8-8. Foods High in Iron

Food Source*	Iron Content (mg)
Organ meats	
Liver	10
Heart of beef	6.7
Other meat	
Beef	3.9
Lean hamburger	4.0
Pork roast	3.9
Eggs (one, 2 oz)	1.1
Clams, raw	6.9
Oysters, raw	13.2
Dark molasses, "black strap" (1 tbsp)	3.2
Dried beans, peas, and nuts	
Navy beans (1 cup, 256 gm)	4.6
Lima beans (1 cup, 192 gm)	4.2
Peas, split (1 cup, 250 gm)	5.6
Almonds (1 cup, 142 gm)	6.7
Cashews, roasted (1 cup, 135 gm)	5.1
Wheat germ (1 cup, 68 gm)	6.4
Dry active baker's yeast (1 oz, 28 gm)	4.6
Enriched cereals	
Corn, rice, or wheat flakes	2.0
Dried fruits	
Apricots (1 cup, 150 gm)	8.2
Dates (1 cup, 178 gm)	5.3
Figs (1 fig, 21 gm)	.6
Green vegetables	
Lima beans (1 cup)	4.0
Mustard greens (1 cup)	2.5
Spinach (1 cup)	4.0

*4 oz, or 112 grams, unless otherwise noted

it is now recommended that food be seasoned to taste so adequate sodium is consumed [14,19].

Vitamin Needs FAT-SOLUBLE VITAMINS

The fat-soluble vitamins (A, D, E, and K) are stored in the liver and therefore are available to meet the needs of the pregnant woman if her dietary intake is inadequate.

Vitamin A. The National Research Council recommends a daily allowance of 1,000 retinal equivalents (RE) during pregnancy, an increase of 200 RE over the nonpregnant state. Vitamin A is important for the growth of epithelial cells, preventing night blindness, the development of the fetal eyes, and the metabolism of carbohydrates and fats.

Both vitamin A and its precursor, carotene, cross the placenta, and fetal storage accounts in part for the recommended increase during pregnancy. Excessive vitamin A intake is believed to be teratogenic. One report associates high vitamin A intake (10 times the RDA) during pregnancy with congenital renal anomalies [1]. Others report excessive vitamin A intake and associated fetal bone malformation, cleft palate, and jaundice. The carotenes, when taken in excess, cause yellow skin. The coloring regresses when intake is reduced. Sources of significant vitamin A include deep green and yellow vegetables, liver and kidney, egg yolk, cream, butter, and margarine.

Vitamin D. The RDA of vitamin D during pregnancy ranges between 10 and 15 milligrams of cholecalciferal (400–600 I.U. vitamin D) or an increase of 5 milligrams (200 I.U.) over the nonpregnant state. Vitamin D is essential for the absorption and use of calcium and phosphorus in skeletal development. Poor intake may compromise development of the enamel of the fetus's primary teeth, while excessive intake (greater than 5–10 times the RDA) may lead to infantile hypercalcemia in which symptoms such as excessive thirst, loss of appetite, vomiting, weight loss, and irritability are seen [30,41]. Dietary sources include fortified milk, margarine, butter, liver, egg yolk, and fatty fish.

Vitamin E (tocopheral). The requirements for vitamin E increase slightly during pregnancy. The role of vitamin E during pregnancy has not been defined; however, its major function in the body is as an antioxidant. By taking on oxygen, it prevents other substances from undergoing chemical change; it therefore has a sparing effect on those substances. It is also essential for the synthesis of nucleic acids required in the formation of red blood cells. Deficiency of vitamin E is related to long-term inability to absorb fats. In animals, deficiency of vitamin E has been associated with abortion. Major sources of the vitamin include vegetable fats and oils, whole grains, greens, and eggs.

Vitamin K. Intake of vitamin K is usually adequate in a well-balanced diet and no increased requirement during pregnancy has been identified. The vitamin's major function is in the synthesis of prothrombin.

WATER-SOLUBLE VITAMINS

The demand for water-soluble vitamins by the mother and fetus during pregnancy increases slightly from the nonpregnant state. Storage of water-soluble vitamins is limited so excess intake results in the extra amounts being excreted in the mother's urine. Because of this minimal storage, there is little protection from dietary inadequacies. In general, water-soluble vitamins are decreased in maternal serum during pregnancy, and high concentrations are found in the fetus.

Vitamin C. The RDA of vitamin C during pregnancy is between 70 and 80 milligrams, an increase of 20 milligrams above that for nonpregnant women. The substance is important for the development of connective tissue and the cardiovascular system, and it is essential in the formation of collagen. If it is deficient, collagen breaks down, cell function and structure deteriorate, and muscular weakness and capillary hemorrhage occur. There are no recognized effects of vitamin C deficiency on the outcome of pregnancy. Excessive ingestion by the mother has been reported to induce fetal dependence on this vitamin so that scurvy may develop in the neonatal period when maternal vitamin C support is withdrawn [3]. Sources of vitamin C include cantaloupe, strawberries, citrus fruit, tomatoes, potatoes, broccoli, and other leafy greens.

B VITAMINS

The B vitamins (folic acid, niacin, thiamine [B_1], riboflavin [B_2], pantothenic acid, B_6, and B_{12}) are important in cell respiration, energy metabolism, and glucose oxidation.

Folic Acid. The RDA of folacin is 800 milligrams during pregnancy, twice the amount recommended for the nonpregnant woman. The increased need for the vitamin results from active DNA synthesis required for growing cells in fetal and maternal tissues. The risk of folic acid deficiency is increased in women with repeated pregnancies, chronic anorexia or dieting, alcohol abuse, diarrheal disorders, anticonvulsants, and poor diet.

Deficiency of folate is associated with abrupto placentae, abortion, fetal malformation, and other late bleeding problems. It has been suggested that folate deficiency causes irreversible damage to the embryo and trophoblast very early in pregnancy [27]. Sources of folates include green leafy vegetables, kidney, liver, food yeasts, and peanuts.

Niacin. An increase of 2 milligrams to a total of 15 milligrams of niacin is recommended during pregnancy. Sources of the vitamin include meat, fish, poultry, whole grains, and enriched breads and cereals.

Thiamine. The requirement for thiamine increases from 1 milligram in the nonpregnant state to 1.4 milligrams during pregnancy. Sources of the vitamin include pork, liver, whole grains, milk, and potatoes.

Riboflavin (B_2). The RDA for riboflavin during pregnancy is 1.5 milligrams, an increase of 0.3 milligrams over that for nonpregnant women. Deficiency results in cheilosis and other skin lesions. Sources of riboflavin include milk, liver, eggs, and whole grains.

Vitamin B_6 (pyridoxine). The RDA of vitamin B_6 is between 2.4 and 2.6 milligrams, an increase of 0.6 milligrams above that recommended for nonpregnant women. Pyridoxal phosphate, the coenzyme form of vitamin B_6, is required for numerous metabolic reactions, most notably nucleic acid and protein synthesis in the growing fetus. Food sources of pyridoxine include wheat germ, yeast, fish, liver, pork, potatoes, and lentils.

Vitamin B_{12}. The capacity to absorb vitamin B_{12} is increased in pregnancy, but a large amount is transferred to the fetus. The RDA of the vitamin is 3 milligrams for nonpregnant women and 4 milligrams for pregnant women.

NUTRITIONAL NEEDS
DURING LACTATION

The breast-feeding mother has additional nutritional requirements, which will vary in relation to the volume of milk she produces. Once she has established her pattern of lactation, she will produce between 500 and 1,000 milliliters of milk each day, although some mothers, such as the mother nursing twins, may produce more [41]. In view of these differences, the RDAs of nutrients needed by the lactating woman must be viewed as general rule-of-thumb guidelines.

Approximately 900 extra calories per day are necessary for the mother to produce 1,000 milliliters of milk. Additionally, the lactating woman has protein needs of 20 grams more than the nonpregnant woman. The amount of calcium, phosphorus, vitamin D, and magnesium recommended is the same as that needed during pregnancy. The mother's need for vitamin A is increased by 200 retinal equivalents over her need during pregnancy. Her needs for vitamins C and E, thiamine, riboflavin, niacin, zinc, and iodine are also increased above pregnancy needs (see Table 8-4).

The woman's increased needs for calories, protein, and calcium (as well as vitamins A and D) can be met by drinking about 3 to 3½ extra cups of whole milk each day. If 2 percent fat or nonfat milk is used, other sources of extra calories may be selected. If the woman has a milk intolerance, alternative dairy products may be chosen, and in some cases nondairy sources of these important nutrients (like soy products) may be preferred [40]. Extra milk, however, will not meet increased requirements for ascorbic acid, vitamin E, vitamin B_6, and folic acid. It is therefore suggested that other foods such as citrus fruits, vegetable oils, whole grain cereals, or legumes be increased slightly in the daily diet.

There are many common beliefs about the relationship of various foods to breast milk. These include the belief that beer improves lactation and that some foods, such as cabbage, onions, and chocolate, pass through breast milk and give the infant gastrointestinal symptoms. There is no basis in fact for either of these assumptions; it cannot be denied, however, that beer would certainly add to the woman's daily fluid and caloric intake [39,40].

WOMEN AT RISK FOR
NUTRITIONAL
DEFICIENCY

While all pregnant or newly delivered women need dietary assessment and counseling, some women need particular attention directed to their nutritional needs. Women who have had a rapid succession of pregnancies (2 or more within 2 years) often have depleted nutrient stores. Those women who have a low prepregnancy weight for their height may experience an increased incidence of hypertensive disorders and prematurity. Women who have very limited weight gains during pregnancy may deliver low birth weight infants. Overweight pregnant women often have diets high in fat and carbohydrate and low in protein, minerals, and vitamins. Women with low incomes or bizarre food choices, those with a history of heavy smoking, alcoholism, drug addiction, or chronic systemic disease [9,12,35], and those whose religious or philosophic beliefs limit their diet to certain foods should have their intakes assessed very carefully. Pregnant girls who are biologically immature also need special guidance [4].

Teenage girls have been cited as having the poorest dietary habits of any group. Their diets have been reported to be inadequate in calories, protein, iron, calcium, and vitamins A and C [16,32]. This deficiency is especially detrimental for girls under 17 years of age, because their growth and development has not been completed. When a pregnancy is superimposed on her own biologic nutritional demands, the pregnant adolescent is competing with the fetus for essential nutrients. Additionally, those girls who mature rapidly and reach menarche early are at a time of peak velocity of adolescent growth, yet their skeletal maturation is less advanced [34], which means that their pelvic capacity has not yet reached adult size. The resulting neonatal and infant mortality for young mothers is often much higher than that for the population in general. The younger the mother, the greater the increase in infant mortality is likely to be.

CULTURAL DIETARY
DIFFERENCES

Prior to assessing the nutritional needs of childbearing women, whether they are at risk for nutritional deficiency or not, it is important for nurses to recognize the cultural, social, and psychologic importance of food for the childbearing woman [20,24].

Most people eat for reasons in addition to physical sustenance. Eating has many meanings that are intimately tied up with an individual's whole way of life. Food habits, like other forms of human behavior, are the result of many personal, social, psychologic, and cultural influences. The meaning and importance they have for the pregnant woman must be kept in mind before nurses or other health workers give diet counseling. The objective is not to change the dietary pattern so that it resembles that of the person doing the counseling but rather to assess the woman's needs and supplement her diet with needed foods acceptable to her. Emphasis should be placed on the desirable features of her diet and on methods of food preparation that preserve food values. Unfamiliar foods and methods of preparation must be assessed before changes are recommended.

Culture develops as a means of interpreting common life experiences and evolves over a long period of time, partially as a result of adaptation to the environment. Attempts to change long-standing cultural habits by someone not familiar with them may be upsetting. Food habits, some of the oldest and most entrenched aspects of culture, exert a deep influence on people's behavior, as noted by Williams [39]. The cultural background determines what will be eaten and when and how it will be eaten. Items considered to be good food in one culture may be viewed with disgust and believed to cause illness in other cultures. In America milk is considered a basic food, while in some other cultures it is rejected and viewed as an animal mucous discharge. In some cultures, such as the Greek culture, bread is the main focus of the meal, with the other foods planned around it. In other cultures, meat serves this purpose. Foods eaten for one meal may be rejected for another: In the western part of the United States, ham, eggs, and fried potatoes are popular for breakfast; in the South grits are popular; and in New England pie is a favorite.

Food is a method of teaching and transmitting many aspects of one's culture. Thanksgiving traditionally involves a turkey; picnic foods are eaten on the Fourth of July. Traditional foods are associated with religious holidays. Food may also serve as an expression of sympathy, sorrow, or support for a family. Cultures that value change lead families or individuals to seek constant variety in diets; because people may want to feel that they are geared for action, they may seek quick-cooking convenience foods [39].

Food is symbolic of sociability, warmth, and friendly gathering. Eating together binds a group or family and builds closeness and solidarity. Special foods closely associated with family sentiments form the most lasting habits throughout life and when eaten in adulthood trigger a flood of childhood memories. Foods may be accepted because they are viewed as having high status or rejected because they carry low prestige.

Religious practices also dictate food habits. Pork is not eaten by Moslems; meat is restricted by Seventh-Day Adventists; strict Hindus or Buddhists eat no meat, while liberal Hindus may eat no beef.

The dietary patterns of American Jews depend on the degree of orthodoxy they practice. Pork in all forms is prohibited by Orthodox Judaism; beef, lamb, goat, and venison are allowed, as are chicken, turkey, goose, pheasant, and duck. All poultry and meat must be freshly slaughtered according to ritual and soaked in salted water (koshered) to remove all traces of blood. Fish must have scales and fins; thus all shellfish are excluded [39]. Eggs, fruits, vegetables, and grain are eaten without restrictions. Milk or milk products and meat are never combined at the same meal or even cooked in the same utensils. The Jewish diet generally includes much fish, poultry (especially chicken), noodles, rye and whole grain breads, rich pastries and cakes, and stewed and canned fruits.

Food habits may also vary according to one's ethnic group. Mexican-Americans use many varieties of beans, as well as rice, potatoes, peas, and some vegetables. Chili pepper is popular and is supposed to bring good health. Little meat or milk is used; however, some calcium is provided by tortillas made from ground whole corn soaked in lime water.

The Puerto Rican diet also does not include much milk. Rice and beans are foods used daily. Salt codfish, chicken, pork, and beef are favorites, as are tomatoes, peppers, onions, and seasonings added to dried peas and beans. Fruits such as bananas and oranges are commonly used.

Italian-Americans use a variety of pastas with various cheeses and sauces, and bread remains an essential part of the meal. Southern Italians use much fish and highly seasoned foods, while their Northern counterparts use more meat and root vegetables. Eggs, cheese, tomatoes, green vegetables, and fruits are used liberally in their diet.

In the diet of those of Middle Eastern extraction, grains (such as wheat or rice) are the major source of calories. Eggs, butter, and cheese are used liberally; lamb is the favorite meat. Sour milk preparations, such as yogurt, are used commonly; sweet milk is seldom used.

The Chinese diet includes meat, fish, eggs, rice, and a large variety of vegetables. The amount of meat eaten is small, although pork is very popular. Fish is used frequently. Grains provide the main source of calories.

Western European and Scandinavian diets include a wide variety of meats, fish, vegetables, fruits, cheese, and grains. Central European diets derive much of the total calories from grains and potatoes. Pork and pork products, cabbage, root vegetables, eggs, fresh milk, sour cream, yogurt, and cheeses are used widely.

Most black Americans have incorporated to some degree dietary patterns of the South. Grits, rice, and potatoes provide the main source of carbohydrate. Dried peas and beans, fried fish, poultry, pork, game, greens, corn, and fruit are commonly eaten. Milk, milk products, and cheeses are not used extensively.

These dietary patterns, like those previously mentioned, are generalizations and much individual variation can be expected. Black Americans born and raised in the North, for example, may have very few of the eating habits of their southern counterparts. Evaluating these variations is essential in assessing dietary patterns prior to providing any dietary counseling.

DETERMINING
DIETARY INTAKE

You may use a number of methods to obtain an overview of a woman's dietary intake. One is to ask the woman to recall foods consumed during the previous 24 hours; another is to ask her to describe her pattern of consumption of certain foods such as meat, etc., for a period of time such as a week. It is helpful to have the dietary intake of several 24-hour periods in order to evaluate nutritional intake and needs [36]. You should also remember that eating patterns on weekdays and weekends often differ significantly. Another method is to ask the mother to record her dietary intake for a different day each week for a period of several weeks. Providing nutritional information (via a daily food guide, a list of food groups, a sample meal pattern, sample menus) and nutritional counseling are important interventions in the care of a pregnant woman [18].

Deskins and Laska [6] suggest to their nursing colleagues that nutritional counseling be approached as follows. During the first trimester evaluate the woman's food intake in a 24-hour period. Assess her nutritional status and the factors affecting the quality of her diet; offer assistance with budgeting and meal planning in keeping with her existing resources and facilities. If the woman needs and is eligible for the WIC program (USDA Supplemented Feeding Program for Women, Infants and Children) help her to enroll. Offer suggestions to relieve any nausea or vomiting she may have.

During the second trimester emphasize the suggestions regarding dietary improvements offered during the first trimester. In addition, explore the possibility of pica, evaluate her weight gain, and stress the importance of the pattern of weight gain as well as total weight gain. Stress that pregnancy is not the time for weight reduction diets. Offer the mother suggestions to alleviate or minimize heartburn and constipation. During the third trimester, in addition to emphasizing diet quality, weight gain, and remedies for discomforts associated with eating, you may begin exploring the woman's feelings regarding the method of infant feeding she wishes to use.

Case Study   Donna Pisarchik

Assess Donna's nutritional status and develop your planned interventions. While not all of the information will be provided by the case study, the outline that follows the case study will serve as a guide in organizing your approach.

Donna Pisarchik is a 24-year-old gravida 2 who is currently 4 months pregnant. She is 5 feet 2 inches tall and prior to becoming pregnant weighed 150 pounds. Thus far she has gained 5 pounds during the pregnancy and now weighs 155. With the exception of being overweight, Donna is in excellent physical condition. She has no chronic medical problems or problems with the pregnancy. Her past pregnancy was uneventful. Donna's hemoglobin is 12, her hematocrit 36. She describes her appetite as good, and she has had no nausea or vomiting thus far during the pregnancy. She is currently taking prenatal vitamins.

The Pisarchiks, both Donna and her husband Albert, are second-generation Polish Americans. Their son, Michael, is 2 years old. Albert is a foreman in a machine shop. They own a seven-room single home in a blue-collar neighborhood. The Pisarchiks own a car, and Albert drives Donna to the grocery store once a week when she purchases the weekly groceries. Facilities for food storage and preparation in the home are good. Donna plans and prepares the meals. The family normally eats three meals a day, with snacks in the evening while they watch television. Albert, who is 6 feet tall and weighs 160 pounds, carries a lunch to work with him.

The following are recordings of the nutritional intake for two typical 24-hour weekday periods for Donna.

Day 1

Breakfast (8:30 A.M.)
Fried egg
White toast (1 slice)
Butter (1 tsp)
Bacon (2 slices)
Coffee (1 cup, ½ tsp
    sugar)

Lunch (11:30 A.M.)
Cream of tomato soup (12 oz)
Hard roll
Butter (1 tsp)
Cottage cheese danish
Coffee (1 cup, ½ tsp
    sugar)

Dinner (5:00 P.M.)
Fried cabbage and noodles
    (1 cup)
Red beets with butter
    (½ cup)
Kielbasa (4 oz)
Canned peaches, medium
    syrup (½ cup)
Coffee (1 cup, ½ tsp
    sugar)

Snacks
2 P.M. Skim milk (8 oz)
7 P.M. Pretzels (6 beer pretzels)
    Skim milk (8 oz)

Day 2

Breakfast (8:00 A.M.)
Cream of Wheat (1 cup)
Skim milk (½ cup)
Sugar (1 tbsp)
White toast (1 slice)
Butter (1 tsp)
Coffee (1 cup, ½ tsp
    sugar)

Lunch (11:30 A.M.)
3 potato pierogies (noodle
    dough filled with 2 tbsp mashed
    potato and 1
    tsp cheese, approx.
    2-in square)
Poppy seed roll
Butter (1 tsp)
Skim milk (8 oz)

Dinner (5:00 P.M.)
3 cabbage rolls
    (stuffed with rice and ground
    pork)
Homemade white bread (2 slices)
Butter (2 tsp)
Pear pie (1 slice)
Coffee (1 cup, ½ tsp sugar)

Snacks
2 P.M. Coffee (1 cup, ½ tsp sugar)
8 P.M. 3 banana fritters
    Skim milk (8 oz)

Assessment Form			
Assessment	Plan	Intervention	Evaluation

I. Clinical Indicators
  A. General appearance
  B. General vitality
  C. Activity level
  D. Eyes
  E. Hair
  F. Skin
  G. Nails
  H. Mouth and gums
  I. Dental health
II. Risk Factors
  A. Smoking
  B. Alcohol consumption
  C. Drug addiction
  D. Pregnancy interval
  E. Pregravid weight
    (underweight, overweight)
  F. Excessive or limited weight
    gain during pregnancy
  G. Age or biologic
    immaturity
  H. Chronic systemic disease
III. Pregnancy Factors
  A. Pattern of weight gain
    1. Gradual and steady (use weight grid)
    2. Sudden excessive increase or decrease
  B. Hb, Hct
  C. Appetite
  D. Nausea or vomiting
  E. Food intolerance
    1. Prior to pregnancy
    2. During pregnancy
  F. Cravings
  G. Bowel habits (diarrhea,
    constipation)
IV. Cultural, Social, Religious,
  and Psychologic Factors
  A. Foods basic to diet
  B. Foods avoided or for-
    bidden and reason
  C. Foods preferred and reason
  D. Foods specific to pregnancy
    according to culture or religion			

Assessment Form			
Assessment	Plan	Intervention	Evaluation

     E. Life-style

   V. Resources

     A. Financial

       1. WIC

       2. Food Stamps

     B. For shopping for food

     C. For storing and preparing food

     D. Person who

       1. Buys food

       2. Plans and prepares meals

     E. Meals

       1. Number eaten per day

       2. Eaten with whom and when

  VI. Special Diet (low salt, low fat, diabetic, etc.)

 VII. Drugs or Vitamin Supplements

VIII. Plans for Infant Feeding

     A. Breast

     B. Bottle

REFERENCES

1. Bernhardt, I. B., and Dorsey, D. Hypervitaminosis A and congenital renal anomalies in a human infant. *Obstetrics and Gynecology* 43:750, 1974.
2. Blackburn, M., and Calloway, D. Basal metabolic rate and work energy expenditure of mature, pregnant women. *Journal of the American Dietetic Association* 69:24, 1976.
3. Cochrane, W. Overnutrition in prenatal and neonatal life. *Canadian Medical Association Journal* 93:893, 1965.
4. Cross, A., and Walsh, H. Prenatal diet counseling. *Journal of Reproductive Medicine* 7:265, 1971.
5. Desforges, J. Anemia complicating pregnancy. *Journal of Reproductive Medicine* 10:111, 1973.
6. Deskins, B., and Laska, M. The community health nurse's nutrition guidelines: A trimester approach for expectant mothers. *American Journal of Maternal and Child Health* 7:202, 1982.
7. Granat, M., Sharf, M., and Cooper, A. Glucose intolerance during pregnancy. *Obstetrics and Gynecology* 53:157, 1979.
8. Hickory, W., Nanda, R., and Catalanotto, F. Fetal skeletal malformations associated with moderate zinc deficiency during pregnancy. *Journal of Nutrition* 109:883, 1979.
9. Hook, D. Dietary cravings and aversions during pregnancy. *American Journal of Clinical Nutrition* 31:1355, 1978.
10. Hytten, F. E., and Leitch, I. *The Physiology of Human Pregnancy.* Philadelphia: Davis, 1971.
11. Jacobson, H. Current concepts in nutrition. *New England Journal of Medicine* 297:1051, 1977.
12. Jacobson, H. Weight and weight gain in pregnancy. *Clinics in Perinatology* 2:233, 1975.
13. Kalkoff, R. D., Jacobson, M., and Lemper, D. Progesterone, pregnancy, and the augmented plasma insulin response. *Journal of Clinical Endocrinology* 31:24, 1970.
14. Kaminetsky, H. Sodium in pregnancy. *Arizona Medicine* 35:401, 1978.
15. King, J. Protein metabolism during pregnancy. *Clinics in Perinatology* 2:243, 1975.
16. King, J. C., Cohenour, S. H., Calloway, D. H., and Jacobson, H. N. Assessment of nutritional status of teenage pregnant girls. *American Journal of Clinical Nutrition* 25:916, 1972.
17. Kitay, D., and Harbort, R. Iron and folic acid deficiency in pregnancy. *Clinics in Perinatology* 2:255, 1975.
18. Korczowski, M., and VanCoevern, S. Strengthen the nurse's role in nutritional counseling. *Nursing and Health Care* 2:211, 1981.
19. Mahan, C. Revolution in obstetrics: Pregnancy nutrition. *Journal of Florida Medical Association* 66:367, 1979.
20. Markesbery, B., and Wong, W. Points for maternity patients. *American Journal of Nursing* 77:1612, 1977.
21. Moghissi, K. Maternal nutrition in pregnancy. *Clinical Obstetrics and Gynecology* 21:297, 1978.
22. Mora, I., deParedes, B., Wagner, M., Navarro, L., Suescum, L., Christiansen, N., and Herrera, M. Nutritional supplementation and the outcome of pregnancy. I. Birthweight. *American Journal of Clinical Nutrition* 38:455, 1979
23. Oakes, G., Chez, R., and Morelli, I. Diet in pregnancy: Meddling with the normal or preventing toxemia. *American Journal of Nursing* 75:1135, 1975.
24. Orr, R., and Simmons, J. Nutritional care in pregnancy: The patient's view. Parts I, II, and III. *Journal of the American Dietetic Association* 75:126, 1979.
25. Osofsky, H. Relationships between nutrition during pregnancy and subsequent infant and child development. *Obstetrical and Gynecological Survey* 30:227, 1975.
26. Philipps, C., and Johnson, N. The impact of quality of diet and other factors on birthweight of infants. *American Journal of Clinical Nutrition* 30:215, 1977.
27. Pitkin, R. Vitamins and minerals in pregnancy. *Clinics in Perinatology* 2:221, 1975.
28. Pitkin, R. M. Obstetrics and Gynecology. In H. A. Schneider, C. E. Anderson, and D. B. Coursin (Eds.), *Nutritional Support of Medical Practice.* Hagerstown, Md.: Harper & Row, 1977.
29. Pitkin, R., Kaminetzky, H., Newton, M., and Pritchard, J. Maternal nutrition: A selective review of clinical topics. *Obstetrics and Gynecology* 40:773, 1972.
30. Purvis, R. Enamel hypoplasia on the teeth associated with neonatal tetany: A manifestation of maternal vitamin D deficiency. *Lancet* 2:811, 1973.
31. Raman, L., Rajalakshmi, K., Kreshnamachari, K., and Sastry, J. Effect of calcium supplementation to undernourished mothers during pregnancy on the bone density of the neonates. *American Journal of Clinical Nutrition* 31:466, 1978.

32. Seiler, J. A., and Fox, H. M. Adolescent pregnancy: Association of dietary and obstetric factors. *Home Economics Research Journal* 1:188, 1973.
33. Sever, L., and Emanuel, I. Is there a connection between maternal zinc deficiency and congenital malformations of the central nervous system in man? *Teratology* 7:117, 1973.
34. Shank, R. A chink in our armor. *Nutrition Today* 5:2, 1970.
35. Smithells, R., Ankers, C., Carver, M., Lennon, D., Schorah, C., and Sheppard, S. Maternal nutrition in early pregnancy. *British Journal of Nutrition* 38:497, 1977.
36. Snowman, M. Nutrition component in a comprehensive child development program. *Journal of the American Dietetic Association* 74:124, 1979.
37. Stein, Z., Susser, M., and Rush, D. Prenatal nutrition and birth weight: Experiments and quasi-experiments in the past decade. *Journal of Reproductive Medicine* 21:287, 1978.
38. Taft, L., Halliday, J., Russo, A. and Francis, B. Serum ferritin in pregnancy: The effect of iron supplementation. *Australian, N.Z. Journal of Obstetrics and Gynaecology* 18:226, 1978.
39. Williams, S. R. *Nutrition and Diet Therapy.* St. Louis: Mosby, 1981.
40. Worthington, B. Nutrition during pregnancy, lactation, and oral contraception. *Nursing Clinics of North America* 14:269, 1979.
41. Worthington, B., Vermeersh, J., and Williams, S. *Nutrition in Pregnancy and Lactation.* St. Louis: Mosby, 1981.

FURTHER READING

Alton, I. Nutritional services for pregnant adolescents within a public high school. *Journal of the American Dietetic Association* 74:667, 1979.

Ancri, G., Morse, E., and Clarke, R. Comparisons of the nutritional status of pregnant adolescents with adult pregnant women. *American Journal of Clinical Nutrition* 30:568, 1977.

Feigenberg, M., and Schiller, R. Nutrition counseling for middle class gravidas. *Journal of Obstetric, Gynecologic and Neonatal Nursing* 6(6):19, 1977.

Hemminki, E., and Starfield, B. Routine administration of iron and vitamins during pregnancy: Review of controlled clinical trials. *British Journal of Obstetrics and Gynaecology* 85:404, 1978.

Henley, E. and Bahl, S. Nutrition across the woman's life cycle: Special emphasis on pregnancy. *Nursing Clinics of North America* 17:99, 1982.

Holey, E. S. Promoting adequate weight gain in pregnant women. *American Journal of Maternal-Child Nursing* 2:86, 1977.

Jelliffe, D., and Vahlquist, B. The mother/child dyad—nutritional aspects. *American Journal of Clinical Nutrition* 31:1425, 1978.

Johnston, E. M., and Schwartz, N. E. Physicians' opinions and counseling practices in maternal and infant nutrition. *Journal of the American Dietetic Association* 73:246, 1978.

Luke, B. Guide to better evaluation of antepartum nutrition. *Journal of Obstetric, Gynecologic and Neonatal Nursing* 5(4):37, 1976.

Luke, B. Lactose intolerance during pregnancy. *American Journal of Maternal-Child Nursing* 2:92, 1977.

Luke, B. Understanding pica in pregnant women. *American Journal of Maternal-Child Nursing* 2:97, 1977.

McDaniel, J. Utilizing the nursing process model to teach nutrition and diet therapy. *Journal of the American Dietetic Association* 74:568, 1979.

Moghissi, K., and Evans, R. R. *Nutritional Impacts on Women Throughout Life with Emphasis on Reproduction.* Hagerstown, Md.: Harper & Row, 1977.

Naeye, R. L. Weight gain and the outcome of pregnancy. *American Journal of Obstetrics and Gynecology* 135:3, 1979.

Nutritional management of obese pregnant women. *PAHO Bulletin* 13:201, 1979.

Sims, L. Dietary status of lactating women. *Journal of the American Dietetic Association* 73:139, 1978.

Slattery, J. S., et al. *Maternal and Child Nutrition: Assessment and Counseling.* New York: Appleton-Century-Crofts, 1979.

The WIC program or "the perils of Pauline." *American Journal of Disorders of Childhood* 133:478, 1979.

Williams, E. Nutrition: Vegetarian diets in pregnancy. *Birth and the Family Journal* 3:83, 1978.

Witti, F. P. Alcohol and birth defects. *FDA Consumer,* 1978.

Zlalnik, F. J. Dietary protein and human pregnancy performance. *Journal of Reproductive Medicine* 4:193, 1979.

Chapter 9 Anticipating Parenthood

Each society has accepted customs surrounding the sexual behavior, marriage, and reproduction of its members. Socially accepted sexual behavior has differed through periods of history, according to one's sex, cultural background, religion, and social class. In many societies the standard of sexual conduct is established as a way to ensure that a man's possessions are passed on only to legitimate heirs.

Likewise, the accepted customs surrounding marriage are influenced by much the same factors as those controlling sexual conduct. While the ceremonies or rites involved may differ from society to society, their function of publicizing the union is the same. The marriage gives the individuals social acceptance to bear children, thus legitimizing them as future parents. The society acknowledges not only the individuals' acceptability as parents, but also their duty to reproduce.

Society is motivated to have its members reproduce since its very survival depends on it, but what about the motivations of the individuals themselves? Often a basic, biologically innate reproductive drive is assumed to be the motivational force, particularly by psychoanalysts. The strongest argument against this theory is that if humans, as other mammals, were motivated solely by such a drive, reproduction would have to continue throughout all of a woman's childbearing years [54]. However, the number of children born to a couple can be a matter of choice in the present day. If the biologic drive were as forceful as is claimed, then the social and personal consequences of having children—strained finances, additional responsibility and work, and restraints on time and freedom—would not have as much influence as they do. For example, the cost of rearing a child has conservatively been set at $80,000. The fact is, however, that the most common reasons for limiting the number of children are the mundane realities involved in having and rearing them. The growth of the "childless by choice" movement testifies to the fact that today's couples are giving serious consideration to the consequences of childbearing.

Most of the psychoanalytic theories of motivation for reproduction begin with Freud. He theorized that a little girl, noticing that she has no penis, wishes to obtain one from her father. The penis becomes equated with a child and therefore she wishes for a child by her father. This wish, suppressed as she grows older, eventually becomes the wish for a child in an adult sexual relationship [17].

Helene Deutsch sees the woman's desire for a child as being related to vaginal sensations and to experiences of eating, holding food inside, and finally expelling it [54]. With maturity, these experiences are synthesized and projected to the image of having a baby.

Therese Benedek believes that the reproductive wish is triggered by the menstrual cycle. She theorizes that the hormonal changes associated with ovulation periodically prepare women for motherhood and constitute the physiologic stimuli for desiring a child [17]. Benedek sees "motherliness" as independent of hormonal control; however, it is through interaction with the hormonal cycle that the ego matures. This is a necessary step in the development of a person's ability to care for others [4, 6].

Motivations formulated by Lerner include gratification of infantile needs for affection and repair of a damaged body image. This is achieved by identification with a perfect fetus and by overcoming a sense of castration with a swelling abdomen. He also contends that with pregnancy women strengthen their sense of female identity by competing with other psychologically significant female rivals, or that women may use pregnancy as a means of self-punishment for guilty thoughts and deeds [17].

In addition to the psychoanalytic theories, a number of other explanations of the motivations of women in bearing children should be examined. In America, like most societies, childbearing is still emphasized by many groups as a primary function of women. This aspect of the feminine role is communicated at an early age, and women who choose not to conform to this expectation often feel guilty, self-doubting and incomplete regarding their feminine role.

Having children can satisfy a number of needs: confirmation of feminine identity, a sense of recognition and adequacy as a mature woman, a substitute for unachieved career aspirations, and a means for easier participation in the activities of friends and relatives who already have children. A couple may look forward to having their own characteristics reflected and passed on in a child. For some parents, childbearing may represent an opportunity to compensate for their own inadequacies by rearing a child who will achieve what they have not been able to accomplish. If their own childhood was not happy, they may look forward to the opportunity of demonstrating their own abilities to be good parents or they may doubt whether they can adequately parent a child. Other individuals may want to reproduce the kind of environment and happy experiences they had as children.

Many people anticipate satisfaction and fulfillment from parenthood. The child may be someone the parent can cuddle, love, nurture, and teach; on the other hand, the child may be thought of as a burden, causing the sacrifice of freedom and a restriction on financial independence.

The appraisal of one's own competence for motherhood or fatherhood affects the decision to have children, as does the relationship with one's younger siblings. Childbearing motivations are also influenced by the relationship with and attitude of one's mate—for example, whether he or she is seen as a potentially good parent and is interested in having children. A couple may anticipate that a child will bring them closer together. Positive influences are provided by the special attention that accompanies pregnancy and the curiosity that is satisfied by it.

An individual's relationship with his own parents is another important consideration. Becoming a parent may symbolize independence from one's own parents; at the same time, it provides an opportunity to satisfy the desire of one's own parents for grandchildren.

Before their reproductive years end, older couples may be highly motivated to have children, as are couples who have been childless because of difficulties in reproducing.

While all of the foregoing factors may be positive motivations for having children, they may have negative aspects that serve as deterrents [17].

ASPECTS OF THE PARENTAL ROLE   Whatever their motivations may be, a couple contemplating having children soon realizes, as Rossi notes, that there are some aspects of this role that are unique when compared to their other major roles as adult members of society, the roles of marriage partner and worker [42]. Educational preparation for parenthood is often minimal. For 12 years, most Americans prepare formally for further education or for employment, spending little or no time learning about how to prepare for parenthood. During this time, some individuals also do reality testing of their future work role, exploring their likes and dislikes as part-time workers before the responsibility of working full time falls upon them.

In the United States most couples date or are engaged for variable periods of time before marriage; during this courtship, aspects of the husband-wife relationship can be tested. This may range from enjoying each other's company for long periods of time, socializing as a couple, and finding housing and buying furniture, to living and loving together. In so doing, many of the assumptions they hold about what it will be like to be married can be verified or rejected; the choice is still open.

Other than babysitting, care of young siblings, or possibly the buying of baby equipment, for prospective parents there is no such preparatory period for reality testing. With the birth of the baby, the transition to parenthood on a 24-hour basis occurs abruptly. The options for rejection of the role at this point barely exist.

According to many authorities, another unique feature of the parental role is the absence of objective standards by which success or failure can be measured during childrearing. Definite criteria exist by which satisfactory role fulfillment as a worker can be judged, and there are popular conceptions of what constitutes a successful marriage, but the objective criteria for parents to judge their success or failure while their children are growing are much more elusive.

Unlike beginning a job or entering into marriage, both of which, for the most part, are entered into voluntarily, pregnancy may be the result of pleasure-motivated sexual activity with no conscious desire to become a parent. Certainly the number of induced abortions, estimated at one million a year, reflects this difference. Likewise, society's attitude toward terminating a potential parental role by abortion differs greatly from its attitude toward terminating one's job or marriage. Certainly this is also true with terminating an actual parental role. Even children who have been legally adopted often become involved in trying to locate or be located by natural parents. The energy and emotion involved here are more intense than that involved in trying to reestablish ties with former mates or jobs.

Society's pressure to assume the parental role is perhaps the common factor that unites the other major adult roles. Women, particularly, are supposed to like children and want babies. Contrary opinions and feelings are still generally met with disapproval. While most people do want children, not all children are wanted. One study [11] of over 200 American mothers from a low-income group reported that slightly over half clearly wanted their children. A Scottish study [43] reported that in a sample of almost 300 primigravidas, 41 percent did not want the pregnancy, 41 percent wanted it, and 18 percent did not mind. In a sampling of over 200 student wives, 64 percent stated they were happy about their pregnancies [39]. Still another study [19] reports that 80 percent of the sampled women were happy about their first one or two children, but only 31 percent were happy about the fourth or more. Other studies reflect higher percentages being happy about the fourth child, but these studies are based on subjects from favored economic groups and also from data obtained sometime after the children were born. Data collected from women while they are pregnant yield more negative responses [45].

FEELINGS DURING PREGNANCY

There have been too few objective large-scale studies to identify common patterns of emotional response in fathers and mothers throughout childbearing. Nevertheless, pregnancy is generally regarded by psychologists and other health care workers as a period of increased susceptibility to crisis. It is a time when preventive intervention can do much to influence the attitudes and functioning of prospective parents.

During childbearing, the couple is faced with the challenges of redefining their present roles, working through old and possibly forgotten conflict relationships, and entering the parent role. In addition, it is a period that can encourage further development of the couple's mutual concern, tenderness, and intimacy. The emotional and physical adjustments required of the parents cause varying levels of stress and anxiety; these may change from one pregnancy to another in the same couple.

Some of the specific factors that contribute to the psychologic response of the parents include body image changes, cultural expectations, relationships with and support of parents and close relatives, emotional security and positive relationships within the marriage, economic security, adequacy of housing, number of other children, and the interval between pregnancies. While pregnancy has been characterized by some as a period of dependency and possibly regression in the mother, this tendency is reduced by a secure life situation, a harmonious environment, and emotional support. In the past pregnant women have frequently been labeled dependent or regressed without a realistic appraisal of the stresses placed on them and of the resources available that might help them cope more effectively.

Much of the empirical research in this area has dealt with anxiety, mood swings, and depression; it has focused on the postpartum period and has considered on a retrospective basis the woman's personality characteristics, whether the pregnancy was wanted, and whether the woman was anxious or insecure. Nilsson, on the basis of a prospective study in which a large number of women were followed until 6 months post partum, inferred that women who have a strong feminine identity have a less tumultuous pregnancy and postpartum period [38]. This theme was echoed in Cohen's research [12]. Cohen also considered the experience of the father and his importance in satisfying his partner's dependency needs. Liebenberg emphasized the sense of stress felt by the father, particularly where his sexual identity was concerned, mainly because of his identification with his pregnant partner [33].

Many researchers have viewed pregnancy as a period of crisis. Bibring [7] postulated that pregnancy is a time when old unresolved conflicts resurface for some reworking and (ideally) resolution. These conflicts may involve issues of dependency, autonomy, and past relationships with the woman's mother. Reworking such conflicts helps the woman to establish her sense of self as distinct from her own mother. Deutsch [54] maintained that childbearing may produce guilt in the woman who feels that she is usurping the prerogatives of her own mother and fears retaliation by her. Therese Benedek [6] also emphasized the importance of a woman's sense of her own mother. How she "received" mothering influences how she will "mother."

Expectant Mother   Because it is a time when so many strange, threatening, and seemingly unpredictable things are happening to her, the pregnant woman has much she would like to talk about yet hesitates to do so for fear of being reprimanded or appearing abnormal or ignorant. According to Caplan [9], there is a shift in the woman's intrapsychic equilibrium; old conflicts and fantasies that were repressed in the unconscious come to the surface. It is as though a weakening of the normal defense forces has occurred, allowing previously unacceptable, irrational thoughts and impulses to surface. The accompanying free-floating anxiety is fixed to various objects and situations in the form of phobias, fearful forebodings, and dreams. The dreams, which may indicate apprehension, involve the infant, misfortunes, environmental threats such as being attacked, and, later in the pregnancy, the process of labor and delivery.

Pregnant women, according to Larsen [31], identify more tangible sources of anxiety in the prenatal period, such as physical discomfort, medical complications, fatigue and irritability, depression, fear of an abnormal baby, and fear for themselves. These anxieties, along with their emotional lability and their thoughts about death and dying, cause them on occasion to question their sanity and their ability to cope. Reassurance that these are normal reactions is an essential part of prenatal care. Pregnant women need an attentive listener, one who displays more than a casual interest in how they are doing, and who will encourage them to verbalize their anxieties.

Every woman must go through the process of adjusting to the reality of the pregnancy, to the fetus as a separate individual, and to the fact that the pregnancy must come to an end. These tasks of pregnancy may be very difficult for the woman who does not have adequate support systems to help her cope with them. Many times the health professional must fill such gaps when they exist. Meeting the needs of the pregnant woman is a team effort, and you may be responsible for seeing that her care is not fragmented.

Kitzinger [29] states that many women have an inability to adjust to the role of pregnancy and motherhood. Even if the baby has been planned, the fact that the pregnancy is a reality still comes as a shock. The woman herself becomes someone different, a subject of interest and concern to society and to health care personnel who ask a variety of personal questions. Some women may be faced with a role that they are unwilling or unable to play, a role that may be unfamiliar and frightening. A woman may indicate that she feels this way if she tries to hide her pregnancy by the clothes she chooses or appears overly concerned that she is losing her figure too soon.

Many times a woman may feel that others are interested in her because she is carrying a baby, not for her own sake. This is reinforced by health care professionals who emphasize the need to protect her baby's health.

The woman may feel alone and unwanted, especially if her partner thinks of pregnancy as a "woman's affair." She may be disturbed by the lack of control she has over the pregnancy process once it has started, the changes in her body image, the changes in her body movements. She will be able to cope with these feelings more successfully if she has a partner who is supportive and affectionate.

Kitzinger [29] points out the woman's need for information and reassurance. Whatever her background and support systems, her relationship with the professionals who provide her health care will affect her outlook on pregnancy. She is especially sensitive to whatever is said to her, and wonders about the meaning of comments like "the baby's a little small," especially when they are not explained to her. It is particularly helpful when the woman's partner is welcomed in the health care agency since the prospective parents are often able to offer each other mutual support.

Kitzinger also emphasizes that as a society we have rather unrealistic ideas about maternal instinct. Many women anticipate having only loving, happy thoughts of babies and motherhood; thus, they are often quite upset to find that they experience as many conflicting emotions about pregnancy and the baby as they do about any other life experience that produces stress and forces them into new patterns of thinking and behaving.

Expectant Father For the expectant father, the changes caused by pregnancy influence his self-concept, his relationship to the woman, and his role in the social world outside the home. While the baby's birth is perhaps the most spectacular moment, a man's psychologic involvement in pregnancy is shown in many ways.

Some men have physical complaints similar to the common symptoms of pregnancy, with the more anxious expectant fathers having the greater number of symptoms. Some have nausea and vomiting, constipation or diarrhea, or headaches and dizzy spells. Studies have shown nausea and vomiting are the most common symptoms, along with loss of appetite and toothache [50]. Symptoms may appear at any time but usually do not appear before the end of the second to the middle of the third month; they are, it is believed, most likely to be the result of feelings of ambivalence toward or identification or empathy with the woman.

Some husbands or partners feel lonely and unwanted as the woman becomes more and more involved in her pregnancy experience. It has been suggested that the man may actually envy the woman's power of bearing children (a counterpart to the woman's penis envy, a theme that appears in some of the literature) [29]. The unconscious desire of the man to share in the pregnancy may actually be expressed in the practice of "couvade," a custom of primitive cultures whereby the husband is treated as if he, and not his wife, were having the baby. He may develop the physical symptoms mentioned above [50].

A man, aware of his strong feelings and desiring to be drawn into the experience, may begin to express extra concern for the pregnant woman. She, unaware of his sense of isolation, may interpret his increased attention as overprotectiveness and grow to resent it. On the other hand, he may withdraw into his own world, asserting his masculine role aggressively. He may pretend to take no interest in his wife's condition or in her feelings about the pregnancy, and consequently she feels hurt at his lack of attention. Couples who prepare together for childbirth and who share the concerns generated by pregnancy are much less likely to grow apart and experience feelings of abandonment [29].

Unfortunately, the impact of pregnancy on men has undergone little investigation in terms of the functional adaptations men make to their new roles. Some studies describe the impact as awakening unresolved conflicts within the man.

The waiting and wondering, combined with a lack of clear responsibilities and roles during the pregnancy, often increase the stress men experience during this period. A number of elements are crucial to the coping abilities of new fathers: the partner relationship and its ability to adjust to the introduction of the new family member; the financial resources of the man and variables that relate to those resources, such as age and education; good support systems, such as family, friends, and work; a commitment to the father role and an effort to prepare for the role; a healthy baby and a healthy mother [49]. Some of these factors are within the control of the man as he nears fatherhood; many, however, are not. The new father must cope with considerable stress as he assumes his new role.

Antle postulates that a man's psychologic involvement in pregnancy may be inhibited by the lack of a clearly defined paternal role, by cultural conditioning, and by a matricentric view of expectant parenthood [5]. As a child, he has been socialized into predominantly occupational roles. During the pregnancy, unlike the woman he has no physiologic changes to reinforce its reality. He gets most of his information secondhand since his partner, and most likely her physician, midwife, or nurse, know what is happening before he does. Antle suggests a prospective father's concerns, emotions, and conflicts relate to four general areas: his protective feelings toward his partner; his anxieties about his role as provider; his fears about the physical vulnerability of his partner and child; and his heightened dependency needs and nurturant or "feminine" emotions. McNall [36] found that the most frequent concern of fathers was their feelings of helplessness and apprehension about labor and delivery. The men in her sample were moderately concerned about the couple's relationship and feelings about impending fatherhood. She suggests that it may be very important for the father to verbally reconstruct his labor and delivery experience in the immediate postdelivery days so that he can relive it and work through it psychologically.

Shannon-Babitz [44] evaluated the needs of eight fathers who wished to participate in their partners' labor and delivery, and her conclusions echo McNall's postulations. Her findings indicate the importance of the father's labor and delivery experiences and the great need he has for support from the nursing staff. This may be provided by reinforcing his participation in the event (suggesting ways that he can help provide physical comfort to his partner), by meeting his physical needs (providing him with a comfortable chair and pillows or suggesting he take breaks when his partner's labor is not very active), and by enhancing his self-esteem (asking if there are any special ways you can help to make the experience more meaningful, praising his contributions to the team effort).

Stresses for the expectant father during pregnancy include coping with the woman's increasing dependency, particularly when the extended family members are far away, and coping with the threat of the loss of the woman's undivided attention and the threat to the couple's economic stability [41]. In addition, as he reflects on and evaluates the role his father played when he was a child, he begins to wonder what kind of a father he will be. Even an expectant father who has other children may feel ambivalence, evaluating his past fathering and projecting what it will be like with an additional child. Thus, pregnancy is frequently a period of insecurity for men.

The most comprehensive review of parents' reactions to childbearing is provided by the Colmans in their book *Pregnancy: The Psychological Experience* [13].

They, as well as other authorities, differentiate the emotions that predominate in each trimester.

First Trimester   The most important task for the woman during the first trimester is accepting the reality of her pregnancy and understanding its implications. Perhaps because of the physical discomforts during this period and the feelings of insecurity about new or additional responsibilities, ambivalence is the primary emotion. Initial positive reactions are more likely to be found in primigravidas. Because initial negative attitudes may be replaced by more accepting ones later in the pregnancy, unplanned babies are not always unwelcomed babies. Likewise, planned babies are not always welcomed once the woman faces the realities of pregnancy and motherhood.

Many factors are involved in the woman's reactions to and ambivalence about the pregnancy. For most women, the focus in the first trimester is on themselves, since there is little tangible evidence of the baby's growth. Physical discomforts and subtle changes within her body demand her attention. She must cope with things such as nausea, vomiting, tender and swollen breasts, irritability, headache, fatigue, depression, and anxiety. The sudden and inexplicable mood swings contribute to the day-to-day difficulties faced by many pregnant women.

In a recent article in a popular woman's magazine, women are quoted as stating that they had not been prepared for the emotional turmoil they experienced during pregnancy—the identity crises, their preoccupations with the health of their babies, their dislike of their own bodies, and the periods of reevaluation of their relationships with their partners. Until recently, many women, thinking they would be labeled as bad mothers, did not share their anxieties with anyone. They are now beginning to talk about their feelings which they believe have been too casually cast aside by others. They resent being told "It's just because you're pregnant, dear," when they believe that a far deeper issue is involved—the fact that their lives are changing and they have little control [48].

One pregnant woman, reflecting on her future responsibilities, stated: I have dreams that the baby doesn't know how to laugh or cry, and I have to guess if it's happy or sick. I wake up in the middle of the night with fears that I won't be a good mother, that I won't know the needs of the different sexes. What gives a boy a strong male identity? Can I raise a girl to be confident about herself? How did my mother know how to raise me? [48].

Another woman, who had recently given birth, said that she felt that she had been involved in a conspiracy of mothers:

Women who have gone through it don't tell someone who has just gotten pregnant and is throwing up every few minutes that she's going to have to sit up to sleep, that she will be so enormous for the last six weeks that she'll find it difficult to breathe, and that she is going to have to work through a bushel of fears and anxieties. Sometimes I think that mothers are like pathological joggers who are always selling the sport. Anybody who has ever jogged knows that it's painful and crazy to go out at seven o'clock in the morning and run five miles. But joggers sell it as being a terrific experience, to get other people to do it [48].

There are other reactions and adjustments required in the first trimester. For some women there is a decrease in sexual desire, perhaps caused by nausea and fatigue or by changes in body image (e.g., breast enlargement and weight increase), which may seem great even at this early stage. Intercourse after conception may produce guilt for those who feel that its purpose is for childbearing. Other reasons for a decrease in sexual desire include fear of injuring the baby, insecurity, and financial and personal worries. However, some women feel more sensual during pregnancy and show an increased sexual drive, wanting to be cuddled, played with, and cared for. Even the most stable relationship may be upset by the changes now taking place. Therefore, it is important for a couple to understand and be prepared for what might happen.

Toward the end of the first trimester and into the second trimester, the primigravida concerns herself with her relationship with her own mother. She now becomes concerned with the kind of mother she will be and begins forming her own maternal identity, incorporating the good qualities to which she has been previously exposed. In doing so, she reviews those facets of her own childhood that produced pleasant and unpleasant feelings. Multigravidas generally review their past experience of mothering in light of an additional child.

For expectant fathers also, the main task during the first trimester is the acceptance of the reality of the pregnancy. This is generally accompanied by mixed emotions. Even those men who dread the responsibility of childrearing may take pride in this proof of their masculinity.

Whatever he feels, his wife will probably be seeking reassurance that he is pleased, that he will not reject her. . . . A husband may at first be pleased with the demands made upon him. . . . But if she is unable to get up every morning or falls asleep each time he wants to make love, it is likely that he will lose his warm protective feelings toward her and become more resentful and demanding [13].

By the end of the first trimester, he begins to feel the responsibilities of fatherhood and questions his competence. He is now involved with the realistic particulars demanded by an enlarging family: need for additional room, financial concerns, and emotional stress and strain. At the same time, he senses the woman's involvement with herself and may feel excluded.

It is still too early for common issues of parenthood to unite husband and wife. If there is to be a mutual alliance during the pregnancy, it must begin to be forged at this stage, before the uniqueness of their experiences creates obstacles too great to be bridged [13].

During the first trimester help the couple to accept the reality of the pregnancy by encouraging them to verbalize their feelings of its unreality. Give them the chance to hear the fetal heartbeat as soon as possible. Counsel them about the emotional changes they may experience [14].

Second Trimester Caplan and other authorities view the second trimester as a time when the mother becomes increasingly introverted, passive, and dependent. Caplan [9] sees the woman as a taker instead of a giver, a situation often requiring family adjustment. Hanford [24] reports that conflicts decline during the second trimester; by this time many women have come to accept the pregnancy. In interpreting data, however, one must remember that acceptance does not necessarily imply happiness. While many women are happy about their pregnancy, some regard it as a stress for as long as six months post partum or longer [38].

The highlight of the second trimester is feeling the baby move, which facilitates awareness of the baby as a separate individual. Perhaps more than in the previous trimester, the woman feels a loss of control as her pregnancy becomes more visible. The fact of intercourse can no longer be hidden; sexually inhibited women may feel shame or disgust. As one woman describes her feelings:

You are quite obviously pregnant; then it is a queer naked feeling to walk along the street and feel no longer anonymous, realizing that there is one secret of your life that everyone who looks can know—that at least one private incident of your past has become almost incredibly public and that you can bear, as it were, the stigma of past passion wherever you go [32].

Figure changes may be awaited with either eagerness or dread. With societal emphasis on a slim appearance, the pregnant woman may experience a reduction in feelings of self-esteem [14]. Jessner [27] points out that few things happen to a woman's body that can compare with the changes produced by pregnancy. Both Jessner and Fawcett [16] comment on the increased amount of space that pregnant women perceive their bodies to occupy; Fawcett noted that fathers may also perceive their own bodies to occupy more space as pregnancy progresses. Carty [10] demonstrated that not only do pregnant women feel dissatisfaction with their bodies but that the feeling may be even greater in the postpartum period. Helping the couple to understand that their feelings of dissatisfaction about body-image change during pregnancy and post partum are usual and to be expected may make it easier for them to cope with the situation. Sometimes allowing them to express feelings of dissatisfaction and reminding them of the transitory nature of the pregnancy can be helpful [16].

Some women may feel more erotic in the second trimester. There is, according to Masters and Johnson [35], a physical basis for this: Vaginal lubrication and the blood flow to the pelvic region increase, which causes the erogenous areas to become engorged more rapidly and excitement to linger after orgasm. This erotic feeling may make the woman more sexually demanding than her partner can cope with, especially with the obstacles of her changing shape and mood swings. Some couples may achieve better sexual relationships; however, if they cannot discuss their sexual feelings, the entire relationship may deteriorate.

The man takes on new importance in the woman's eyes during this trimester, and she becomes very concerned for his safety. The woman's closeness to her partner is more evident if her mother or other close relatives or friends are not available to help care for her or plan for the baby.

Feeling the baby move is also a dramatic high point for the expectant father, intensifying the reality of his coming fatherhood. He may become preoccupied with childhood memories about his mother's or a relative's pregnancies, or even dream of becoming pregnant himself. He may become upset as he recognizes his own nurturant qualities or feels envy or jealousy toward the mother of his child. The woman's dependence on him and her concern about him and his safety may be a threat to his independence. In an effort to cope with these increased demands, expectant fathers may now develop new hobbies or devote more time to their work.

Third Trimester   During the third trimester, women feel a sense of accomplishment as well as anxiety about the coming labor and delivery. The anxiety shows a definite increase in the last half of the third trimester, according to Grimm [21]. In several studies [31, 52] multigravidas show higher anxiety levels than primigravidas; therefore, as the Colmans note, it is not valid to assume that multigravidas feel they have proved themselves or know what it is all about [13].

In addition to labor and delivery, the baby becomes the pregnant woman's main focus in the last trimester. Much of her time and thoughts are consumed with making the final preparations for the baby, naming him, and dreaming of how he will appear. The end of pregnancy can be a very sentimental time as she thinks of the special privileges that have been hers for the past months. Despite this, she looks forward to the end of pregnancy, for it is more difficult to sleep, eat, and carry out many of her daily activities. Another source of concern at this time for some pregnant women is that careers are temporarily interrupted as they are forced to leave their jobs.

Kitzinger [29] reports that many women suffer from depression about six weeks or a month before delivery. This is a time when their self-confidence is lowest, when their fears become dominant, and when they become most impatient with their pregnancy. Sometimes little morale-lifters can be very helpful to the woman. If she is prepared to expect this let-down feeling, it may be easier for her to accept the fact that she must adjust to her new slower body rhythms and allow herself more rest. It is at this time that she will be most tempted to rebel against her self-imposed disciplines, to eat and drink whatever she desires, to forget her exercises, to forget her pregnancy.

Kitzinger [29] also comments on the fear that many women have that their baby will be malformed or dead, especially if they have been smoking, drinking, or taking drugs. This fear may also be felt by women who considered abortion when they found out that they were pregnant, as though they might be punished for having had such negative feelings. Such fears are particularly common after the fifth month of pregnancy when the baby becomes more of a reality to the mother. If she expresses fears of this nature, mere explanations by the health professional that few babies are born malformed are not so helpful as further exploration of her feelings and thoughtful listening.

Sherwen [46] points out that fantasies during the third trimester of pregnancy are quite common. Themes that were predominant among the women in her sample were fantasies about having an abnormal infant, being attacked, being enclosed or drowning, forgetting or losing things, and being unprepared. Sherwen offers the following suggestions for nursing colleagues in helping the woman to cope with her fantasies: Encourage the discussion of day or night dreams that the woman has found disturbing; listen to her with a nonjudgmental attitude; help her to understand that her fantasies are not unique; supply missing factual information where appropriate to alleviate some of the woman's concern.

The third trimester is a time when the pregnant woman especially questions her self-image since she seems so large and her shape is so different. She needs reassurance that she is still loved. Attempts at intercourse may now pose a problem:

The wife's abdomen may present an insurmountable obstacle for a couple whose sex practices have always been conservative. Guilt or regression may result from experimentation with alternate modes of gratification which rely on exotic postures or oral and manual manipulation [13].

It is especially important that the couple be close and communicate well with each other because of the experimentation that lovemaking may require or the fact that abstinence may be the choice of some couples.

By the third trimester the expectant father has had to cope with some of the problems brought on by the pregnancy. Men who have avoided dealing with the pregnancy in the past will continue to do so, spending their time and energies at work, with hobbies, or perhaps with other women [26].

Men actively involved with the pregnancy are drawn into practical activities such as helping with final preparations for the baby, planning for the trip to the hospital, and dealing realistically with financial issues. Some expectant fathers may participate in childbirth education classes with the woman and learn specific ways to care for her. Some may share the woman's increasing anxiety, and, in working together, their relationship may become more intense. Since some men may feel a sense of responsibility for the pregnancy, they may feel more tender or protective toward the woman. A man's own ideas about fathering now become more concrete.

A New Approach by Clinicians

Recently some attention has been given to the use of drawings to help health professionals come to a better understanding of some of the perceptions and attitudes held by men and women who are going through the pregnancy experience. One such attempt by Lumley has shed some light on how women view their fetuses during the first trimester [34]. Only nine of the 30 women in the sample thought the fetus was a real person at this point in pregnancy. Most women grossly underestimated the size and development of the fetus as well as its activities, attributing formless, unattractive, and animal-like features to it. In another report of drawings done by pregnant couples [25], the researchers state that such drawings many times offer an avenue for the couples to express the negative side of ambivalent feelings when it would not be otherwise acceptable.

FAMILY SUPPORTS

In our society the nuclear family (mother, father, and children) is the best known family form. The Industrial Revolution has been considered the turning point from which the nuclear family evolved from the extended family, although some historical evidence indicates that it was the prevailing residential unit long before that time [20]. The nuclear family has been considered the center of emotional support, responsible for the growth of privacy in the family, and a way of better training the young in an isolated and controlled setting [20].

Within the nuclear family, members are not influenced as much by the limits and standards of older generations but rather have the opportunity to test things on their own. Stereotyped masculine and feminine roles are not as workable, since both partners must work together as an intimate team. Of necessity, the myriad of family needs are satisfied by few family members. In the nuclear family the pregnant woman has her husband for support. Unless she has sufficient money or close friends or relatives nearby, her support system may be limited to him.

The nuclear family has been criticized for the above reasons, and also because of the intense relationship that develops among the family members and the fact that its children have few adult role models. Some critics feel that society has gradually usurped many of the functions of the nuclear family, e.g., as a recreational facility, as a socializing group for children, and for personal fulfillment of its members.

The extended family (mother, father, children, and one or more relatives) has a number of advantages. The daily work may be shared, as well as the economic cost of maintaining the household. According to some authorities, children who are cared for by several loving adults may be able to relate more easily to others. They may develop their male or female identities with less difficulty because they have been exposed to more role models. In general, they receive better socialization than those confined to two parents in the nuclear family. For some adults, the extended family provides security; for others, it requires conformity, limiting the opportunity to develop new life-styles [40].

The resurgence of the communal movement in America represented an attempt to allow for new ways of living and approaches to problem-solving, while incorporating the more positive aspects of the extended family. The communal movement in urban as well as rural settings has assumed a number of different forms. In some instances, the commune retains nuclear family units within it, and couples simply live in the same residence. In other communes, there are no identifiable smaller family units and everything is shared in common. Members may or may not hold jobs outside the commune.

The more stable, longer-lived communes are usually highly structured and tend to be centered around a common ideology, values, and goals. Decision-making is usually done by the group according to majority rule; responsibility for daily work, expenses, and childrearing is shared. Less stable communes seem to lack a strong cohesiveness and organization. While their members espouse a philosophy of closeness and involvement, they function fairly independently, often leaving group conflicts unresolved and work unfinished [28].

Home delivery with the father and midwife or doctor present is popular in some communes, since it reduces medical intervention and allows the childbirth experience to be shared more fully. The child is with the mother from the moment of birth and may be breast-fed for several years. In more radical communes birth certificates may be scorned, since the individual is then registered and will become a likely candidate for taxation and compulsory public education [47].

THE SINGLE PARENT   In contrast to the support offered in the extended family and some communal systems, the responsibilities of family life in the one-parent family fall for the most part on a lone individual [30]. Single-parent families result from single-parent adoptions, loss of one parent through death or divorce, or unwed parenthood, a major source of single-parent families in the United States today. One of five children under the age of 18 in America today lives in a one-parent family. For blacks the proportion is about one in two, according to new Census Bureau reports. The 1980 figures contrast sharply with those from 1960 when only 12.4 percent of children lived in single-parent households [37a].

This increase in single-parent families is a striking social development of the past generation. About 19 percent of all families with children, and more than 38 percent among black families alone, are now headed by a single parent. Single parenthood, poverty, and dependency on public welfare are often linked. There is some speculation about why the figures are so much higher for black families. Low earnings, lack of economic security, and relatively high unemployment among black men have been cited as factors that may discourage marriage by women who become pregnant. Since marriage is economically unappealing or impractical, many women will bear and care for their babies alone [37a].

A small but growing number of single-parent families result from the change in adoption policies since the mid-1960s. These changes took place in response to the difficulties in finding homes for children with physical handicaps, older children, and children of a minority or mixed race. It is now recognized that a single parent can adequately raise children if given sufficient support from the parent's friends, relatives, and community resources.

In the past one of the concerns of adoption agencies about single individuals adopting children was the lack of a suitable role model for the development of sexual identity. Today they look for a male or female figure in the adopting single parent's circle of friends or relatives. Even without one, they recognize that with an emotionally mature mother or father, a child can be expected to develop an appropriate sexual identity.

Single individuals adopting children appear to be emotionally mature, self-aware, self-confident, and able to tolerate a great deal of frustration. They tend to pursue an independent life and are not overly concerned about what other people think. While they do not have to be well educated, studies show that they are intelligent. They are motivated more by what they can contribute to the child's normal development than by the fulfillment of their own needs [8].

Single-parent families resulting from divorce, desertion, separation, or death must cope with a number of problems. Because the remaining parent must develop a different life-style, he is initially faced with a period of adjustment. He has to adjust to parenting for 24 hours a day without the assistance of the other parent that he once had. Other problems involve finding day-care centers and housekeepers and a need both to work and to provide the additional emotional support to the child that was formerly supplied by the other parent. According to the Eglesons [15], the children often react by developing closer ties and being more sympathetic to the remaining parent. However, some children resent the fact that the parent's job requires that they assume more responsibility at home.

ADOPTION   Adoption has a long history. Early Romans, Egyptians, and Greeks used adoption as a means of providing an heir or successor. The Bible mentions the adoption of Moses and Esther. It is only since the 1850s in the United States that adoption has had legal restrictions placed on it [2]. Before that time couples took parentless children into their homes, often treating them as second class citizens and using them to provide extra help. Until the beginning of the twentieth century adopted children were still expected to work harder than biologic children to show their gratitude to the adoptive parents. Gradually adoption came to be seen as a means of satisfying the emotional needs of the infertile couple. In more recent years adoption has been viewed more as a way of meeting the child's needs as well as the prospective parents' needs.

Table 9-1 reflects the steady increase in adoptions until 1971. Complete national statistics are not available after 1971 when a decline in adoptions began, but figures available for those states reporting between 1972 and 1975 continue to reflect a decrease in total adoptions completed. The number of black children placed has declined most precipitously [37].

Type of Adoption	1955	1960	1965	1968	1970	1971
By relatives	45	49	65	80	86	86
By nonrelatives	48	58	77	86	89	83
Placed by social agencies	27	33	53	64	69	66
Total number of adoptions	93	107	142	166	175	169

Source: Modified from U.S. National Center for Health Statistics. *Vital Statistics of the United States*. Washington, D.C. (published annually).

In spite of the decline in completed adoptions, statistics indicate that the demand for adoptions continues to rise. The supply of white babies available for adoption has greatly decreased, mainly because of better birth control methods, liberalized abortion laws, and the increasing number of unmarried mothers who decide to keep their babies. Fewer than 30 percent of the babies born to unmarried mothers in a year are adopted. As a result in the United States the patterns of adoption are changing. Policies are becoming somewhat more flexible and the number of single-parent adoptions is increasing. Children with handicaps, older children, and children of all minority groups are being placed more frequently. Although they remain only a fraction of total U.S. adoptions, adoptions of children born in foreign countries have increased each year [37]. This has been particularly true since the mid-1970s when many Vietnamese children were adopted by American families. As the number of nonwhite or mixed race children adopted by white families has increased, critics have expressed concern that these children might lose their racial identity and be forced to cope with a host of other related problems. Subsequent research has failed to support these predicted consequences.

It is suggested that more black families might adopt if there were not misunderstandings of adoption requirements regarding age, economic status, and proof of sterility. Other deterrents have included a reluctance to be questioned about personal matters, the expectation of rejection, anxiety about filling out required forms, and inability to meet the legal fees [1, 18, 23].

About half of the children adopted each year are adopted by relatives. Of the other 50 percent, well over half involve children born out of wedlock. About 80 percent of these adoptions by nonrelatives are arranged by social agencies, while the other 20 percent result from independent adoptions [37]. In the latter instance, the child is placed directly with the adoptive parents, either by the mother herself or through an unlicensed intermediary, such as a physician, lawyer, or minister.

In agency adoptions, the child is first placed with an agency and from there with the adoptive parents. While agency adoptions seem to be more controlled, there are still a number of associated problems. Often there are unnecessary delays, long waiting lists of up to 3 years, and restrictive policies. Substandard legal and health services may be a problem if there is inadequate legal and medical staff supervision [2]. An agency adoption is usually completed in about 2 years after the process is initiated.

A service provided by some agencies is the collection of detailed information about the natural father as well as the mother, which they can make available to the adoptive parents. This effort is directed toward providing adopted children with a realistic and more complete picture of their biological heritage and with the reasons their natural parents chose adoption for them [3].

Problems associated with independent adoptions are far more numerous. This type of adoption can foster a "black market" in baby-selling. There is no assurance that the intermediary is competent or willing to do the studies of prospective parents usually completed by agencies. It is also unlikely that the natural mother will receive casework help, and there is a greater likelihood that she will try to get her baby back. Frequently the child is not legally free for adoption at the time he is placed and at the time the adoption should be completed [2]. Independent adoptions, which are usually completed in about 6 months to 1 year, have been outlawed in five states [37].

The best professional service is provided when lawyers, social workers, and doctors work cooperatively to represent the best interests of the child, whose rights supersede those of the natural or adoptive parents. It is paramount in importance that the child is placed in a family evaluated by qualified persons as having emotional, physical, mental, financial, and spiritual qualities that will best implement the child's maximum development [53].

At the same time the natural mother has the right to medical, legal, religious, and financial assistance during her pregnancy, delivery, and recovery. She also has the right to decide about the disposition of her child under a minimum of pressure. When the parents are not married, generally only the mother's consent is necessary for purposes of adoption. Once she has relinquished the child for adoption, she may lose her right to participate in decisions about the child's future, except to ask that he be placed in a family whose religion is similar to hers. (This exception seems to be becoming less common [22].) Recent court cases have challenged the concept that the mother's decision is irrevocable, however, and the flexibility of the "withdrawal of consent" statutes varies from state to state.

The general rule has been that the mother's right to the child supersedes the father's, but the father's right is superior to that of all other persons. While historically only the mother had to consent to an adoption, since 1972 the father of the child must be afforded the right to notice of any adoption, custody, or termination proceeding concerning the child. Since the Supreme Court did not indicate the form or extent of the notice required nor clarify the extent of the father's role in such proceedings, state courts and legislatures have differed in their interpretations of the ruling [37].

The adoptive parents have a right to know the physical, social, mental, and emotional makeup of the natural parents of the child. They also have a right to be protected against the possibility that the natural parents might change their minds about the adoption. The child must reside in the adoptive home for a period of 6 to 12 months before legal adoption can take place. Once the adoption has been finalized, the child and the adoptive parents have the same legal rights as any other family.

Research by Walker [51] indicates that adoptive parents have information needs (about normal growth and development, helping the child adapt to a new environment), feeling needs (for encouragement), and judgment needs (how to fit the child into existing patterns of living, how to handle problem behavior in the child). Mothers who had adopted children as their first or second child reported more informational and judgment needs relating to parenting than other adoptive parents. Walker emphasizes that nurses can be a valuable and nonthreatening resource to new adoptive parents in helping them to gain skill and confidence. Well-child examinations might provide an ideal time for you to spend extra time with the parents, listening to them, answering their questions, and complimenting them on the good job they are doing as parents. A valuable referral resource might be a self-help group of other adoptive parents where they might share common concerns. If no such group exists, you might be instrumental in organizing one.

Problem Situation   Anticipating Parenthood

Bob and Laura Brown are 27-year-old graduate students who are having their first baby. Although the baby was unplanned, the couple decided to proceed with the pregnancy. When Laura comes for a check-up at the beginning of her second trimester, you notice that she appears somewhat reticent. When you share this observation with her, you learn that she is still not sure that she and Bob have made the right decision. She states that one minute she feels happy and the next minute she starts crying. She has sensed at times that Bob just does not understand why she is behaving as she does. She herself feels that she is "losing her mind."

What additional assessments would you want to make before addressing the current needs of Bob and Laura? What elements would you be sure to include in your nursing care?

REFERENCES

1. Adoption, 1975. *Contemporary Obstetrics/Gynecology* 5:35, 1975.
2. American Academy of Pediatrics. *Adoption of Children.* Evanston, Ill., 1967.
3. Anglim, E. The adopted child's heritage—Two natural parents. *Child Welfare* 44:339, 1965.
4. Anthony, E. J., and Benedek, T. (Eds.). *Parenthood: Its Psychology and Psychopathology.* Boston: Little, Brown, 1970.
5. Antle, K. Psychologic involvement in pregnancy by expectant fathers. *Journal of Obstetric, Gynecologic and Neonatal Nursing* 4(4):40, 1975.
6. Benedek, T. The organization of the reproductive drive. *International Journal of Psychoanalysis* 41:1, 1960.
7. Bibring, G. Some considerations of the psychological processes in pregnancy. *Psychoanalytic Studies of the Child* 14:113, 1959.
8. Branham, E. One parent adoptions. *Children* 17:103, 1970.
9. Caplan, G. Psychological aspects of maternity care. *American Journal of Public Health* 47:25, 1957.
10. Carty, E. My, you're getting big! *Canadian Nurse* 66(8):40, 1970.
11. Cobliner, W. G. Some maternal attitudes toward conception. *Mental Hygiene* 49:550, 1965.
12. Cohen, M. Personal identity and sexual identity. *Psychiatry* 29:1, 1966.
13. Colman, A., and Colman, L. *Pregnancy: The Psychological Experience.* New York: Herder and Herder, 1971.
14. DeGarmo, E., and Davidson, K. Psychosocial Effects of Pregnancy on the Mother, Father, Marriage, and Family. In L. McNall and J. Galeener. (Eds.), *Current Practice in Obstetric and Gynecologic Nursing,* Vol. 2. St. Louis: Mosby, 1978.
15. Egleson, J., and Egleson, J. *Parents Without Partners.* New York: Dutton, 1961.
16. Fawcett, J. Body image and the pregnant couple. *The American Journal of Maternal-Child Nursing* 3:227, 1978.
17. Flapan, M. A paradigm for the analysis of childbearing motivations of married women prior to birth of the first child. *American Journal of Orthopsychiatry* 39:402, 1969.
18. Gallagher, U. Adoption resources for black children. *Children* 18:49, 1971.

19. Gordon, E. M. Acceptance of pregnancy before and since oral contraception. *Obstetrics and Gynecology* 29:144, 1967.
20. Gordon, M. *The Nuclear Family in Crisis.* New York: Harper & Row, 1972.
21. Grimm, E. Psychological tension in pregnancy. *Psychosomatic Medicine* 23:520, 1961.
22. Gustin, K. The Adopting Family. In D. Hymovich and M. Barnard (Eds.), *Family Health Care.* New York: McGraw-Hill, 1973.
23. Hammons, C. The adoptive family. *American Journal of Nursing* 76:251, 1976.
24. Hanford, J. Pregnancy as a state of conflict. *Psychological Reports* 22:1313, 1968.
25. Harris, R., Dombro, M., and Ryan, C. Therapeutic uses of human figure drawings by pregnant couples. *Journal of Obstetric, Gynecologic and Neonatal Nursing* 9:232, 1980.
26. Jarvia, W. Some effects of pregnancy and childbirth on men. *Journal of the American Psychoanalytical Association* 10:689, 1962.
27. Jessner, L. The Development of Parental Attitudes During Pregnancy. In E. Anthony and T. Benedek (Eds.), *Parenthood: Its Psychology and Psychopathology.* Boston: Little, Brown, 1970.
28. Kanter, R. Communes. In M. Gordon (Ed.), *The Nuclear Family in Crisis.* New York: Harper & Row, 1972.
29. Kitzinger, S. *The Experience of Childbirth* (4th ed.). New York: Penguin Books, 1978.
30. Klein, C. *The Single Parent Experience.* New York: Walker, 1973.
31. Larsen, V. Stresses of the childbearing year. *American Journal of Public Health* 56:32, 1966.
32. Lewis, A. *An Interesting Condition.* New York: Doubleday, 1950.
33. Liebenberg, B. Expectant fathers. *American Journal of Orthopsychiatry* 37:358, 1967.
34. Lumley, J. The image of the fetus in the first trimester. *Birth and the Family Journal* 7(1):5, 1980.
35. Masters, W. H., and Johnson, V. E. *Human Sexual Response.* Boston: Little, Brown, 1966.
36. McNall, L. Concerns of Expectant Fathers. In L. McNall and L. Galeener (Eds.), *Current Practice in Obstetric and Gynecologic Nursing.* St. Louis: Mosby, 1976.
37. Meezan, W., Katz, S., and Russo, E. *Adoption Without Agencies.* New York: Child Welfare League of America, 1978.
37a. Nationally the family is fragmenting. *The Philadelphia Inquirer,* May 12, 1982.
38. Nilsson, A. Para-natal emotional adjustment: A prospective investigation of 165 women. Part 1. *Acta Psychiatrica Scandinavica* 220 (Supplement):9, 1970.
39. Poffenberg, S., Poffenberg, T., and Landis, J. T. Intent toward conception and the pregnancy experience. *American Sociological Review* 17:616, 1952.
40. Rayner, E. *Human Development.* London: Allen & Unwin, 1970.
41. Retterstol, N. Paranoid psychoses associated with impending or newly established fatherhood. *Acta Psychiatrica Scandinavica* 44:51, 1968.
42. Rossi, A. S. Transition to Parenthood. In I. L. Reiss (Ed.), *Readings on the Family System.* New York: Holt, Rinehart, & Winston, 1972.
43. Scott, E. Illsley, R., and Biles, M. E. A psychological investigation of primigravidae. Part 3. Some aspects of maternal behavior. *Journal of Obstetrics and Gynaecology of the British Commonwealth* 63:494, 1965.
44. Shannon-Babitz, M. Addressing the needs of fathers during labor and delivery. *American Journal of Maternal-Child Nursing* 4:378, 1979.
45. Sherman, J. *On the Psychology of Women.* Springfield, Ill.: Thomas, 1971.
46. Sherwen, L. Fantasies during the third trimester of pregnancy. *American Journal of Maternal-Child Nursing* 6:398, 1981.
47. Smith, D., and Sternfield, J. The hippie communal movement: Effects on childbirth and development. *American Journal of Orthopsychiatry* 40:527, 1970.
48. Stukane, E. What nobody ever tells you about being pregnant. *McCalls,* January, 1981, p. 91.
49. Tonti, M. Fatherhood. In P. Ahmed (Ed.), *Pregnancy, Childbirth, and Parenthood.* New York: Elsevier, 1981.
50. Trethowan, W. H. The Couvade Syndrome. In J. G. Howells (Ed.), *Modern Perspectives in Psycho-Obstetrics.* New York: Bruner/Mazel, 1972.
51. Walker, L. Identifying parents in need: An approach to adoptive parenthood. *American Journal of Maternal-Child Nursing* 6:118, 1981.
52. Winokur, G., and Werhoff, J. The relationship of conscious maternal attitudes to certain aspects of pregnancy. *Psychiatric Quarterly 30* (Supplement):61, 1956.
53. Wolff, S. The fate of the adopted child. *Archives of Disease in Childhood* 49:165, 1974.
54. Wyatt, F. Clinical notes on motives of reproduction. *Journal of Social Issues* 23:29, 1967.

FURTHER READING

Anderson-Courchene, T. Adoption or assimilation. *Canadian Nurse* 74:38, 1978.

Ballou, J. *The Psychology of Pregnancy.* Lexington, Mass.: Lexington Books, 1978.

Carter-Jessop, L. Promoting maternal attachment through prenatal intervention. *American Journal of Maternal-Child Nursing* 6:107, 1981.

Collier, P. Understanding couvade. *American Journal of Maternal-Child Nursing* 7:114, 1982.

Cranley, M. Development of a tool to measure maternal attachment during pregnancy. *Nursing Research* 30:281, 1981.

Devaney, S., and Lavery, S. Nursing care for the relinquishing mother. *Journal of Obstetric, Gynecologic and Neonatal Nursing* 9:375, 1980.

Fishbein, E. The couvade: A review. *Journal of Obstetric, Gynecologic and Neonatal Nursing* 10:356, 1981.

Hill, R. *Informal Adoption Among Black Families.* Washington, D.C.: National Urban League, 1977.

Joe, B. *Public Policies Toward Adoption.* Washington, D.C.: Urban Institute, 1979.

Josten, L. Prenatal assessment guide for illuminating possible problems with parenting. *American Journal of Maternal-Child Nursing* 6:113, 1981.

Lamb, G., and Lipkin, M. Somatic symptoms of expectant fathers. *American Journal of Maternal-Child Nursing* 7:110, 1982.

Lockhart, B. When couples adopt, they too need parenting classes. *American Journal of Maternal-Child Nursing* 7:116, 1982.

Macfarlane, A. *The Psychology of Childbirth.* Cambridge, Mass.: Harvard University Press, 1977.

Marguart, R. Expectant fathers: What are their needs? *American Journal of Maternal-Child Nursing* 1:32, 1976.

May, K. Active involvement of expectant fathers in pregnancy: Some further considerations. *Journal of Obstetric, Gynecologic and Neonatal Nursing* 7(2):7, 1978.

McRae, M. An approach to the single parent dilemma. *American Journal of Maternal-Child Nursing* 2:164, 1977.

Oakley, A. *Women Confined.* New York: Schocken Books, 1980.

Rubin, R. Attainment of the maternal role: Part II. Models and referrents. *Nursing Research* 16:342, 1967.

Rubin, R. Cognitive style in pregnancy. *American Journal of Nursing* 70:502, 1970.

Rubin, R. Maternal tasks in pregnancy. *American Journal of Maternal-Child Nursing* 4:143, 1975.

Sorosky, A., Baran, A., and Pannor, R. *The Adoption Triangle.* New York: Anchor Press, 1978.

Sorosky, A. Identity conflicts in adoptees. *American Journal of Orthopsychiatry* 45:18, 1975.

Spezzano, C. Prenatal psychology. *Psychology Today* 15(5):49, 1981.

Stichler, J., Bowden, M., and Reimer, E. Pregnancy: A shared emotional experience. *American Journal of Maternal-Child Nursing* 3:153, 1978.

Tizard, B. *Adoption: A Second Chance.* New York: The Free Press, 1977.

Ward, M. The relationship between parents and caseworker in adoption. *Social Casework* 60:96, 1979.

Weinberg, J. Body image disturbance as a factor in the crisis situation of pregnancy: A review. *Journal of Obstetric, Gynecologic and Neonatal Nursing* 7(2):18, 1978.

Wolff, S. The fate of the adopted child. *Archives of Diseases of Children* 49:165, 1974.

Zimmerman, B. The exceptional stresses of adoptive parenthood. *American Journal of Maternal-Child Nursing* 2:191, 1977.

Chapter 10　Education for Childbirth

Organized childbirth education has been a relatively recent development. The great scientific advances of the nineteenth and early twentieth centuries brought about a change of location for childbirth—from the home to the hospital. This change was accompanied by a change in attitude toward the birth process itself. Formerly, birth was associated with the company of family and friends and with normal health, despite the dangers. However, in the modern era birth has been more associated with the hospital, the doctor, and illness, despite the increased safety. Increasingly, in recent years consumers have been seeking a combination of the safety afforded by the hospital setting and the supportive presence of family members and friends. The result has been the formation of alternative settings for birth, such as birthing rooms in the hospital and community birthing centers.

HISTORICAL BACKGROUND

The history of childbirth education also reflects the influence of consumers of maternity care. Childbirth education evolved along two different paths as a result of two different types of needs, a need to teach and a need to participate. Today both of these concepts are embodied in the educational programs offered to consumers.

In the early 1900s public health personnel became increasingly aware of the need to teach mothers about hygiene and good health practices. The first organization to act on such a need was the American National Red Cross, which in 1908 offered a class on mother and infant care as part of its home health course. The Red Cross promoted the idea nationally in 1913 [11].

In the 1920s the Maternity Center in New York began urging women to seek early prenatal care and to attend general classes on health during pregnancy. By the 1930s the pregnant couple had become the focus of the educational endeavors of the Maternity Center.

Influence of Grantly Dick-Read

In 1932 in England, Grantly Dick-Read [4] began to speak and write in opposition to much of the medical intervention in childbirth, such as the use of forceps and anesthesia, and formulated a philosophy on which he based a method of natural delivery. Dick-Read proposed that, through the ages, fear and anxiety were introduced by society into pregnancy and childbirth. Negative experiences related by family members and friends were reinforced by scenes in literature and motion pictures.

Dick-Read wrote that fear and anticipation of pain arouse natural protective tensions in the body, both psychic and muscular. Unfortunately, these muscle tensions tend to oppose dilatation of the birth canal during labor and make the outlet rigid. This resistance causes pain by exciting nerve endings in the uterus that respond to excessive tension. Thus, a process that Dick-Read referred to as the fear-tension-pain syndrome is set in motion. To break the circular reaction, Dick-Read advocated overcoming fear, eliminating anxiety and tension, and replacing them with calmness and relaxation.

To this end, Dick-Read held antepartal courses in education for childbirth, aimed at eliminating fear and overcoming ignorance. He also devised a series of physical and respiratory relaxation exercises designed to reduce mental and physical tensions. The physical exercises were largely influenced by Helen

Heardman, a physiotherapist in England. These exercises included tailor sitting, squatting, and the pelvic rock (Fig. 10-1); their aim was to increase the elasticity of perineal muscles, mobilize the joints of the pelvis and back, and foster general improvement of circulation in the pelvic area.

Dick-Read's followers were taught to control their breathing by four respiratory exercises. These are integrated with different phases of labor to demonstrate to the woman how they will help her and to motivate her to practice them. The exercises included deep respiration for relaxation during the latent phase of the first stage of labor, more rapid respirations (25 per minute) for distraction during contractions in the active phase, breath-holding for pushing, and short panting respirations (40 per minute) at the time of delivery.

It is now recognized that excessive panting may result in improper alveolar ventilation. Some think that the respiratory alkalosis produced by hyperventilation may contribute to increased maternal suggestibility and some amnesia [2]. By disturbing the acid-base balance, severe hyperventilation can be detrimental to the fetus [13].

Dick-Read advocated learning relaxation by concentrating on each part of the body separately, from the toes toward the head, contracting and then relaxing the muscles. He believed that the best way to support the mother in labor was based on the three Ps and the three Cs—patience, peacefulness, personal interest, confidence, concentrated observation, and cheerfulness. It was important that the woman never be left alone, since loneliness generated fear. If she had a consistent coach, particularly one who believed in the value of the method of preparation being used, the woman would be able to cope with her labor very well.

Dick-Read believed in showing the baby to the mother immediately after delivery so that she might fully experience the great moment of giving birth and a profound sense of achievement. Although Dick-Read's philosophy included the use of analgesics when necessary, the thrust of his writing emphasizes the avoidance of these "unnatural aids," as he called them. Dick-Read's method was introduced to the United States under the direction of Dr. Thoms of Yale University.

Figure 10-1. Pelvic rocking exercise to relieve back pain. The woman first allows her back to sag while holding her head up; then she lets her head drop and arches her back.

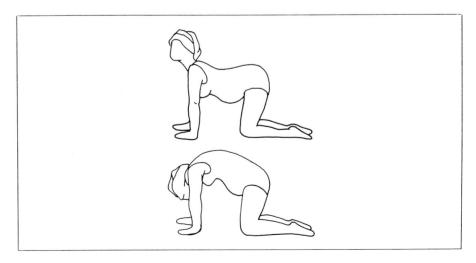

While the Western world was contemplating the merits of the Dick-Read method, the Russians were applying a different approach based on Pavlovian psychology, which was presented in 1950 at a World Congress of Gynecology held in Paris. A French obstetrician, Dr. Fernand Lamaze, became so interested that he later traveled to the Soviet Union to learn more about it. He and his colleague, Pierre Vellay, were responsible for popularizing this method of preparation for childbirth in the Western world.

According to the Pavlovian philosophy, the degree of discomfort caused by uterine contractions is influenced by two important factors: (1) the actual physiologically transmitted discomfort (the strength of the pain signal to the brain) and (2) the behavioral response to this signal once it has been interpreted. The exercises taught by the Lamaze method are based on the theory that conditioned reflexes minimize the strength of the signal received in the brain and alter the behavioral response to whatever signal is received.

This method takes advantage of the fact that the brain can accept, integrate, interpret, and transmit only one set of signals at a time. If the strongest set of signals arriving at the brain comes from the uterus and is interpreted as a labor pain, the behavioral response is likely to be one of discomfort. If, however, at the time of the uterine contraction, a series of actions begins that requires for its successful execution stronger signals than those the uterus sends, then the uterine signals assume second place and the conscious perception of the uterine contraction diminishes markedly. The exercises of Lamaze (psychoprophylaxis) provide the strong stimuli necessary to take precedence over signals from uterine contractions. In addition, in this method the total preparation for childbirth involves learning what the process of having a baby entails, removing superstition and misinformation, and absorbing correct information. Such knowledge allows a woman to work effectively with her labor [8].

The Lamaze, or psychoprophylactic, method was popularized in the United States by the late Marjorie Karmel in her book *Thank You, Dr. Lamaze* [6]. In 1960 interested laymen and health professionals founded the American Society for Psychoprophylaxis in Obstetrics (ASPO), which has been growing ever since. This is related, no doubt, to the satisfaction of the many mothers who have delivered using the Lamaze technique and their belief that others should have the opportunity to learn about the method.

Women who are educated by the Lamaze method are instructed to time Braxton Hicks' contractions during the last weeks of pregnancy and to do shallow fast breathing during the contractions. This establishes a relationship between these painless uterine contractions and the type of respiratory pattern to be used later during labor, thus building a favorable conditioned reflex that excludes the feeling of pain.

Pain-reducing procedures that are a part of the Lamaze training include slow breathing for the first part of labor, effleurage of the abdominal wall when active labor begins, pressure on the anterior-superior iliac spine to reduce abdominal pain, and pressure on the rhomboid triangle to reduce back pain when contractions are stronger. The mother must also be coached in muscle relaxation, best achieved in a half-sitting position with knees slightly flexed over a pillow. Carrying out all of these exercises in detail requires a great deal of concentration and a lot of encouragement from a good coach. Lamaze emphasized two periods when support is most needed by the woman in labor: when her cervix becomes completely dilated and when her perineum becomes completely distended.

Actually the Dick-Read and Lamaze methods of prepared childbirth are very similar in philosophy, techniques, and principles of management. Both depend on education to reduce apprehension and fear, to decrease anticipation of pain, and to decrease the pain sensation. Both methods offer respiratory exercises to achieve distraction and teach relaxation techniques to diminish pain.

Childbirth Education Association

About the same time that the Lamaze method gained popularity, another organization began to grow out of the belief on the part of women who had had satisfying childbirth experiences that they should band together, sometimes with the assistance of professionals, to offer information and training to other interested women. These groups eventually consolidated into a federation of groups, the International Childbirth Education Association (ICEA), which still serves as a core for a variety of philosophies and approaches represented in its local groups.

The local groups of the ICEA seem to advocate a less zealous approach than either Dick-Read or Lamaze, though they use the same general techniques. Although their philosophy does not lead parents to expect a "painless labor" nor one necessarily conducted without analgesia or anesthesia, they do emphasize the point that prepared parents usually require less medication, a finding recently emphasized in the nursing research of Timm [15]. One of their aims is to foster in parents a sense of responsibility for their experience and provide them with ways in which they can participate in the birth of their baby. Affiliated with the LaLeche League International, they also try to help those mothers who wish to breast-feed to do so successfully for as long as they wish. To this end, through nursing mothers' groups, they offer information as well as practical suggestions and emotional support.

The Maternity Center Association in New York continues to be active in promoting programs for childbirth education. An increasing number of such programs are developing throughout the United States.

GENERAL APPROACHES

Combinations of techniques for coping with pregnancy and labor are usually presented in childbirth education classes in this country. Generally the benefits enjoyed by the mother-participants are enhanced when more involvement is encouraged for their "significant others" during childbirth classes and labor and delivery. The presence of a support person other than the husband, such as a male friend, parent, relative, or other close friend, should be openly supported by the nursing staff.

Interpersonal relationships between the woman, her coach, and the attending nursing and medical staff form the foundation for a psychologic analgesia that can result from effective use of a prepared childbirth method. It is dependent on the interplay of elements of suggestion, motivation, emotions, attention, and distraction. It is therefore important that all maternity personnel be aware of the basic principles of the method being used, so that they can offer reassurance and careful explanations of the sensations the mother is experiencing.

It is generally accepted that decreased apprehension, fear, and anxiety are of psychologic and physiologic value to the mother and to the progress of her labor. The work of nurse researcher Lederman and colleagues has demonstrated significant correlations in the active phase of labor between plasma epinephrine and anxiety, and among epinephrine, uterine activity, and the length of labor [9]. Additionally, well-executed childbirth education programs will enable certain women to experience childbearing with deep emotional satisfaction. Research [5] indicates that the more prepared women are for labor and delivery, the higher their level of awareness at delivery and their ability to cope successfully with it will be. This success is strongly associated with positive reactions to the infant and may also reflect the fact that individuals choosing childbirth education are already generally very interested and highly motivated to make the childbearing experience as positive as possible.

A significant disadvantage of childbirth education can occur if the director of the educational program insists on the importance of avoiding analgesic medications. In this situation, if the woman feels that she must have some medication in order to continue, she is left to cope with her resulting guilt feelings. Research studies [2, 18] thus far report contradictory findings regarding differences in the effects of childbirth education methods and various forms of regional or general anesthesia on duration of labor, incidence of complications, blood loss, use of cesarean birth, and postpartum complications. The use of prepared childbirth techniques does not exclude the use of analgesics since the combination of the two leads to a worthwhile goal. The woman gets the benefit of both a well-planned educational program during her antepartal period and analgesia during labor if and when she needs it.

All childbirth techniques use principles of relaxation, which sometimes must be consciously achieved. The key to relaxation is correct basic posture and proper breathing. Relaxation is especially important during pregnancy, when body reserves are already taxed and fatigue readily accompanies increased tension. In labor, relaxation reduces muscular tension that may actually impede progress.

Research by Worthington and colleagues indicates that a combination of structured breathing, attention focal points, and coaching produces the most effective strategies for coping with the tension of labor [17]. Controlled breathing provides one of the easiest ways to relax once correct posture is achieved. The exact rhythm is not so important as the comfort it provides. The Maternity Center Association advocates that a complete breath be used periodically during relaxation, followed by slow, quiet, easy respirations. With a complete breath (deep inspiration slowly exhaled under pressure) there is a more complete exchange of oxygen and carbon dioxide. Decreased muscular tension is accomplished when groups of muscles are systematically tightened and loosened. As a part of antepartal preparation, women are taught to contract their abdominal muscles and those of their pelvic floor.

Controlled breathing and relaxation techniques are taught for use during labor. During the first stage, deep breathing is done with a complete breath at the beginning and the end of each contraction. Approaching transition, the woman in labor uses modified deep breathing—a complete breath at the beginning and end, and quiet shallow throat breathing at the peak of each contraction. If she becomes dizzy or lightheaded, she is instructed to breathe more slowly. During transition she continues modified deep breathing, but blows out gently as she exhales on every third or fourth breath. In the second stage, pushing and panting are used as indicated. (For a more detailed discussion of this topic see Chapter 12.)

The woman's partner (father of the child or other supportive person) provides her with practical assistance, close emotional support, and encouragement to go on. During early labor, he (or she) can encourage her to sleep and can provide information for the staff regarding how the woman is reacting to her labor and what she is finding distracting or helpful. He assists her to assume the positions she has practiced during labor, reminds her about her breathing patterns, times her contractions, and helps her to relax when he notices signs of tension (such as clenched fists, curled feet, or a wrinkled brow). If she has a backache, he can apply firm pressure during contractions. Effleurage brings relief for aching in her lower abdomen or thighs. He helps to keep her lips and mouth moistened with mouthwash, ice chips, or fruit-flavored candy drops. His firm coaching, assistance with pushing, and frequent reassurance provide valuable support for the woman. As long as the staff remains certain that she and the baby are safe, they should adopt an attitude of support but should not interfere with the relationship between the mother and her coaching partner. His involvement throughout the pregnancy and during labor helps to make him an integral part of the birth process.

Until fairly recently, many obstetricians and hospital administrators objected rather strongly to the father's presence in the delivery room in the belief that he would probably contaminate the sterile drapes or that he might faint. Some even suggested that the experience might result in the man's impotence. Experience has indicated that these fears were groundless. The number of fathers who choose to be with their partners during the actual delivery, either vaginal or cesarean birth, continues to grow larger.

The presence of siblings at birth is a topic of current controversy. Objections of some health professionals range from the usual fear of contamination to the fear of psychologic trauma to the child. Research done in more permissive birth settings seems to indicate that these fears are groundless as well [1].

Successful programs of prenatal education for children and children attending the birth of their siblings have been reported by several nurses. Sweet teaches prenatal classes especially for children [14]. The children, usually between 2 and 10 years old, are referred for the instruction by other maternity clinic nurses, prepared childbirth educators, physicians, or midwives. The children's parents review the class content before the actual session, which includes the entire family. Parents' attendance, according to Sweet, is essential since most children will ask questions at home about the material introduced in class. To reinforce the learning, parents must be prepared to answer these questions even if they were covered in detail in class. Questions often asked include: How did the baby start in Mommy's tummy? How did the seed get in there? How does the baby come out? What does the baby eat inside? How does the baby go to the bathroom?

Teaching methods used include a birth atlas, a film, and life size models which the children may take apart to explain development and birth of a baby. Sweet encourages mothers to have the children listen to the baby's heartbeat through a stethoscope and to let them see and feel the baby kick. She encourages using correct terminology with an explanation at a level the child will understand. Children tour the hospital's maternity area and are shown where their mothers might stay. The telephone is pointed out, and children are assured that they can call their mother when she is in the hospital. The classes are individualized for each family and generally last 1 hour. A fee is charged for families who can afford to pay. Evaluation occurs by having the parents complete two questionnaires, one following the session and the second three weeks after the birth of the baby. Results indicate that the classes give children an understanding of the development and birth of a baby, reduce their anxiety about their mothers' hospitalization, and make them feel involved in the pregnancy [14].

Paulina Perez, from her experience with children attending birth in a hospital's alternative birth center, offers suggestions for working with children who will be present at birth [10]. She suggests beginning with the question "What do you think about having a new baby?" during the family's orientation to the birthing area and hospital. The child's answers will tell much about how he thinks his role in the family will change. As the family is familiarized with the birth room environment, she suggests assessing the knowledge base of each child. She advises asking such questions as, "What do you think will happen in labor and in delivery? Have you seen movies of birth? What did you think of them? How does the baby get out of the mother's body? Does it hurt? What does the mom look like when she is pushing the baby out? Do you want to be here when the baby is born? What do you want to do during the birth? Do you want to help?" Most important is listening to the child to find out what he wants out of the experience.

During labor it is most helpful to have a support person especially for the child, someone he knows and likes. It may be helpful to have the child bring books, games, cards, and snacks from home since even in a flexible atmosphere labor may be boring to a child. The child can also be an active participant, getting juice or ice chips for his mother, rubbing her back or walking with her. Older children may even join in doing breathing techniques. Perez notes that it is also wise to make sure the child knows that pushing is hard work and that his mother may be tired between pushes.

Before delivery the child must scrub his hands and put on a gown. Anyone entering the room should be introduced to the child and the child should be positioned so he can see the birth if he wants to. In her experience, Perez reports, children are usually eager to hold the infant as soon as possible, and are fascinated with the looks of the placenta. Discussing the events of the day with the child after the delivery can be most revealing. Comments made by children have included: "The baby looked at me when he was first born. I think he likes me," and "Now whenever I hold my little sister, I think about my experience in the birthing room. You know, I don't think I would love my sister like I do if I hadn't seen her being born" [10].

ROLE OF HEALTH PROFESSIONALS

Occasionally it is difficult for hospital personnel to accept the fact that the woman or couple are capable of exercising control over the birth process. Personnel who react in this way need the support of their peers in examining the range of possible outcomes when couples make decisions about and exercise control over their care. As a consequence it might be easier for these health personnel to see the situation as less threatening. Fortunately couples who use prepared childbirth techniques are more readily accepted now than in the past, as preparation for childbirth has become more popular across the country, particularly among well-educated, middle-class consumers [12].

Health professionals must recognize the need to provide an experience that will meet the consumer's needs and must work toward increasing the flexibility of hospital policies surrounding childbirth. Otherwise, consumers will seek those experiences in settings that do not offer the safety features of an in-hospital or birthing center delivery.

PLANNING A CHILDBIRTH EDUCATION PROGRAM

Developing a program of childbirth education raises several questions: What will be the philosophy and goals of the program? What content needs to be taught and when during the childbearing process and how should it be taught? Who should do the teaching and where should the classes be held? Finally, how will the childbirth educator know if the learning has occurred and if the program goals have been met?

Philosophy and Overall Program Goals

The philosophy and goals of the program of childbirth education will dictate the content and much of the conduct of the program. If the philosophy and goals of the program are based on the assumption that childbearing couples, as consumers, need to be informed of the variety of health care options open to them and that once they are aware of their options they are capable of making independent decisions regarding their care, the content of the program will generally be broad based and often issue oriented. If the objective is to advise the couple about the options available to them in a given agency or institution with the assumption that the childbearing clients will choose their options with the guidance of the health care team, the content of the program will generally be more narrow.

Despite differences in philosophical approaches to childbirth education, most programs include among their goals education regarding the childbearing process and preparation for the new roles and responsibilities of parenthood.

General Content and Class Objectives

What will actually be taught depends upon the philosophy and goals of the program. Generally, content concerning pregnancy, the birth process, parenthood, and early childhood is divided and offered according to the concerns of expectant parents during various stages of the childbearing process. During early pregnancy the focus is on the validation of pregnancy, understanding physical changes, and recognition of the normal emotions of pregnancy. In midpregnancy, clients are especially receptive to information about fetal growth and development and maintenance of their own and their growing fetus's health. During later pregnancy, clients are concerned with the upcoming period of labor and delivery, preparing for the baby's arrival, infant behavior, and child care such as feeding, bathing, and handling newborns. The actual choice of topics and the time devoted to each topic will vary according to the needs of the clients and the time available. (Topics commonly covered in childbirth education classes are presented in Table 10-1.)

Before presenting the topics chosen, objectives for each class that are more specific than the overall program objectives need to be developed. These objectives should focus on the learner rather than the educator and represent the client behaviors desired as a result of the learning process. The objectives should be realistic and should be developed so that they can be used to evaluate the client's learning and ultimately the program goals.

While some educators prefer to use broad objectives in teaching clients, most educators find that more specific behavioral objectives give focus to their teaching and to clients' learning (Table 10-2). For example, the objective of having the client "be familiar with the changes of pregnancy" is very broad and open to many

Table 10-1. Topics Taught in Childbirth Education Classes

Pregnancy
Anatomy and physiology of the reproductive system
Physical changes in pregnancy
Common discomforts of pregnancy and relief measures
Nutrition
Exercises
Psychologic changes in pregnancy—impact on the family unit
How the husband or significant other can help and how they also need help
Fetal development
Preparing for the hospital or birth center

Labor and Delivery
Signs and symptoms of labor
Hospital or birth center admission procedures
Tour of labor and delivery area or slides and description of unit and equipment
Husband and siblings in the labor and delivery unit
Hospital birthing rooms
Stages of labor
    Physical changes
    Breathing and relaxation techniques
    Other coping and comfort measures
    Role of labor coach or support person
    Delivery positions
Anesthesia and analgesia
Episiotomy
Induction of labor
Forceps
Cesarean births
    Reasons for cesarean births
    Types of surgical procedures
    Husband or significant other present during delivery
    Anesthesia and analgesia
    Postdelivery course and procedures
    Implications for future childbearing

Postdelivery Adjustments
Immediate reactions to childbirth—attachment and emotional preparation for parenting
Care in the recovery room
Physical and emotional changes
Going home
Resuming sexual and social relationships
First postdelivery checkup for mother and infant
Care of the newborn
    Immediate postdelivery care
    Needs and characteristics—physical, developmental, temperamental
    Breast or bottle feeding
    Handling, bathing, and appropriate clothing

Parenting
Community resources available for new or expectant parents and their infants

interpretations. How would the educator measure the learner's success in achieving this objective? More specific objectives of the client being able "to identify common discomforts during the first trimester of pregnancy and to identify helpful relief measures" are much easier to evaluate in relation to the client's learning.

Method of Presentation
The actual conduct of the classes depends in part upon the learner, the topic, the educators, the time available, and the physical facilities.

Learners differ in their capacity to learn, in their goals, interests, attitudes, life

Table 10-2. Verbs for Use in Stating Cognitive Objectives

Knowledge	Comprehension	Application	Analysis	Synthesis	Evaluation
Define	Discuss	Apply	Analyze	Propose	Evaluate
Record	Describe	Use	Differentiate	Formulate	Rate
List	Explain	Demonstrate	Compare	Construct	Score
Recall	Report	Practice	Contrast	Organize	Select
Name	Review	Illustrate	Diagram	Prepare	Estimate

Source: Modified from Johnson & Johnson. *Assuring Learning with Self-Instructional Packages*. Self-Instructional Packages, Inc., 1973.

experiences, living habits, perceptions, age, and education. All of these factors need to be considered in deciding upon teaching methods for each sequence of classes. One group may be composed of well-educated individuals who learn best through written materials and group discussion. Another group may normally read little (or be unable to read) but watch a great deal of television; this group may learn best through audiovisual materials such as large charts, posters, slides, videotapes, or movies. Delafleur and Payne have used role playing most successfully as another method [3]. The clients' goals in attending the classes and what it is that they want to learn should also be assessed prior to or at the beginning of a series of classes.

To some extent the topic will dictate how the material or class is presented. Topics involving psychomotor skills such as exercises in preparation for labor are best learned through demonstration and practice. Topics such as physiologic changes of pregnancy, which are understood by cognitive skills, may be presented most effectively through lecture, discussion, and the use of audiovisual aids. Topics involving affective learning such as role changes are often best handled through group discussion.

Woolery and Barkley use several techniques to help couples enhance their relationships [16]. One critical component of childbirth educational programs is a discussion of the normal emotional changes associated with the childbearing year. During an early class, they open such a discussion by dividing the men and women into separate groups. Women list the physical changes they are experiencing in their pregnancy while men are requested to list the emotional changes they have been noticing in their wives and themselves since pregnancy began. Both lists are posted and the discussion begins with the physical changes. The instructor leads the groups together in a discussion of possible causes for some of the emotional changes.

Couples usually are relieved to find out their emotional changes are normal, temporary, and usually explainable. Husbands become more understanding and patient with irritable wives, and wives become more tolerant and patient with busy and seemingly indifferent husbands. Because the group shares the experience of pregnancy, they relate well to each other's needs.

Toward the end of the childbirth preparation series, Woolery and Barkley lead the group into a discussion of transition to parenthood. New parents, they comment, tend to consider the baby's needs first and then their own. Yet each individual needs to feel good about himself and herself in order to be a loving spouse and parent. Couples are assigned homework in which they list five things they would like to do for themselves, as a couple and as a family, to nurture children, and the five things they want in a marriage [16]. The techniques used in education for childbirth have results beyond the childbearing period, and help couples through early parenting and toward an open, loving relationship.

Some topics are best approached using a variety of methods. Childbirth educators have taught nutrition by having pregnant women prepare and eat lunch together while using the opportunity to discuss dietary patterns. Some programs for childbirth education provide videotapes featuring topics on postpartum exercises, infant feeding, and bathing, which can be viewed by women in their hospital rooms during their postpartum stay. The women may practice while viewing the tapes.

In addition to the type of learner and the topic, the conduct of the classes is dependent upon the teachers, time, and the physical facilities available. Most educators have not only interest and expertise on certain topics but preferred methods of presentation. Whenever possible, a variety of members of the health care team and community should be called upon to offer topics in their areas of competence. Childbirth education often remains an isolated component of care to childbearing families when the teaching is limited to one or two people without involving others who will participate in the care of the family. The nutritionist can provide invaluable information on the dietary patterns of the clients. A social worker can often provide a cultural, socioeconomic, and age profile of the group in addition to knowing community agencies and resources available. Nurses in a clinic, labor and delivery area, or postpartum and in nursery facilities can provide information on topics that need to be taught, and are often willing to participate in the teaching and to reinforce what has been taught in their individual units.

Principles of Teaching and Learning

Once the educator is clear on the program philosophy and goals, topic areas needed to meet the program goals, specific learner objectives for the classes, and methods to be used in teaching and has assessed the needs of the clients, a review of basic principles of teaching and learning is helpful.

Learning must be active—that is, the individuals must be involved in the process. If the discussion focuses on common discomforts of pregnancy, begin by asking members of the group what discomforts they have experienced, and then each may be discussed, rather than presenting a prearranged lecture on that subject. Discomforts that do not come up in discussion can be addressed at the end.

A second basic principle of teaching is that the learning must be meaningful. The nurse as educator must address "where the learner is now," that is, the learner's current life situation. Show the individual that the learning has a purpose and will facilitate more intelligent adjustments in the future. Teaching a woman to increase the iron in her diet, for example, might focus on the effects it will have on her and the baby. Her current dietary habits, including cultural and socioeconomic factors, and her individual likes and dislikes must be explored. The changes in her diet must have meaning for her before she will follow through. This illustrates a third principle to remember: Learners are different and have different capacities, goals, interests, attitudes, life experiences, and perceptions, as well as different educational and cultural backgrounds. All of these factors must be considered in order to make the learning meaningful. Knox, for example, notes that adults are more interested in changing their performance levels than in learning information per se [7].

Another principle helpful to the nurse educator is that the learner must be motivated. Most childbearing families are well motivated to learn about the process. They want the pregnancy to result in a healthy baby and a good experience for each of them. The learner must also be physically and mentally ready to learn. Timing is important: The exhausted mother in the active stage of labor is hardly ready to learn about child care. Remember that the more an individual accepts the goal, the more meaningful and effective the learning will be. The woman who cannot accept the fact that she is pregnant will learn little until that conflict is resolved.

As an educator, the nurse should make the learner feel comfortable. This can be accomplished by controlling the environment so that physical comfort is possible and by avoiding direct questions that may threaten the individual within the group. Periods of stress, anxiety, or pain will interfere with learning. Remember that learning feeds on success. The woman who contributes something to the discussion should be recognized for her contribution. The learner should be helped to identify and apply previous learning. Likewise, the learning that has taken place should be reinforced, which can be done by the nursing staff in the clinic, labor and delivery rooms, and postpartum and nursery units, even though they may not have been directly involved in the initial teaching. It is important that a record of the teaching plan be made, so that it can accompany the mother's chart as she enters the other units.

Group Teaching   While some childbirth educational teaching is done with individual clients, most often childbirth education is carried out through group teaching (Fig. 10-2). The advantages of group teaching are that it saves time for those teaching, individuals within the group may become aware of common problems, and the questions raised may be questions that less vocal members would hesitate to raise. There is also a mutual sharing of ideas and experiences.

Prior to the first group session, the objectives and plan are developed. The setting should be clean and bright, with the chairs in a circle so each person can be seen and heard. During the first session introduce all of the people and try to learn their names. The purpose of the sessions should be discussed from the nurse's perspective, and the expectations of the group should be elicited.

If discussion is the method chosen, it should begin with general, nonthreatening questions so that individuals will respond and gain confidence in answering and speaking in front of the group (learning feeds on success). The questions should be directed toward the group, so that no individual feels "put on the spot." This approach will maximize spontaneity and make members feel more secure (individuals must be secure for learning to take place). Members should be encouraged to talk about their particular experiences (learning must be meaningful to them). As the group begins talking, your role changes from an active participant to an active listener (learning should be active). Your role now may be to keep the group's discussion on the original topic, to correct misinformation or misunderstanding, to encourage all to participate, making sure the quiet individuals have a chance to express their views, and to summarize the important points.

Evaluation   Evaluation should be made of each class and of the total program. This process may provide educators with some degree of satisfaction as well as direction for

Figure 10-2. Physician and nurses participate in childbirth preparation class. Their relaxed manner puts the group at ease. (Courtesy of Pennsylvania Hospital, Philadelphia, Pa.)

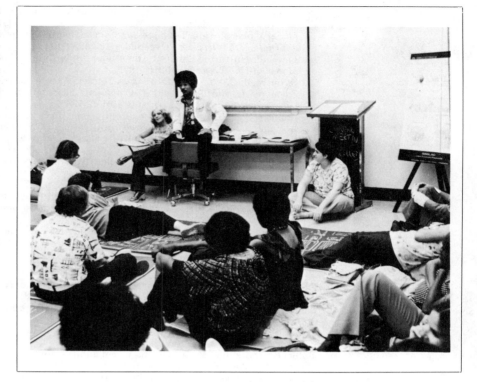

changes and improvements. Evaluations of the effectiveness of the class may be made directly by observing changes in the woman's or family's behavior. The evaluation may also be made through discussions with the women and their families. A written evaluation form may be used after a class or a group of classes. During class, nonverbal communication, such as facial expressions of anxiety, confusion, or boredom, can be validated by questions; this provides for reassessment and redirection.

Statistics may also provide some indication of program effectiveness. If women in the community had been coming to receive their initial prenatal care during the later months of pregnancy and now are doing so earlier, the educational program may be a factor; this assumption can be validated by discussion with them. While some research has been completed, further research is needed to identify how childbirth education improves the outcomes of pregnancy and the transition to parenthood.

REFERENCES

1. Anderson, S. Siblings at birth: A survey and study. *Birth and the Family Journal* 6:80, 1979.
2. Bonica, J. J. *Principles and Practice of Obstetric Analgesia and Anesthesia.* Vol. 1. Philadelphia: Davis, 1967.
3. Delafleur, T., and Payne, J. Role playing in childbirth education classes. *American Journal of Maternal and Child Health* 6:333, 1981.
4. Dick-Read, G. *Childbirth Without Fear.* New York: Harper & Row, 1953.
5. Doering, S., and Entwisle, D. Preparation during pregnancy and ability to cope with labor and delivery. *American Journal of Orthopsychiatry* 45:825, 1975.
6. Karmel, M. *Thank You, Dr. Lamaze.* Philadelphia: Lippincott, 1959.
7. Knox, A. *Adult Development and Learning.* San Francisco: Jossey-Bass, 1977.

8. Lamaze, F. *Painless Childbirth*. London: Burke, 1958.
9. Lederman, R., Lederman, E., Work, B., and McCann, D. Relationship of maternal anxiety, plasma catecholamines and plasma cortisol to progress in labor. *American Journal of Obstetrics and Gynecology* 132:495, 1978.
10. Perez, P. Nurturing children who attend the birth of a sibling. *American Journal of Maternal-Child Nursing* 4:215, 1979.
11. Sasmore, J. *Childbirth Education: A Nursing Perspective*. New York: Wiley, 1979.
12. Sasmore, J., and Grossman, E. Childbirth education in 1980. *Journal of Obstetric, Gynecologic and Neonatal Nursing* 10:155, 1981.
13. Shnider, S. The Hyperventilation Controversy. In S. Shnider and F. Moya (Eds.), *The Anesthesiologist, Mother and Newborn*. Baltimore: Williams & Wilkins, 1974.
14. Sweet, P. Prenatal classes especially for children. *American Journal of Maternal-Child Nursing* 4:82, 1979.
15. Timm, M. Prenatal education evaluation. *Nursing Research* 28:338, 1979.
16. Woolery, L., and Barkley, N. Enhancing couple relationships during prenatal and postnatal classes. *American Journal of Maternal and Child Health* 6:184, 1981.
17. Worthington, E., Martin, G. and Shumate, M. Which prepared-childbirth coping strategies are effective? *Journal of Obstetric, Gynecologic and Neonatal Nursing* 11:45, 1982.
18. Zax, M., Sameroff, A., and Farnum, J. Childbirth education, maternal attitudes, and delivery. *American Journal of Obstetrics and Gynecology* 123:185, 1975.

FURTHER READINGS   Allen, E., and Mantz, M. Are normal patients at risk during pregnancy? *Journal of Obstetric, Gynecologic and Neonatal Nursing* 10:348, 1981.

Anderson, C. Enhancing reciprocity between mother and neonate. *Nursing Research* 30:89, 1981.

Avant, K. Anxiety as a potential factor affecting maternal attachment. *Journal of Obstetric, Gynecologic and Neonatal Nursing* 10:416, 1981.

Balik, B., and Foley, M. Developing a community-based parent education support group. *Journal of Obstetric, Gynecologic and Neonatal Nursing* 10:197, 1981.

Bampton, B., Jones, J., and Mancini, J. Initial mothering patterns of low-income black primiparas. *Journal of Obstetric, Gynecologic and Neonatal Nursing* 10:174, 1981.

Bing, E. *Adventure of Birth*. New York: Simon & Schuster, 1970.

Block, C., and Block, R. The effect of support of the husband and obstetrician on pain perception and control in childbirth. *Birth and the Family Journal* 2:43, 1975.

Bowen, S., and Miller, B. Paternal attachment behavior as related to presence at delivery and preparenthood classes: A pilot study. *Nursing Research* 29:307, 1980.

Brown, B. Maternity-patient teaching—A nursing priority. *Journal of Obstetric, Gynecologic and Neonatal Nursing* 11:11, 1982.

Buxton, C. L. *Study of Psychophysical Methods for Relief of Childbirth Pain*. Philadelphia: Saunders, 1962.

Cadwell, K. Improving nipple graspability for success at breastfeeding. *Journal of Obstetric, Gynecologic and Neonatal Nursing* 19:277, 1981.

Carey, J. First-trimester prenatal counseling in private practice. *Journal of Obstetric, Gynecologic and Neonatal Nursing* 10:336, 1981.

Carter-Jessop, L. Promoting maternal attachment through prenatal intervention. *American Journal of Maternal and Child Health* 6:107, 1981.

Cranley, M. Development of a tool for the measurement of maternal attachment during pregnancy. *Nursing Research* 30:281, 1981.

Dooher, M. Lamaze method of childbirth. *Nursing Research* 29:220, 1980.

Felton, G., and Segelman, F. Lamaze childbirth training and changes in belief about personal control. *Birth and the Family Journal* 5:141, 1978.

Fishbein, E. The couvade: A review. *Journal of Obstetric, Gynecologic and Neonatal Nursing* 10:356, 1981.

Gay, J. A conceptual framework of bonding. *Journal of Obstetric, Gynecologic and Neonatal Nursing* 10:440, 1981.

Gaziano, E., Garvis, M., and Levine, E. An evaluation of childbirth education for the clinic patient. *Birth and the Family Journal* 6:89, 1979.

Gottlieb, L. Maternal attachment in primiparas. *Journal of Obstetric, Gynecologic and Neonatal Nursing* 7:39, 1978.

Hall, L. Effect of teaching on primiparas' perceptions of their newborn. *Nursing Research* 29:317, 1980.

Halstead, J., and Fredrickson, T. Evaluation of a prepared childbirth program. *Journal of Obstetric, Gynecologic and Neonatal Nursing* 7(3):39, 1978.

Harris, R., Dombro, M., and Ryan, C. Therapeutic uses of human figure drawings by the pregnant couple. *Journal of Obstetric, Gynecologic and Neonatal Nursing* 9:232, 1980.

Hart, G. Maternal attitudes in prepared and unprepared cesarean deliveries. *Journal of Obstetric, Gynecologic and Neonatal Nursing* 9:243, 1980.

Hassid, P. *Textbook for Childbirth Educators.* New York: Harper & Row, 1978.

Hott, J. Best laid plans—pre and postpartum comparison of self and spouse in primiparous Lamaze couples who share delivery and those who do not. *Nursing Research* 29:20, 1980.

Howley, C. The older primipara: Implications for nurses. *Journal of Obstetric, Gynecologic and Neonatal Nursing* 10:182, 1981.

Jimenez, S. Education for the childbearing year. *Journal of Obstetric, Gynecologic and Neonatal Nursing* 9:97, 1980.

Josten, L. Prenatal assessment guide for illuminating possible problems with parenting. *American Journal of Maternal-Child Nursing* 6:107, 1981.

Kitzinger, S. *Experience of Childbirth.* New York: Taplinger, 1972.

Petrowski, D. Effectiveness of prenatal and postnatal instruction in postpartum care. *Journal of Obstetric, Gynecologic and Neonatal Nursing* 10:386, 1981.

Preparation for Childbearing. New York: Maternity Center Association, 1972.

Reiser, S. A tool to facilitate mother-infant attachment. *Journal of Obstetric, Gynecologic and Neonatal Nursing* 10:294, 1981.

Roberts, F. A model for parent education. *Image* 13:86, 1981.

Sherwen, L. Fantasies during the third trimester of pregnancy. *American Journal of Maternal-Child Nursing* 6:398, 1981.

Simchak, M. Childbirth education in China—A sharing of skills. *International Childbirth Education Association News* 21:2, 1982.

Smith, E. Group process and childbirth education. *Journal of Obstetric, Gynecologic and Neonatal Nursing* 7(4):51, 1978.

Stevens, R. Psychological strategies for management of pain in prepared childbirth. I. A review of the research. *Birth and the Family Journal* 3:157, 1976.

Stevens, R. Psychological strategies for the management of pain in prepared childbirth. II. A study of psychoanalgesia in prepared childbirth. *Birth and the Family Journal* 4:4, 1977.

Taubenheim, A. Parent-infant bonding in the first-time father. *Journal of Obstetric, Gynecologic and Neonatal Nursing* 10:261, 1981.

Trabert, C. Prenatal tactile intervention can be encouraged. *American Journal of Maternal and Child Health* 6:108, 1981.

Vellay, P. *Childbirth Without Pain.* New York: Dutton, 1960.

Whitley, N. A comparison of prepared childbirth couples and conventional prenatal class couples. *Journal of Obstetric, Gynecologic and Neonatal Nursing.* 8:109, 1979.

Windwer, C. Relationship among prospective parents' locus of control, social desirability, and choice of psychoprophylaxis. *Nursing Research* 26:96, 1977.

Women's reactions toward childbirth. *Science News* 107:72, 1975.

Zacharias, J. Childbirth education classes—Effects on attitudes toward childbirth in high risk indigent women. *Journal of Obstetric, Gynecologic and Neonatal Nursing* 10:265, 1981.

Zwirn, E., Fry, L., Reed, D., and Martin, R. Childbirth education: The Indianapolis experience. *Birth and the Family Journal* 6:105, 1979.

Chapter 11 Adolescent Pregnancy

Throughout the world, pregnancy and childbearing are occurring at younger ages than in the past, with undesirable health, demographic, and social consequences. In developing countries the concept of adolescence as a time of gradual transition from childhood to adulthood is often relatively new; traditionally, initiation rites, puberty, or child marriage marked the abrupt acquisition of adult status. Only recently in some countries has this distinct group of individuals been recognized as psychologically and physiologically different from children and adults [1]. A definition of adolescence formulated by the World Health Organization in 1974 [42] included such reference points as the period from the development of secondary sex characteristics to the development of sexual maturity; the period when psychologic processes change to those of an adult; and the period during which relative socioeconomic independence is achieved.

Historically most cultures have attempted to control the sexual activity of their young people. In Asia and many parts of Africa adolescent marriages have encouraged adolescent childbirth but it has occurred within a socially accepted pattern. Some African cultures allow premarital adolescent sexual activity but discourage pregnancy by methods such as coitus interruptus (withdrawal). If pregnancy occurs, the result may be a forced marriage, legal action, ostracism, abortion, or even infanticide. In some other parts of the world, such as parts of Latin America and the Caribbean, adolescent sexual activity and childbearing are common and culturally acceptable. In some of these areas there is often a history of unofficial marriage, or consensual union, where the young couple lives together. It may be that more than half of all births in these places are to mothers (adolescent and older) who are unmarried or involved in a consensual union [1].

Current trends indicate that across the world there is a growing percentage of births to young married and unmarried mothers compared with other age groups. Three factors suggest that these trends will probably continue: Teenagers in many countries are sexually mature, sexually active, and capable of reproduction at a younger age than their parents were; couples are marrying at older ages; and urbanization and the life-styles associated with it provide many more opportunities for the development of sexual relationships at the same time that the effectiveness of traditional social restraints is weakened [1].

*Earlier Menarche and
Later Marriage* The trend toward earlier menarche has been well documented in developed countries, and there is evidence of a similar trend in the developing countries. Sexual maturation is not only occurring earlier, but couples are getting married later, thereby lengthening even more the period of nonmarital fertility. Since adolescents spend more time in school, enter the labor market later, and marry later, the gap between sexual and social adulthood has continued to widen.

Urbanization With increased urbanization, traditional mechanisms to control adolescent sexuality are less effective. Social controls, such as segregation of the sexes and the presence of chaperones, are far more difficult to enforce. Modern adolescents have greater personal freedom and are less willing to be guided by community and family pressures.

DEMOGRAPHIC CONSEQUENCES OF EARLY CHILDBEARING

Family planning programs in developing countries traditionally have concentrated on serving older couples who already have children, encouraging them to prevent additional unwanted births. Emphasis has not yet been placed on making these services available to the adolescent population [1]. It is postulated that the population under 20 years of age, including children under 10, who will be adolescents during the 1980s constitutes more than half the total population in many developing countries. It might be assumed that a potentially serious population growth problem might be averted if these teenagers were offered options to early parenthood through family planning services and provided with sex education [1].

SOCIAL CONSEQUENCES OF EARLY CHILDBEARING

The social consequences of early childbearing vary from culture to culture. As previously mentioned, adolescent birth can be common and socially acceptable. In most countries, however, this is not the case. In Malaysia, the pregnancy of an unmarried girl is regarded as a sin and a disgrace to her entire family. Strong social pressure may result in forced marriage or illegal abortion, or even cause the pregnant girl to commit suicide. The unmarried adolescent who has a child may also find that her prospects for marriage are limited [1].

Throughout the world, the child of an unmarried adolescent may face social and legal discrimination and economic difficulty. With the advent of urbanization, the child is even more likely to be subject to neglect or abandonment since the extended family members may not be close enough to care for the child if the mother cannot.

In countries where society frowns on the unmarried mother, marriage is viewed as a necessary consequence of adolescent pregnancy. Although this course of action may permit the girl to avoid social disapproval or discrimination, it does not help her to avoid the increased health risks or interrupted education. In addition, in many cultures forced marriage has been shown to be less stable than planned marriage, and the failure rate is high [1].

HEALTH CONSEQUENCES OF EARLY CHILDBEARING

Pregnant adolescents throughout the world face a greater risk of reproductive problems. Although research reports are not always in agreement concerning physiologic complications, rather consistent mention is given to premature delivery [11,46], anemia [17,30], preeclampsia [1,5,17,37], and a higher maternal mortality [32].

The death rate from complications is 35 percent higher for those from 15 to 19 years old and 60 percent higher for adolescents 14 and under [2]. The death rate for infants born to teenagers under 18 is almost twice that for infants born to women in their early twenties. The incidence of low birth weight among infants is estimated to be twice as high in teen mothers as in women in their twenties [2].

FAMILY PLANNING SERVICES

Provision of family planning services to adolescents is restricted by legal and social limitations. In some countries availability of contraception is limited by age regardless of marital status or by rules that married adolescents must have their husbands' consent for contraception services. Similar restrictions are placed on abortion services in many regions of the world. The few family planning services that are available for adolescents are often a part of postabortion or postpartum programs [1].

Anecdotal reports and fragmentary data suggest that in most developing countries couples are not usually encouraged to use contraception until they have had at least one and frequently more children. Access to free or inexpensive contraception from official sources appears to be especially limited in the developing countries of Asia, which have traditionally emphasized premarital virginity. In other cases provision of contraceptive services is hindered by some physicians' and midwives' reluctance to prescribe contraception for unmarried minors [1].

Unmarried teenagers also often have difficulty obtaining abortions, since the abortion laws of many countries require parental permission. In Taiwan, where abortion is illegal, an unmarried adolescent may obtain an abortion, but often at a much higher price than a married woman. On the other hand, in some countries abortion is easier for young or unmarried women to obtain; for example, the Finnish Abortion Act permits abortion without a doctor's certificate for women under 17 and over 40 years of age. The current trend in developed countries is to allow teenagers improved access to contraception and abortion services and to avoid setting age limits when new laws relating to family planning are established [1]. Currently in the United States the trend seems to be toward a more restrictive birth control program.

ADOLESCENT USE OF CONTRACEPTIVES

Although there are limited comparative data on contraceptive knowledge and use in developing countries, anecdotal information suggests that only a small percentage of sexually active adolescents use contraceptives. In developed countries as well there is substantial ignorance about birth control as well as lack of contraceptive use among adolescents. In the United States, for example, only half of sexually active adolescent girls knew when they were theoretically fertile and safe [1].

Withdrawal has been a traditional method of birth control in many cultures and has sometimes proved to be successful. Generally, however, it is regarded as an unreliable method and is very difficult to practice.

Even though oral contraceptives are the most effective method of birth control, many physicians will not prescribe them until a regular menstrual pattern has been established for one to two years. This may be due to the fact that estrogen given to the very young girl before puberty may alter her future growth rate. In addition, because of systemic side effects associated with the pill, physicians may be reluctant to prescribe oral contraceptives for the teenager who is not sexually active on a regular basis [1]. It is also difficult for many teenagers to remember to take a daily pill, and contraceptive failure may result. As far as the teenager is concerned, the unmarried girl who asks for oral contraceptives admits an interest in sexual activity, a fact she may not want known.

As with the oral contraceptive, the adolescent girl who seeks an intrauterine device (IUD) is admitting that she contemplates sexual activity. Although retention rates are better in the young nulligravida with the newer, smaller IUDs, because of its systemic effects the IUD would not be the contraceptive of choice for the teenager who is not sexually active on a regular basis.

The diaphragm may be difficult for the teenager to use since it requires planning, preparation for each intercourse, skill in insertion, and facilities for washing and storage. It has not been widely used and is not available in many developing countries, but in the United States some studies have reported high contraceptive effectiveness rates for young women using diaphragms. On that basis some family planners have recommended greater use of diaphragms in adolescent programs [1].

Condoms are widely used by young people to prevent pregnancy and are especially suitable for the adolescent because they are inexpensive and accessible. It is also safer for the boy to use a condom than for the girl to use oral contraceptives, especially if they are not sexually active on a regular basis. Studies in the United States have suggested that young men are increasingly willing to share in family planning when they are given the opportunity. In many countries, condoms are the birth control method that is most readily available. They are particularly valuable in many developing countries where other contraceptives are often difficult to obtain [1].

ABORTION
The number and percentage of total abortions performed on adolescent girls have increased in most countries. Adolescent abortions account for about 25 percent of the total abortions performed in England, Scotland, Wales, and Sweden, and about 33 percent of total abortions in Canada and the United States [1]. Medical and psychologic consequences of abortion seem to be similar for both young and older women. Unfortunately, adolescents tend to request abortions when their pregnancies are advanced and therefore require more complicated termination procedures. Many times adolescents have difficulty in recognizing and/or accepting that they are pregnant. They may be unaware of where to go for advice and help or may be reluctant to ask for guidance from adults in general. In addition, adolescents are less likely to have the money necessary to pay for the abortion and may hesitate seeking one for that reason.

SEX EDUCATION
At present few countries provide organized sex education for adolescents. Several major obstacles to sex education in the school setting are noted in an international study of population and sexuality education; they include taboos and customary laws, religious objection, fears of promoting sexual promiscuity, objections by parents and school officials, and difficulties in recruiting and training teachers. The present trend seems to be toward greater acceptance of such programs, and both developed and developing countries are beginning to enter the sex education field [1].

SCOPE OF THE PROBLEM IN THE UNITED STATES
Pregnancy among adolescents is an increasingly serious problem in the United States. It carries with it tremendous medical, social, economic, psychoemotional, educational, and vocational risks for the mother and baby. Currently there are more than twenty million females between the ages of 10 and 19, and 50 percent of those between 15 and 19 are sexually active [5,35]. It is estimated that almost one million teens will become pregnant this year, and about 600,000 will carry their pregnancies to term. This constitutes 20 percent of all births in the United States [34].

Because the decline in the fertility rate among older women has been greater than that among adolescents, births in the younger age group now account for a larger proportion of all births in the United States [13,35]. Although the actual birth rate among teens has declined somewhat in recent years, this has had an effect only on the 15- to 19-year-old group; rates are still rising for young

Table 11-1. Estimated Number (in Thousands) of Live Births to Unwed Mothers in the United States, by Race and Age of Mother

Race and Age	Number of (thousands) Births to Unwed Mothers					
	1945	1950	1960	1965	1970	1977
By race of mother						
White	56.4	53.5	82.5	123.7	175.1	220.1
Nonwhite	60.9	88.1	141.8	167.5	223.6	295.5
By age of mother						
Under 15	2.5	3.2	4.6	6.1	9.5	10.1
15–19	49.2	56.0	87.1	123.1	190.4	239.7
20–24	39.3	43.1	68.0	90.7	126.7	168.6
25–29	14.1	20.9	32.1	36.8	40.6	62.4
30–34	7.1	10.8	18.9	19.6	19.1	23.7
35–39	4.0	6.0	10.6	11.4	9.4	8.8
40 and over	1.2	1.7	3.0	3.7	3.0	2.3
Total number	117.4	141.6	224.3	291.2	398.7	515.7
Percent of all births	4.1	3.9	5.3	7.7	10.7	15.7

Source: Modified from U.S. National Center for Health Statistics. *Vital Statistics of the United States*. Hyattsville, Md., 1981.

adolescents (under 15) [2]. The largest such increase has been among young white girls (Table 11-1).

Research by Zelnick and Kantner [44] reveals a sharp increase in the proportion of females among both whites and blacks who have had sexual intercourse at each age. Although the overall level of intercourse is lower among white adolescents, the rate of increase is faster than among black adolescents (Table 11-2).

In the United States, the general increase in births to teens has been attributed to the decrease in age of menarche [43], the increase in the number of adolescents in the population, a reported increase in sexual activity among young people, and inadequate use of contraceptives, especially by younger teens [44]. In 1976 an estimated 83 percent of unintended first pregnancies among adolescents occurred in the absence of contraception [2].

Obviously not all teenage pregnancies end in the birth of a baby. In 1977 approximately 400,000 legal abortions (one-third of the total number of such abortions in the United States) were performed for women under 20 years of age

Table 11-2. Percent of Metropolitan Area Females Aged 15–19 Who Were Sexually Active Before Marriage, by Race, 1979, 1976, and 1971.

Marital status, age	1979			1976			1971		
	Total	White	Black	Total	White	Black	Total	White	Black
All women	49.8	46.6	66.2	43.4	38.3	66.3	30.4	26.4	53.7
Ever married	86.7	86.2	91.2	86.3	85.0	93.9	55.0	53.2	72.7
Never married									
Total	46.0	42.3	64.8	39.2	33.6	64.3	27.6	23.2	52.4
15	22.5	18.3	41.4	18.6	13.8	38.9	14.4	11.3	31.2
16	37.8	35.4	50.4	28.9	23.7	55.1	20.9	17.0	44.4
17	48.5	44.1	73.3	42.9	36.1	71.0	26.1	20.2	58.9
18	56.9	52.6	76.3	51.4	46.0	76.2	39.7	35.6	60.2
19	60.0	64.9	88.5	59.5	53.6	83.9	46.4	40.7	78.3
15–17	36.3	32.6	55.0	30.2	24.5	55.0	20.5	16.2	44.8
18–19	63.0	58.8	82.4	55.5	50.1	80.1	43.1	38.1	69.3

Source: Adapted from M. Zelnik, and J. F. Kantner. Sexual activity, contraceptive use and pregnancy among metropolitan-area teenagers: 1971–1979. *Family Planning Perspectives* 12:230, 1980.

Year	Total Abortions	Abortions to Women 15–19		Abortions to Women Under 15	
		Number	Percent of Total	Number	Percent of Total
1978	1,410	419	29.7	15	1.1
1977	1,320	398	30.1	16	1.2
1976	1,179	363	30.8	16	1.3
1975	1,034	325	31.4	16	1.5
1974	899	278	31.0	14	1.5
1973	745	232	31.2	12	1.6
1972	587	191	32.6	n.a.	n.a.

Source: *Factbook on Teenage Pregnancy.* New York: Alan Guttmacher Institute, 1981.

(Table 11-3). Data indicate that about 30 to 40 percent of adolescents 15 to 19 years old and 42 percent of those 14 or younger terminate their pregnancies through abortion (Table 11-4) [14].

CAUSES OF THE PROBLEM—SOME SPECULATIONS

Everyone from psychiatrists, psychologists, and sociologists to the man on the street has attempted to characterize and in many cases stereotype young women who have become pregnant. A recurrent theme is that adolescent pregnancy reflects an underlying family pathology; the problem may be a lack of love, understanding, and security at home, a broken home, a poor parent-child relationship, conflict between parents, or a dominating mother or father [36]. Other theories emphasize the young woman's immature personality; they suggest that her increased dependency needs, emotional disturbances, rebellion against authority, and weak ego have resulted in sexual acting-out. Each of these theories has been taken to task. Wimperis [41] points out that premarital intercourse is fairly common; should all who have sexual relations be regarded as emotionally disturbed, or would this designation apply only to those who have a child as a result? Older studies by Clark Vincent [38] show that many young mothers apparently have mature personalities and come from stable homes with good parent-child relationships. A girl may be more apt to come from a broken home if she happens to come from a lower socioeconomic class, where broken homes occur more frequently. Emotional deprivation is not inevitable for a person from a broken home, since there are often strengths in the situation that compensate for the absence of a parent.

Other theories attribute unwed motherhood to the young woman's need to be pregnant and to have a child. Sometimes teens fear and doubt their femininity

	Total			Currently Married			Unmarried		
	Total	White	Non-white	Total	White	Non-white	Total	White	Non-white
Total <20	38.0	39.1	35.4	6.4	5.4	13.8	54.6	64.5	38.8
15–19	37.6	38.8	34.7	6.4	5.4	13.9	54.6	64.6	38.2
18–19	36.6	37.2	34.9	7.4	6.1	16.8	57.3	67.2	39.5
15–17	39.3	41.6	34.4	3.7	3.8	2.7	51.2	61.0	36.8
15	51.1	54.4	48.4	0	0	0	54.2	61.0	49.0

Source: *Factbook on Teenage Pregnancy.* New York: Alan Guttmacher Institute, 1981.

and even question their ability to produce children. Pressure from the peer group may also be a powerful influence in causing adolescent pregnancy. However, in other cases peer group contacts may be limited, with few social interactions, few permanent friendships, and few male contacts; this deprivation may cause the girl to feel a need to establish a close relationship with someone.

Another belief is that the rate of births out of wedlock reflects a decrease in religious conviction. In one study [6], however, one-third of a group of Canadian unwed mothers considered themselves fairly religious or strongly religious, which is similar to the proportion of religious adherence in the general population. In addition, Cutright [8] notes that in the United States church membership rose from 49 to 64 percent between 1940 and 1965; during that same period the illegitimacy rate more than doubled.

Thus, pregnant adolescents have been described as promiscuous, emotionally disturbed, products of troubled families. Their pregnancies have been attributed to loose morality, lower class status, or behavior that is acceptable to a minority group. Low academic achievement and desire for recognition and self-esteem have also been associated with adolescent pregnancy [47].

RELATIONSHIP TO
ADOLESCENT
DEVELOPMENT

Socially and emotionally, adolescents develop both a sense of themselves as individuals and a sense of identification with group ideals. The development of an adolescent's personal identity involves the evolution of continuity between his perception of himself from one moment to the next and the congruity of his perception of himself with others' perceptions of him [20]. Part of that self is his sexual identity, including gender roles, sexuality, and capacity for intimacy.

The exploration of one's identity requires taking risks, experimenting with different roles, and testing personal relationships. For the first time adolescents are aware that they have a personal destiny. But even though they are beginning to feel some commitment to making contributions to their future through mastery of significant tasks, society continues to view them as childlike and denies them the opportunity for such ego growth. For example, at the first sign of adolescents' seeking peer relationships instead of parental companionship, parents may overreact with extreme parenting styles, thus pushing the adolescents farther away [20]. (In the past even though adolescents were biologically younger, society considered them to be socially older as they were a desirable addition to the labor force. Today because of child labor laws and compulsory education requirements, adolescents are considered to be socially younger even though they are biologically older.)

Adolescence is a time of great intellectual growth and change. The beginning of the ability to think abstractly makes it possible for adolescents to see themselves as others see them. Elkind [10] points out that this may lead to typical adolescent egocentric behavior, a great self-conscious concern about how others (their "imaginary audience") actually see them. It may also lead to a sense of privateness based on the assumed uniqueness of their personal feelings—their "personal fable." A personal fable is a belief that contradicts what an individual has learned to be true; for example, a sexually active girl may truly believe that she herself cannot become pregnant although she knows how pregnancy occurs. The "imaginary audience" concept refers to the adolescent's believing that he attracts everyone's attention. He is often self-conscious about walking into a room full of people, thinking that everyone is staring at him. His perception of how he looks to others is of the utmost importance, and his self-esteem may be somewhat fragile.

It has been suggested that pregnancy in some middle-class adolescents results from problems peculiar to their stage of development. These include attempting to break the bonds of a dependent mother-daughter relationship, steering a boyfriend into a more committed relationship, rebellion, desire for peer affection and acceptance, need for a personal possession, or assurance of fertility.

SPECIFIC PROBLEMS AND APPROACHES TO SOLUTIONS

Adolescent pregnancy and its associated problems began receiving national attention in the early 1970s. The Children's Bureau and later the Office of Education stimulated demonstration programs across the country aimed at ameliorating the problem. With the help of the National Alliance Concerned with School Age Parents, they also undertook a major information dissemination and technical assistance effort, which helped many communities realize the magnitude of their adolescent pregnancy problem and find ways to attempt to solve it [35]. More recently, additional governmental funds have been made available for comprehensive community services for these adolescents under Public Law 95-626 passed in November 1978. Such major program developments occurred after the number of births to females from 15–19 years of age began to decrease. As abortion statistics became more reliable, it was obvious that the numbers of pregnancies had not declined: By 1977, among females 14 years of age and under there were more abortions than births [35].

Adolescent sexuality, pregnancy, and parenthood are multidimensional experiences and therefore demand multidimensional responses on the part of service providers. Recognition of this fact has led in the past 10 years to the establishment of more programs for adolescents, although not many are truly comprehensive. Most do include some health, education, and social services but not to the extent that all the adolescents' needs are met.

A 1970 survey of services provided for pregnant adolescents in 150 U.S. cities of 100,000 population or more indicated a need for day care for infants, contraception and abortion services, and services for unwed fathers [39]; a repeat survey in 1976 showed that the same needs remained unmet to a great extent [13]. The results of these surveys are consistent with general descriptions of major problems related to the access of pregnant adolescents to health services: The population at risk has not been reached adequately; the impact of maternal-child health programming has not been documented/evaluated; programs for teenage mothers are underfinanced and understaffed; many members of the at-risk group have no health insurance coverage; and existing programs have been characterized by a lack of planning and coordination.

HEALTH CARE

Pregnancy in young mothers is associated with distinct hazards, including higher rates of prematurity, increased susceptibility to complications of pregnancy, and a resulting increased infant and maternal mortality. The age, parity, and social conditions of many girls in this group may be, in part, responsible for the increased risks. Whatever the reason, the fact remains that this high-risk group is in need of early and continuous prenatal care.

A number of deterrents prevent many young women from receiving the care they need. Some of them postpone seeking care; they conceal their pregnancy out of fear, guilt, or denial. Others neglect to seek assistance because of inadequate information about resources available to them, the cost of health care, or disillusionment with medical clinics and the response of many personnel. If staff members fail to recognize that their own values and standards may not be the same as the teenager's, they may make erroneous assumptions about her feelings and react in inappropriate ways. The needs of the girl are often not met because health personnel are concerned only with the needs they have identified.

Effective nursing care of the pregnant adolescent depends on the establishment of effective communication with her [28]. Open-ended questions and clear descriptions at the individual's level of understanding are helpful. Listening to the adolescent express her thoughts, fears, and misconceptions is a fruitful beginning. Try to create a stable, secure atmosphere by offering accurate consistent responses to the adolescent's questions, planning discussion topics in advance, encouraging the adolescent to select topics for discussion, and meeting on a regular basis. Give her individual attention and enhance her self-image by encouraging her and praising her in the presence of her peers. Be available at specific times in case the adolescent seeks clarification about certain topics [28].

Copeland's research [7] supports the notion of the adolescent's participation in her own care. The 14 adolescents in her study preferred group-discussion-oriented classes and chose the topics for discussion. Mercer [23] suggests that finding out how the adolescent perceives the role in which she finds herself, whom she perceives as being helpful to her in that role, and how she views her infant will give clues as to how to effectively plan her care.

Often, care in existing medical facilities is still fragmented, depersonalized, and so time-consuming that it frustrates even the most mature adult. In an attempt to counteract this deficiency, some agencies have made efforts to personalize their patient care by instituting an appointment system, having the adolescents relate to the same staff members at each visit, and arranging clinic time to include evening hours.

Other attempts to improve care include establishment of comprehensive programs, such as Young Mothers' Educational Development (YMED) in New York State, Delaware Adolescent Program in Wilmington, Yale–New Haven's Young Mothers' Program, and the federally funded Maternal-Infant Care (MIC) Project. The health services of all of these programs generally include prenatal care, hospital care, postpartum checkups to mothers, newborn care in the hospital, and well-baby care for varying periods after birth.

CONTRACEPTIVE
SERVICES—
ACCESSIBILITY

Family planning clinics have grown from 214,000 to 1.5 million between 1969 and 1978. Many states permit adolescents to consent on their own to contraception and abortion services at a lower age (14–16) than the age of majority; some states have no age limit. Some states permit adolescents to give their own permission if they can be considered "emancipated minors" (the definition varies but generally requires that the adolescent be married, pregnant, or a parent already, living apart from parents, supporting herself in part or managing her own finances, or in the armed forces [9]). In any case, contraception is not used on a regular basis by most teenagers. In one study almost 70 percent of the sample of 15- to 19-year-olds had never used a contraceptive method because they did not think they would get pregnant, did not worry about it, were afraid to ask for it, or

Reason for Delay	Percentage
Didn't get around to it	39.5
Afraid family would find out	32.4
Thought birth control dangerous	28.4
Afraid of examination	25.5
Waiting for closer relationship with partner	24.3
Thought it cost too much	18.8
Didn't think had sex often enough to get pregnant	18.4
Didn't know where to get birth control	16.2
Never thought of it	15.4
Didn't expect to have sex	14.0
Thought had to be older to get birth control	13.5
Too young to get pregnant	11.4
Thought birth control wrong	9.8
Thought wanted pregnancy	9.5
Partner objected	9.4
Thought birth control I was using was good enough	8.8
Forced to have sex	1.7
Had sex with relative and didn't want to talk	0.8

Note: Table excludes patients who came to the clinic before they had sex or within a month of first intercourse.
Source: Unpublished tabulations from L. S. Zabin and S. M. Clark, Johns Hopkins University School of Medicine, 1980. In *Factbook on Teenage Pregnancy*. New York: Alan Guttmacher Institute, 1981.

felt that it made intercourse too planned. The remaining teens thought that they were too young to get contraception or were not aware of its availability [45] (Table 11-5).

EDUCATION

For many teenage mothers, in addition to the medical risks of pregnancy, there is the added problem of the interruption of their education, which decreases the likelihood of their ultimate independence. Many drop out of high school because of personal embarrassment, family pressure, and school policy.

Educational repercussions of adolescent pregnancy are a troubling social problem. Pregnancy is the major cause of school attrition among young girls and may contribute significantly to the dropout ratio among boys. As many as eight out of 10 teenagers pregnant at age 17 or younger may never finish high school; as many as four out of 10 teenagers pregnant under age 15 may never go beyond the eighth grade. Of young women who are under 16 when they first become pregnant, perhaps 60 percent will have another child while still of school age. All of this has implications for the teenager's future preparedness for entry into the job market as well as her realization of her potential [35]: Adolescent mothers must develop marketable skills so that their futures will be as productive as possible, but they often cannot take advantage of opportunities for job training and employment because they lack basic education and because child care services are next to nonexistent (at present about 93 percent of adolescents giving birth are keeping their babies).

SEX EDUCATION

A major problem facing youth today is the contradictory messages they receive from society: On one hand, it is chic and desirable to be sensual and sophisticated, with an emphasis on having fun and developing one's sexual responses; on the other hand, part of the sophistication is knowing when to stop or what to do so that one does not become a parent before being ready to fill the role. It would seem that adolescents are expected to learn how to achieve the appropriate balance by some kind of magic. Sex education in schools is required or encouraged by only a handful of states. Fewer still encourage teaching about birth control or abortion. Most states still let the local school boards decide how to implement sex education programs. Arnold [4] aptly notes that "legislators and schools say 'it' should be taught at church or at home. Church and home 'pass the buck' back to the school. Consequently sex education is taught by anyone a year older than the one learning or by those who can sneak into X-rated movies."

For the most part, no one cares to deal with the affective component of sexual relations and methods of coping with the emotions involved. Young people are left to determine for themselves how to deal responsibly with sexual drives, either by controlling situations that could end in unplanned pregnancy or by using birth control measures to prevent pregnancy. Studies reflect a frightening lack of knowledge on the part of young people of the function of their reproductive system, of the consequences of unprotected intercourse, and of the magnitude of the pregnancy experience, as well as a lack of acceptance of responsibility.

SOCIAL SERVICE
Sociologically, the pregnant adolescent has been described as suffering from a syndrome of failure [40]: the failure to fulfill functions of adolescence, failure to remain in school, failure to limit the size of her family, failure to be self-supporting, and failure to have healthy infants. This "adolescent trap" appears to be difficult to break out of without supportive services. Therefore, the teenage mother is often in need of practical assistance in dealing with the stresses of daily life and the plans that must be made for her and the baby's future. In one study [29], mothers identified their needs as housing, financial aid, baby care, employment or job training, help with personal or social adjustment, medical care, and legal aid. Health care workers felt that the mothers also had implicit needs for friendship, an independent life, and the respect of others for their personal worth.

Social service agencies attempt to help girls solve their personal problems that may have led to or been caused by their pregnancy, thereby increasing their potential for a more satisfying future. These agencies also provide assistance with practical aspects of housing, finances, and baby care centers if the girl will not be living at home. Finding adequate housing can be a particular problem for unmarried mothers: Managers of public housing may be reluctant to give her space, viewing her as a social liability, and landlords may exploit her situation [31].

UNMARRIED FATHERS
Unlike the unmarried adolescent mother, who has been the focus of research and comprehensive supportive programs, the unmarried father remains virtually ignored. Vincent [38] cites several reasons for this. The double standard has led to a harsher judgment for the female than the male for sexual misbehavior. The presumption of innocence until proved guilty offers more protection for the male. Sexual misbehavior that threatens the mores supporting legitimacy is very evident in the female; therefore, her behavior is censured. Since the unmarried mother and her child constitute a potential economic burden for society, they generate more public interest. Unwed mothers also are easier to identify and study as a group than are unwed fathers.

The most comprehensive work that has been reported was done at Vista Del Mar Child Care Service in Los Angeles by Ruben Pannor and his associates [26]. Data were collected on 222 unmarried mothers and 96 unmarried fathers. Contrary to the widely held stereotype, the relationship between the mother and father was more than a casual one. When the pregnancy became known, most of the fathers were very willing to take part in the mother's planning and decision-making, especially when she requested it. Pannor's data reinforced other findings that the fathers and mothers were approximately the same age and from a similar social, economic, cultural, and educational background.

Interviews of the fathers revealed seemingly contradictory ideas. Although most subscribed to the "sex is fun" ethic, many reported their actual experiences to be unsatisfactory, leaving them feeling guilty, depressed, and scared. The majority of the fathers and mothers did not use contraception, although they were knowledgeable about it and did not feel they would have difficulty in obtaining it. Almost 50 percent of the fathers stated that they did not like contraceptives; 24 percent stated that intercourse was not planned; 12 percent acted on the faith that nothing would happen. A recurring comment was to the effect that the use of contraceptives debased the act: "She wasn't that kind of girl."

There appeared to be a widespread lack of concern for the consequences to the partner: "When neither sexual partner possesses a strong identity and neither is responsible and mature, each reinforces the other to satisfy personal needs" [26].

Pannor and associates [26] list ways in which the unmarried father can best participate when pregnancy becomes a reality:

1. Giving support to the unmarried mother. This lends some dignity to the relationship and is important to the mother.
2. Helping to plan for the child's care and future.
3. Acknowledging and meeting financial responsibility. (Fathers in the study were willing to do this.)
4. Looking at the problems revealed by the pregnancy.
5. Understanding the meaning and responsibilities of marriage and parenthood.
6. Examining his attitude toward the child's mother.
7. Identifying his attitude toward sex and understanding the meaning of sexual relations.
8. Understanding his attitude toward fatherhood. (Holding their babies after birth helped the fathers toward this goal.)

The fathers in Pannor's study had the social workers' help in working toward the above goals. When the fathers were involved throughout the pregnancy, the final decision about the child's future either was made jointly by the father and mother or, as in most of the other cases, was made by the mother and reinforced by the father. This seemed to leave both parents with a more positive feeling about their choice.

Parents of the unwed couples also were participants in the study since Pannor and his associates felt that they had a right and a responsibility to assert themselves. The couples needed to be aware of their parents' thoughts and feelings, as well as the extent of the practical support that they were willing to offer. In addition, the parents needed to help in understanding and coping with the situation.

RELINQUISHING THE BABY

Whether or not to keep the baby is a decision that is made by the mother alone or with the support of the baby's father, relatives, or friends. In some cultural groups it is the accepted norm to keep the baby; in these cases, for the most part, the decision is ready-made. When a mother decides to place her baby for adoption, she should have explored all the alternatives open to her and have chosen the one that is best for her. It is important that she be supported in her decision by health care personnel; the mother should not have the additional burden of having to cope with the expression of opposing attitudes and values of the staff. As one young mother stated, "I found myself giving support to nurses who would say, 'I don't see how you can give up such a beautiful baby,' or 'I can't be here when you leave. It will be so sad because I know you're giving up the baby.' "

The first few days after delivery can be particularly trying as additional details concerning adoption procedures must be finalized at a time when the mother feels fatigued, isolated, and unable to make decisions. Following the relinquishment of the baby, the mother may begin to feel guilt and loneliness. She may undergo a grieving process as she works through what the separation from the baby has meant to her. For some, this will take a considerable amount of time.

IMPLICATIONS FOR THE FUTURE

The statistics reported in Table 11-6 indicate that health care planners (including nurses) involved in future multidisciplinary efforts to address the problem of adolescent pregnancy should pay increased attention to some specific issues. More consideration needs to be given to pertinent services—either primary or secondary prevention [16]. Family life and sex education for adolescents who are not yet sexually active would be the ideal starting point for primary prevention, but this is easier said than done, considering the opposition experienced by health

Table 11-6. Teenage Pregnancy—An Overview

Births to Teenagers	Health Risks
Teenagers have nearly one in five babies born in the United States; two-fifths of these births are to unmarried girls.	The death rate from complications of pregnancy and childbirth is 13 percent greater for 15- to 19-year-olds and 60 percent greater for teenagers 14 or younger compared with women in their early 20s.
Pregnancy	
One in six teenage girls who have premarital intercourse becomes pregnant.	Babies born to teenagers are two to three times more likely to die before their first birthday than babies born to women in their early 20s.
One in 10 teenage girls aged 15–19 becomes pregnant each year.	**Contraception**
Six in 10 teenage pregnancies end in live births, nearly three in 10 are terminated by abortion, and one in 10 ends in spontaneous abortion.	Only three in 10 sexually active teenage girls use contraception consistently.
One-third of all legal abortions performed in the United States are performed on teenagers.	Among sexually active teenage girls who do not use contraceptives, seven in 10 think that they cannot become pregnant.
	The condom, withdrawal, and the pill account for more than three-fourths of all birth control methods used by teenagers.
	Half of all sexually active teenage girls are not receiving family planning services from clinics or private physicians.

Source: Adapted from C. Green, and K. Potteiger. *Teenage Pregnancy: A Major Problem for Minors.* Washington, D.C.: Zero Population Growth, 1977.

educators who have tried to introduce such subjects into elementary and secondary school curricula. Research needs to be done to provide data on adolescent learning patterns in relation to sexuality and health care and on ways to make primary prevention programs accessible and acceptable to the adolescent population as a whole.

When sexually active adolescents in the pursuit of either primary or secondary prevention enter the system of comprehensive services (for pregnancy testing, contraception, or abortion), it is important that they not be lost to follow-up. Some person or agency in each community should be readily identifiable as a source of help and should assume responsibility for the coordination and continuity of care for each teenager. Transportation to needed services should be an option provided for each adolescent client.

Some evaluation of current programs has been done, but the studies have been on a short-term basis and have been mainly concerned with the numbers receiving services rather than with the service's effectiveness or suitability [3]. To facilitate evaluation, program goals and objectives should be stated at the beginning of the planning process, and an evaluation model should be built in so that evaluation of progress toward goals is continuous. Continued program effectiveness should be a condition for financial support. Mechanisms should be explored by both public and private funding agencies to consolidate resources and provide the best use of available monies. Research needs to be done on the cost of such comprehensive service programs to society as well as to the individual, and some standardization of accessibility and eligibility requirements is also in order. Flexibility and inconsistency in state definitions for eligibility have caused a denial of health care and other services to adolescents. In some states women may be excluded from Medicaid unless there is a dependent child already in the home. Since states develop their own plans for the provision of many services, they may or may not include support for pregnant adolescents.

It has taken a long time for the law to recognize the rights of adolescents and many gray areas still remain [9]. As progress is made toward the goal of uniformity of laws regulating the provision of reproductive health services with or without parental consent, there is finally emerging a coherent body of law based on two fundamental principles: the constitutional right of mature minors to obtain reproductive health services on their own consent and the constitutional right of all minors to have an alternative to parental involvement in implementing their decisions about such health care [27]. This does not diminish the need for programs to include other family members as well as the adolescent father in the comprehensive antepartal services provided. Research needs to be done on the total effect of reproduction on the adolescent mother, the adolescent father, the baby, and the extended family. Data are only beginning to be gathered on the adequacies or inadequacies of adolescents as parents [23]. In addition, there is a need to look at the effect of long-range hormonal contraception and abortion on adolescents' future childbearing potential [21].

The adolescent should be an active participant in the learning and caretaking process during childbearing. She should be involved in planning for her individual care and needs to be recognized by the staff as someone who is capable of making valuable and responsible suggestions in this regard [7]. The adolescent should be encouraged to make some self-assessment of her health status since research indicates a significant correlation between perceived health and psycho-physiologic symptoms, perceived stressfulness of life, and current health status [12]. Such data would have an impact on planning for that individual's care, might offer an explanation for her subsequent acceptance or rejection of offered services, and might yield significant preventive health benefits. Such data would also provide clues to the adolescent's perception of pregnancy as an illness or a normal event [22].

It is obvious that the attitudes of health care professionals toward the pregnant adolescent can exert a potent influence on the success of her participation in the program of care. It is unfortunate that many times she is treated in a punitive fashion or viewed as having a lower social desirability because of her socioeconomic status [24]. Perhaps self-awareness programs should be a part of the inservice education of those who will be working with this highly specialized population.

Development of mutual participation between the adolescent and the caregiver in a one-to-one sustaining relationship appears to be effective; several reports comment specifically on the positive relationship between successful outcome and the role played by the nurse in a primary nursing milieu [14, 19, 25, 33]. It also appears advisable that the relationship extend beyond the normal six-week postpartum period in order to assure maximum effectiveness. Klein has emphasized the critical nature of the period six months after delivery when many additional high school dropouts occur [18]; if the caregiver is still there to offer necessary support, the dropout rate during this crisis period may not be so high.

Planners of reproductive health programs have not always paid sufficient attention to the program evaluation research that has already been done. Such study results can indicate how to improve programs in order to cope more effectively with the problem of adolescent pregnancy. The most recent publication by the Alan Guttmacher Institute [35] suggests that programs for pregnant teens need to emphasize the following: realistic sex education; nonjudgmental personnel; adequate pregnancy counseling; adequate health care for the teenager and her baby; education, employment, and social services for adolescent parents; national health insurance coverage for all health services related to adolescent pregnancy; expansion of research efforts to discover new safe and effective methods of contraception to meet the needs of teenagers; and earlier provision of education in the areas of family life and health by parents and the school, even as early as the third grade.

Adolescent Pregnancy

Problem Situation

Kim Jackson is a 16-year-old high school senior who is 18 weeks pregnant. She lives in a six-room home with her mother, father, a 19-year-old sister, and a 14-year-old sister. Kim's father is 50 years old, suffers from hypertension, and is employed as a printer with the local newspaper. Kim's mother is 54 years old and a housewife. Kim's 19-year-old sister is a student at a local community college and her 14-year-old sister is a high school freshman at Kim's high school. The Jacksons are a church-going family and are active in the affairs of their community. They expect their girls to complete college.

Kim claims that the father of her baby is Nate Smith although Nate denies this and wants nothing to do with Kim. Kim did not want to carry the pregnancy and was about to have an abortion when her parents found out and stopped her. They wanted her to deliver the baby and then place it for adoption. Kim now feels if she carries the baby to term she will keep him or her. She is not sure if she wants to finish high school, although she has passing grades. Her current plan is to deliver the infant and move from her parent's "gospel" home into an apartment of her own. Many details of her plan are vague, including her future income. Kim's best girlfriend is also pregnant. She is marrying the 18-year-old father of the baby.

Thus far in her pregnancy Kim has gained 2 pounds. She is 5'3" and weighs 115 pounds. She admits to smoking occasionally and to drinking beer on occasion. She doesn't eat breakfast, has a couple of sweet rolls for lunch, and has dinner with her family.

Her hemoglobin is 10.5, her hematocrit 31.5. Kim also insists that she wants to deliver at a birth center, not a hospital. She has just registered at the local hospital's prenatal clinic where you will be her primary nurse.

What would be your initial response to Kim? Identify the essential elements of the nursing care you will provide to Kim. Questions to consider:

1. What are some of the actual or potential health care problems in Kim's situation?
2. How may the developmental tasks of adolescence affect Kim's childbearing experience?
3. How may family roles, expectations, and support systems affect Kim's childbearing experience?
4. What are the high school and community resources in your town that could be used to support Kim and her family?
5. Identify how the care you provide to Kim differs from that of other members of the health care team.

REFERENCES

1. *Adolescent Fertility, Risks and Consequences.* Population Reports, Series J, No. 10, July, 1976.
2. American College of Obstetricians and Gynecologists. *Adolescent Perinatal Health: A Guidebook for Services.* Chicago, 1979.
3. American College of Obstetricians and Gynecologists. *Statement of Policy: Adolescent Reproductive Health Care.* Chicago, 1979.
4. Arnold, L. Teenage pregnancy. *Journal of the Tennessee Medical Association* 64:1054, 1971.
5. Baldwin, W. Adolescent pregnancy and childbearing—growing concerns for Americans. *Population Bulletin* 31(2):2, 1976.
6. Clamen, A., Williams, B., and Wogan, L. Reaction of unmarried girls to pregnancy. *Canadian Medical Association Journal* 101:328, 1969.
7. Copeland, D. Unwed adolescent primigravidas identify subject matter for prenatal classes. *Journal of Obstetric, Gynecologic and Neonatal Nursing* 8:248, 1979.
8. Cutright, P. Illegitimacy: Myths, causes, and cures. *Family Planning Perspectives* 3:26, 1971.
9. Dowben, C., and Bunch, P. Legal Aspects of Adolescent Pregnancy. In P. Smith, and D. Mumford, *Adolescent Pregnancy.* Boston: G. K. Hall, 1980.
10. Elkind, D. Egocentrism in adolescence. *Child Development* 38:1025, 1967.
11. Erkan, K. Juvenile pregnancy: Role of physiologic maturity. *Maryland State Medical Journal* 20:50, 1971.

12. Garrity, T. Factors influencing self-assessment of health. *Social Science and Medicine* 12:77, 1978.
13. Goldstein, H., and Wallace, H. Services for and needs of pregnant teenagers in large cities of the United States, 1976. *Public Health Reports* 93(1):46, 1978.
14. Hayes, L., and Crovitz, E. Adolescent pregnancy. *Southern Medical Journal* 72:869, 1979.
15. Hibbard, L. Maternal mortality due to acute toxemia. *Obstetrics and Gynecology* 42:263, 1973.
16. Jekel, J. Primary or secondary prevention of adolescent pregnancies. *Journal of School Health* 47:457, 1977.
17. Jovanovic, D. Pathology of pregnancy and labor in adolescent patients. *Journal of Reproductive Medicine* 9(2):61, 1972.
18. Klein, L. Early teenage pregnancy, contraception, and repeat pregnancy. *American Journal of Obstetrics and Gynecology* 120:249, 1974.
19. Klerman, L., and Jekel, J. *School-age Mothers: Problems, Programs, and Policy.* Hamden, Ct.: Linnett Books, 1973.
20. Lipsitz, J. Adolescent Psychosexual Development. In P. Smith, and D. Mumford, *Adolescent Pregnancy.* Boston: G. K. Hall, 1980.
21. McAnarney, E. Adolescent pregnancy—a national priority. *American Journal of Diseases of Children* 132:125, 1978.
22. McKinlay, J. The sick role—illness and pregnancy. *Social Science and Medicine* 6:561, 1972.
23. Mercer, R. Teenage motherhood: The first year. *Journal of Obstetric, Gynecologic and Neonatal Nursing* 9:16, 1980.
24. Osofsky, H. Some social-psychologic issues in improving obstetric care for the poor. *Obstetrics and Gynecology* 31:437, 1968.
25. Osofsky, H. A program for pregnant schoolgirls. *Adolescence* 3:89, 1968.
26. Pannor, R., Massarik, F., and Evans, B. *The Unmarried Father.* New York: Springer, 1971.
27. Paul, E., and Pilpel, H. Teenagers and pregnancy: The law in 1979. *Family Planning Perspectives* 11:297, 1979.
28. Petrella, J. The unwed pregnant adolescent. Implications for the professional nurse. *Journal of Obstetric, Gynecologic and Neonatal Nursing* 7(4):22, 1978.
29. Sauber, M., and Rubinstein, E. *Experiences of the Unwed Mother as Parent.* New York: Community Council of Greater New York, 1965.
30. Scher, J., and Utian, W. Teenage pregnancy—an inter-racial study. *Journal of Obstetrics and Gynecology of the British Commonwealth* 77:259, 1970.
31. Singer, A. A program for young mothers and their babies. *Social Casework* 52:567, 1971.
32. Stickle, G. Pregnancy in adolescents: scope of the problem. *Contemporary OB/GYN* 5(6):85, 1975.
33. Tatelbaum, R. Management of teenage pregnancies in three different health care settings. *Adolescence* 13:713, 1978.
34. *Teenage Pregnancy—A Major Problem.* Washington, D.C.: Zero Population Growth, 1977.
35. *Teenage Pregnancy—The Problem That Hasn't Gone Away.* New York: Alan Guttmacher Institute, 1981.
36. Young, L. *Out of Wedlock.* New York: McGraw-Hill, 1954.
37. Youngs, D. Experience with an adolescent pregnancy program. *Journal of Obstetric, Gynecologic and Neonatal Nursing* 50:212, 1977.
38. Vincent, C. *Unmarried Mothers.* New York: Free Press, 1961.
39. Wallace, H. A study of services and needs of teenage pregnant girls in the large cities of the United States. *American Journal of Public Health* 63:5, 1973.
40. Waters, J. Pregnancy in young adolescents: A syndrome of failure. *Southern Medical Journal* 62:655, 1969.
41. Wimperis, V. *The Unmarried Mother and Her Child.* London: Allen & Unwin, 1960.
42. World Health Organization. Pregnancy and abortion in Adolescence: a report of a WHO meeting, Geneva, June 24–28, 1974. Geneva, 1975.
43. Zacharias, L. Sexual maturation in contemporary American girls. *American Journal of Obstetrics and Gynecology* 108:833, 1970.
44. Zelnick, M., and Kantner, J. Sexual and contraceptive experience of young unmarried women in the United States, 1976 and 1971. *Family Planning Perspectives* 9(2):55, 1977.
45. Zelnick, M., and Kantner, J. Reasons for nonuse of contraception by sexually active women aged 15–19. *Family Planning Perspectives* 11:289, 1979.

46. Zlatnik, F., and Burmeister, L. Low gynecologic age: An obstetric risk factor. *American Journal of Obstetrics and Gynecology* 128:183, 1977.

47. Zonkler, C. The self concept of pregnant adolescent girls. *Adolescence* 12:477, 1977.

FURTHER READING

Abernathy, V. Illegimate conception among teenagers. *Nursing Digest* 4(2):8, 1976.

Adams, B. N. The pregnant adolescent—a group approach. *Adolescence* 11:467, 1976.

Ambrose, L. Misinforming pregnant adolescents. *Family Planning Perspectives* 10(1):51, 1978.

American Academy of Pediatrics statement on teenage pregnancy. *Pediatrics* 63:795, 1979.

Anderson, C. The lengthening shadow: A case study in adolescent out of wedlock pregnancy. *Journal of Obstetric, Gynecologic and Neonatal Nursing* 5(4):19, 1976.

Anthony, E. Nutrition crucial for pregnant adolescents. *CEA News* 20:2, 1981.

Baldwin, W. The children of teenage parents. *Family Planning Perspectives* 12(1):34, 1980.

Beric, B. Obstetric aspects of adolescent pregnancy and delivery. *International Journal of Gynecology and Obstetrics* 15:491, 1978.

Brandt, C. L. Pregnant adolescents: Some psychosocial factors. *Psychosomatics* 19:790, 1978.

Burst, H. V. Adolescent pregnancies and problems. *Journal of Nurse Midwifery* 24(2):19, 1979.

Coddington, R. D. Life events associated with adolescent pregnancy. *Journal of Clinical Psychiatry* 40:180, 1979.

Cooper, J. C. Pregnancy in adolescents: Helping the patient and her family. *Postgraduate Medicine* 64(12):60, 1978.

David, H. P. International trends: Pregnancy and the unmarried girl. *Journal of Psychiatric Nursing* 15(2):40, 1977.

Dickerson, P., and Ouellette, M. Prenatal education for adolescents in a delinquent youth facility. *Journal of Obstetric, Gynecologic and Neonatal Nursing* 11:39, 1982.

Elster, A. B. Medical and psychosocial risks of pregnancy and childbearing during adolescence. *Pediatric Annals* 9(3):89, 1980.

Factbook on Teenage Pregnancy. New York: The Alan Guttmacher Institute, 1981.

Fischman, S. H. Adolescent unwed motherhood: Implications for a national family policy. *Health Social Work* 3(2):30, 1978.

Furstenberg, F., Lincoln, R., and Menken, J. *Teenage Sexuality, Pregnancy and Childbearing.* Philadelphia: University of Pennsylvania Press, 1981.

Gabbard, G. O. The unwed pregnant teenager and her male relationship. *Journal of Reproductive Medicine* 19:137, 1977.

Hardy, J. B. Long range outcome of adolescent pregnancy. *Clinical Obstetrics and Gynecology* 21:121, 1978.

Hendry, J. M. Pre and postnatal care sought by adolescent mothers. *Canadian Journal of Public Health* 71:112, 1980.

Hollingsworth, D. R. Sounding board. Teenage pregnancy solutions are evolving. *New England Journal of Medicine* 303:516, 1980.

Hutchins, F. L., Jr. Experience with teenage pregnancy. *Obstetrics and Gynecology* 54:1, 1979.

Jarrett, G. Childrearing patterns of young mothers: Expectations, knowledge, and practices. *American Journal of Maternal-Child Nursing* 7:119, 1982.

Kandell, N. The unwed adolescent pregnancy: An accident? *American Journal of Nursing* 79:2112, 1979.

Kinard, E. M. Teenage parenting and child abuse: Are they related? *American Journal of Orthopsychiatry* 50:481, 1980.

Levenson, P. Serving teenage mothers and their high risk infants. *Children Today* 7(4):11, 1978.

Merritt, T. A. The infants of adolescent mothers. *Pediatric Annals* 9:100, 1980.

Naeye, R. L. Teenaged and pre-teenaged pregnancies: Consequences of the fetal maternal competition for nutrients. *Pediatrics* 67:146, 1981.

Nakishima, I. C. Teenage pregnancy—its causes, costs, and consequences. *Nurse Practitioner* 2(7):10, 1977.

Phipps-Yonas, S. Teenage pregnancy and motherhood: A review of the literature. *American Journal of Orthopsychiatry* 50:403, 1980.

Ruszala, J. Adolescent pregnancy. *Nurse Practitioner* 5(2):22, 1980.

Steinman, M. E. Reaching and helping pregnant adolescents. *American Journal of Maternal-Child Nursing* 4:35, 1979.

Taylor, D. A new approach to contraceptive teaching for teens. *American Journal of Maternal-Child Nursing* 1:378, 1976.

Thompson, R. J., Jr. et al. Neonatal behavior of infants of adolescent mothers. *Developmental Medicine in Child Neurology* 21:474, 1979.

Tietze, C. Teenage pregnancies: Looking ahead to 1984. *Family Planning Perspectives* 10:205, 1978.

Turner-Woodson, E. Improving parenting practices among adolescents. *American Journal of Maternal-Child Nursing* 7:122, 1982.

PART 3 LABOR AND DELIVERY

Chapter 12   The Birth Process

ONSET OF LABOR   Labor consists of the regular, rhythmic contractions of the uterus, resulting in the birth of the infant and the delivery of the remaining products of conception. The mechanism responsible for the initiation of labor is unknown; theories that have been advanced include uterine stretch, oxytocin sensitivity, and progesterone blocking. Currently the prostaglandin and fetal cortisol theories are receiving much research attention.

Uterine Stretch Theory   According to the uterine stretch theory, labor is initiated because the uterus functions as any other viscous organ. The more the uterine wall is stretched as pregnancy advances, the more irritable it becomes and the more easily it will contract. It is also theorized that as pregnancy advances, the intrauterine pressure increases, perhaps causing local ischemia and aging of the placenta, thus reducing the pregnancy-stabilizing factors. This theory is receiving little research focus currently.

Oxytocin Theory   Proponents of the oxytocin theory note that as pregnancy advances the uterus becomes more sensitive to oxytocin. The levels of endogenous oxytocin do not appear to be increased during the course of pregnancy but concentrations in venous blood have been found to be elevated during labor [19,21]. One of the weaknesses of this theory is that pregnant women who have had hypophysectomies have a normal onset of labor. Research has also shown that hormones previously believed to be produced in the pituitary may actually arise in the hypothalamus; this is the case with oxytocin [24,30].

Evidence continues to accumulate that fetal oxytocin may affect uterine activity, especially during labor [14]. If this is the case, the oxytocin is probably infused into the myometrium across the fetal membranes rather than into the mother's circulation via the placenta. The placenta is an important source of enzymes (oxytocinase in particular) that destroy oxytocin. Many researchers believe that oxytocinase helps to keep the pregnancy intact through prompt inactivation of oxytocin which may be released suddenly into the maternal circulation, thereby preventing excessive uterine activity. However, its clinical importance is still unproven [14].

Progesterone-blocking Theory   Progesterone has been cited as a blocking agent to uterine activity. This theory holds that the estrogen effects that increase myometrial contractility are counteracted by the influence of progesterone in effecting hyperpolarization of the cell membrane, thereby blocking electrical conduction. The degenerative changes that take place in the placenta cause a withdrawal of the progesterone and its relaxant effects on the uterus [12,13].

Most research has not produced conclusive evidence that progesterone levels necessarily fall before labor [54]. However, studies by MacDonald [40], Schultz [57], and Schwarz [58] suggest that as pregnancy progresses, there is a decrease in metabolism of progesterone by fetal membranes, which makes cellular lysosomes unstable and results in the release of phospholipase A. This enzyme works to make the prostaglandin precursor, arachidonic acid, more available for use [54].

Prostaglandin Theory   Prostaglandins have also been implicated as the initiators of labor since they are able to induce abortion and labor. Prostaglandin formation by the fetal membranes and uterine decidua vera may be the final step that occurs before the onset of labor contractions. It has been shown that prostaglandins administered intravenously or intra-amnioticly will cause myometrial contractions at any time during gestation, suggesting that prostaglandins play an important role in the initiation of contractions. Further support for this theory is the observation that levels of prostaglandins increase in the amniotic fluid of women in labor [54]. Metabolic products of prostaglandins also are increased in the maternal peripheral blood just before and during labor. Other evidence supporting the prostaglandin theory is that the administration of large amounts of aspirin has been shown to inhibit the conversion of arachidonic acid to prostaglandin and has resulted in prolonged gestation. [11].

Fetal Cortisol Theory   One currently prominent theory is that the fetus at term produces increased levels of cortisol which inhibit progesterone production from the placenta. With an anencephalic fetus whose pituitary hypofunction causes adrenal hypofunction, labor may be delayed and pregnancy prolonged. Research in sheep shows that stimulation of the fetal adrenal gland can provoke premature labor. Some research, however, suggests that elevated levels of cortisol found in fetal blood may be the result of labor, not the cause of it [53].

Combined Effect   Most of the prior research concerning the initiation of labor has been concerned primarily with the placenta and the uterus; now the fetus and fetal membranes are being considered as the main source of such a signal. A sequence of events might begin with an increased rate of fetal cortisol secretion because of some unknown stimulus, which acts on the placenta in some way to reduce the secretion of progesterone and to increase the secretion of estrogen and prostaglandins. Progesterone usually inhibits the synthesis and release of prostaglandins and thus a decrease in progesterone would augment the prostaglandin effect. The myometrium responds to prostaglandins with an increased sensitivity to oxytocin, which may lead to the onset of contractions without an actual change in oxytocin levels [39].

Ultimately the stimulus for uterine contractions must act on the contractile elements of the uterus, especially the myometrium. This mechanism probably requires an increased intracellular concentration of free calcium to cause the contraction of the smooth muscle of the uterus, just as free calcium is necessary to cause contractions in striated muscle. Prostaglandins and oxytocin appear to inhibit the ATP-dependent binding of calcium to the sarcoplasmic reticulum, thus increasing the concentration of free calcium, which may act with the muscle cell to produce a contraction. Uterine relaxation is associated with the translocation of calcium back to a stored form [39].

Nursing Intervention   Gay [20] emphasizes some points about these theories that have relevance for nurses. Women who are at risk for repeated spontaneous abortions or premature deliveries are often advised by their physicians to abstain from intercourse for varying periods of time. If you are aware of the relationship between the onset of labor and prostaglandins (found in semen), you can use this information to clarify the physician's counseling and make it more meaningful and perhaps more acceptable to the woman and her partner.

If the woman is in premature labor, you should be aware of the possibility that frequent cervical exams could stimulate oxytocin release via Ferguson's reflex. Therefore, these exams should be kept at a minimum. Also, the effect of the fetal stress and ACTH-cortisol relationship requires that nursing care be directed at minimizing maternal and fetal stress [38]. Nursing research by Lederman and others [35,36] has demonstrated that psychologic variables such as conflict and anxiety affect plasma catecholamine and cortisol production which in turn affects uterine activity (inhibited or uncoordinated contractions) and progress in labor (longer length of time). Her work underscores the woman's need for educational preparation to cope with labor as well as support from significant others, nurses, and physicians during the labor process.

MECHANICAL FACTORS AFFECTING LABOR

Pelvic Dimensions

The success of a woman's labor depends on a number of mechanical factors, including a pelvis with adequate dimensions, normal size and presentation of the fetus, and adequate uterine contractions. The woman's pelvis will already have been evaluated for adequate dimensions prior to the beginning of labor (see Chap. 7), but reevaluation generally takes place as labor begins. In addition, the dimensions of the pelvis are capable of changing slightly during the process of labor [49].

Fetal Dimensions

The fetus is well prepared for labor during the last trimester. His head is capable of changing its dimensions in order to accommodate itself to the woman's bony pelvis. While the skull bones of some fetuses are firmly ossified and capable of little change in shape, generally these bones remain relatively soft and able to change their shape and dimension. This is possible not only because the bones are soft but also because they are not united, remaining separated by membranous spaces known as *sutures*. The most important are the frontal (between the two frontal bones), the sagittal (between the two parietal bones), the coronal (between the frontal and parietal bones), and the lambdoid (between the back of the parietal bones and the margin of the occipital bone). With the exception of the temporal suture, these sutures can be felt by vaginal examination during labor (Fig. 12-1).

Where two or more sutures meet, an irregular space is formed on the fetal head, known as a *fontanelle*. The two most important fontanelles are the anterior, a diamond-shaped area formed by a meeting of the sagittal and coronal sutures, and the posterior, a triangular area formed by a meeting of the sagittal and lambdoid sutures. Less important are the two temporal fontanelles formed by the junction of the lambdoid and temporal sutures, and the sagittal fontanelle, a space sometimes found midway between the anterior and posterior fontanelle. The sutures and fontanelles allow the fetal skull bones to overlap or override in order to pass through the woman's bony pelvis. This overlapping is known as molding and is the reason for elongation of the fetal head at birth.

During birth it is important not only that the fetal skull bones are able to override but also that the fetus's head passes through the birth canal with the smallest diameters presenting. When the head is fully flexed, the suboccipito-bregmatic diameter enters the woman's pelvis (this diameter is measured from

Figure 12-1. Fetal head bones, sutures, and fontanelles.

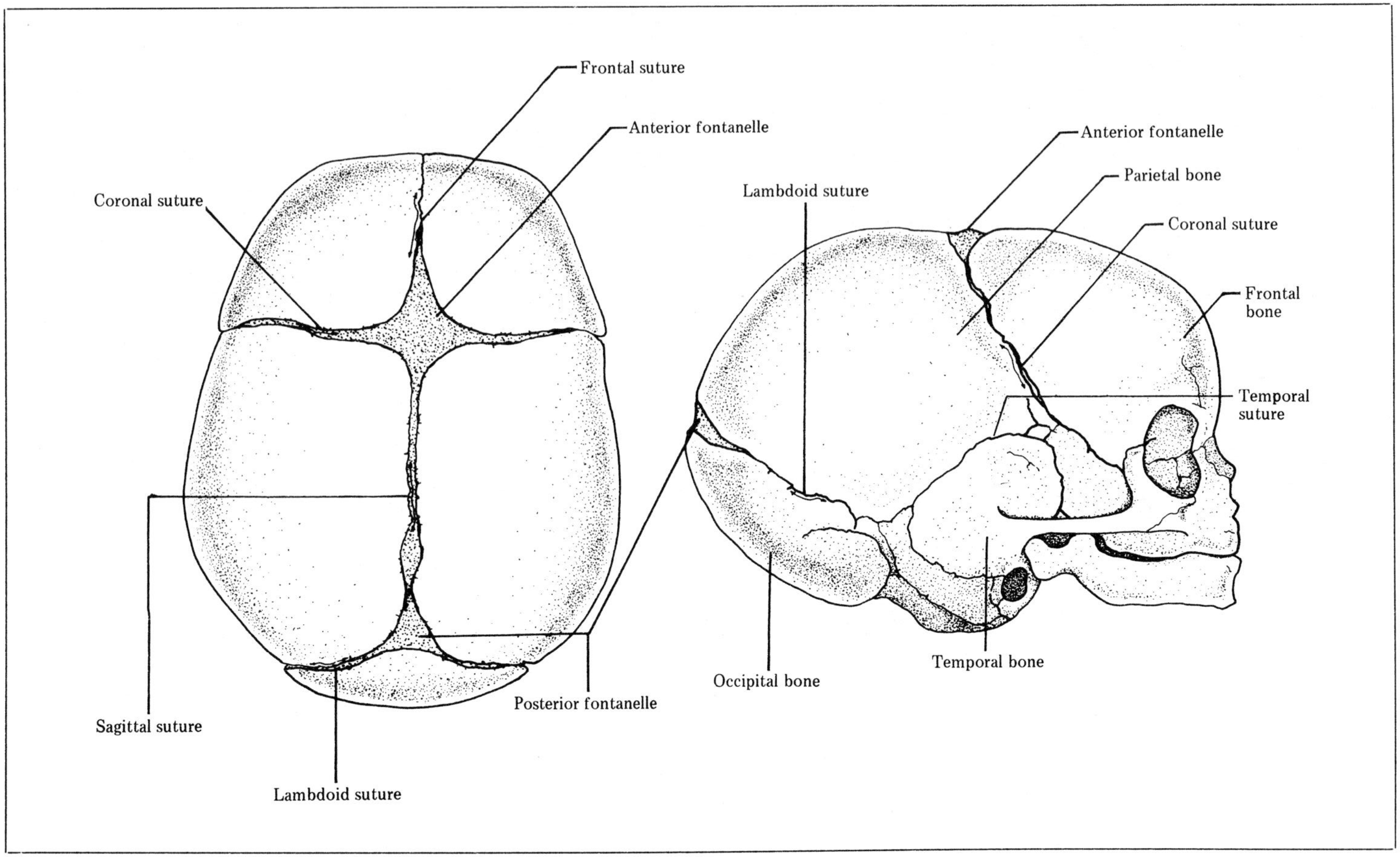

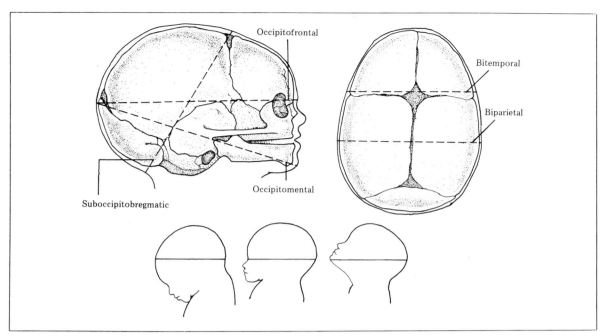

Figure 12-2. Presenting diameters of the fetal head.

the middle of the large fontanelle to the undersurface of the occipital bone; it averages 9.5 centimeters, or 3.7 inches). As the fetal head assumes various extended positions, other diameters become important. With moderate extension the occipitofrontal diameter presents (this diameter extends from just above the root of the nose to the most prominent portion of the occipital bone; it averages 11.8 centimeters, or 4.6 inches). With marked extension the occipitomental diameter presents (this diameter extends from the chin to the most prominent portion of the occiput; it averages 13.5 centimeters, or 5.3 inches). Two additional measurements often evaluated during pregnancy or labor are the biparietal diameter (the greatest transverse diameter of the head, averaging 9.3 centimeters, or 3.6 inches) and the bitemporal diameter (the greatest distance between the two temporal sutures, averaging 8.0 centimeters, or 3.1 inches) (Fig. 12-2).

Fetal Posture   During the last weeks before delivery, the fetus assumes a characteristic posture, or attitude, that is partially an attempt to accommodate himself to the space inside the uterus (Fig. 12-3). Generally the fetus tries to conform to the shape of the uterine cavity by folding his extremities and bending his back. The head is sharply flexed, the chin almost resting upon the chest; the thighs are flexed over the abdomen; the legs are bent at the knee joints; and the arms are folded across the chest or are straight down at the sides. This whole posture is characteristically referred to as *fetal attitude* or *fetal habitus*.

Fetal Lie   The fetus also assumes a *lie* (i.e., a comparison of his long axis and that of his mother), which can be either transverse or, more commonly, longitudinal (99 percent of fetuses at term). When the fetus assumes a longitudinal lie, either his head will present (cephalic presentation) and be felt on vaginal examination, or

Figure 12-3. Fetal posture in utero in a vertex presentation.

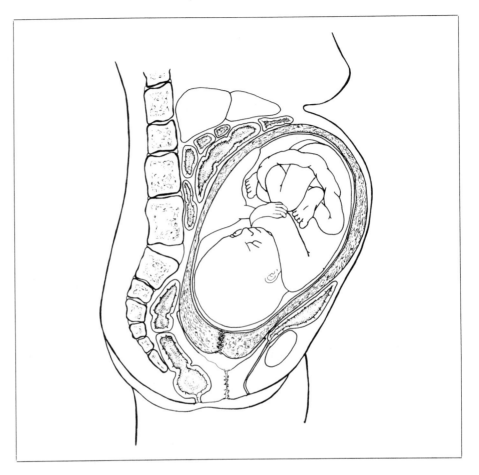

his buttocks or feet will present (breech presentation). In a transverse lie the shoulder will present.

Fetal Presentation and Position

Whichever portion of the infant is deepest in the birth canal and is felt on vaginal examination is referred to as the presenting part; this determines the presentation of the fetus. Cephalic presentations are classified according to the relation of the head of the fetus to the body. When the head is sharply flexed so that the chin rests on the thorax, the occipital area of the skull (vertex) is the presenting part (vertex presentation). Less commonly the head may be sharply extended, with the occiput in contact with the back; in this instance the face is felt on vaginal examination (face presentation). When the head is partially flexed, the large fontanelle is felt on vaginal examination (sincipital presentation), and when the head is partially extended, the brow can be felt upon vaginal examination (brow presentation) (Fig. 12-4).

Breech presentations are classified according to the position of the thighs and legs of the fetus. When the thighs are flexed on the abdomen and the legs extended up onto the chest, the presentation is known as a single, or frank, breech. When the thighs of the fetus are flexed on the abdomen and the lower legs

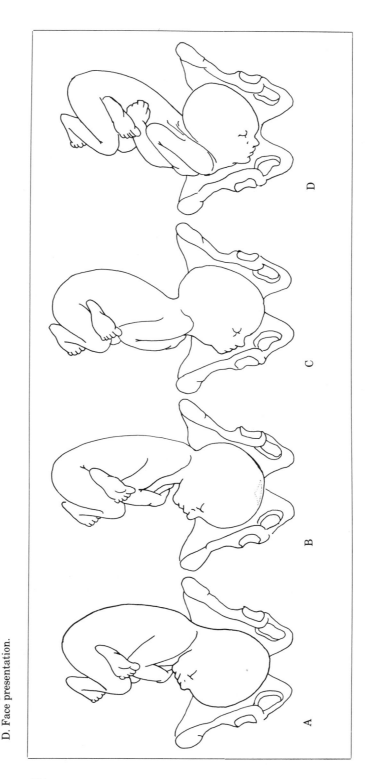

Figure 12-4. Types of cephalic presentation.
A. Vertex presentation.
B. Sincipital presentation.
C. Brow presentation.
D. Face presentation.

Figure 12-5. Breech presentations. A. Full or complete breech, with thighs flexed on abdomen and legs flexed on thighs. B. Single or frank breech, with legs extended over anterior surface of body. C. Incomplete or footling breech; if both feet present, as shown here, this is known as a double footling presentation.

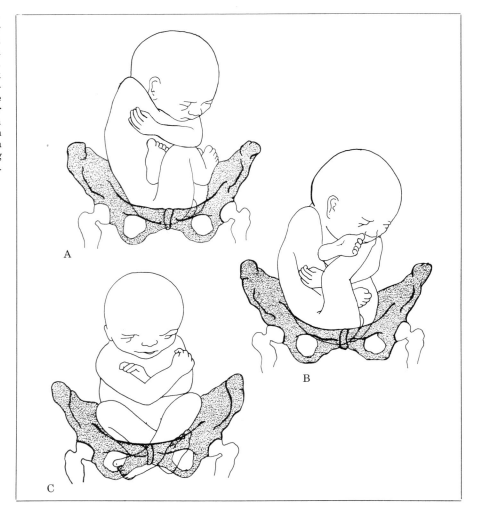

rest flexed on the thighs, the presentation is a full, or complete, breech. If one or both feet present first in the birth canal, the presentation is an incomplete breech of the type known as a single or double foot, or footling. Another form of incomplete breech presentation involves one or both knees presenting first (Fig. 12-5).

With each presentation, a landmark has been designated on the presenting part to help identify the type of fetal presentation during vaginal examination. The landmark designated for identification on breech presentations is the sacrum; in vertex presentations, the occiput; in face presentations, the chin (mentum); in shoulder presentations, the scapula (acromium).

In addition to identifying the landmark, and thus the type of fetal presentation, it also becomes essential during the course of labor to identify the position of that landmark in relation to the right or left side of the maternal pelvis. The identification of this position enables the midwife or physician to determine the

Figure 12-6. Positions of the fetus in utero. A. Left occipital anterior (LOA) position. B. Right sacral posterior (RSP) position.

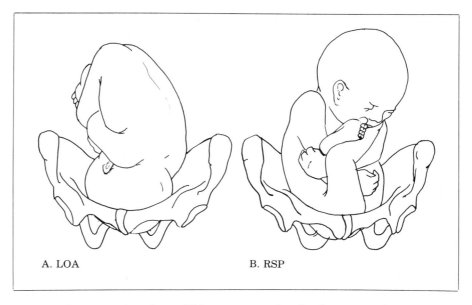

A. LOA   B. RSP

movements or rotation that will be necessary for the fetus to undergo prior to delivery.

The woman's pelvis is divided into four quadrants: a right and a left anterior quadrant and a right and a left posterior quadrant. A transverse position has also been designated as the position that divides the anterior and posterior portions of the pelvis.

On vaginal examination the landmark is identified, and a determination is made of the fetal position on the right or left side of the woman's pelvis and of its position in the anterior, transverse, or posterior portion of the woman's pelvis. For example, a vertex presentation with the fetus's occiput on the left side of the woman's pelvis and directed anteriorly would be designated as a left occipital anterior (LOA) position. Likewise, a breech presentation with the sacrum on the right side of the woman's pelvis and directed posteriorly would be designated as a right sacral posterior (RSP) position (Fig. 12-6).

As term approaches, the incidence of vertex presentations is approximately 95 percent, breech 3.5 percent, face 0.5 percent, and shoulder 0.5 percent. About two-thirds of all vertex presentations are on the left side of the woman's pelvis and one-third on the right side. The fetal occiput is usually directed transversely. The incidence of breech presentations is much higher earlier in pregnancy; one study notes an incidence of 7.2 percent at 34 weeks [54]. As pregnancy advances, it is believed that the fetus takes advantage of the diminishing room within the uterus by positioning himself so that the bulkier buttocks and flexed legs are accommodated within the fundus. For the same reason, many fetuses with hydrocephalus are born in breech presentation.

DETERMINING FETAL PRESENTATION AND POSITION
As discussed in Chapter 7, you may determine the presentation and position of the fetus by abdominal palpation using Leopold's maneuvers. Another method of determining fetal position and presentation is auscultation. In the later months of

pregnancy and during labor you will hear fetal heart sounds best a short distance from the midline if the fetus is in an occipitoanterior position, since the heart sounds are heard best through the fetus's back. With the fetus presenting in an occipitotransverse position you will hear the fetal heart sounds lateral to the midline; in an occipitoposterior position they are found in the woman's flank. Generally in cephalic presentations you will hear the fetal heart sounds best below the woman's umbilicus; in breech presentations they are most clearly heard at or slightly above the woman's umbilicus.

The use of x-rays is sometimes needed to determine fetal position and presentation. However, ultrasonography, which is also used for this purpose, offers the advantage of locating fetal position and parts without the hazards of radiation. (Other uses of ultrasonography in obstetrics include detection of early pregnancy, estimation of gestational age, identification of optimal sites for amniocentesis, localization of intrauterine contraceptive devices, and diagnosis of twin pregnancy, hydatidiform mole, intrauterine fetal death or growth retardation, placenta previa, fetal abnormalities, and ectopic pregnancy.)

Ultrasonography involves little preparation of the woman; the only requirement is that her bladder be full, since that will lift her uterus up and will provide a fluid-filled medium to aid in the transmission of sound. Oil or aqueous jelly is placed on the woman's abdomen so that the transducer can be moved back and forth with continuous airless contact between the transducer and her abdomen. The woman experiences no discomfort or problems and usually enjoys seeing the fetal parts and movements on the screen or photographic printout [16].

During labor when the cervix has dilated, fetal presentation and position can be identified on vaginal examination. If you are the examiner, using a sterile glove, introduce the index and middle finger of either hand into the woman's vagina. Upon palpation of the presenting part, identify the appropriate landmarks. You will feel the sutures and fontanelles in a vertex presentation, the nose, mouth, and other portions of the face in a face presentation, and the sacrum and ischial tuberosities in a breech presentation. With a vertex presentation, pass your fingers behind the symphysis pubis and then in a sweeping movement pass them toward the sacrum [54]; this will cause you to cross the sagittal suture, which you can then follow to locate the fontanelles.

Uterine Contractions   Successful labor depends on adequate uterine contractions as well as appropriate pelvic size and position of the fetus. There are a number of characteristics that can be noted of uterine contractions during labor. The contractions are involuntary and are usually associated with some degree of discomfort. During the contractions of labor, the actively contracting upper portion of the uterus becomes thicker, while the lower uterine segment (isthmus and cervix) becomes very thin. These changes divide the uterus into two distinct zones, an upper portion, which is actively contracting, and a lower portion, which is passive.

At the completion of a contraction of the upper uterine segment, the cells of that segment do not resume their original length but become fixed at a shorter length. While this occurs in the upper segment, the lower uterine segment becomes stretched with each contraction. Upon completion of the contraction, the cells in the lower segment remain stretched and fixed at a longer length; this is called receptive or postural relaxation. As the cells become stretched, this portion of the

Figure 12-7. A. Lower uterine segment thick; upper uterine segment contracting. B. Later in labor. The upper uterine segment thickens, pushing the fetus downward. The lower uterine segment thins and relaxes, allowing the fetus to pass through that portion.

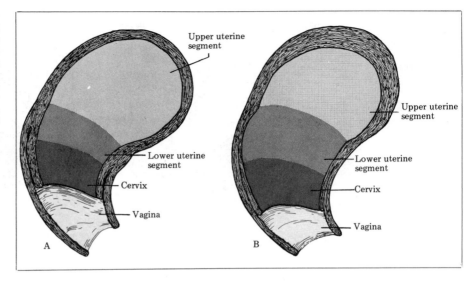

uterus and cervix becomes thinner (Fig. 12-7). (If this phenomenon did not occur, the fetus would not be pushed farther into the birth canal.) The round ligaments also contract with each uterine contraction, elevating the fundus and aligning the fetus more directly with the curve of the birth canal.

MECHANISMS OF LABOR

If the woman's pelvis is of adequate size, the uterine contractions adequate, and the size and position of the fetus appropriate, the fetus will make adaptive movements enabling him to progress through the birth canal. The movements are caused by the involuntary uterine contractions during the first stage of labor, together with voluntary abdominal muscle contractions during the second stage. The positional and rotational changes of the fetus are also effected by the resistance offered by the woman's bony pelvis, cervix, and surrounding tissues of the birth canal. The events of engagement, descent, flexion, internal rotation, extension, external rotation, and expulsion do not occur separately but rather overlap in time (Fig. 12-8).

Engagement

When the fetal head enters the pelvic inlet, the biparietal diameter, which is the narrowest presenting diameter, will go through the narrowest diameter of the pelvis. The occiput will rotate to the widest portion of the pelvis. Since the widest diameter of the pelvic inlet is the transverse diameter, the fetal head most often enters the inlet in a transverse position. Engagement is often defined as having occurred when the biparietal diameter of the fetal head has passed through the pelvic inlet. Other clinicians prefer to define it as having occurred when the biparietal diameter has reached the level of the ischial spines. In primigravidas, the fetal head may sink into the pelvis enough during lightening to constitute engagement. In most multigravidas engagement occurs during labor.

Descent

Fetal descent occurs throughout labor and is essential for the rotational movements that must occur prior to birth. It is accomplished through the force of the uterine contractions on the amniotic fluid, or, after rupture of the membranes, on

Figure 12-8. Mechanisms of labor. A. Cervical effacement complete; head flexed; descent begins. B. Descent continues; cervix dilating; internal rotation begins. C. Internal rotation complete. D. Extension. E. External rotation. F. Posterior shoulder delivered.

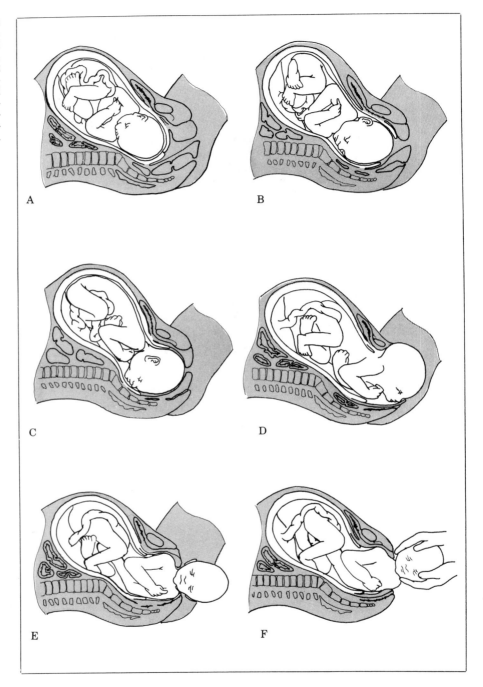

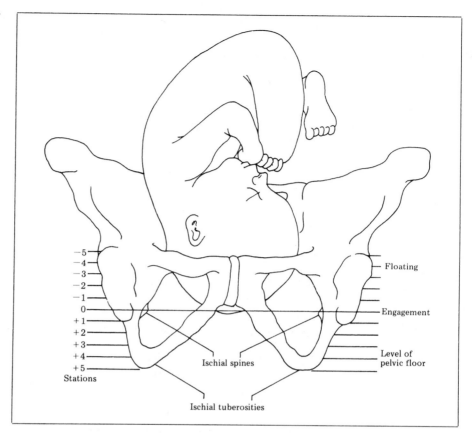

Figure 12-9. Stations of
the pelvis. Station 0 is
the level of the ischial
spines.

the portion of the fetus occupying the fundal area in the uterine cavity. During the second stage the efforts of the mother in bearing down increase intra-abdominal pressure and help effect expulsion of the fetus.

The degree of fetal descent may be described as floating, fixed, engaged in the midpelvis, or on the pelvic floor. Descent of the fetal presenting part is also described in relation to the ischial spines and is evaluated by stations. Station 0 is at the level of the ischial spines (engagement); stations −1, −2, −3, and −4 refer to 1, 2, 3, and 4 centimeters above the spines. When the presenting part is at station −4, the presenting part is floating. When the presenting part is 1, 2, 3, or 4 centimeters below the level of the spines, the station is referred to as +1, +2, +3, and +4. When the presenting part is at station +4, it is on the pelvic floor (Fig. 12-9).

Flexion   Flexion is an important movement in the mechanism of labor, since it aids accommodation of the fetal head to the birth canal by effecting presentation of the smallest fetal head diameter, the suboccipitobregmatic diameter (9.5 centimeters). Pressure is exerted on the fetus by the uterine fundus; as the fetal head meets resistance from the lower uterine segment, cervix, or pelvic floor, it is tipped forward so that the chin lies close to the chest.

Internal Rotation   In accommodating to the birth canal, the fetal occiput rotates from its original position anteriorly toward the symphysis. This movement results from the shape of the fetal head, the amount of space available in the midpelvis, and the sling shape of the perineal muscles. The ischial spines project into the midpelvic cavity, causing the anterior segment to be larger than the posterior and the anteroposterior diameter larger than the transverse. Since the occipital portion of the fetal head is larger than the frontal and sincipital areas, the occiput comes to occupy the anterior portion of the cavity. By doing this, the most flexible part of the fetal body, the nape of the neck, adapts to the curve of the birth canal.

Extension As the fetal head descends farther in the birth canal, it meets resistance from the perineal muscles and is forced into extension. The fetal head becomes visible at the vulvovaginal ring; its largest diameter is encircled (crowning), and it emerges from the vagina.

External Rotation Following delivery of the head, the occiput rotates to the position it occupied prior to internal rotation. The anterior shoulder also rotates so that it comes to lie under the symphysis. When the shoulder rotation takes place, the occiput rotates further so that the head and shoulders return to their normal alignment.

Expulsion Following delivery of the infant's head and internal rotation of the shoulders, the infant's anterior shoulder comes to rest beneath the symphysis pubis. The posterior shoulder is then delivered, followed quickly by the anterior shoulder, which slips from beneath the pubic arch. In some instances the anterior shoulder is delivered first. The remainder of the infant's body follows shortly.

The mechanisms above are descriptive of the delivery of the occiput anterior presentation. For a description of the delivery process of other presentations, see Chapter 19.

EVENTS PRELIMINARY TO LABOR
Prior to the onset of labor, several events occur. In nulliparas, approximately 2 weeks before the onset of labor, the fetal head drops into the pelvic inlet, thus causing descent of the uterus. In multiparas, this phenomenon, known as *lightening*, generally occurs with the onset of labor. After lightening, the woman may experience more leg cramping and difficulty in walking as a result of increased pressure in the lower pelvic region. Urinary frequency also follows lightening, while breathing generally becomes easier.

As labor approaches and as the cervix begins to dilate and efface, the plug of mucus that filled the cervical canal during pregnancy is discharged along with a very small amount of blood from the surrounding capillaries. The discharge, referred to as *show* (or *bloody show*), usually precedes labor by a few hours or days. This discharge also commonly follows vaginal examination during the later weeks of pregnancy, and often there is an increase in the discharge following vaginal examination during labor. Occasionally, the membranes will rupture prior to the onset of labor.

False labor contractions, which may occur as early as 3 to 4 weeks prior to delivery, are an exaggeration of Braxton Hicks' contractions, which occur during pregnancy. They can be differentiated from true labor contractions in a number of ways (Table 12-1).

THE COUPLE AND LABOR
The experience of labor and delivery is accompanied by varying degrees of stress for prospective parents, whether they have been prepared for the experience or not. How they are able to cope with and exercise control over their labor and

Table 12-1.
Differentiation of False
Labor from True Labor
Contractions

True Labor Contractions	False Labor Contractions
Result in progressive cervical dilatation and effacement	Do not result in progressive cervical dilatation and effacement
Occur at regular intervals	Occur at irregular intervals
Interval between contractions decreases	Interval between contractions remains the same or increases
Intensity increases	Intensity decreases or remains the same
Located mainly in back and abdomen	Located mainly in lower abdomen and groin
Generally intensified by walking	Generally unaffected by walking
Not affected by mild sedation	Generally relieved by mild sedation

delivery experience has far-reaching effects on their self-images, and on their relationships with each other and with their newborn.

Health services to the couple throughout childbearing and especially during this period of stress can do much to foster or inhibit the personal growth of each family member and of the family as a unit. Delivery of services must focus on the consumer's needs and desires supported by the expert knowledge of health care providers. As a nurse, your expert knowledge, your skills as a liaison between health care disciplines, and your skills as a client advocate will be particularly important during this period.

In the past 10 years in response to consumer needs and desires, numerous alternatives to traditional approaches to the labor and delivery experience have developed. These include birth centers, home deliveries, in-hospital birthing rooms, and changes in traditional hospital policies and approaches to care. As a part of their education for childbirth, consumers should be informed of the variety of alternatives available to them so that they might choose the one that best meets their needs.

The approach to care that follows is one that is general and can be applied to many settings. As an advocate for the consumer, remember that even within a given institution there are a variety of alternatives you can make available to the woman and her partner so that their experience of giving birth is satisfying and growth producing.

WHEN LABOR BEGINS

Regardless of the type of health provider or birthing facility the couple has chosen, they are generally advised to contact their midwife or physician when contractions are 5 to 10 minutes apart if the woman is a primigravida or when contractions have established a regular pattern if she is a multigravida. Both primigravidas and multigravidas are also asked to notify the midwife or physician immediately if they have vaginal bleeding or if their membranes rupture, since the incidence of intrauterine infection rises significantly when membranes have been ruptured more than 24 hours.

When the couple or woman arrives at the birth facility or hospital, your first action is to introduce yourself if you haven't met them before. This establishes the initial tone of the interaction and communicates to the couple that they are welcome. Initial impressions are generally long lasting, especially those established during times of stress.

In beginning your assessment, explain to the couple that it will be necessary to find out how far the woman's labor has progressed, and that to do so, you will be asking a number of questions, followed by a vaginal examination to see how much cervical dilation has occurred. You may begin your questioning with: What is the woman's gravidity, parity? When did contractions begin? How strong are they? How far apart are they? How long do they last? Has the woman noticed mucus or bloody vaginal discharge? If so, what is the color, consistency, amount? Have her membranes ruptured? If so, what is the color, consistency, amount, and odor? Rupture of membranes can be verified by placing a nitrazine-treated tape or swab in a pool of the fluid in her vagina. The presence of alkaline fluid will result in a positive test.

As you begin asking questions, observe the amount of discomfort the woman is experiencing. If she appears to be in obvious discomfort and is having contractions 2 or 3 minutes apart or if she shows any signs of wanting to bear down, it is essential that she be examined vaginally almost immediately.

If she is not in acute discomfort, next take her vital signs, including temperature, blood pressure, pulse, respiration, and fetal heart sounds. Take the woman's blood pressure between contractions; during and immediately after a contraction, the blood pressure reading is higher. Take the fetal heart rate also between contractions and count it for a full minute. You may also want to listen to the rate during a contraction and, immediately following one, to evaluate the fetal response to the stress of a contraction.

In recording the woman's vital signs, also time the *duration*, *intensity*, and *interval* of her contractions. The duration is timed from the beginning to the end of the contraction. The interval is measured from the beginning of one contraction to the beginning of the next. Each contraction has three phases: *increment*, *acme*, and *decrement*. Increment is the period of increasing intensity; acme, the period when the contraction is strongest; decrement, the period of decreasing intensity. The intensity of the contraction is measured by your ability to indent the uterus. With your fingertips on the woman's fundus, a mild contraction feels like a tense muscle, a moderate contraction is more firm, and a strong contraction cannot be indented by pressure of your fingertips (it may be described as being as hard as wood).

Next a vaginal examination will indicate the amount of cervical dilatation. Usually the woman will remain or be sent home on the basis of the extent of cervical dilatation and your evaluation of the woman's contractions.

If she is to go home, tell the woman or couple that they were correct in coming. This is usually a discouraging time and couples often feel guilty and foolish. Reassure the couple that the evaluation was useful, and introduce them to some of the staff members with the explanation that it would be good for them to meet, since they may be working together when the woman or couple returns. You might also take this opportunity to orient them to the surroundings if this has not already been done. If they have traveled a distance, you might suggest that they have a beverage or snack before going home to provide an opportunity for them to discuss the events and relieve the tension of the past few hours before driving in traffic.

If the woman is to remain, in some instances she may be given an enema and/or have her pubic hair shaved. An enema may be given to evacuate the colon and thus provide more room in the pelvic cavity; a full colon is believed to impede the progress of labor [65]. Also, feces from a full colon may be expelled during delivery and, if not wiped away, may contaminate the area unnecessarily [64]. However, many women who have had an enema prior to delivery have more difficulty establishing regular bowel movements following delivery. If the woman's membranes have ruptured, enemas are generally contraindicated to prevent infection of the birth canal.

Some midwives and physicians feel that a pubic shave makes episiotomy and its repair easier and aids in keeping the perineum clean. Some prefer a partial pubic shave (pubic hair removed from the top of the labia to the anus); a few prefer all pubic hair removed. Landry and Kilpatrick [34] and Young [65] point out that perineal shaving is not necessary in labor and delivery care since there are no significant differences between amounts of perineal skin bacteria with or without shaving. Lack of awareness of the relevant research, personal feelings, or discomfort with change may be some of the reasons why perineal shaves are still performed.

Following initial admission procedures, show the woman to a labor area. Orient her and her partner to the surroundings, explain the equipment and introduce them to the staff and the other women or couples who might be sharing the labor area. As Shannon-Babitz notes, this is the time when you can indicate to the couple how you can be of assistance to them during labor. During the discussion it is important for you to emphasize your collaborative role with the parents during the birth process [59].

Having made your initial assessment, you now want to turn your attention to a number of other items.

Much of the woman's essential history, such as history of previous labors, past medical history, and history of this pregnancy, already will have been collected through the nursing history and nursing assessments done throughout the woman's pregnancy. Access to the woman's prenatal nursing care plan will enable you to provide continuity of care if you are not the primary care provider or the woman's primary nurse who already knows her and her history. If this information is not available, you will need to collect these data during or immediately after the admission process.

The beginning of labor represents the culmination of 9 months of preparation by the woman and her partner for the arrival of their infant. It is a time when their anxiety may be at its highest level, when they are most in need of support by health care personnel, and when events have a profound impact on their future relationship. As you begin to develop a relationship with the woman and her partner, you will make several other assessments which will enable you to plan their care more effectively.

What is the woman's (or couple's) chief concern at this time?

What has been her (their) preparation for labor (type, by whom, when)?

What is her (their) understanding of the labor process? Is it perceived to be painful? What are the woman's expectations of the labor and delivery process? Partner's expectations? Family's expectations?

What are the woman's (partner's) needs? Do they have a need to be in control? Are they assuming a dependent role? How are they attempting to cope with the situation? What effective support resources are they using? What is the quality of their relationship? Intimate? Restrained? Interactive? Withdrawn? Anxious?

What type of communication are they using? Verbal? Nonverbal?

How fatigued do they appear to be? How much sleep have they had recently?

Have they experienced any stressful life changes recently?

This is a time to focus on the father's needs as well as on the mother's. Many men strongly identify with the expectant mother and their active participation in the birth of their children is extremely important to them. Wapner found that over 56 percent of the first-time fathers he studied felt "like we are both pregnant" [63]. He concluded that these men did not recognize themselves primarily as support persons for their partners but felt that they themselves were actively involved in an important life experience. Indeed, men may experience actual physical symptoms (nausea, weight gain, abdominal distension) known as the "couvade syndrome" as well as psychological changes during their wives' pregnancies. As Shannon-Babitz notes, merely allowing the father to attend the birth is not enough to make the experience of childbirth all that it can be for him and ultimately for the mother and child as well. She urges nursing colleagues to focus on the needs of the father as well as those of the mother throughout the birthing process [59]. Being aware of the needs and wishes of the couple includes an awareness of their feelings regarding technology used during labor.

FETAL MONITORING IN LABOR
Issues Involved in the Use of Monitoring

The use of fetal monitoring for assessing the progress of a woman's labor pattern and the condition of her fetus is controversial. While most consumers and health care professionals agree upon the value of using this technology with women who are clearly at risk of having a poor pregnancy outcome, routine monitoring of all women has raised several issues. What, if any, value does it hold for women with normal pregnancies? Does increased use of fetal monitoring increase the rate of cesarean births? What are the feelings and perceptions of the mothers on whom the technology is used? While more research is needed to address these issues, some data are available.

The intrapartum death rate for infants of women at risk during labor is lower in monitored women than in women who have not been monitored during labor, as reported in a number of studies. Paul and Hon [50] reported the results of a 3-year study of 6,686 high-risk monitored women: The intrapartum death rate for infants over 1,500 grams was 0.6 per 1,000 for the monitored group and 1.4 per 1,000 for the unmonitored women.

Several other studies [62] have been carried out to determine the effect of electronic fetal monitoring during labor on perinatal death rates. Some studies have suffered from small sample size [25], while a number of others have randomly assigned women to a monitored or nonmonitored group without analyzing risk factors for any of the women. Results from one of the largest studies to determine the benefit of fetal monitoring indicated that monitoring provided an absolute benefit of 1.5 lives saved per 1,000 babies monitored [50]. A subsequent study [47] of almost 16,000 live-born infants assessed the effect of electronic fetal monitoring on neonatal death rates: The crude neonatal death rate was 1.7 times higher in unmonitored infants than in those monitored. The researchers then adjusted the results for risk factors. When this was done, in the highest risk group 109 newborn lives might be saved for every 1,000 babies monitored. In the lowest risk group (babies at term with no associated risk factors) the neonatal death rate is about 1 per 1,000, approximating that of previous studies. Results such as these on routine monitoring of women not at risk provide data for arguments against routine monitoring of this group.

Opponents of fetal monitoring often indicate that auscultatory monitoring of the fetal heart rate by a nurse every 15 minutes is as effective as electronic monitoring. Benson et al. [3], however, in a computerized evaluation of 24,863 deliveries concluded that no single reliable auscultatory indicator of fetal distress exists in terms of fetal heart rate, save in extreme degree. Under optimal conditions in the labor and delivery unit, if one listens to the fetal heart every 15 minutes for a duration of 30 seconds, only 3 percent of the available information is gathered. Also, the rate is averaged over a time interval of 30 seconds, and baseline variability cannot be determined.

There have been reported associations between increased use of fetal monitors and increased rates of cesarean birth operations [1,7,46]. This association, however, has raised additional issues that require further research to answer adequately. What, if any, difference in newborn outcome can be documented? If an increased number of cesarean operations is associated with fetal compromise as documented by fetal monitoring, is subsequent neurologic impairment decreased in this group of infants? What are the legal implications for the physician and nurse if fetal monitoring indicates fetal compromise and a cesarean operation is not performed? These are but a few of the issues currently raised by consumers and health care personnel alike.

Attitudes Toward Fetal Monitoring

The feelings and perceptions regarding electronic monitoring of women who have been monitored vary according to the group studied. In a 1972 nursing study by Beck [2] of 50 women interviewed post partum to elicit their responses to having been monitored, it was reported that none had a positive initial response, whereas 31 had negative initial responses. The study replicated in 1977 reported that 11 women had negative initial responses and 28 had neutral initial responses. In a similar study, Dulock and Herron [17] studied the pre- and postnatal responses of 31 women who were monitored. Prenatally, 39 percent reported a positive attitude toward possibly being monitored during labor; however, after delivery, 85 percent reported a positive monitoring experience. Neutral attitudes were decreased from 29 to 15 percent, and no woman who was monitored reported negative attitudes following delivery. Shields [60] reports similar positive reactions to monitoring in the group she studied.

Much of the attitude change and positive response to fetal monitoring in all studies appears to depend upon the preparation and teaching about the technology prior to and during labor and delivery. The most consistent negative comments from mothers being monitored externally were that the abdominal straps were uncomfortable, the belts interfered with effleurage, and they had difficulty in getting comfortable. When internal monitoring was used, the most frequent complaints were fears that the fetal scalp clip would injure the baby, panic when the scalp clip slipped off and the fetal heart rate stopped, and discomfort during vaginal examinations to insert fetal scalp electrodes and uterine catheters.

Positive reactions to monitoring reported by McDonough, Sheriff, and Zimmel [41] and previously cited studies included feeling a sense of security when listening to the fetal heart beat. This allowed mother and father to relax. Additionally, mothers and fathers reported that the fetal monitor readout helped them with the woman's breath control since they knew when a contraction was starting. Mothers who had cesarean births because the fetus was in distress thought that if the monitor had not been used their babies might have died or been born very ill. Fathers reportedly felt mothers and babies received better care because the fetal monitor was used.

Clearly for some consumers and health care workers the issues raised by use of increased technology in childbirth, including fetal monitoring, will not be resolved by the results of research alone The use of technology in an area as intimate and closely associated with feelings of self-image and self-esteem has a strong emotional overlay. Thus, informing consumers about the results of research on all sides of the issues, as well as providing information on the various childbirth services available to them in the community and the various options available at each site, is an essential part of helping the future parents feel satisfied and ultimately experience personal growth during this time in their lives. For health care professionals, fetal monitoring is a tool for providing the best care possible to childbearing families. As any tool, it can be used appropriately or inappropriately and is only as helpful and effective as the individuals who use it.

External Monitoring   Recordings of fetal heart rate (FHR) and uterine contractions can be obtained by external or internal monitoring. In external monitoring an external tokodynamometer is strapped to the mother's abdomen to transmit uterine contractions and an external ultrasound transducer is attached similarly to transmit fetal heart rate patterns. In order to assure adequate uterine recordings, the pressure-sensitive tokodynamometer must be placed over the most contractile portion of the upper uterine segment. As labor progresses and the uterus descends, the tokodynamometer has to be lowered. If not readjusted, it may slip off the fundus and begin recording the woman's respiratory pattern and rate. The uterine contraction recording from an external tokodynamometer is accurate only for the frequency of the uterine contractions and semiaccurate for evaluation of duration of uterine contractions; estimation of the intensity of uterine contractions is inaccurate and is significantly altered by tension of the abdominal belt, maternal position changes, and obesity of the woman. Contractions that appear flat-topped on the tracing may indicate that the abdominal belt is too tight. In external monitoring the baseline level of the uterine contraction pattern is merely an arbitrary setting and bears no relationship to the actual resting tone of the uterine musculature (Fig. 12-10).

The external ultrasound transducer is applied to the mother's abdomen over the area of clear fetal heart sounds. The fetal signal used in this method relies on the mechanical opening and closing of the mitral and aortic valves. The method's limitations include loss of the signal source outside the transducer's range such as in maternal or fetal position change, maternal obesity, or excessive amniotic fluid (Fig. 12-11).

Figure 12-10. External fetal monitoring.

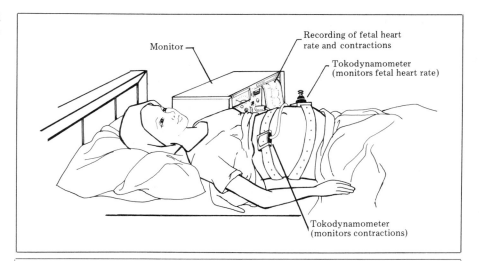

Monitor

Recording of fetal heart rate and contractions

Tokodynamometer (monitors fetal heart rate)

Tokodynamometer (monitors contractions)

Figure 12-11. Midwife assessing the progress of the woman during labor. (Courtesy of Pennsylvania Hospital, Philadelphia, Pa.)

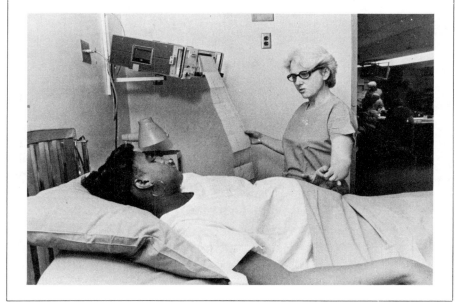

Internal Monitoring   Internal monitoring involves attaching a spiral electrode to the fetal presenting part, usually the fetal scalp, in order to transmit fetal heart signals (Fig. 12-12), and the placement of a water-filled catheter beyond the presenting part into the uterine cavity to record changes in uterine pressure. Uterine contractions cause the intrauterine pressure to increase and are represented in tracings by elevations in intrauterine pressure to 60 millimeters of mercury. Resting tone of 5 to 15 millimeters of mercury is normal.

The uterine contraction pattern is evaluated for frequency, intensity, and duration of contractions. Uterine contractions during the course of labor should show a regular pattern, with intervals of at least 2 minutes, durations of less than 90 seconds, and peak pressures of greater than 40 millimeters of mercury. In the

Figure 12-12. Internal fetal monitoring.

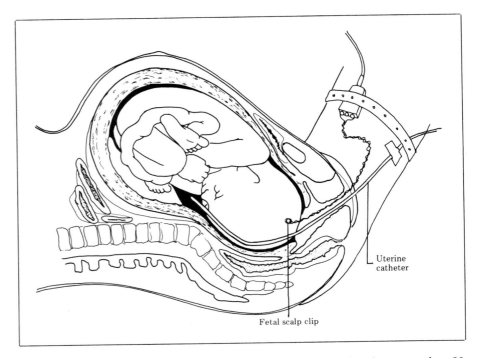

Uterine catheter

Fetal scalp clip

later phase of the first stage of labor (active labor), the amplitude approaches 60 millimeters of mercury. Adequate contractions also should be well-rounded and symmetrical in appearance on the tracing produced by the monitor. Uterine contractions with intervals of more than 3 minutes and durations of less than 45 seconds may be associated with slow progress in labor. Contractions with sharp peaks may be the result of oxytocin infusion. With excessive oxytocin administration, a pattern of one large contraction followed by a smaller one may develop. A similar pattern may occur in a persistent occiput posterior presentation (Fig. 12-13).

BASELINE FHR PATTERNS

Fetal heart rate patterns are evaluated for baseline patterns and periodic patterns. The FHR that occurs between contractions is known as baseline. Evaluation of patterns of baseline FHR includes evaluation of rate and variability. A baseline FHR is obtained by taking the average FHR over a tracing of several minutes. Normal FHR falls between 120 and 160 beats per minute. A rise in the FHR above 160 beats per minute for 10 minutes or longer is known as baseline tachycardia (Fig. 12-14). A fall in the baseline FHR below the 120 beats per minute level for 10 minutes or longer is known as baseline bradycardia.

Fetal baseline tachycardia may result from immaturity of the fetal autonomic nervous system, maternal fever from amnionitis, maternal anemia, and minimal fetal hypoxia. It may also be seen if the mother has received atropine or scopolamine. Tachycardia associated with late or prolonged variable decelerations indicates fetal distress.

Bradycardia may be caused by severe fetal hypoxia or maternal hypothermia. Baseline FHRs that are consistently low over a period of weeks are associated

Figure 12-13. Variations in uterine contractions. A. Normal uterine contractions. B. Long intervals, short contractions. C. Flat-topped contractions. D. Oxytocin contractions.

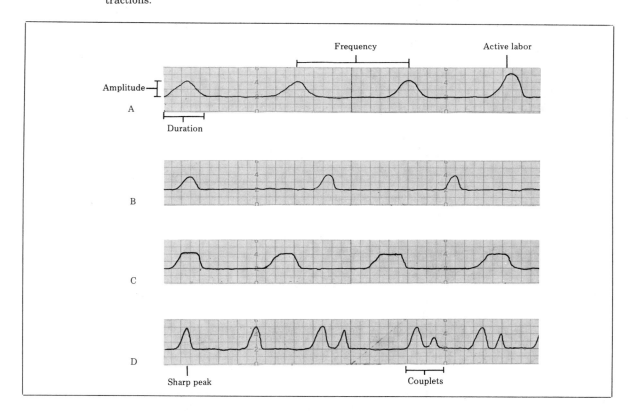

Figure 12-14. Baseline changes in fetal heart rate. Top tracing shows tachycardia (161–180 beats per minute). Bottom tracing shows bradycardia (100–119 beats per minute).

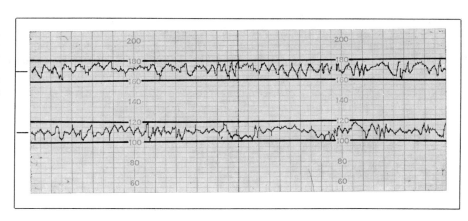

with congenital heart lesions. If, during labor, low FHRs are also accompanied by marked FHR decelerations, the newborn will usually be depressed.

In addition to assessing the rate of the fetal heart, assessing the fluctuations in the baseline rate or beat-to-beat variability is a most important measurement. The interaction between vagal and sympathetic tone causes variations of 3 to 10 percent of the baseline FHR. Variability may be categorized as reduced or absent, normal or average, and increased or exaggerated. Minimal or absent variability ($\leq$ 5 bpm) may indicate fetal nervous system depression or damage due to hypoxia, immaturity of the autonomic nervous system as seen in the preterm infant, "sleep" or reduced activity states of the fetus, or the pharmacologic vagal blocking action of drugs such as atropine, or drugs such as narcotics, tranquilizers, barbiturates, and alcohol which depress the nervous system. Diminished variability is often encountered in maternal disorders such as fever, preeclampsia, and diabetes.

Normal or average variability ranges between 6 and 25 beats per minute and is thought by many clinicians to be the most reliable indicator of a normal fetus.

Increased or exaggerated variability is greater than 25 beats per minute. Fluctuations of more than 25 beats per minute may represent fetal overcompensation following recurrent late or variable deceleration and may be a forerunner of hypoxia. Most often, this type of variability is associated with an intact fetus and normal newborn [51].

PERIODIC FHR PATTERNS

The FHR response during the period of a uterine contraction is known as periodic FHR. A FHR increase during a uterine contraction is called an acceleration; a transient decrease in FHR associated with a uterine contraction is known as a deceleration.

Accelerations are often associated with breech presentation, immature central nervous systems, maternal use of atropinelike drugs, partial cord compression, and fetal stimulation such as manipulation and sound. Acceleration appears to represent a sympathetic response in a well-integrated cardiovascular system.

When the FHR begins to drop with the onset of the contraction and returns to its baseline rate as the contraction ends, the response is called early deceleration, or type I dip (Fig. 12-15). The FHR during this deceleration remains above 100 beats per minute. The decrease is caused by compression of the head during the contraction. The resulting pressure alters intracranial pressure, resulting in altered blood flow and vagal stimulation. Stimulation of the vagus causes release of acetylcholine at the sinoatrial (SA) node, with resultant slowing of the fetal heart. Early deceleration also can be elicited by digital pressure on the fetal head during vaginal examination or by the pressure of forceps during delivery. Since this pattern is mediated through the vagus, it will not be affected either by giving the mother oxygen or by changing her to a position lying on her side. Early decelerations are considered innocuous and are not associated with fetal compromise, deteriorating acid-base status, or low Apgar scores.

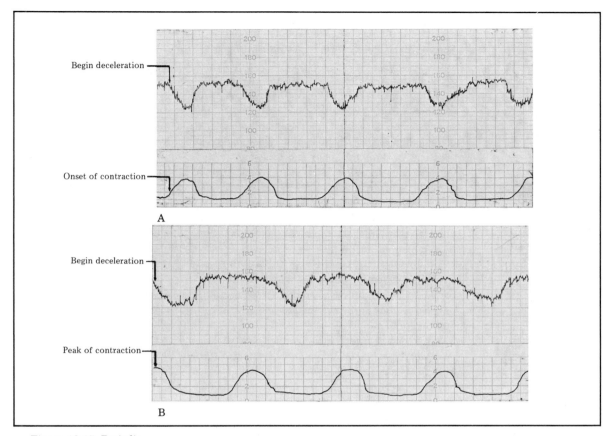

Figure 12-15. Periodic changes in fetal heart rate. A. Early deceleration, or type I dip. B. Late deceleration, or type II dip.

A late deceleration, or type II dip, occurs when the FHR begins to drop approximately 20 seconds or more after the beginning of the contraction, bottoms after the peak of the contraction, and returns to baseline after the end of the contraction. Late decelerations may be categorized into mild (< 15 bpm fall), moderate (15–40 bpm fall), and severe (> 40 bpm fall), depending upon their drop from FHR baseline. This pattern is found with impaired uteroplacental exchange and is considered ominous because it is related to fetal hypoxia. Each uterine contraction impedes uterine blood flow, imposing periodic stress on the fetus.

The three major clinical factors associated with uteroplacental insufficiency are excessive uterine activity, maternal hypotension, and decreased exchange surface area of the placenta. It is not known whether this pattern reflects asphyxia to the central nervous system or a direct effect on the fetal myocardium. The pattern is modified by the administration of oxygen, a change of maternal position so that the woman is lying on her left side, and increased intravenous fluids. Since patterns of late deceleration lasting for longer than 30 minutes are associated with fetal hypoxia, Hon suggests that the labor be terminated if the pattern persists this long after therapeutic measures are initiated [29].

Some FHR decelerations vary in relation to the onset of uterine contractions and may begin before, with, or following the contractions' onset. Commonly the deceleration is characterized by a sharp angularity of the deceleration with a rapid fall in FHR to below 100 beats per minute. While sharp angularity is a common form of variable deceleration, the deceleration is nonuniform and has several shapes (Fig. 12-16). Variable decelerations can be caused by umbilical cord compression. Total compression of the umbilical cord acutely raises the pressure in the fetal aorta and left heart, which stimulates baroreceptors. These baroreceptor impulses activate a vagal response, causing acetylcholine release near the fetal SA node with a reflex-evoked FHR deceleration. Incomplete vessel compression is likely to evoke varying FHR responses. In addition to the pressure-related effects, interference with fetal blood flow produces blood gas alterations. Thus, varying degrees of hypercapnia, hypoxemia, and increased hydrogen ions stimulate chemoreceptors with resultant vagal activation and FHR slowing [51]. Changes in the woman's position may alter the pattern.

While patterns of early, late, and variable decelerations may be found singularly, patterns including a mixture of each may also be observed. When a mixed pattern is found, it is managed according to the pattern indicative of the worst outcome.

A pattern of unrelenting, prolonged, variable or late decelerations associated with decreased baseline variability suggests that fetal oxygenation is precarious and that operative delivery may be necessary. Additional information can be obtained by means of scalp blood sampling, a technique that is especially helpful in the case of an infant who shows a pattern suggesting hypoxia. In this

Figure 12-16. Variable decelerations.

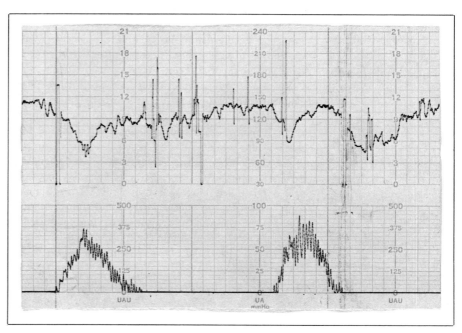

procedure, fetal acid-base status is evaluated. Under endoscopic visualization, the fetal scalp is cleaned, made hyperemic with ethyl chloride, coated with a silicone gel to promote formation of a blood globule, and incised with a stab blade; capillary blood is then collected. When placental function is limited, fetal asphyxia is revealed by increased carbon dioxide partial pressure and decreased oxygen pressure, pH, and base excess, all of which result in metabolic acidosis. Reduced pH and reduced base excess reflect breakdown of glycogen to pyruvate and lactic acid by anaerobic pathways. Most authorities consider pH values of less than 7.20 and a base deficit of 7 to be critical. While a single value may reflect maternal acidosis seen in prolonged labor, progressive decrease in serial pH determinations is an ominous sign.

STAGES OF LABOR

The woman in true labor progresses through the stages of labor. The first stage begins with the onset of true labor contractions and ends with full cervical dilatation; the second stage begins with full cervical dilatation and ends with the birth of the baby; and the third stage begins after the birth of the baby and ends with the delivery of the placenta. The immediate postpartum period is sometimes referred to as the fourth stage of labor.

The First Stage of Labor

The first stage of labor is the longest of the three stages (Table 12-2) and is divided into three phases (Fig. 12-17). During this stage the woman's cervix thins (effacement). The cervical canal changes from a structure of approximately 2 centimeters in length to a circular orifice with paper-thin edges. During this process the muscular fibers around the internal os are pulled upward and incorporated into the lower uterine segment. In primigravidas effacement occurs prior to the beginning of cervical dilatation. In multigravidas the process occurs simultaneously with cervical dilatation (Fig. 12-18).

The external cervical os progresses by dilatation from an opening a few millimeters in diameter to an opening large enough to allow birth of the fetus. When the cervical os has reached a diameter of 10 centimeters, it is referred to as being in the state of full or complete cervical dilatation. During the latent phase cervical dilatation progresses from 0 to approximately 4 centimeters.

Dilatation is accomplished by uterine pressure exerted on the amniotic sac (hydrostatic pressure) or, if the mother's membranes have ruptured, on the presenting part (fetal axis pressure). The amniotic sac or presenting part then serves as a wedge to effect cervical dilatation. As the cervix dilates, a reflex that further stimulates myometrial activity (Ferguson's reflex) [54] is activated.

ASSESSMENT AND INTERVENTION DURING THE LATENT PHASE
During the latent phase of the first stage of labor, the woman is generally comfortable. Her contractions are generally 20 to 40 seconds in duration and occur at intervals of 5 to 10 minutes. At this point it would be helpful for you to suggest diversionary activity, perhaps watching television, reading, or a walk around the area, provided the woman's membranes have not ruptured. If the

Table 12-2. Average Duration of Labor

Pregnancy	First Stage	Second Stage	Third Stage
Primigravida	12½ hours	80 minutes	10 minutes
Multigravida	7½ hours	30 minutes	10 minutes

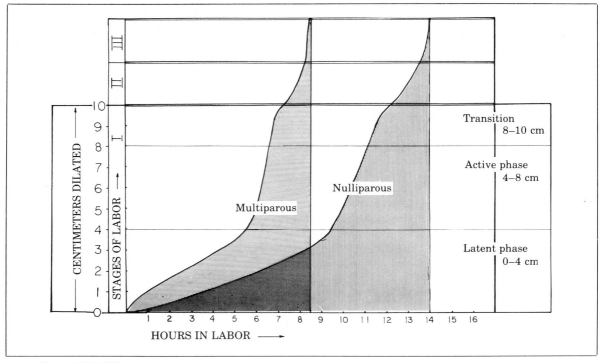

CENTIMETERS DILATED

STAGES OF LABOR

HOURS IN LABOR

Multiparous

Nulliparous

Transition
8–10 cm

Active phase
4–8 cm

Latent phase
0–4 cm

Figure 12-17. Time curves for normal labor in multiparous and nulliparous women.

woman's membranes have ruptured, she may still be encouraged to walk around if the presenting part is far enough down in the pelvis that the umbilical cord cannot slip by and become wedged between the bony pelvis and the presenting part.

The freedom to move during labor is both psychologically and physically important. Some obstetric procedures, such as fetal monitoring, often make ambulation difficult but should not serve as an absolute contraindication. A new technique, radiotelemetry, provides for continuous monitoring while the woman is fully mobile, wearing a portable monitoring device. Flynn [18] has reported the benefits of ambulation during labor, noting that the women who ambulated had shorter labors, lower incidence of FHR abnormalities, and a decreased use of oxytocin for labor augmentation. Hodnett [28] reported that women monitored with radiotelemetric fetal monitoring spent more time out of bed during labor, required less anesthesia, and related more positive labor experiences and feelings of control than women using standard monitoring.

During the latent phase of labor you can further assess the woman's feelings about the pregnancy and labor. The woman is likely to want to talk about the time of labor's onset and how it is progressing. The events of the present are predominant in her mind, although she may express concern for the immediate future—e.g., what her partner will do, what pain relief she may require. It is likely that she will be relieved that labor has begun and will alternate feelings of apprehension with excitement and happiness [26].

If the woman or couple have attended classes in preparation for childbirth, this

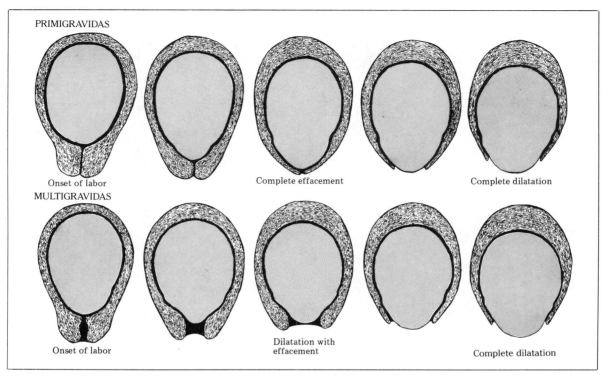

PRIMIGRAVIDAS

Onset of labor
Complete effacement
Complete dilatation

MULTIGRAVIDAS

Onset of labor
Dilatation with effacement
Complete dilatation

Figure 12-18. Dilatation and effacement in primigravidas and multigravidas. Primigravidas reach complete effacement prior to dilating. Multigravidas undergo effacement and dilatation simultaneously.

is a time when you might ask them to describe and demonstrate the techniques they were taught. In this way you can assess their understanding and performance of them. If the woman has not attended classes, you can teach the techniques of breathing and pushing that will help her in the succeeding stages of labor (Table 12-3, Fig. 12-19). During this time find out the expectations that the woman or couple have for their experience during the woman's hospital stay. Assess any specific cultural practices used during birth (Table 12-4).

If the woman is accompanied by a support person assess their interaction and

Table 12-3. Breathing Techniques During Labor

Stage of Labor	Breathing Technique
Early First Stage	Relax, cleansing breath. Breathe deeply, slowly, rhythmically through contraction, then cleansing breath.
Late First Stage	Assume comfortable position. Cleansing breath. Regular breathing to more shallow. With stronger contractions, accelerate breathing (very light throat breaths). Cleansing breath.
Transition	Concentrate on breathing control. Cleansing breath. Breathe fairly deeply at beginning of contraction. Shallow breathing. Puff out on every third, fourth, or fifth breath if urge to push. Cleansing breath.
Second Stage	Push toward vaginal opening as directed. Catch breath as needed. Relax pelvic floor. Go limp between contractions. Pant during contraction. Push gently as directed.

Source: Reproduced, with permission, from *Preparation for Childbearing*, published by Maternity Center Association, New York, 1972.

Figure 12-19. Nurse teaches the mother breathing techniques.

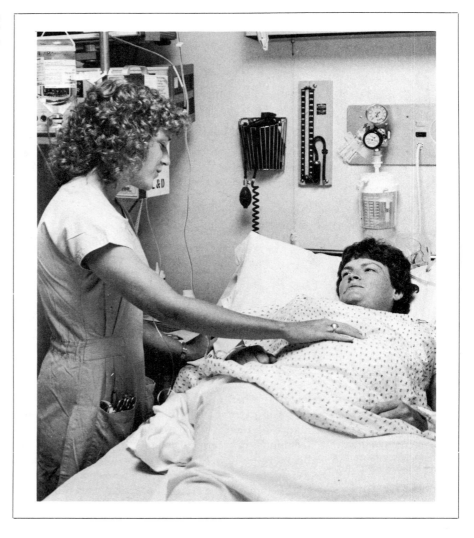

ability to work together. Whenever possible, assist the woman's partner in helping her if he so wishes, teaching him techniques to increase her comfort during labor. However, do not abandon him; remember the normal sights, sounds, and smells of a laboring woman are foreign to most men, and in fact can be overwhelming and frightening experiences for even the best-prepared father. Reassurances that he is doing well and that all is normal can be of great help in decreasing his anxiety. The couple should be allowed the privacy they need. When direct care is necessary, do it without physically coming between them or breaking their eye contact (Fig. 12-20). Intervene when the partner needs support or a break, perhaps by saying that he looks tired and that he might like to get coffee. Tell the partner that you will stay with the woman until he returns. Both partners need support and encouragement during labor. Support persons, especially fathers, should feel that they have played a vital role in the birth of the

Table 12-4. Cultural Practices During Birth

Ethnic Group	Cultural Practices
Arab	Pregnancy is considered the greatest opportunity for woman to actualize her potential. Woman's status is improved and acceptance by her husband's family is enhanced when she bears male children. Verbal agreements are respected; the written word, including consent forms for delivery, is distrusted. Decision making is relegated to the husband. Pain tolerance may be low, experienced in a diffuse and generalized way, and expressed verbally. Breathing and relaxation techniques are not readily accepted; epidural and spinal anesthesia is avoided.
American Indian	Variations among tribes. Women may deliver in a local hospital or at home in the presence of a midwife. The Laguna Pueblo Indian woman is given a belt that has been blessed and hangs onto it instead of using analgesics. The Navajo Indian custom holds that delivery is an affair for all the family to view. Following delivery the placenta is buried, a common practice among many Indian tribes.
Mexican American	Women delivered in hospitals by midwives or physicians. Prior to 1950 many were delivered by a folk midwife called a *partera*. Immediately following delivery of the infant the woman's legs were placed together to prevent air from entering the uterus. The midwife dipped her thumb in olive oil and pressed on the infant's palate to prevent "falling of the fontanelle." The placenta was burned or buried. If the placenta was eaten by an animal it was believed the mother would experience afterpains.
Puerto Rican	Most women deliver in hospitals. The husband may not be with the woman during labor due to the modesty traditionally attributed to Puerto Rican women.
Vietnamese	Women deliver in hospitals (urban areas) and at home (rural). Husbands usually not present. Women may be shy about their husbands seeing them during birth when they may not "look right" to their husbands. Women do not cry out to avoid embarrassing their family. In traditional rural areas a bamboo bed is constructed for delivery.
Filipino	Presence of the family during birth is important in the traditional culture, especially elderly family members.

Sources: A. Clark, *Culture Childbearing Health Professionals.* Philadelphia: Davis, 1978; A. Hollingsworth, L. Brown, and D. Brooten. The refugees and childbearing: What to expect. *RN* 43:44, 1980; A. Meleis, and L. Sarrell. Arab American women and their birth experiences. *American Journal of Maternal-Child Nursing* 6:171, 1981; P. Stern. Solving problems of cross-cultural health teaching: The Filipino childbearing family. *Image* 13:47, 1981; L. Todd. Indochinese refugees bring rich heritages to childbearing. *International Childbirth Education Association News* 21:2, 1982.

child. When this is communicated, family relationships are strengthened as well as relationships with this particular child.

Both prepared and unprepared women in labor have certain needs, which they have identified for nurse researchers [37]. These needs include the relief of pain, the support of another human being, the assurance of their own safety and that of the baby, and the acceptance by those around them of their attitudes toward labor and their behavior during it. As you support and coach parents through the process of labor, you will develop a strong rapport with them and help determine how well they are able to cope with the experience. Through your warmth and prompt response to needs, you can make the parents feel that they are very important. This help is even more important when the laboring mother is solely dependent on you for support.

Figure 12-20. Midwife examines the woman but does not impose herself physically between the couple. (Courtesy of Booth Maternity Center, Philadelphia, Pa.)

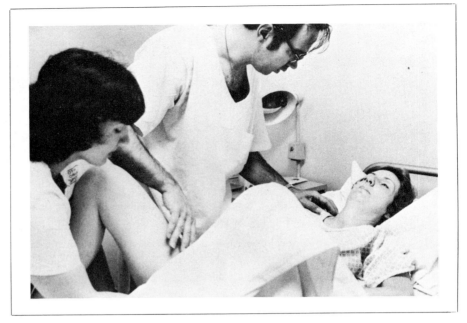

In one nursing research study by Shields [61], with specific reference to the labor and delivery experience, the sustaining presence of the nurse was the most frequently cited element leading to patient satisfaction with care. The second most frequently cited measure was an explanation of what was occurring. Generally the expressed needs of the 80 patients in this study were categorized as maintenance of control, realization of expectations, and maintenance of self-esteem. In Butani and Hodnett's study of 50 women [6], the nurse researchers found that the same items generally were specified as determinants of satisfaction with the childbirth experience. Norr et al. [48] and Klein et al. [32] have also cited social support as a critical factor in improving birth experiences for women.

Your support can either make analgesia unnecessary for the woman in labor or greatly enhance its effects.

In providing this support, reinforce whatever antepartal preparation the mother has had and reassure her that what she is experiencing is common and that medication is available if she needs it. Use a straightforward approach in explaining what is happening. Since mothers in labor are especially sensitive to their environment, they are very aware of the tone of voice, facial expression, disinterest, or false enthusiasm of those around them. They tend to interpret most of what they see and hear with reference to themselves. In spite of this fact, staff members will sometimes have casual conversations among themselves within a woman's hearing, discussing other women's conditions, or laughing, with little realization that the mother may see herself as the topic of their discussion or laughter.

Because the mother is so open to suggestion during labor, she is likely to follow commands regarding breathing patterns, for example, even though she may say that it is impossible for her to do so. If you are coaching a mother through labor, you can use this fact to great advantage; you should be careful to avoid anxiety-provoking terms like *pain*, using the more neutral term *contraction* instead.

During the latent phase of the first stage of labor, the woman may have a clear liquid diet, since the maintenance of fluid and glucose levels aids in the effectiveness of uterine contractions. Since it is the early stage of labor, her stomach should be empty by the time of delivery, which reduces the chance of her aspirating stomach contents. In high-risk centers physicians may prefer to give intravenous dextrose and water to maintain fluid and glucose levels during labor rather than allow the woman to take anything by mouth. In either case, cracked ice is usually allowed by mouth and is appreciated by the woman during this period. Monitor and record the woman's fluid intake and urinary output.

During the excitement of labor, especially if under the influence of analgesics, women often forget to void. A full bladder during labor can impede progress, cause pain, and lead to urinary retention after delivery. It is a good idea for you to explain this to the mother and to remind her to void about every 2 hours during labor to avoid distention. Also remind her that perineal pads (sanitary napkins) are not worn during labor in order to prevent contamination of the vaginal area by fecal matter.

As part of your assessment during this period of labor, monitor the woman's vital signs every hour: blood pressure, pulse, and respiration, as well as contractions and FHR (which should range between 120 and 160 beats per minute). Take blood pressure and FHR between contractions because of the changes that occur during a contraction. Listen occasionally to FHR during a contraction to assess fetal response and heart rate changes during the stress of a contraction. Check the woman's temperature every 4 hours during this phase unless a deviation is noted, in which case her temperature is taken more frequently, perhaps every hour. The woman's temperature is also checked more often if her membranes have been ruptured for more than 12 hours.

ASSESSMENT AND INTERVENTION DURING THE ACTIVE PHASE

With the beginning of the second or active phase (4–8 centimeters' dilatation) of the first stage of labor, the woman has completed one-half to two-thirds of the length of the first stage. This fact can be a source of real encouragement to the father and to the mother who has labored for so many hours with so little progress in terms of cervical dilatation. During the active phase, dilatation proceeds much more rapidly; the woman is usually more uncomfortable, because the intensity of the contractions has increased. Her contractions are now generally between 30 and 50 seconds in duration and are occurring at intervals of 2 to 5 minutes. The woman now needs continuous evaluation.

Monitor her vital signs, including blood pressure, pulse, respiration, contractions, and FHR from every 30 minutes in the beginning of this phase to every 15 minutes at its end. Time the uterine contractions rather than relying on information from the woman, since contractions begin about 10 seconds before there is any subjective feeling of discomfort. Occasionally a woman will appear to be having strong, painful contractions yet your evaluation does not coincide with the mother's reactions. Often the woman's anxiety level has greatly exaggerated her perception of the pain. Once you are able to decrease the woman's anxiety through encouragement and comfort measures, her subjective pain tends to coincide more with your objective evaluation.

The fetus must also be carefully monitored. Bradycardia, an increase in fetal activity, and meconium-stained amniotic fluid in a vertex presentation may be signs of compromised fetal oxygenation and distress. If any of these occur, the physician should be notified and the fetus monitored very closely.

Fetal position can often be predicted by the location of the mother's discomfort and the position she assumes. When the woman complains of severe backache and is unable to lie on her back, the vertex may be in the posterior position. In this instance, the fetal heart tones are heard in her flank, and the contraction pattern may show a long contraction followed by one or two shorter ones. Chest (or costal) breathing may decrease the woman's discomfort [43].

If the woman is restless and rolls back and forth in the bed with equal discomfort in the back and front, the occiput may well be in a transverse position. In either the transverse or posterior position, vertex rotation may be speeded by having her lie on her side opposite the fetus's back. Lying on her side also keeps her uterus from compressing the inferior vena cava and permits better circulation.

When the fetus is in one of the anterior positions, the woman tends to lie on her back with the backrest elevated; the discomfort is generally concentrated over the symphysis and down into the groin area. The contractions are generally long and strong, but she may benefit by abdominal breathing. If the fetus is in a breech position, raising the backrest may make her more comfortable.

In giving direct care or in working through the woman's support person you can use a number of comfort measures to help the mother cope with labor. Since women react differently to labor, comfort measures helpful to some women may not be helpful to others. When you care for a woman in labor you must continually evaluate the woman's response to the measures being used; if one measure is not effective, another may be substituted.

Back pain may be relieved by applying pressure with the heel of the hand or some firm object such as a tennis ball to the small of the back (Fig. 12-21). Some women get relief from a hot-water bottle applied to the back, while others find relief with an ice bag. Many women find relief from discomfort by lying on their side with the bed elevated or by doing pelvic rocking.

Figure 12-21. Applying sacral pressure.

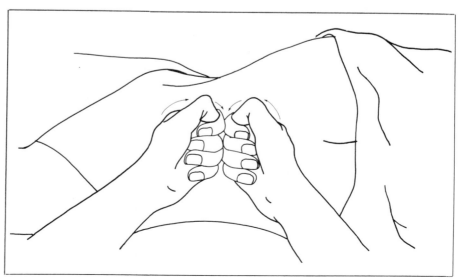

Some women find that brushing their teeth or rinsing their mouths with mouthwash is very refreshing. Moistening the lips with a wet gauze pad or lemon and glycerine, sucking a piece of hard candy, or chewing gum are also helpful.

Another important comfort measure is to make sure the woman's perineum is clean and that she is resting on dry linens. She may also rest more comfortably if her feet are kept warm. A superficial circular stroking of the abdominal skin (effleurage) is comforting to some women.

Creating an environment that is conducive to rest is at least as important as the physical care you can offer. The room should have soft lighting (keeping the overhead light on tends to make women more restless). Noise should be kept to a minimum. Women also find this period easier to cope with when someone is with them continuously.

Occasionally a woman becomes uncomfortable and cannot decide what will make her comfortable; at such times she needs direction. Often having her turn on her side, close her eyes, and try to rest between contractions while someone rubs her back is all that is needed. When this is done, many women are able to get considerable rest between contractions. Help the father rest while his wife does. Provide him with pillows and juice or coffee. Suggest that you relieve him for a break.

If the woman needs or requests analgesics she should receive them, provided that she is dilated approximately 4 to 5 centimeters if she is a primigravida, 4 to 6 centimeters if she is a multigravida. Analgesics given before this time can slow the progress of labor. Often a woman who requests analgesics early in labor can be made comfortable by other measures, and the amount of analgesic necessary can be decreased considerably. Whenever analgesics are administered, the woman's vital signs (including the FHR) should be checked just before administration. This will serve as a baseline should the woman or the fetus experience side effects from the analgesic.

During the active phase the woman places increased emphasis on events of the present moment. She may talk about the duration of labor but with little focus on events beyond delivery. As she becomes more introspective she may speak only in reply to questions. Her apprehension begins to increase and she begins to rely more heavily on the supportive presence of a companion. Her emotions may range from seriously doubting her ability to deal with contractions to a strong desire to use prepared childbirth techniques to cope with them. The woman and her partner may be ready and eager for explanations about how they can maintain control over the experience [26] (Table 12-5).

ASSESSMENT AND INTERVENTION DURING TRANSITION

The third phase (8–10 centimeters' dilatation) of the first stage of labor is known as transition (deceleration phase); it is generally the most difficult of the phases of the first stage. The woman's contractions are usually between 50 and 60 seconds in duration, with an interval of approximately 2 minutes. Women need a great deal of encouragement and support at this point. They will be encouraged to hear that labor is almost over, since this stage usually averages 10 contractions or 20 minutes for multigravidas, and 20 contractions or 40 minutes for primigravidas [43].

During the transition phase the woman automatically rests or sleeps between contractions; this is known as partial amnesia. During a contraction, pressure

Table 12-5. Assessment and Intervention During Labor and Delivery

Assessment	Intervention
Expectations for labor and delivery	Reinforce realistic expectations
Coping ability during labor	
Mother	Provide supportive measures
	Early labor: Use diversionary activities—walking, television, magazines; review breathing techniques; provide fluids and glucose
	Active phase: Work with woman or through her support person (nurse or other person remaining with woman); help with breathing techniques, back rub and sacral pressure for backache, mouth care, dry linens, change of position, adequate hydration, frequent voiding, analgesics when necessary, consistent encouragement, monitor vital signs; encourage rest between contractions, periods of privacy for the couple, quiet environment
Father	Encourage periodic breaks for the father or support person, recognition for his supporting role
Reaction to infant	Provide time and opportunity for parents to interact with each other and the infant; brief physical exam for infant, allowing close examination by parents—note normal newborn variations and unique features of their infant

and massage to the sacral area helps to ease discomfort, as does rapid shallow breathing. Since the woman perspires more now, she will be more comfortable if her face and brow are wiped with a cool cloth.

During transition a number of signs and symptoms appear that should alert you to the beginning of the second stage. These include an increase in bloody show, irritability, restlessness, and anxiety. Some women prefer not to be touched during this period. Women perspire much more at this stage and may develop hiccups or nausea and vomiting (a reflex sign of rapid cervical dilation). As the presenting part of the fetus descends, the woman will probably complain more of low back pain and pain in her upper thighs. Because of the pressure, she may experience involuntary leg shaking or involuntary bearing down. As the presenting part of the fetus reaches the perineal floor and presses on the rectum, the woman may complain of needing to have a bowel movement.

The woman's membranes may rupture now if they have not ruptured before (while this may occur at any time in labor, it is most frequent during this period). When the membranes rupture, take the FHR immediately, since on rare occasions the cord is washed down the canal with the fluid (prolapsed cord) and becomes wedged between the bony pelvis and the presenting part, compromising the fetal oxygen supply. Note and record the character and amount of amniotic fluid since meconium-stained fluid may be a sign of fetal distress.

During this stage you or the supporting person should breathe with the woman during her contractions and apply sacral pressure and massage. Keep her perineum clean and the sheets or pads under her dry.

At this time the woman concentrates her energies on internal activities. She becomes more apprehensive, more irritable, unwilling to be touched, more frustrated. She is unable to cope if left alone at this point and may be unable to follow directions readily. Her attention span is short, and she has no energy for lengthy explanations. She welcomes comments that she is doing well and that labor is nearing an end, as does the father.

The Second Stage of Labor—Assessment and Intervention

The second stage of labor, which extends from full cervical dilatation to the birth of the infant, is a period that most women find less stressful than the first. Now the woman can increase the effectiveness of the uterine contractions by pushing.

At the beginning of a contraction help the woman lean forward, flex her legs on her abdomen, and grasp them just below the knee (Fig. 12-22). Have her take a deep breath, blow it out, take another deep breath, hold it and bear down using her abdominal muscles.

FHR patterns, intrauterine pressure, and maternal blood pressure have been recorded by Caldeyro-Barcia [8] with a variety of maternal bearing-down efforts. Efforts that lasted longer than 5 seconds resulted in late decelerations of the FHR, a decrease in maternal systolic and diastolic blood pressure, and delayed recovery of the FHR. In some cases where bearing down lasted longer than 15 seconds there was fetal hypoxia and acidosis. This can be avoided when women are not urged to bear down long and hard since their spontaneous efforts are usually 5 to 6 seconds in duration, well within physiologic limits. With this shorter spontaneous bearing down, the second stage of labor is lengthened somewhat, allowing the perineum to stretch more slowly and decreasing the need for episiotomy.

Assess the woman's ability to bear down with a contraction and, if improvement is necessary, work with the woman directly or through her support person to improve her pushing. If fecal material is expelled during the bearing down, remove it at once and keep the perineal area clean. Between contractions have the woman close her eyes and rest. Check fetal heart tones frequently, possibly

Figure 12-22. Woman in labor pushing with the coaching of her husband. (Courtesy of Booth Maternity Center, Philadelphia, Pa.)

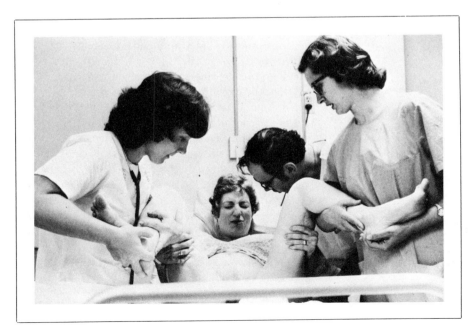

after every other contraction. Check the woman's vital signs approximately every 15 minutes.

The second stage is usually completed with an average of 20 contractions for a primigravida and 10 contractions for a multigravida. Since the second stage is short for a multigravida, if she is going to be transferred to a delivery room, she is usually transferred during the transition phase. In general, a primigravida is transferred when a portion of the fetal head approximately the size of a 50-cent piece can be seen at the perineum between contractions.

In a traditional delivery room, the woman is positioned on the delivery table usually with her legs placed in stirrups. This continues to occur in spite of research that indicates that labor and delivery may occur more efficiently in the lateral, upright, semirecumbent, or inclined positions [4, 9, 42, 44]. The upright position has been found to facilitate progress of labor and delivery by increasing the strength of contractions, decreasing their pain, and increasing the rate of cervical dilatation. The principle of giving birth in an upright squatting or semireclining position dates back thousands of years. (Having the mother deliver from a reclining position was introduced into Western civilization as late as the eighteenth century, when an obstetrician of the Queen of France proposed the method in order to facilitate his efforts—not those of the mother.) A more modern version of the original birthing chair recently has been added to the labor and delivery rooms of some health care settings (Fig. 12-23). A variety of birthing beds also have been placed in birthing rooms to facilitate delivery in other than the traditional dorsal lithotomy position.

As a rule, consumers have seldom been offered a choice in positions for labor and delivery. They need to be informed of the benefits of various positions (Table 12-6) and encouraged to discuss various options with their physicians and midwives. Many women automatically assume that labor means that they must go to bed and remain supine. Since change from the traditional is often difficult, education of consumers as well as health professionals is necessary to institute various options in labor and delivery.

Prior to delivery, the mother is usually draped in some fashion with sterile linens and her perineum is cleansed with an antiseptic solution.

Before the crowning of the fetal head, the midwife or physician may perform an episiotomy. This is an incision of the woman's perineal skin, vaginal mucosa, urogenital septum, constrictor cunni, and transversus perinei muscles, fascia, and a few fibers of the puborectal portion of the levator ani muscle. An episiotomy enlarges the vaginal outlet, avoiding perineal tears (Table 12-7), which do not heal as well as a repaired straight-edged incision, and it allows the infant to be born with less effort. It also avoids prolonged and severe stretching of the muscles supporting the bladder and rectum, preventing later stress incontinence and vaginal prolapse. In addition, it reduces the duration of the second stage of labor and decreases pressure on the fetal head, which is especially important in delivery of premature infants.

The incision may be made in the midline of the perineum (median episiotomy), or it may be made on an angle directed laterally away from the rectum of the right or left side of the mother's perineum (mediolateral episiotomy) (Fig. 12-24). Usually infiltration with a local anesthetic precedes the incision, although some clinicians state that when the perineum is stretched, the pressure on the nerve

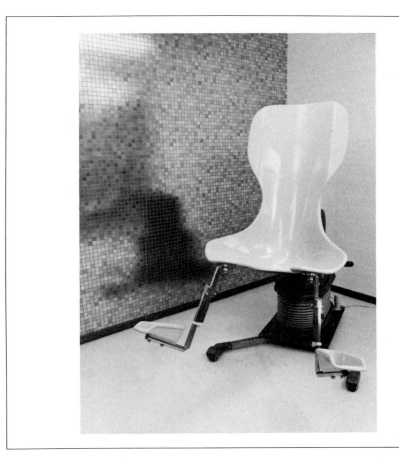

endings at the height of a contraction makes anesthesia unnecessary. Some mothers state otherwise!

The mediolateral episiotomy avoids the anal sphincter if further enlargement is necessary, but many women find it very uncomfortable during healing. The median episiotomy may necessitate further incision into the anal sphincter, but it is generally more comfortable for the woman during the healing process. Advocates of the latter method also state that it is easier to repair well and that it heals better with fewer complications.

After the head is delivered (Fig. 12-25), blood and mucus are wiped from the infant's face, and his nose and mouth are suctioned, usually with bulb suction. Following delivery of the remainder of the infant's body, he is held below the level of the mother's body, and his nose and mouth are suctioned further. His cord is clamped with two Kelly clamps and then cut between them. Some clinicians prefer to wait until the umbilical cord has stopped pulsating before it is clamped and cut; in this way the infant receives approximately 100 milliliters of additional blood from the placenta. Critics of this procedure argue that the infant does not need the additional blood and, in fact, becomes more likely to develop higher levels of bilirubin as the extra blood is broken down (Figs. 12-26, 12-27).

*Table 12-6. Advantages
and Disadvantages of
Various Positions for
Labor and Delivery*

Position	Advantage	Disadvantage
Labor		
Left side-lying	Increased intensity and regularity of contractions; less danger of vomitus aspiration; prevention of supine hypotensive syndrome	Difficulty in continuous electronic fetal monitoring
Left lateral Sims	Increased comfort in addition to advantages listed above	Difficulty in continuous electronic fetal monitoring
Upright—sitting or standing	Increased intensity and regularity of contractions; increased comfort; shorter labor; no undesirable effect on fetus; facilitates entrance of fetal presenting part into inlet and more direct application to cervix; optimum pelvic diameters achieved prior to engagement	Squatting prior to engagement may prevent descent
Supine	Easy to maintain continuous electronic fetal monitoring	Increased risk of supine hypotensive syndrome; contractions weaker, more irregular
Kneeling	Encourages rotation of fetal head if persistent posterior	
Delivery		
Traditional dorsal lithotomy	Easier to maintain asepsis, monitor fetal heart rate, administer anesthesia, repair episiotomy and tears	Hypotensive syndrome; thrombosis or nerve lesions from leg supports; back pain; resentment of posture; narrowed and tightened introitus as thighs are flexed; contractions weaker, more irregular; more frequent episiotomies as increased tension placed on stretching tissue; increased force necessary to give birth since push is against gravity
Left lateral Sims	"Comfort" position assumed; hypotension controlled; efforts to push not inhibited; extension and expulsion of head more precisely encouraged by digital pressure behind anus to fetal maxilla; temptation to apply fundal pressure avoided; placental separation not delayed; fewer episiotomies—perineum looser	Difficult to apply forceps; difficult to do episiotomy; more inconvenient for practitioner
Squatting	Enlarges pelvic outlet in second stage; allows for more efficient bearing-down efforts	Technically difficult to control birth process, administer anesthesia, apply forceps, and hear fetal heart tones
Sitting (birth chair or adaptation)	Increased uterine contractions	
Table with use of a back rest and lower stirrups or no stirrups	Shortened second stage due to enlarged pelvic dimensions; shortened delivery time; more efficient pushing with gravity; easier viewing of newborn; increased comfort	

Source: Adapted from S. McKay. Maternal position during labor and birth: A reassessment. *Journal of Obstetric, Gynecologic and Neonatal Nursing* 9:288, 1980.

Table 12-7. Lacerations of the Birth Canal

Degree of Laceration	Extent of Damage
First degree	Involvement of the fourchet, perineal skin, and mucous membrane of the vagina. No muscle involvement
Second degree	Involvement of perineal skin, vaginal mucous membrane, and muscles of the perineal body. No rectal sphincter involvement
Third degree	Involvement of perineal skin, vaginal mucous membrane, muscles of the perineal body, and rectal sphincter
Fourth degree	Sometimes used to designate involvement of the anterior rectal wall, in addition to the above areas

After the cord is clamped and the infant is breathing on his own, he is generally placed on his mother's abdomen or chest so that new relationships within the family unit may begin (Figs. 12-28, 12-29). Some physicians have expressed concern that when the baby is not placed immediately in a heated crib, he becomes excessively chilled. However, nurse researchers Britton [5], Gardner [19], Hill and Shronk [27], and Phillips [52] have found that full-term infants held by their mothers in the delivery room or placed on their mother's undraped abdomen are able to maintain body heat well within an acceptable range (Fig. 12-30). In most settings the infant then receives routine newborn care.

Newborn Care
The following is a general description of newborn care. The sequence of the procedures may differ from one birth setting to another. In traditional settings, the care is often carried out immediately after the infant's birth. In other settings it is performed after the parents have had an hour or more to become acquainted with their newborn.

Figure 12-24. Sites for episiotomy incisions.

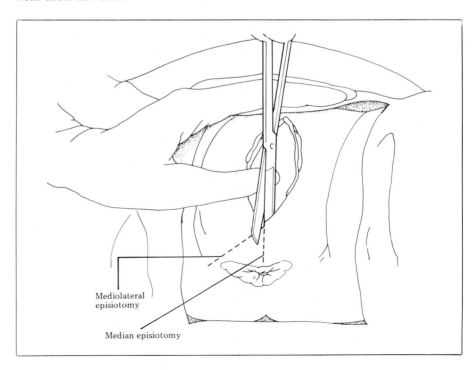

Mediolateral episiotomy

Median episiotomy

Figure 12-25. Birth of infant's head. A. Head distends the perineum, anus flattens. B. Perineum much distended by the head, a process called crowning. C. Fetal head extended, perineum slipping back over the infant's face. D. Fetal head delivered, perineum retracted under chin. (From J. P. Greenhill and E. A. Friedman. *Biological Principles and Modern Practice of Obstetrics.* Philadelphia: Saunders, 1974.)

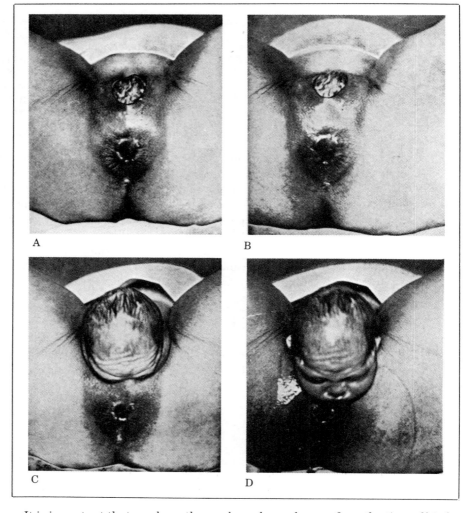

It is important that you keep the newborn dry and warm from the time of birth. Wipe off blood and amniotic fluid to prevent fluid evaporation from chilling the infant. The chilling can easily increase his metabolism and consequently his need for oxygen, which would cause him to use his readily available glucose and induce an acidosis or aggravate the degree of metabolic acidosis already present. Metabolic acidosis in turn causes higher levels of bilirubin, since the binding of bilirubin to albumin is decreased. Moore [45] stresses the amount of heat loss and notes that

A wet, small newborn loses up to 200 calories per kilogram per minute in the delivery room through evaporation, convection, and radiation. Realizing that an adult at full compensation generates only about 90 calories per kilogram per minute makes it easier to appreciate the severity of this heat loss.

Wiping the infant dry cuts this heat loss in half. Chilling also makes it more difficult for the infant's body temperature to increase and then stabilize after birth.

Although the newborn does not have the shivering mechanism of the adult for

Figure 12-26. Father participating in the delivery of his newborn by clamping her umbilical cord.

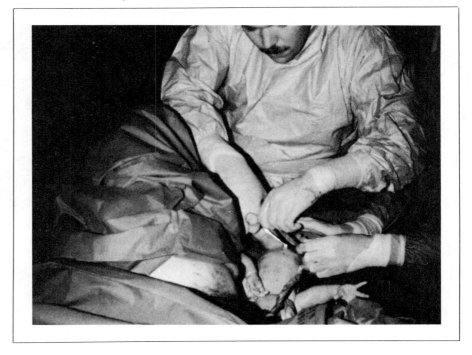

Figure 12-26. Father participating in the delivery of his newborn by clamping her umbilical cord.

compensation, he does have brown fat, a source of heat that is unique to neonates. Brown fat, which accounts for 2 to 6 percent of body weight in newborns, contains fat vacuoles, mitochondria, and an abundant blood and sympathetic nerve supply. Deposits are found between the scapulas, around the neck and thorax, behind the sternum, and around the kidneys and adrenals. Brown fat is believed to warm blood flowing through it, thus contributing to body heat. It is believed to hypertrophy after birth and then disappear several weeks later.

The newborn has a large body surface in comparison to his weight; because of this he experiences more heat loss than an adult. Perhaps to compensate in some degree, his extremities remain flexed immediately after birth, which decreases the exposed skin surface. While all of these factors contribute to heat loss in a normal newborn, in a low birth weight baby the heat loss problems are intensified. He has less subcutaneous fat to insulate him, a larger surface area in relation to his weight, a less flexed position, and small glycogen stores to be used when his metabolic rate increases. Therefore, it is especially important that he be dried and warmed immediately.

Newborn care includes an Apgar score, cord care, eye care, a vitamin K preparation, and an identification bracelet. The infant is also weighed, footprinted, and assessed for gestational age. If internal fetal monitoring was used, an antibiotic ointment may be applied over the area where the fetal scalp clip was inserted.

APGAR SCORE

The Apgar score was developed in 1952 by Virginia Apgar, M.D., as a means of evaluating the physical condition of an infant after birth [55]. Apgar scoring of heart rate, respiratory effort, muscle tone, reflex irritability, and color is done at 1

Figure 12-27. Crying newborn, cord not yet cut.

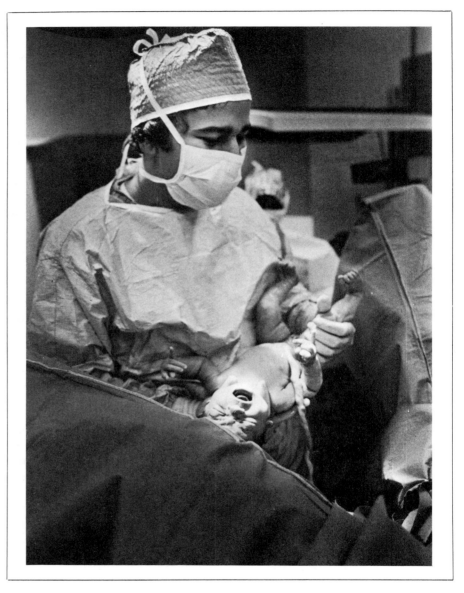

minute and 5 minutes after birth (Table 12-8). The heart rate is generally regarded as the most important of the five items scored. You can count it by using a stethoscope on the infant's chest wall, by feeling the pulsations in the cord, or by placing two fingers on the infant's chest wall and counting for 30 seconds. A heart rate below 100 beats per minute is associated with asphyxia.

Respiratory effort is next to heart rate in importance, and a vigorous cry with regular respirations is given a score of 2. Muscle tone is scored according to the degree of flexion in the extremities. Normally the newborn keeps his extremities flexed, resisting extension; as you extend a limb and then release it, the healthy infant's response is to bring it back into a flexed position; this response merits a score of 2.

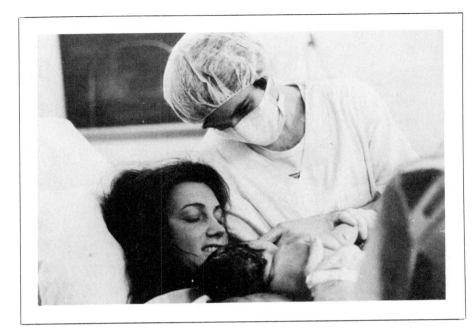

Figure 12-28. Parents meeting their newborn.

Test reflex irritability by flicking the sole of the infant's foot. If he responds by crying, he receives a score of 2, while a weak cry or change in facial expression merits a score of 1.

Evaluate color according to the degree of cyanosis; if there is no cyanosis in the body or in the extremities, the infant receives a score of 2.

Infants who score between 0 and 3 are severely depressed, those scoring from 4 to 6 are moderately depressed, and those who score from 7 to 10 are free of immediate stress. Infants with low Apgar scores, particularly on a 5-minute test, have a significantly higher mortality and a higher incidence of neurologic defects.

CORD CARE

Routine cord care consists of tying off the cord 2 or 3 centimeters (approximately 1 inch) from the abdominal wall and then cutting it. The cord is tied with a rubber band, a cotton cord tie, or one of a variety of plastic or metal clamps. Make sure

Table 12-8. Apgar Scoring

Sign	Score		
	0	1	2
Heart rate	Absent	Below 100	Over 100
Respiratory effort	Absent	Slow, irregular	Good, crying
Muscle tone	Flaccid	Some flexion of extremities	Active motion, flexed extremities
Reflex irritability	No response	Weak cry, facial grimace	Vigorous cry
Color	Pale, cyanotic	Pink body, extremities blue	Completely pink

Figure 12-29. Mother and father becoming acquainted with their newborn.

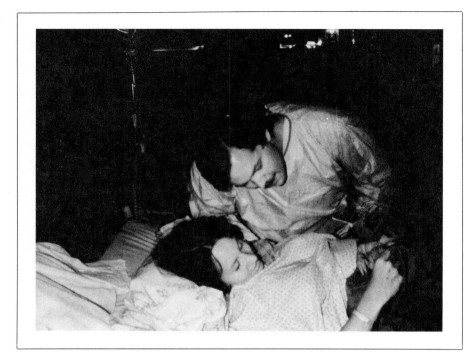

the cord is securely tied or clamped to prevent blood loss. Examine the cord for the presence of three vessels—one large vein and two smaller arteries. Some hospital routines require that an antiseptic solution be applied over the cord stump.

EYE CARE

The infant's eyes may become infected as his head passes through the vagina. Routine eye care is performed as prophylaxis against ophthalmia neonatorum, which causes a purulent inflammation of the conjunctiva and cornea. While the gonococcus is usually the organism responsible, pneumococcus, *Corynebacterium diphtheriae,* and other organisms can cause serious conjunctivitis.

Prophylaxis may be carried out according to modifications of Credé's method, which calls for the use of a silver nitrate solution in the eye. Generally two drops of a 1% silver nitrate solution are put in the conjunctival sac of the infant's eye. One minute later, sterile saline or water is used to flush out the eye. The irrigation should be directed so that the stream of irrigating fluid flows from the bridge of the nose and tear duct to the outer corner of the eye, serving to wash material away from the duct.

Some clinicians prefer to irrigate the eyes before as well as after the instillation of the silver nitrate; in this way any blood or mucus is removed from the area. Others prefer not to irrigate the eyes at all, noting that the incidence of chemical conjunctivitis as a reaction to silver nitrate is no higher in infants who do not have their eyes irrigated after instillation of the silver nitrate. The Committee on Ophthalmia Neonatorum of the National Society for the Prevention of Blindness does not recommend irrigating the eyes following silver nitrate administration

Figure 12-30. A growing family unit. (Photograph by Shelly Harrison.)

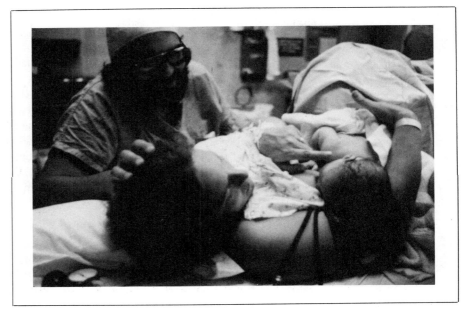

[45]. Since silver nitrate administration may disrupt the quiet alert gaze of the infant, some practitioners feel that this may interfere with the initial attachment process. Therefore they recommend that the administration of silver nitrate be delayed until later in the first hour of life.

In some hospitals antibiotics such as penicillin or tetracycline are used for eye care instead of silver nitrate. However, this treatment carries with it the risk of the infant's developing a sensitivity to the antibiotic or the organisms' developing a resistance to it.

Greenberg and Vandow [23] questioned whether any single drug is really effective in preventing gonococcal ophthalmia; they reported the incidence of this infection with the use of a number of regimens. With no prophylaxis there were 25.5 cases per 100,000; using silver nitrate, 6.6; using saline, 7.4; using antibiotic ointments, 11.2; and using parenteral penicillin, no cases.

VITAMIN K
As part of routine newborn care, 1 milligram of vitamin K may be administered either in the delivery room or in the nursery, since the newborn is unable to manufacture vitamin K on his own due to inadequate intestinal flora immediately after birth. Vitamin K administration prevents decreases in plasma prothrombin levels and thus decreases hemorrhagic disease in the newborn. Larger amounts of the vitamin predispose the infant to the development of hyperbilirubinemia and carry no therapeutic advantage.

IDENTIFICATION
Identification of the newborn is generally done by putting identification bracelets on both the mother and newborn and by footprinting the infant. The bracelets applied to the infant and mother should have matching identification numbers

and note the mother's name, the infant's sex, and the date and time of birth. The bracelet put on the infant should be tight enough that it will not slip off in the nursery, but not so tight as to be constricting.

When taken properly, footprints can be a good source of identification [22]. The sole of the infant's foot should first be cleaned gently and dried (rigorous cleaning may well make the infant's skin peel). The sole is then pressed against the ink plate of the footprinter. Cradle the infant's foot between your thumb and index finger and place the infant's foot, heel first, on the footprint paper. By gently turning your wrist, the ball of the foot and the toes will be pressed between the paper and the back of your hand (Fig. 12-31). The paper should be attached to a clipboard for stability and to provide a hard surface. Check the footprint to see if the ridges are distinct. The mother's thumbprints are also placed on the identification sheet.

ASSESSMENT

Immediately after birth examine the infant to determine maturity and any anomalies. The full-term infant will have sparse lanugo, cartilage present in his ears, formed nipples, creases over more than one-third of the soles of his feet, and relatively thick, smooth skin. The mature male infant will have rugae on his scrotal sac and descended testes, while the mature female infant will have labia majora that cover the labia minora. (For a more thorough physical assessment of

Figure 12-31. Footprinting the newborn (see text for details).

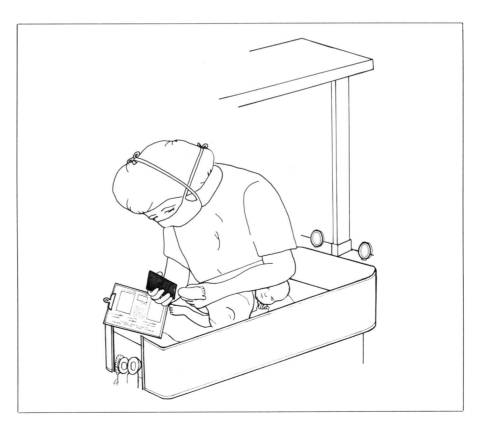

the newborn and assessment of gestational age see Chaps. 16, 21). This postnatal assessment is important, since if the infant is preterm, postterm, or small for gestational age, he is likely to experience a number of disturbances after birth.

CIRCULATORY AND RESPIRATORY CHANGES

During fetal life, the lungs are filled with fluid that keeps them partially inflated. In a vertex delivery, part of the fluid is squeezed out through the infant's nose and mouth. The blood vessels and lymphatics surrounding the lungs pick up the remaining fluid. If the birth is breech or cesarean, the fluid is not as easily expelled; in this case the infant may breathe rapidly for several days (transient tachypnea of the newborn). The vital lung capacities reach values proportional to those of the adult within 8 to 12 hours after birth.

With the onset of respiration, a number of changes occur in the infant's circulatory system. Alveolar expansion at birth results in decreased resistance in the pulmonary vessels, perhaps due to an increase in arterial PO_2, which causes a decrease in the right atrial pressure as the blood flows through the lungs. The increased blood flow from the lungs causes an increase in pressure in the left atrium, which in turn closes the foramen ovale. As the arterial PO_2 rises, the wall of the ductus arteriosus begins to constrict and close; it is usually obliterated by approximately 2 weeks of age, and most are sealed by 2 months [33]. The ductus venosus and umbilical arteries and vein become obliterated by 2 months of age.

If hypoxia occurs, the resistance in the pulmonary vessels increases and the blood flow through the lungs diminishes, changing pressures within the atria and opening the foramen ovale. The ductus arteriosus stops constricting and again shunts blood away from the lungs.

Occasionally an infant will be slow to breathe immediately after birth even though his heart rate is normal. This may happen as a result of undue pressure on the fetal head with a forceps delivery, abnormally long uterine contractions, or administration of large amounts of analgesia or anesthesia to the mother. Delay in respiration may also result from low maternal blood pressure or other factors that cause fetal distress. Often, rubbing the infant's skin when drying him and further suctioning of the upper airway [56] provide enough stimulation that he begins regular respirations and manages a lusty cry or two (Fig. 12-32). He should also respond to a flick of the finger on the sole of his foot or gentle stroking of his back from his waist to his neck while he is held in the Trendelenburg position. If his respirations are still irregular, the infant will often respond after a very brief period of oxygen delivered via face mask.

RESUSCITATION OF THE NEWBORN

If after a minute the infant remains moderately depressed, appears limp and cyanotic, and has shallow, irregular, or gasping respirations but maintains a heart rate above 100, he needs ventilatory assistance. A laryngoscope is passed, the airway cleared of any mucus or particles, and an airway inserted. Oxygen is then administered via a face mask attached to a hand-operated bag. The infant's chest should rise with each insufflation, and breath sounds should be heard in each lung. If the infant's respiration and color do not improve shortly, or if his

Figure 12-32. Suctioning the newborn.

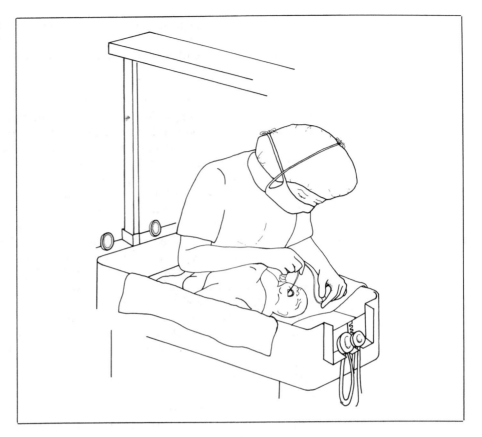

heart rate drops below 100, endotracheal intubation is performed and he is given oxygen through a bag attached to the endotracheal tube.

If the heart beat remains depressed, external cardiac massage is started, using the index and middle fingers over the left side of the infant's sternum (Fig. 12-33). The heart is compressed at a rate of approximately 120 times per minute, and oxygen is administered by bag after every three cardiac compressions. The external massage is continued until the heart rate recovers.

Prolonged hypoxia is accompanied by a metabolic acidosis, which is treated with administration of a 7.5% solution of sodium bicarbonate through the umbilical vein, provided that cardiac activity is adequate. When heart action is absent or depressed, the solution is infused into the infant's liver via the ductus venosus and remains there [33]. The infant also receives additional sugar, usually a solution of 10% dextrose. During resuscitation, the infant must be kept warm in order to ensure more rapid recovery.

Throughout the procedure, you must consider the parents' feelings. When their infant fails to cry, their anxiety may be overwhelming. Tell them what is happening in a manner that does not increase their anxiety further and inform them of any improvement as soon as it occurs. There is no better way of reassuring them and decreasing their anxiety than to have them see, touch, and hold their infant as soon as possible after his condition has stabilized. This can be

Figure 12-33. External cardiac massage of the newborn (see text for details).

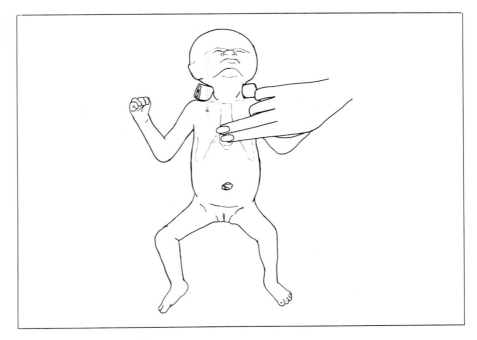

done simply by moving the crib unit close to the delivery table and giving the parents some time with their infant. If the infant is transferred to the intensive care unit, the parents should be kept informed of his progress, and the father should be encouraged to be with the infant as soon after transfer as possible.

The Third Stage of Labor—Assessment and Intervention

When the baby is born, the uterine cavity is obliterated. The uterus itself is almost a solid mass of muscle, with walls that are several centimeters thick; the fundus is usually just below the level of the umbilicus. With the decrease in size of the uterus, there is also less space available for placental attachment. To accommodate to the smaller area, the placenta first increases in thickness but is soon forced to fold on itself. The resulting tension causes the weakest layer of the decidua, the spongiosa, to break away, and the placenta begins to separate at that point. As a result of this continuing process, a hematoma forms between the separating placenta and the remaining decidua basalis; this hematoma may function in accelerating further separation. Usually placental separation occurs within a few minutes after delivery, 6 to 7 percent of the time within the first or second postpartum contractions.

After the separation of the placenta, the uterus becomes globular instead of discoid in shape. If the placenta remains in the uterus after separation, the fundus will rise up to or above the umbilicus or above the original position of the fundus. At the same time, a slight bulge appears just above the symphysis pubis, while the umbilical cord protrudes about 10 to 12 centimeters (4–5 inches) more than previously from the vulva. All of these signs indicate that the placenta has moved to the lower uterine segment or the upper part of the vagina. Because the formerly collapsed lower uterine segment becomes distended by the placenta, it mechanically lifts the tightly contracted body of the uterus to a higher level.

Studies have shown the periphery of the placenta to be the most adherent portion, so separation usually begins in a more central location. With central separation, the hematoma is thought to push the placenta toward the uterine cavity, where it becomes inverted; it descends, weighted with the hematoma. Surrounding membranes that are still attached to the decidua are dragged after it, and the shiny fetal surface of the placenta presents at the vulva. This type of placental presentation (Schultze's placenta) occurs over 70 percent of the time, usually accompanied by a gush of blood.

In the other method of separation (Duncan's placenta), the process begins at the periphery, with the result that blood collects between the membranes and the decidua and trickles from the vagina. The placenta descends to the vagina sideways, and the rough maternal surface appears first at the vulva. As can be surmised, with the continuous loss of blood in a Duncan separation, total blood loss may be greater. Fetal membranes usually remain in place until separation of the placenta is practically completed; they are then pulled off the uterine wall, partly by further contraction of the myometrium and partly by traction exerted by the separated placenta.

In some cases the placenta may be expelled by an increase in intra-abdominal pressure if the mother is coached to bear down. It is thought that this not only is less traumatic for her but also permits less fetal blood from the placenta to enter her circulation, which is particularly important in prevention of Rh sensitization. Unfortunately, women in the supine position can expel the placenta spontaneously only about 15 to 20 percent of the time. Since the figure is probably even lower when the woman has received anesthesia, artificial means of terminating the third stage of labor are generally necessary.

The usual method for delivering the placenta involves the midwife or obstetrician using manual pressure over the contracted fundus, thus using the uterus as a "piston" to expel the placenta, with the umbilical cord as a guide (Fig. 12-34). If the placenta is not expelled quickly following separation, blood may be lost unnecessarily. On the average, blood loss during and after vaginal delivery is around 600 milliliters. If you are caring for a mother after delivery, you should be aware of what her estimated blood loss is so that you might assess its effect on the woman. Signs and symptoms of hypovolemic shock include pallor, tachypnea, air hunger, restlessness, euphoria, and vertigo.

Attempts to deliver the placenta prior to complete separation are not only futile but also dangerous, and excessive traction or pulling on the cord is never done, since part of the placenta may tear away and remain inside the uterus, predisposing the mother to hemorrhage and infection. However, manual removal of the placenta is sometimes necessary if bleeding is heavy and the placenta cannot be delivered otherwise.

The placenta is delivered carefully to prevent the membranes from being torn off and left inside the uterus; it is routinely examined for completeness and for the number of fetal vessels in the cord. As mentioned previously, retained placental fragments or membranes can easily cause postpartum hemorrhage by preventing adequate myometrial contraction.

The First Postdelivery Hour (Fourth Stage of Labor)

Sometimes the mother is extremely fatigued by the time she gets to the recovery room, so schedule care to allow for her maximum rest and to ensure privacy for

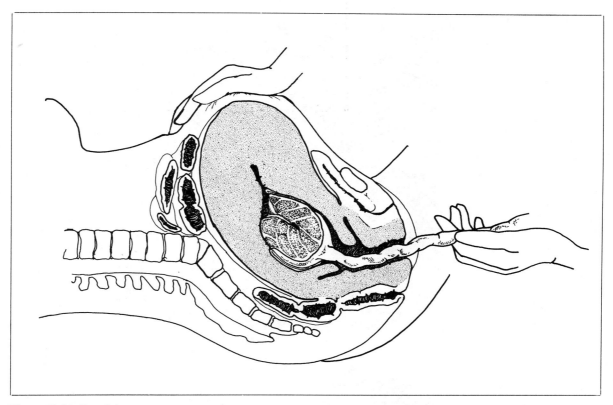

Figure 12-34. Expulsion of the placenta (see text for details).

the parents and their infant. Whenever possible, transfer the baby to the recovery room in the mother's or father's arms. The new family interaction has already been initiated (Fig. 12-35).

If the parents have not had adequate opportunity to see their newborn while in the delivery room, time in the recovery room can be used to great advantage in helping them get acquainted. Since they may be apprehensive about handling their infant, stay with them, offering support, until they are comfortable. This also, of course, provides you with an opportunity to make pertinent observations that should be added to the care plan that will be passed on to other personnel who will care for the new family unit in succeeding days.

The first postdelivery hour, sometimes referred to as the fourth stage of labor, is a very critical period for the mother. It is the time that postpartum hemorrhage is most likely to occur as a result of uterine relaxation. After the baby and placenta are delivered, hemostasis is achieved at the placental site through vasoconstriction produced by the contraction of the myometrium. Oxytocin (Pitocin, Syntocinon), ergonovine (Ergotrate), and methylergonovine (Methergine) may be used during the third and fourth stages of labor, principally to stimulate myometrial contractions and minimize blood loss. The tetanic effect of ergonovine is ideal for the prevention and control of postpartum hemorrhage, but it must be used carefully, since hypertension is a common side effect.

During the first postdelivery hour the mother is usually in the recovery room, where you can monitor her closely. Check her vital signs and the condition of her

Figure 12-35. Family interaction continues in the recovery room.

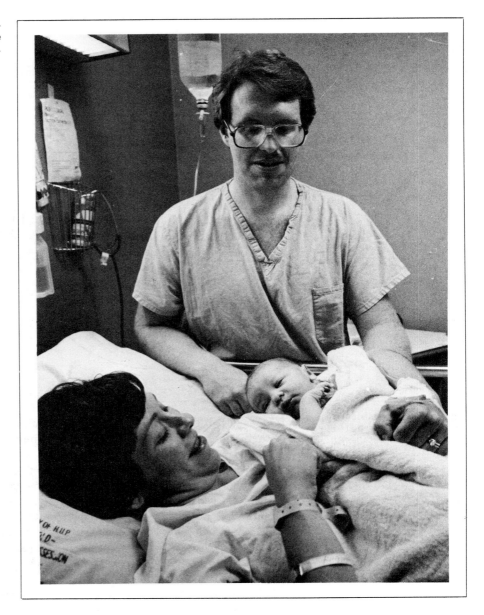

fundus and lochia (vaginal discharge after delivery) at least every 15 minutes. The fundus should remain firmly contracted, since even with slight relaxation it can quickly fill with blood and be unable to contract. If this occurs, massage the fundus and expel the blood that has collected in the uterine cavity.

In preparation for fundal massage ask the mother to flex her legs and allow them to fall apart. Palpate the mother's fundus by placing the side of one hand on top of and slightly cupped under the fundus while the other hand is placed over the symphysis pubis, exerting slight pressure (Fig. 12-36). The fundus is usually felt in the midline, at or below the umbilicus. If it is boggy, rub it lightly until it contracts firmly; it is important not to overmassage or overstimulate it, since the muscle may become fatigued and consequently relax. If blood has collected within the uterus, slight downward fundal pressure after the fundus is firm is usually all that is necessary to expel the blood.

In the recovery room mothers often are given intravenous fluids, commonly containing 10 units of oxytocin to promote uterine contraction. The intravenous fluids also result in rapid filling of the bladder, which may become distended and inhibit contractions by pushing the uterus high in the abdomen and displacing it to the right or left. A distended bladder may easily be seen and felt as a spongy, fluid-filled mass below the uterus and above the symphysis. If the mother has had block anesthesia that has not yet worn off, she may be totally unaware of the distention and may, in fact, be unable to void. In that case she will need to be catheterized (her voiding or catheterization is, of course, included in the nurse's notes).

Inspect the mother's perineum for swelling, or unusual tenderness when touched, or ecchymosis, all signs of a perineal or vaginal hematoma. Application of an ice bag may be helpful to lessen perineal edema and numb the area as anesthesia wears off. Keep the mother's perineum clean and dry, with regular changes of perineal pads and linen. Routinely check her lochia for color, amount, odor, and presence of clots. Since the discharge often pools under the mother's buttocks instead of collecting on the perineal pad, each examination should be a thorough one. If the lochia is excessive and the uterus is not remaining well contracted, or if there is a continuous bright red trickle, indicative of an unrepaired laceration, place the mother on a pad count and notify her physician.

During the first hour after delivery the mother's vital signs should return to their prenatal base. Be particularly alert for an increase in the mother's temperature (dehydration, infection), an increase in blood pressure (preeclampsia), or an increase in pulse rate followed by a decrease in blood pressure (hemorrhage). Remember that blood pressure and pulse rate usually do not show marked fluctuations in hemorrhage until after a large amount of blood has been lost and the circulatory system is unable to compensate for the decrease in volume.

Nursing care of the mother in the recovery room includes measures to increase

Figure 12-36. Fundal massage (see text for details).

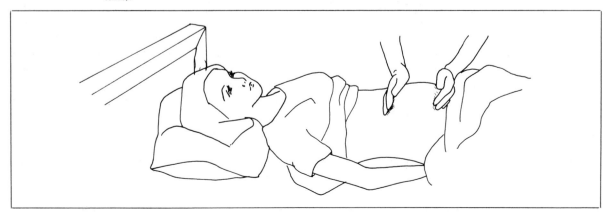

the mother's comfort such as a clean gown, a cup of coffee or tea, ice water, or whatever she wishes to eat if she is not nauseated. She may experience a postpartum chill and require an additional blanket, preferably already warmed. The cause of the postpartum chills is uncertain, but it may result from a nervous reaction, imbalance between external and internal body temperature due to muscular exertion, the sudden release of intra-abdominal pressure, or even infection.

Depending on the mother's condition, the recovery room can be a good place to educate her. You may, for example, teach the mother how to palpate her own fundus and massage it until it is firm.

EMERGENCY CHILDBIRTH

Any nurse whose background includes an understanding of the essentials of adequate antepartal care, the conduct of labor and delivery, and the immediate care of the newborn should be able to apply that knowledge to situations outside of a prepared, organized environment [31]. Some general principles are important in providing the mother and child with adequate protection and safety in an emergency delivery. The mother and baby should be considered as a unit, with the father or family involved as much as possible if they are present. Everything possible should be done to prevent infection, injury, and hemorrhage in the mother and baby. All necessary steps should be taken to ensure an adequate airway and the establishment of respiration in the newborn. For medical and legal purposes the time and location of birth should be recorded, as well as the names of the parents and any problems encountered.

Wherever the emergency delivery occurs, assessment of the general situation is the first priority. What is the condition of the mother and the fetus? How close is the delivery? How much time and what facilities exist for planning? Who will handle the delivery? Who will seek help? Who will prepare needed equipment?

Whatever circumstances surround the delivery, basic medical asepsis is observed as much as possible. Since the baby is not born through an aseptic passage, no delivery is really sterile, but cleanliness remains an essential consideration. All care is directed toward maintaining physical and emotional reserves, interpreting progress to the mother and father, and providing rest, fluids, and support.

During the second stage of labor, observe the mother constantly for signs of complications and exhaustion and give encouragement as necessary. As the delivery becomes imminent, wash your hands and then wet the mother's perineum with a towel and liquid soap, if possible. As the baby's head crowns, instruct the mother to pant during her contractions, since this may give an additional 3 to 5 minutes for extra planning before the actual delivery and decrease the possibility of a perineal tear. Support and protect the woman's perineum with a clean towel (a sterile towel, if available). If there is no clean material, do not touch the birth canal and surrounding perineum, and instruct the woman to keep her hands away from these areas.

Delivery of the Infant

Apply gentle pressure against the baby's head as it emerges so that it is not delivered too rapidly; however, do not hold it back. If membranes are still present, remove them. Slip the umbilical cord over the baby's head if it is looped around his neck. Wipe mucus and amniotic fluid from the infant's mouth and nose by stroking the nose downward and "milking" the throat with an upward movement on the neck and under the chin.

After the head is delivered, it usually turns spontaneously to one side or the other; occasionally it has to be gently rotated, in which case it should be turned in whichever direction it tends to go toward more easily. This motion will bring one shoulder anteriorly behind the symphysis pubis. With the baby's head in both of your hands, you can deliver the anterior shoulder by exerting gentle steady pressure downward. When the upper portion of the arm can be seen, the direction of traction should be reversed upward to deliver the posterior shoulder over the mother's perineum. This is done slowly and carefully, since there is no need to rush at this point.

As the baby's body is delivered, support it and then wrap it in a warm towel or clean cloth. After the parents have seen their newborn, place the baby on the mother's abdomen with the head low so that the mucus will drain out. If he does not cry immediately, stimulate respiration by gently rubbing his back.

If proper equipment is available, tie the infant's umbilical cord in two places after it has stopped pulsating. Make the ties about 8 centimeters (3 inches) from the abdomen and 5 centimeters (2 inches) farther up. Cut the cord between the ties if it can be done under aseptic conditions; otherwise it should not be cut, since the risk of infection is too great. In this case or if transportation is available, wrap the cord and placenta with the baby. The cord will be cut later when the baby and mother are in more favorable circumstances. No harm will result even in the extreme event that the cord is never cut, since the cord will dry naturally and fall off. Common household equipment can be sterilized to tie and cut the cord, including such items as wool, or string and a kitchen knife, scissors, or a new razor blade.

Delivery of the Placenta

Following the baby's delivery, observe the mother for signs of placental separation. Once this has occurred, the mother may be able to help push the placenta out. If not, gentle pressure on the contracted fundus toward the vaginal outlet will aid in placental delivery. Do not exert excessive traction on the cord, since it may snap or a placental fragment may break off and be left in the uterus. The entire placenta can stay in the uterus for several hours without harm to the mother if you monitor her carefully for bleeding [14].

Once the placenta and membranes are delivered, examine them thoroughly for completeness. If the mother's uterus is soft and bleeding, massage it to promote contractions. Start the baby on breast-feeding to stimulate the release of natural oxytocin to achieve the same effect. Make the mother as comfortable as possible, give her nourishment (such as hot tea with honey, or salty broth), encourage her to void, and allow her to rest. If she is to be transferred to a medical facility, it might be better to give her no fluids, since anesthesia may be necessary for repair of lacerations or for uterine exploration.

Care of the Newborn

Two important aspects of the routine care of the newborn are identification and warmth; also important are cleanliness (especially when dealing with the cord stump), gentle handling, and pertinent observations of the infant's condition.

Sometimes improvised methods of identification become necessary during wide-scale emergencies. The infant may be kept warm by wrapping him in lightweight blankets and placing him either next to his mother's skin (they can be wrapped together in the blankets) or in a warm place, such as in a box near an oven turned to a low heat.

The infant will also need food. Breast-feeding is preferable, but it should never be forced on the mother. A suitable formula can be prepared from powdered infant formula or dried skim milk. If there is no refrigeration, the formula should be made immediately prior to the feeding. Canned evaporated milk, diluted 1 part milk to 2 parts water, may also be used. If no bottles are available, milk may be placed in a teaspoon on the baby's lower lip or dropped on the inside of his cheek with a medicine dropper.

Other Situations of
Emergency Childbirth

Emergency care of the pregnant woman may be necessary in her home, en route to the hospital, during local or national disasters, or even in the hospital itself. If the mother delivers precipitously in the hospital, there is usually an emergency delivery kit and sterile gloves in each labor room. The kit commonly includes two Kelly clamps, a plastic cord clamp, scissors, sterile towels, sponges, a bulb syringe, and a basin for the placenta. After the cord is cut, the baby and mother are usually transferred to the delivery room, where the placenta is delivered, the uterus is examined, and any lacerations are repaired.

If the delivering mother is en route to the hospital in an automobile or taxi, she should be on the back seat with something under her buttocks (blanket, coat, skirt) to avoid contact with the seat, which has been used by many other people. When she reaches the hospital, usually she and the baby are taken directly to the delivery room. There the cord is cut, the placenta is removed, her uterus is explored, and any lacerations are repaired. The infant is usually taken to the isolation-observation nursery, where he can be closely watched for signs of trauma, fever, intracranial hemorrhage, or infection. Both mother and baby may be given prophylactic antibiotics.

If the mother in labor is at home and is on the floor, several thicknesses of heavy material (towels) should be placed under her buttocks to give a little more space for delivery of the baby's shoulders. If possible, she should be moved to a bed (or table) and positioned so she is lying crosswise with her buttocks slightly off the edge. She may place her hands under her thighs to support herself, or rest her feet on the backs of two chairs. If it is at all possible, the furnishings should be protected by newspapers, a plastic shower curtain or table cloth, towels, or old sheets.

In actual large-scale disaster situations, principles of triage for obstetric patients will most likely be observed. Pregnant women who only need reassurance that their pregnancy is unthreatened and that they are not in active labor, in premature labor, or aborting are classified as requiring *minimal treatment*. Multiparas may be assigned duties in maternal areas and, with proper guidance, may be called on to assist in delivery or even to perform a delivery themselves. *Immediate treatment* is required for those mothers who are ready to deliver or who are actively aborting. Oxytocics may not be available, and unless hemorrhage is a major threat, no manipulation or instrumentation is even considered. Treatment may have to be *delayed* for women in active labor or with minor complications of pregnancy requiring nursing care; these women are allowed to progress until some spontaneous outcome is reached. *Expectant casualties* include those women in whom no normal spontaneous outcome can be expected (e.g., those requiring a cesarean birth); treatment for these women will have to be deferred until more advanced obstetric care is available.

For disasters and other emergency situations in which prior planning has been done, delivery kits are usually available. If there has been no time for planning, materials for meeting certain priorities of care should be gathered: for cleansing—liquid soap, alcohol, or vinegar; for adequate airway—bulb syringe, meat-basting syringe, a plastic straw, or rubber tubing of a small diameter; for padding and protection—newspapers, plastic bags, or old sheets and towels; for warmth—blankets, towels, clean sheets, shirts, or diapers; for a baby bed—a carton or box; for food—bottles and milk powder. The major concern in this situation, as in any childbearing experience, is as healthy an outcome as possible for mother, baby, and family.

Case Study   Joan Mitchell

As Joan's primary nurse, develop a plan of care for the Mitchells including your interventions aimed at helping them through labor and delivery and the transitional period. Each of you will develop your own approach and style in providing care to laboring couples; applying the nursing process to the outline following the case study will serve as a guide in organizing your approach to the family during labor and delivery.

Joan Mitchell is a 22-year-old college senior who has 6 more months of school before she will graduate. Five months ago Joan married Thomas Mitchell, also a college senior, at the urging of both Tom's and her own parents when they found out Joan was pregnant. Although they are very fond of each other, Joan and Tom admit they have many adjustments to make and problems to iron out. They are currently living in two rooms on the third floor of Tom's parents' home. Both Tom's and Joan's parents are contributing to the couple's financial needs. Tom works after classes and weekends at a local bookstore. He hopes to go to law school after graduation but isn't sure this will be possible with the expenses of his new family. His parents aren't sure how much they can or are willing to contribute to his plans after graduation. Tom's father is a plumber, his mother a housewife. Tom, 22, has a younger brother Joe, 14. Joan's mother is also a housewife; her father owns a hardware store. Joan is an only child. Both sets of parents were initially angry about the pregnancy but have now accepted it and are supporting "the kids."

Joan had few difficulties during her pregnancy. She was very nauseated and vomited almost daily during the first trimester. Her hemoglobin was 9.4 grams early in pregnancy but with iron therapy is now 10.2 grams per 100 deciliters at term. Her hematocrit is 30.6. Joan gained only 14 pounds during pregnancy. She attributes this to her inability to eat in the early months and her dislike of her new mother-in-law's cooking later in pregnancy. Other than these difficulties, Joan's pregnancy was normal and the fetus appears to have grown normally. She did not attend prenatal classes. Joan has no significant existing health problems.

Joan went into labor a week prior to her EDC and came to the hospital when her contractions were 5 minutes apart. The contractions were 40 seconds in duration and of moderate intensity. Joan's membranes were intact and she had minimal bloody show. The fetal heart rate was 134 and found below and to the right of Joan's umbilicus. Her temperature, blood pressure, and pulse were within normal range.

It is now 3 hours later. Joan's cervix is 100 percent effaced, 4 centimeters dilated, O station, and the fetus is in an ROA position. Tom and Joan's mother are waiting in the family waiting room. Tom doesn't want to be with Joan during the labor and delivery; he is afraid he won't be able to take it and will faint. "I won't be much help to her," he states.

Joan's contractions are now 50 seconds in duration, 3½ to 4 minutes apart, and of moderate intensity. FHR is 140. External fetal monitoring is being used. Joan is thrashing about in bed, groaning with discomfort, and asking for her mother.

Assessment Form

Assessment	Plan	Intervention	Evaluation
I. Significant factors from pregnancy			

I. Significant factors from pregnancy
   A. Specific problems during current pregnancy
      1. Planned or unplanned
      2. Bleeding
      3. Hypertension
      4. Severe nausea or vomiting
      5. Weight gain
      6. Anemia
      7. Infections
   B. Problems during previous pregnancies
   C. Previous or existing health problems
   D. Childbirth education preparation
      1. Type
      2. Length
      3. Educator

II. Admission
   A. Gravida, para
   B. EDC
   C. Membranes ruptured—color, amount, odor
   D. Bloody show
   E. Vital signs
      1. Temperature
      2. Pulse
      3. Respirations
   F. Fetal heart rate
   G. Contraction pattern
      1. Duration
      2. Frequency
      3. Intensity
      4. When did contractions begin
      5. Amount of discomfort
   H. Cervical dilation and effacement
   I. Blood type and RH
   J. Allergies

III. Labor progress
   A. Physical changes
      1. Vital signs—temperature, blood pressure, pulse, respirations

Assessment Form			
Assessment	Plan	Intervention	Evaluation

2. Contraction pattern
   (a) Duration
   (b) Frequency
   (c) Intensity
3. Cervical dilation and efface-ment—normal progress accord-ing to normal labor curve (graph)
4. Rupture of membranes—color, amount, odor
5. Fetal heart rate
   (a) Baseline rate
   (b) Variability
   (c) Response to uterine contrac-tions
6. Fetus
   (a) Lie
   (b) Presentation
   (c) Position and rotation
   (d) Station and descent

B. Comfort measures
   Mother
   1. Positioning
   2. Mouth care
   3. Back rub and sacral counterpres-sure
   4. Effleurage
   5. Pain relief
      (a) Breathing techniques
      (b) Analgesia
      (c) Anesthesia
   6. Safety precautions
   7. Hydration
   8. Urinary elimination
   9. Perineal hygiene
   10. Restful environment, soft lights
   11. Sponge bath (face, neck, upper chest)

   Father or support person
   1. Rest
   2. Nutrition

Assessment Form

Assessment	Plan	Intervention	Evaluation
3. Relief from support role			
C. Woman's expectations regarding:			
1. Labor			
2. Delivery			
3. Type of delivery			
4. Type of anesthesia			
5. Fetal monitoring			
6. Position for delivery			
7. Episiotomy			
8. Support person during			
(a) Labor			
(b) Delivery			
9. Interaction and time with infant following delivery			
10. Breast or bottle feeding			
D. Father's or support person's expectations regarding above			
E. Couple's need for information regarding:			
1. Labor			
2. Delivery			
3. Institutional routines and alternatives			
4. Unforeseen emergency measures			
F. Behavioral			
1. Coping of mother			
2. Coping of father or support person			
3. Communication pattern—verbal, nonverbal			
4. Dependent functioning			
5. Need for control			
6. Measures to enhance self-esteem of mother and father:			
(a) Information to make informed choices			
(b) Reassurance			
(c) Praise			
(d) Help to achieve expectations and goals			
G. Needs identified by			
1. Mother			
2. Father			

Assessment Form			
Assessment	Plan	Intervention	Evaluation

IV. Delivery
    A. Preparation for:
        1. Physical
        2. Informational
    B. Vital signs
    C. Contractions
    D. Fetal heart rate
    E. Mother's ability to push
    F. Parents' ability to:
        1. View delivery process
        2. See and hold newborn

V. Recovery period
    A. Vital signs
    B. Uterus
        1. Position
            (a) Height in relation to umbilicus
            (b) Midline
            (c) Firmly contracted
    C. Lochia
        1. Amount
        2. Character
    D. Perineum
        1. Episiotomy
        2. Swelling
        3. Ecchymosis
    E. Comfort measures
        1. Adequate warmth
        2. Hydration
        3. Voiding
        4. Relief of
            (a) Pain
            (b) Nausea or vomiting
        5. Restful environment
    F. Opportunity and privacy to interact with:
        1. Newborn
        2. Each other
    G. Opportunity to have questions answered

REFERENCES

1. Applegate, J., Haverkamp, A., Orleans, M., and Taylor, C. Electronic fetal monitoring: Implications for obstetrical nursing. *Nursing Research* 28:369, 1979.
2. Beck, C. Patient acceptance of fetal monitoring as a helpful tool. *Journal of Obstetric, Gynecologic and Neonatal Nursing* 9:350, 1980.
3. Benson, R., Shubeck, F., Deutschberger, J., Weiss, W., and Berendes, H. Fetal heart rate as a predictor of fetal distress. *Obstetrics and Gynecology* 32:259, 1968.
4. Bond, S. Reevaluating positions for labor—lateral vs. supine. *Journal of Obstetric, Gynecologic and Neonatal Nursing* 2(6):29, 1973.
5. Britton, G. Early mother-infant contact and infant temperature stabilization. *Journal of Obstetric, Gynecologic and Neonatal Nursing* 9:84, 1980.
6. Butani, P., and Hodnett, E. Mothers' perceptions of their labor experiences. *Maternal-Child Nursing Journal* 9:73, 1980.
7. Caire, J. Are current rates of Cesarean justified? *Obstetrical and Gynecological Survey* 34:34, 1979.
8. Caldeyro-Barcia, R. The influence of maternal bearing-down efforts during second stage on fetal well being. *Birth and the Family Journal* 6:17, 1979.
9. Caldeyro-Barcia, R. The influence of maternal position on time of spontaneous rupture of membranes, progress of labor, and fetal head compression. *Birth and the Family Journal* 6:7, 1979.
10. Coch, J., Brovetto, J., Cabot, H., Fielitz, C., and Caldeyro-Barcia, R. Oxytocin-equivalent activity in the plasma of women in labor and during the puerperium. *American Journal of Obstetrics and Gynecology* 91:10, 1965.
11. Collins, E., and Turner, G. Maternal effects of regular salicylate ingestion in pregnancy. *Lancet* 2:335, 1975.
12. Csapo, A. Function and regulation of the myometrium. *Journal of New York Academy of Medicine* 75:790, 1959.
13. Csapo, A., Pohinka, O., and Kaihola, H. Progesterone deficiency and premature labor. *British Medical Journal* 1:137, 1974.
14. Danforth, D. Physiology of uterine action. In D. Danforth (Ed.), *Obstetrics and Gynecology* (3rd ed.). New York: Harper & Row, 1977.
15. Dickason, E., and Schult, M. *Maternal and Infant Care.* New York: McGraw-Hill, 1975.
16. Doust, B. The role of ultrasound in obstetrics and gynecology. *Hospital Practice* 8:143, 1973.
17. Dulock, H., and Herron, M. Women's response to fetal monitoring. *Journal of Obstetrics, Gynecologic and Neonatal Nursing* 5s: 68s, 1976.
18. Flynn, A. Ambulation in labor. *British Medical Journal* 2:591, 1978.
19. Gardner, S. The mother as incubator—after delivery. *Journal of Obstetric, Gynecologic and Neonatal Nursing* 8:174, 1979.
20. Gay, J. Theories regarding endocrine contributions to the onset of labor. *Journal of Obstetric, Gynecologic and Neonatal Nursing* 7(5):42, 1978.
21. Gibbens, D., Boyd, N., and Chard, T. Spurt release of oxytocin during labor. *Journal of Endocrinology* 54:53, 1972.
22. Gleason, D. Footprinting for identification of infants. *Pediatrics* 44:302, 1969.
23. Greenberg, M., and Vandow, J. Ophthalmia neonatorum: Evaluation of different methods of prophylaxis in New York City. *American Journal of Public Health* 51:836, 1961.
24. Greenhill, J., and Friedman, E. *Biological Principles and Modern Practice of Obstetrics.* Philadelphia: Saunders, 1974.
25. Haverkamp, A., Thompson, H., and McFee, J. The evaluation of continuous fetal heart rate monitoring in high-risk pregnancy. *American Journal of Obstetrics and Gynecology* 125:310, 1976.
26. Highley, B., and Mercer, R. Safeguarding the laboring woman's sense of control. *American Journal of Maternal-Child Nursing* 3:39, 1978.
27. Hill, S., and Shronk, L. The effect of early parent-infant contact on newborn body temperature. *Journal of Obstetric, Gynecologic and Neonatal Nursing* 8:287, 1979.
28. Hodnett, E. Patient control during labor, effects of two types of fetal monitors. *Journal of Obstetric, Gynecologic and Neonatal Nursing* 11:94, 1982.
29. Hon, E. Electronic evaluation of fetal heart rates. *American Journal of Obstetrics and Gynecology* 83:333, 1962.
30. Jacobsen, G. Gross Anatomy of the Female Reproductive Tract, Pituitary and Hypothalamus. In D. Danforth (Ed.), *Obstetrics and Gynecology* (3rd ed.). New York: Harper & Row, 1977.
31. Jennings, B. Emergency delivery: How to attend one safely. *American Journal of Maternal-Child Nursing* 4:148, 1979.

32. Klein, R., Gist, N., Nicholson, J., and Standley, K. A study of father and nurse support during labor. *Birth and the Family Journal* 8:161, 1982.
33. Korones, S. *High Risk Newborn Infants.* St. Louis: Mosby, 1976.
34. Landry, K., and Kilpatrick, D. Why shave a mother before she gives birth? *American Journal of Maternal-Child Nursing* 2:189, 1977.
35. Lederman, R. P. Relationship of maternal anxiety, plasma catecholamines and plasma cortisol to progress in labor. *American Journal of Obstetrics and Gynecology* 132:495, 1978.
36. Lederman, R. P., Lederman, E., Work, B., and McCann, D. Relationship of psychological factors in pregnancy to progress in labor. *Nursing Research* 28:94, 1979.
37. Lesser, M., and Keane, V. *Nurse Patient Relationships in a Hospital Maternity Service.* St. Louis: Mosby, 1956.
38. Levinson, G., and Shnider, S. Catecholomines. The effects of maternal fear and its treatment on uterine function and circulation. *Birth and the Family Journal* 6:167, 1979.
39. Little, A. Endocrinology. In S. Romney, M. Gray, A. Little, J. Merrill, E. Quilligan, and R. Stander, *Gynecology and Obstetrics: The Health Care of Women* (2nd ed.). New York: McGraw-Hill, 1981.
40. Macdonald, P. Initiation of human parturition. *Obstetrics and Gynecology* 44:629, 1974.
41. McDonough, M., Sheriff, D., and Zimmel, P. Parents' responses to fetal monitoring. *American Journal of Maternal-Child Nursing* 10:32, 1981.
42. McKay, S. Maternal position during labor and birth: A reassessment. *Journal of Obstetric, Gynecologic and Neonatal Nursing* 9:288, 1980.
43. *Mechanism of Normal Labor.* Columbus, Ohio: Ross Laboratories, 1970.
44. Mendez-Bauer, C. Effects of standing position on spontaneous uterine contractility and other aspects of labor. *Journal of Perinatal Medicine* 3:89, 1975.
45. Moore, M. L. *Newborn, Family and Nurse.* Philadelphia: Saunders, 1981.
46. Neutra, R. Effect of fetal monitoring on cesarean section rates. *Journal of Obstetrics and Gynecology* 2:175, 1980.
47. Neutra, R. Effect of fetal monitoring on neonatal death rates. *New England Journal of Medicine* 229:324, 1978.
48. Norr, K., Block, C., Charles, A., Meyering, S., and Meyers, E. Explaining pain and enjoyment in childbirth. *Journal of Health and Social Behavior* 18:260, 1977.
49. Ohlsen, H. Moulding of the pelvis during labor. *Acta Radiologica: Diagnosis* (Stockholm) 14:417, 1973.
50. Paul, R., and Hon, E. Clinical fetal monitoring. V. Effect on perinatal outcome. *American Journal of Obstetrics and Gynecology* 118:529, 1974.
51. Paul, R., and Petrie, R. *Fetal Intensive Care,* Vols. I, II, III. North Haven, Conn: William Mack Co., 1979.
52. Phillips, C. Neonatal heat loss in heated cribs vs. mother's arms. *Journal of Obstetric, Gynecologic and Neonatal Nursing* 3(6):11, 1974.
53. Pokoly, T. The role of cortisol in human parturition. *American Journal of Obstetrics and Gynecology* 117:549, 1973.
54. Pritchard, J., and Macdonald, P. *Williams Obstetrics* (16th ed.). New York: Appleton-Century-Crofts, 1980.
55. Querec, L. Apgar score in the United States, 1978. *National Center for Health Statistics Monthly Vital Statistics Report* 30:1, 1981.
56. Roberts, J. Suctioning the newborn. *American Journal of Nursing* 73:63, 1973.
57. Schultz, F. Initiation of human parturition. *American Journal of Obstetrics and Gynecology* 123:650, 1975.
58. Schwarz, B. Initiation of human parturition. *Obstetrics and Gynecology* 46:564, 1975.
59. Shannon-Babitz, M. Addressing the needs of fathers during labor and delivery. *American Journal of Maternal-Child Nursing* 4:378, 1979.
60. Shields, D. Maternal reactions to fetal monitoring. *American Journal of Nursing* 78:2110, 1978.
61. Shields, D. Nursing care in labor and patient satisfaction. *Journal of Advanced Nursing* 3:535, 1978.
62. Tutera, G., and Newman, R. Fetal monitoring: Its effect on the perinatal mortality and cesarean section rates and its complications. *American Journal of Obstetrics and Gynecology* 122:750, 1975.
63. Wapner, J. The attitudes, feelings and behaviors of expectant fathers attending Lamaze classes. *Birth and the Family Journal* 3:7, 1976.
64. Whitley, N., and Mack, E. Are enemas justified for women in labor? *American Journal of Nursing* 80:1339, 1980.

65. Young, D. Predelivery shaving and enema—Are there any benefits? *International Childbirth Education Association News* 21:1, 1982.

FURTHER READINGS

Blair, C., and Mahoukis, C. Comparing notes: The nurse as patient/the nurse as labor coach. *American Journal of Maternal-Child Nursing* 5:102, 1980.

Bonica, J. *Obstetric Analgesia and Anesthesia.* Amsterdam: World Federation of Societies of Anaesthesiologists, 1980.

Carmack, B., and Corwin, T. Nursing care of the schizophrenic maternity patient during labor. *American Journal of Maternal-Child Nursing* 5:107, 1980.

Carr, K., and Walton, V. Early postpartum discharge. *Journal of Obstetric, Gynecologic and Neonatal Nursing* 11:29, 1982.

Cranston, C. Obstetrical nurses' attitudes towards fetal monitoring. *Journal of Obstetric, Gynecologic and Neonatal Nursing* 9:344, 1980.

Gray, J. Nursing care for monitored women in labor. *American Journal of Nursing* 78:2104, 1978.

Hawkins, J., and Higgins, L. *Maternity and Gynecological Nursing.* Philadelphia: Lippincott, 1981.

Howe, C. Physiologic and psychosocial assessment in labor. *Nursing Clinics of North America* 17:49, 1982.

Jennett, R., Warford, H., Kreinick, C., and Waterkotte, G. Apgar index: A statistical tool. *American Journal of Obstetrics and Gynecology* 119:775, 1974.

Johnson, J. Teaching self-hypnosis in pregnancy, labor and delivery. *American Journal of Maternal-Child Nursing* 5:98, 1980.

Jolivet, A., Blancher, H., and Gantray, J. Blood cortisol variations during late pregnancy and labor. *American Journal of Obstetrics and Gynecology* 119:775, 1974.

Jones, C. Father-to-infant attachment: Effects of early contact and characteristics of the infant. *Research in Nursing and Health* 4:193, 1981.

Keirse, M., Anderson, A., and Gravenhorst, J. *Human Parturition.* Leiden, Netherlands: Leiden University Press, 1979.

Kunst, W., and Cronenwett, L. Nursing care for the emerging family: Promoting paternal behavior. *Research in Nursing and Health* 4:201, 1981.

Lum, S-B, Lortz, R., and Barnett, E. Reappraising newborn eye care. *American Journal of Nursing* 80:1602, 1980.

Mahoney, R. *Emergency and Disaster Nursing.* New York: Macmillan, 1969.

Norr, K., Block, C., Charles, A., and Meyering, S. The second time around: Parity and birth experience. *Journal of Obstetric, Gynecologic and Neonatal Nursing* 9:30, 1980.

Paukert, S. Maternal-infant attachment in a traditional hospital setting. *Journal of Obstetric, Gynecologic and Neonatal Nursing* 11:23, 1982.

Quilligan, E. Maternal factors influencing the onset of labor. *Clinical Obstetrics and Gynecology* 16:150, 1973.

Shnider, S. Choice of anesthesia for labor and delivery. *Obstetrics and Gynecology* 58:24s, 1981.

Standley, K., and Nicholson, J. Observing the childbirth environment: A research model. *Birth and the Family Journal* 7:15, 1980.

Tucker, S. *Fetal Monitoring and Fetal Assessment in High Risk Pregnancy.* St. Louis: Mosby, 1978.

Wagner, P. Continuous fetal tissue pH monitoring—A preliminary experience. *Journal of Obstetric, Gynecologic and Neonatal Nursing* 10:164, 1981.

Whitley, N. Uterine contractile physiology: Applications in nursing care and patient teaching. *Journal of Obstetric, Gynecologic and Neonatal Nursing* 4(5):54, 1975.

Wiley, J. The nurse's legal responsibility in obstetric monitoring. *Journal of Obstetric, Gynecologic and Neonatal Nursing* 5s:77s, 1976.

Yunek, M., and Lojek, R. Intrapartal fetal monitoring. *American Journal of Nursing* 78:2102, 1978.

Chapter 13 Pain Relief in Labor

The experience of childbirth is interpreted individually by each woman or couple. This interpretation is colored by many factors including their expectations of the experience, the amount of discomfort and anxiety the woman experiences, the amount of control she feels over her situation, the amount of support she receives from her partner, the amount of support he is capable of giving, and the support they receive from nursing personnel. It is generally believed that preparation for childbirth can diminish such anxiety, subsequently reduce the need for anesthetic and analgesic medications during labor and delivery, and increase the couple's enjoyment of the childbirth experience. As you shall see, you can play an important role in helping the couple reach the goal of a safe and growth-producing childbirth experience.

Since it is known that pain, fear, and anxiety all cause a significant increase in the basal metabolic rate, reflex irritability, and oxygen demand [1], it is important to decrease each of these elements as much as possible. Fear and anxiety can be lessened with knowledge; parents who approach labor having attended childbirth education classes are usually able to cope with the situation more successfully. Unprepared women, on the other hand, tend to feel discomfort much more acutely and at an earlier phase of labor. In either case, the pattern of the woman's reactions depends not only on her present emotional state but also on her interpretation of pain in light of her past life experiences and the symbolic meaning of pain to her.

The analgesic techniques of childbirth education, psychoprophylaxis, and hypnosis are usually effective in the first stage of labor. Properly applied, each technique produces complete pain relief in 10 to 20 percent of laboring patients; these patients will require no anesthesia for delivery. In another 30 to 50 percent, pain will be decreased, and these women will need less medication than the unprepared patient. In the remainder of patients, the degree of pain does not seem to be affected [1].

Pregnant women approach anesthesia with the same fears as persons facing surgery; the most serious and most powerful fear, of course, is the fear of death. Fear of loss of consciousness and loss of control are closely related to each other. Also present are the fear of pain and fear of possible complications, such as paralysis due to spinal anesthesia. In addition, women may have heard about many unpleasant, if not terrifying, experiences from relatives and friends. There are also women who approach labor with the conviction that to request anything for relief of discomfort is an admission of failure. If it becomes necessary for them to be medicated, they often feel guilt or even depression following delivery.

PAIN DURING LABOR AND DELIVERY
The pain of uterine contractions travels along afferent fibers via the posterior roots of the eleventh and twelfth thoracic nerves (sympathetic nervous system) to the spinal cord. Pain due to cervical dilatation and stretching of the birth canal travels via the roots of the second, third, and fourth sacral nerves (parasympathetic nervous system) to the spinal cord. Perineal pain is conducted via the pudendal nerve.

The exact mechanism that produces the pain of childbirth is a controversial issue. It is generally thought that the pain of the first stage of labor is primarily a result of cervical dilatation. This is corroborated by the fact that there is often an interval of about 15 to 30 seconds after the onset of a contraction before pain is experienced. It takes this long for the amniotic fluid pressure to increase to 15 millimeters of mercury, the minimum pressure needed to distend the lower uterine segment and cervix, resulting in dilatation. (Pain is also felt when the cervix is dilated with an instrument or manually in pregnant or nonpregnant women [1].)

Pain is also probably caused by the contraction of the myometrium itself; the myometrium becomes ischemic or puts pressure on the nerve endings between the muscle fibers of the uterus. Perhaps the most severe pain of labor is produced by the distention of the pelvic outlet, vulva, and perineum, resulting in stretching (and possibly tearing) of the fascia, skin, and subcutaneous tissue of these structures. Other factors that contribute to the pain of childbirth include tension in the supporting uterine ligaments, pressure on the adnexa and peritoneum, and pressure on and stretching of the bladder, urethra, and rectum. Discomfort from these accessory structures is conveyed by sensory nerves associated with the ovarian plexus via the posterior roots of the tenth thoracic nerve.

The intensity of the perceived pain depends on the preparation of the woman for labor and the support she receives from her coach and health personnel. It also depends on the intensity and duration of uterine contractions; the degree of cervical dilatation and how quickly it is reached; the degree of distention of the perineum; the woman's condition, age, parity, and anxiety level; and the size of the infant and the birth canal. As a rule, labor in the younger primigravida (under 30) is neither as long nor as painful as that in the older primigravida (35 or older), but it is longer than that of the multigravida [1].

During the first stage of labor most of the pain is caused by uterine contractions and cervical dilatation. As the fetal head begins to descend into the pelvis, pain is caused by the stretching of structures in the pelvis and the perineum. Pain of contractions and cervical dilatation is referred to the lower abdominal wall and skin and to the soft tissue over the lower lumbar spine and upper sacrum. With more intense stimulation, the pain spreads to the upper thighs, midsacral area, and the umbilical region. During the second stage of labor, the pain is intense in the area of the vulva and perineum; however, during the third stage pain may again result from uterine contractions and from dilatation of the cervix by passage of the placenta.

| PAIN RELIEF DURING THE BIRTH PROCESS | In the middle 1800s anesthesia was used when Queen Victoria gave birth to Prince Leopold, and from that time the medical profession and lay public began to see it as having great potential in obstetric practice. Research results in the past quarter century have added greatly to the knowledge and techniques of the relief of labor pain [1]. |

When considering analgesic and anesthetic needs, certain elements distinguish women in labor from persons facing surgery. A major difference is that anesthesia is not an absolute necessity for labor and delivery and there are two individuals to be cared for when a mother is in labor. The respiratory center of the newborn is highly vulnerable to sedative, analgesic, and anesthetic drugs. Also, a pregnant woman usually has little time to be prepared physically for anesthesia and often begins labor with some food in her stomach. Another difference is that some continuous methods of regional anesthesia permit the agent to be given throughout labor and thus over a longer period of time than most surgery lasts. Another very important consideration is that if the analgesia or anesthesia is begun too early in labor, it may stop progress entirely.

All methods of pain relief for the mother in labor and delivery have three essential criteria: fetal homeostasis, simplicity, and safety. Some methods of pain relief are associated with sustained or repeated maternal hypotension and thus reduce the PO_2 gradient across the placenta. Under this type of stress, fetal homeostatic mechanisms become increasingly less competent, since they depend on the maternal concentration of inhaled oxygen, uterine blood flow, and the umbilical blood flow. Impaired fetal oxygenation is most often the result of either compression of the umbilical cord or repeated or prolonged decreases in placental blood supply. The latter may be caused by hypertonic uterine contractions, severe pregnancy-induced hypertension, hemorrhage from premature separation of the placenta, or maternal hypotension from spinal or epidural anesthesia. It is also known that potential complications increase in a direct relationship with the complexity of the method used for pain relief.

No completely safe and satisfactory method of analgesia and anesthesia has yet been developed in obstetrics. Probably the one that satisfies the three criteria best is proper psychologic support throughout the antepartal period and during labor. This not only provides a natural sedative for the mother but also reduces her fears and anxieties. She tends to develop a feeling of confidence in her support person, the nurses, and the midwife or obstetrician. In this context, anesthesia really begins with the first prenatal visit!

When the use of additional methods becomes necessary, usually they are not begun until there is evidence of progressive effacement and dilatation of the cervix. Usually the cervix is 4 to 5 centimeters dilated in the primigravida and 4 to 6 centimeters dilated in the multigravida before medication is given. Since labor may be prolonged if medication is given too early, it is probably better if the mother receives it only when she is clearly in the active phase of labor [1].

The choice of technique depends on many factors, most important of which is the woman's choice, her condition, and the condition of her fetus. Has she eaten recently? Is she hypotensive or hypertensive? Is she dehydrated? Other significant variables include the stage of labor she is in, the rapidity of the progress she is making, and the expertise of the personnel who will administer her anesthesia.

Methods of Pain Relief   Traditionally, methods for pain relief during labor and delivery have been sedatives, ataractics, and analgesics during the first phases of labor. These have been followed by the use of anesthetic techniques such as spinal anesthesia, pudendal block, or general anesthesia for the delivery process. More recently, certain regional anesthetic techniques, such as epidural and caudal blocks, have been used. The advantage of these types of anesthesias is that they can be used continuously for the first stage of labor as well as for the second stage.

SEDATIVES AND ATARACTICS

Sometimes during labor, mothers are given sedative doses of barbiturates to produce a feeling of well-being and increased susceptibility to suggestion;

however, sedatives do not produce analgesia. If they do not have the desired calming effect, occasionally a tranquilizer might be necessary.

For over 70 years scopolamine was used to potentiate the sedative effects of barbiturates and narcotics and to produce amnesia. Currently it is rarely used, since there are many better sedatives and tranquilizers available; in addition many mothers prefer to participate in their infant's birth and want to remember as many details of the event as possible.

NARCOTIC ANALGESICS

Narcotics are probably the most widely used analgesics for labor and the most simple to administer; they decrease fear and anxiety and promote physical relaxation and rest between contractions. However, they may slow the progress of labor if given before the active phase of labor and are specific depressants of neonatal respiration (Table 13-1). The narcotic has its peak depressing effects on the fetus 2 hours after administration; to avoid the occurrence of that peak at the time of delivery (when the infant is under the most stress), the mother should be given the last injection 3 hours before the predictable time of delivery. She can also be given an injection if the delivery is expected in less than an hour [1].

The most commonly used narcotics are meperidine (Demerol), pentazocine (Talwin), and fentanyl (Sublimaze). Respiratory depression is the most significant maternal side effect of narcotic administration. Some narcotics such as Sublimaze produce a peak respiratory depression of much greater magnitude

Table 13-1.
Pharmacologic Agents
Used in Labor

Drug	Maternal Side Effects	Effect on Labor	Placental Transmission	Effect on Newborn
Narcotics	Respiratory depression, bradycardia, orthostatic hypotension, nausea and vomiting, urinary retention	With optimum dose, none. If dose is excessive or given too early, slows progress of labor	Rapid	With proper use, mild depression; with excessive use, severe depression
Sedatives, hypnotics, and ataractics	Sleep, sedation, tranquilizing action, antiemetic; respiratory depression is dose-dependent	With optimum dose, none; may enhance contractions. Excessive dose may slow labor	Rapid	Possible depression; may contribute to narcosis by potentiating narcotics
Anesthetic agents Pudendal block	If poor, no pain relief, apprehension, and tachycardia	May eliminate urge to bear down	None	None, unless injected into maternal vessels; then results in fetal depression
Paracervical block	None	If given in latent phase, may arrest labor	Readily	Transient bradycardia
Epidural block	Hypotension, due to vasodilatation	Initial decrease in intensity of uterine contraction; urge to push interrupted	None	If maternal hypotension occurs, fetal distress results
Spinal block	Hypotension	Urge to push interrupted	None	If maternal hypotension occurs, fetal distress results

Source: J. J. Bonica. Principles and Practice of Obstetric Analgesia and Anesthesia, Vols. 1, 2. Philadelphia: Davis, 1972.

than equal doses of other narcotics. Another potentially serious side effect of all narcotics is orthostatic hypotension from peripheral vasodilation. This is particularly true if women who have been horizontal are allowed to ambulate or sit up or are moved too vigorously. Therefore the blood pressure of women receiving narcotics should be monitored [10].

The drugs also may produce nausea and vomiting, probably by direct stimulation of the trigger zone in the medulla. Narcotics also decrease gastric motility, intensifying this effect in the laboring woman and increasing the likelihood that any food already in her stomach will remain there throughout labor. Usually it is better to administer the narcotic in smaller doses more frequently than to give large doses less often. Occasionally a narcotic and an ataractic will be administered together in the hope that the effect of the narcotic will be potentiated so that smaller doses may be used.

Promethazine (Phenergan), hydroxyzine (Vistaril), and propiomazine (Largon) are three ataractics that are commonly used during labor in conjunction with a narcotic. Despite rapid placental transfer and decrease in beat-to-beat variability of the fetal heart rate, these drugs in recommended doses do not seem to cause neonatal depression.

The use of diazepam (Valium) in obstetrics is not without controversy. It rapidly crosses the placenta, with maternal and fetal blood levels reaching equal proportions very quickly. Beat-to-beat variability of the fetal heart rate is decreased even with small doses. At birth neonatal blood levels may actually exceed maternal levels. If the mother has received more than 300 milligrams during labor, the drug and its metabolite remain active in the neonate for at least a week, resulting in hypotonia, lethargy, decreased feeding, and hypothermia. Therefore, it is very important to maintain a warm environment for this infant. Sodium benzoate, a powerful bilirubin-albumin uncoupler, is used as a buffer in the injectable form of diazepam, thus subjecting the neonate to increased risk of hyperbilirubinemia and kernicterus [10].

REGIONAL ANESTHETICS

Regional anesthesia is used to anesthetize a specific area of the body. The anesthetic agent is deposited around a particular nerve or nerve pathway so that the transmission of nerve impulses to receptors in the central nervous system is blocked. The most common types of regional anesthesia used in obstetrics are subarachnoid blocks (spinal and saddle), pudendal block, and extradural blocks (caudal and lumbar epidural) (Table 13-2). Caudal and lumbar epidural blocks can be used during labor as well as delivery. Regional anesthesia has many advantages: In contrast to narcotics it produces complete relief of pain, and it causes no maternal or neonatal depression, provided that there are no complications. If the techniques used during labor are administered when the mother's labor is in the active phase, they will not impede the progress she is making. They may be continued for her delivery and may even be modified for a cesarean birth if necessary.

Regional anesthesia permits the mother to remain awake during labor and delivery so that she can actively participate in the birth of her infant. The use of regional anesthesia for delivery generally produces no respiratory depression or other effects harmful to the mother and newborn. Since uterine tone is main-

*Table 13-2. Regional
Anesthetic Agents*

Agent	Advantages	Disadvantages
Ester-Linked Agents (usually rapidly broken down in the bloodstream; end product crosses placenta but does not cause fetal depression)		
Chloroprocaine (Nesacaine)	One of safest agents for use in obstetrics. Speed of breakdown very fast; therefore, unlikely to reach fetus in appreciable amounts. Fast onset, good quality anesthesia. First stage labor = 1.5–2.0% concentration. Perineal analgesia and C-section = 3% concentration	Short duration of action. Often lasts only 35–50 minutes in plain solution and 50–65 minutes when epinephrine added. Repeated injections necessary if anesthesia prolonged
Tetracaine (Pontocaine)	Long duration of action. One of most effective and popular drugs for subarachnoid block in late first stage labor or second stage	Poor choice in epidural. By this route, produces profound motor block but less than average analgesia
Dibucaine (Nupercaine)	Very potent and long lasting. Used extensively for epidural block in first stage labor. Excellent for subarachnoid block	Not a successful agent for local infiltration
Amide-Linked Agents (most powerful and effective local anesthetics; broken down in the liver; long half-life)		
Mepivacaine (Carbocaine)	Effective agent. Slightly longer action than lidocaine	Of all amide-linked agents, most likely to show greatest degree of placental transfer. Long half-life in neonate (9 hours); use has declined in obstetric practice
Lidocaine (Xylocaine)	Excellent epidural analgesia. Duration of action 60 minutes without epinephrine and 75 minutes with epinephrine. Good for subarachnoid block in second stage labor. Carbonated solution is ideal agent for C-section under epidural block	Placental transfer appreciable. Half-life in neonate less than 3 hours. Losing popularity in obstetrics because of observed neurobehavioral changes in newborn
Bupivacaine (Marcaine)	Quality of analgesia high in relation to motor block. Duration long, especially when epinephrine added. Heavily protein bound, so less placental transfer. Therefore, most reliable amide local anesthetic agent (0.75% concentration) for epidural in labor and delivery	

Source: Adapted from P. Bromage. Choice of Local Anesthetics in Obstetrics. In S. Shnider and G. Levinson, *Anesthesia for Obstetrics.* Baltimore: Williams & Wilkins, 1979.

tained, blood loss is usually less than with inhalation anesthesia. Since regional anesthesia is a more complicated method than systemic drugs or inhalation agents, it requires greater skill to administer and the chance of failure (inadequate anesthesia) is greater. Complications can occur, notably maternal hypotension. Those techniques that produce perineal muscle paralysis (i.e., continuous epidural and caudal blocks) interfere with the mechanism of internal rotation and tend to increase the incidence of persistent posterior positions of the fetus [1].

Paracervical Block (Uterosacral Block).   In a paracervical block the anesthetic agent is placed along the base of the broad ligament and lateral walls of the lower uterine segment (Fig. 13-1) and is injected submucosally into the vaginal fornix lateral to the cervix. It blocks the afferent sympathetic pathways (hypogastric plexus) as they pass through the uterovaginal plexus in the parametrium, relieving the pain of the first stage of labor but not the perineal pain of the second and third stages. Thus, it is not an anesthetic for delivery; at that point it is usually used in conjunction with a pudendal block. Analgesia occurs in 3 to 5

Figure 13-1. Paracervical block (see text for details).

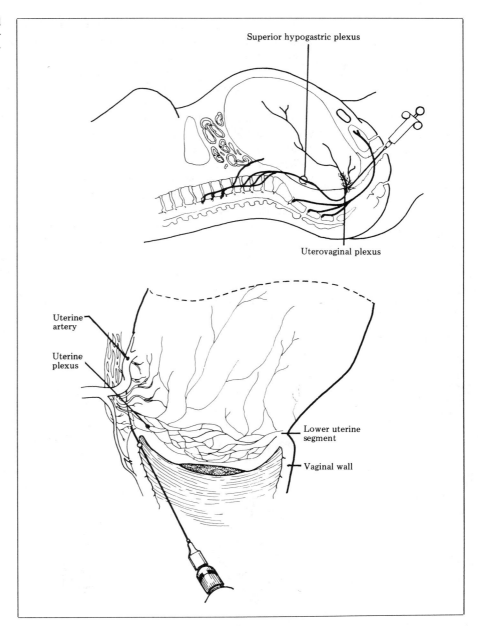

minutes and lasts 1 to 2 hours. The paracervical block may be repeated and seems to work best when given in the latter half of labor. It does not interrupt the mother's ability to push with her contractions.

The major disadvantage of this type of anesthesia is the relatively high frequency of fetal bradycardia following the block. The bradycardia has been associated with fetal acidosis and an increased chance of neonatal depression. The cause is uncertain but it is felt that it may result from decreased uterine blood flow from uterine vasoconstriction from the local anesthetic or from fetal absorption perhaps by diffusion across uterine arteries [10].

Since fetal bradycardia is indicative of fetal distress, paracervical block probably should not be used in cases of uteroplacental insufficiency or when there is pre-existing fetal distress. It is usually used with caution when the mother's cervix is 8 centimeters dilated or more, since there is the chance that the anesthetic may be injected accidentally into the fetal scalp [11]. Monitor maternal vital signs and fetal heart rate continuously for at least 10 minutes following the administration of a paracervical block.

Extradural Blocks (Caudal and Lumbar Epidural Blocks).   Many women who have had continuous caudal or lumbar epidural anesthesia during labor consider it the ultimate in pain relief. These techniques can be used on most mothers with normal uncomplicated labor. Since they can provide complete pain relief, they promote a feeling of calmness and well-being in the mother. Since she has to work less, her metabolism and oxygen consumption tend to decrease. Both caudal and epidural anesthesia may produce maternal hypotension, however, since they interrupt enough vasomotor segments to decrease peripheral resistance, venous return, and cardiac output.

Figure 13-2. Continuous caudal block (see text for details).

In a continuous caudal block, the anesthetic is injected through a small catheter into the sacral canal (peridural space) via the sacral hiatus (Fig. 13-2). In

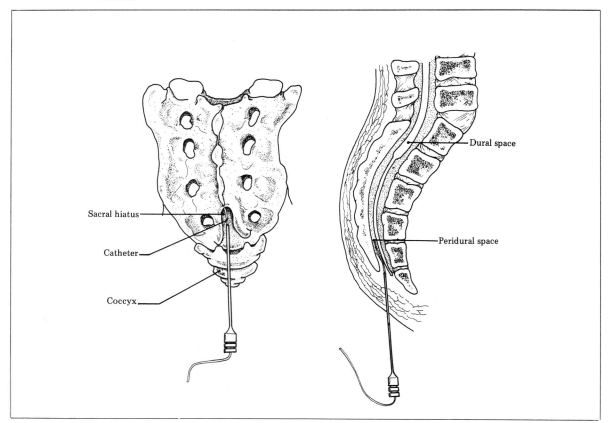

the sacral canal it anesthetizes a rich network of sacral nerves that emerge from the dural sac about 6 to 9 centimeters above. In an epidural block the anesthetic is injected in the lumbar or lower thoracic peridural space (usually L4–L5), also through a small catheter (Fig. 13-3). The standard epidural block provides pain relief from T10 to S5 within 3 to 5 minutes.

Compared with an epidural block, a caudal block requires more local anesthetic, the onset of pain relief is slower, and the chances of failure are greater. In addition, there is more risk of infection because the skin over the sacral hiatus is more difficult to keep clean than that over the lumbar region [1]. In both caudal and epidural blocks the catheter may remain in place throughout labor, and the anesthetic agent is reinjected as necessary to continually block pain impulses.

Women who have had continuous extradural blocks during labor may receive a reinjection just before delivery, usually with a greater concentration of the drug. The dose is commonly administered with the woman in a sitting position ("sitting dose"), so that the effect of gravity results in adequate perineal anesthesia. This usually takes about 15 minutes to achieve and can permit a calm, unhurried,

Figure 13-3. Epidural block (see text for details).

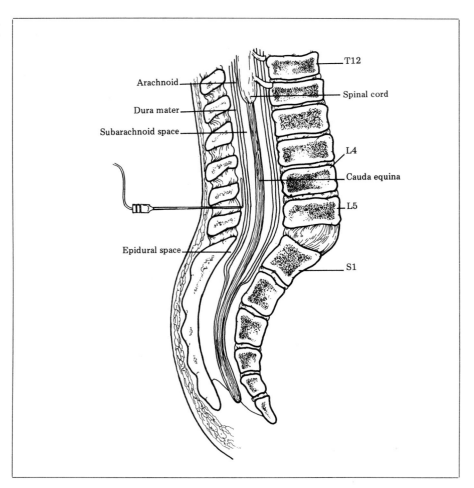

well-controlled delivery. The anesthesia may also be used for a cesarean birth.

If the block is successful, the mother's legs will become warm and may tingle. Even though hypotension occurs less frequently and to a lesser degree than with a subarachnoid block (spinal), the mother should have intravenous fluids running well before the procedure is started. Because it may take 15 or 20 minutes for hypotension to develop, monitor the mother's blood pressure and fetal heart rate very frequently (every 2 minutes) for 20 minutes after each injection. If her blood pressure is below 100 millimeters of mercury or decreased by 20 percent in a hypertensive woman, prompt treatment should be begun. In a normotensive woman, turning her to her left side (relieving pressure on the inferior vena cava) may be all that is necessary; however, it may be necessary to place her in the Trendelenburg position, increase the flow of intravenous fluids, and provide her with extra oxygen [1]. However, use of the Trendelenburg position without turning the woman on her left side may actually aggravate the hypotension by shifting the uterus farther back into the vena cava and aorta, thus restricting blood flow. The incidence and severity of the hypotension depends on the height of the block, maternal position, addition of epinephrine to the local anesthetic, physical status of the woman, and measures taken to avoid hypotension.

If the drug is inadvertently injected into a blood vessel the woman may experience tinnitus, light-headedness, circumoral numbness, tingling, and a metallic taste in her mouth. This may be followed by a convulsion. Should these symptoms occur, give the woman oxygen, keep her airway open, call for a physician, and monitor the fetal response.

Both caudal and epidural anesthesia, if begun too early in labor, may block Ferguson's reflex and decrease uterine contractions. For this reason they are not usually administered until the woman's labor is well established: cervical dilation of 6 to 8 centimeters in the nullipara or 4 to 6 centimeters in the multipara, with strong contractions lasting 1 minute and occurring every 3 minutes. They may also relax the perineal muscular sling enough to decrease the forces of internal rotation and may eliminate the mother's urge to bear down during contractions in the second stage, in which case you will need to coach her to do this in order to avoid a low forceps delivery. The mother may also experience bladder distension because of increased intravenous fluids and decreased sensation. Both caudal and epidural blocks, when properly used and when complications have not occurred, have no direct effect on the fetus and cause no residual depression of the newborn.

Subarachnoid Block (Spinal and Saddle). Subarachnoid block is thought to be the most widely used regional technique to produce terminal anesthesia for vaginal delivery. Its advantages include simplicity of induction and minimal side effects; the major disadvantages are maternal hypotension and postanesthetic headache. Usually this type of anesthesia is given to a multigravida at the beginning of the second stage of labor or when she is 8 centimeters dilated if her labor is progressing rapidly. The effects of the anesthesia usually last for about an hour [1]. Occasionally the anesthesia interferes with the woman's ability to bear down.

In a low spinal block (saddle block) the agent is usually introduced into the cerebrospinal fluid in the subarachnoid space between L4 and L5. (Spinal blocks are usually introduced at the level of L3–L4—Fig. 13-4.) Generally a hyperbaric solution (specific gravity greater than spinal fluid) is injected into the woman's subarachnoid space while she remains in a sitting position, which enables the solution to gravitate to the lower part of the dural sac. She usually remains sitting for 1 to 3 minutes, depending on the amount of solution used, and then is placed flat on her back with two pillows under her head. Any change in intra-abdominal pressure during bearing down or any active effort to change position may cause a disturbance in cerebrospinal fluid pressure, enhancing the spread of the anesthetic solution. Instruct the woman to remain as quiet as possible during the procedure as you support her in the correct position (Fig. 13-5). Some physicians will advise the woman not to elevate her head for 6 to 8 hours (or as ordered) after delivery to avoid a postspinal headache. It is believed these headaches are due to spinal fluid leakage through the puncture site in the dura, causing a decrease in spinal fluid pressure and subsequent traction on pain-sensitive structures within the cranial cavity. (To prevent this, smaller gauge needles are now used in administering anesthesia.)

Pudendal Block.   A pudendal block provides relaxation and analgesia to the

Figure 13-4. Spinal block (see text for details).

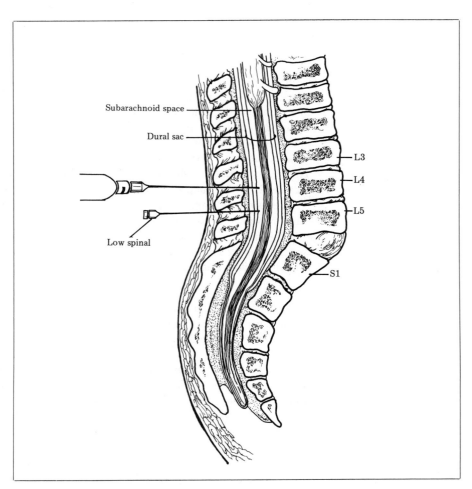

Figure 13-5. Sitting position for spinal anesthesia.

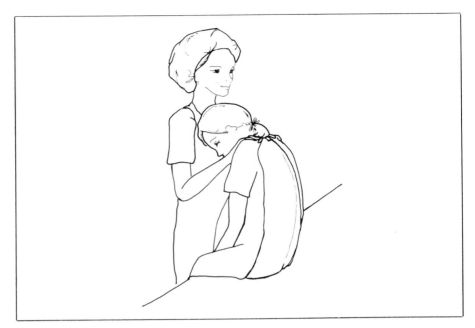

woman's perineum without disturbing uterine contractions or having harmful effects on the baby. However, it may eliminate the mother's urge to bear down. Since pudendal blocks are more difficult and time-consuming to give, they are followed by a higher incidence of failure (inadequate anesthesia) than subarachnoid blocks, and they provide no relief from the discomfort of contractions [1].

Each pudendal nerve is blocked in its position near the ischial spine (Fig. 13-6). The transvaginal route provides less risk of infection and less discomfort than the transperineal approach. Transvaginal pudendal blocks must be done before the fetal presenting part completely fills the vagina; otherwise the transperineal route becomes necessary.

If the block is improperly done, the inadequate pain relief may increase the woman's apprehension, anxiety, and fear. Possible maternal complications are hematoma formation and rectal puncture.

INHALATION ANESTHESIA

If continuous regional anesthesia during labor is contraindicated for some reason, the mother during labor may administer inhalation anesthetic agents to herself as necessary. The most common agent used in this manner is trichloroethylene (Trilene).

The agent is given by mask (Fig. 13-7), and the woman is instructed in its proper use when she is in early labor. At the beginning of a contraction she applies it to her face, allowing no gaps for air to enter and dilute the anesthetic. She breathes deeply until the pain disappears, and then the mask is removed. A mechanism on the inhaler makes it possible to regulate the anesthetic concentration to produce analgesia without loss of consciousness. If trichloroethylene has been used during the first stage of labor, the mother is usually given a pudendal block to eliminate the perineal pain of the second stage. Trichloroethylene may

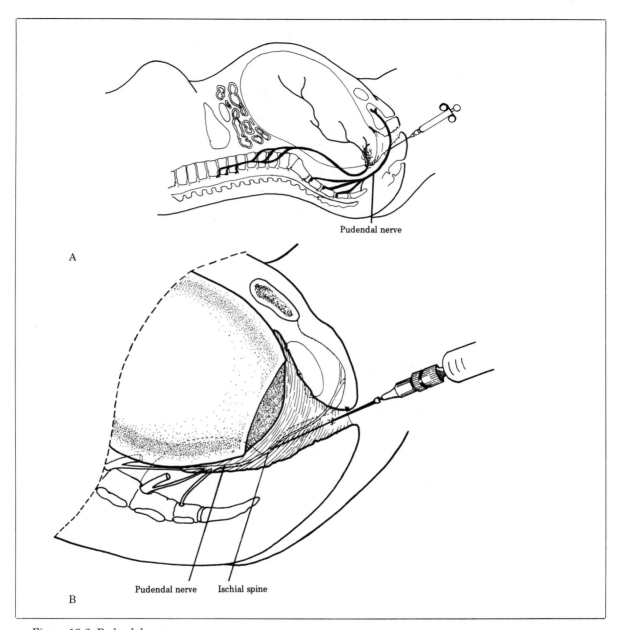

Pudendal nerve

A

Pudendal nerve   Ischial spine

B

Figure 13-6. Pudendal anesthesia administered by the transperineal route (A) or by the transvaginal route (B) (see text for details).

then be continued throughout the delivery. The major risk is inadvertent anesthetic overdose with loss of protective mechanisms so that, if vomiting should occur, respiratory obstruction and asphyxia may result [4].

LOCAL ANESTHETICS
Absorption of the anesthetic, once it is injected into tissues, depends on the vascularity of the part and the solubility and concentration of the drug. Local anesthetics cause local vasomotor paralysis, thus increasing local blood flow and

Figure 13-7. Use of the
trichloroethylene mask
(see text for details).

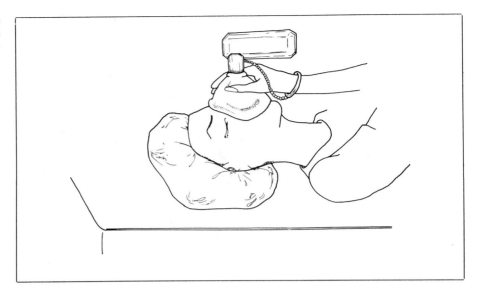

enhancing absorption. As a result, they are often administered with a vasoconstrictor (epinephrine), which prolongs the duration of action, increases the potency, and permits the use of smaller concentrations of the drug [1].

Local infiltration of the perineum for episiotomy repair has been used for many years. It is simple, effective, and practically free of maternal or fetal complications. It has no systemic effect on either the mother or the infant.

GENERAL INHALATION ANESTHESIA
Inhalation anesthesia used in approximately one-third of all vaginal deliveries in the United States has the advantages of providing greater control of the depth and duration of the anesthesia, a rapid smooth induction, and a quick recovery [4]. Certain obstetric problems, such as tetanic uterine contraction and impending uterine rupture, and procedures such as internal version can only be handled with transient deep inhalation anesthesia. A serious disadvantage is the danger of aspiration of stomach contents, which is one of the major reasons that the complications of obstetric anesthesia rank fourth or fifth among the causes of maternal mortality. Consequently, inhalation anesthesia is contraindicated in women who have recently eaten, women who have acute respiratory infections or other respiratory diseases, and women with severe diabetes, kidney or liver disease, or severe hypertension. It is also contraindicated when the infant is thought to be preterm. Another disadvantage of inhalation anesthesia is that it usually results in neonatal depression if given for longer than 5 minutes [1].

Nitrous oxide is a popular inhalation agent used for normal vaginal deliveries. Usually 40% nitrous oxide with 60% oxygen is satisfactory until the actual delivery of the baby, when 70% nitrous oxide with 30% oxygen produces adequate analgesia. Whatever the concentration, there must always be at least 20% oxygen in the combination. The main drawback of nitrous oxide is its lack of potency as a true anesthetic agent in concentrations that allow adequate fetal oxygenation.

Cyclopropane has a pleasant, rapid induction and recovery and can be used with high concentrations of oxygen. A major disadvantage is its flammability and explosiveness; in addition, it can produce occasional cardiac arrhythmias and has a tendency to cause fetal and maternal respiratory depression if deep anesthesia is required.

Ether is still considered useful by a limited number of practitioners, since it is inexpensive and easy to administer and has a wide margin of safety. However, it contributes to a high incidence of nausea and vomiting, and it also irritates the respiratory tract [1]. *Halothane,* a potent relaxant, is used when deep uterine relaxation is required, as in tetanic contractions, retained placenta, and breech delivery.

The presence of a significant volume of gastric juice or a very low gastric pH cannot be excluded in any laboring woman. Routine administration of oral antacids before induction of general anesthesia has therefore been recommended and is routine in many units. It is postulated that the overall safety of inhalation analgesia and anesthesia would be increased if all recipients were to receive 15 to 30 milliliters of antacid every 3 hours throughout labor [4].

Placental transfer of all inhalation anesthetics occurs rapidly. Anesthetic levels rise rapidly in the fetal brain, and in general the degree of fetal and neonatal depression that can be expected is directly related to the depth and duration of maternal anesthesia.

General anesthetics depress uterine contractility and myometrial tone. This may result in an increased blood loss following delivery.

EFFECTS OF PAIN RELIEF METHODS ON THE NEWBORN
Drugs administered to the mother in labor and delivery may result in subtle and prolonged effects in the newborn, even if his Apgar scores are normal at birth [2, 3]. Such effects have taken the form of poorer sucking responses for as long as 4 days after birth in infants of mothers medicated just before delivery [9]; a lag of 2 days in the establishment of breast-feeding in infants of mothers who were heavily medicated in labor [2]; and depressed visual attentiveness for as long as 4 days after the administration of narcotics or barbiturates to the mother within 1½ hours of delivery [12].

Neurobehavioral assessment techniques used by most researchers have been criticized as being subjective and therefore less meaningful than "biochemical" data. These techniques are only one method of evaluating the newborn and should be used along with the history, Apgar score, and biochemical parameters in a continuing evaluation. Until more knowledge is acquired regarding the long-term effects of maternal medication on the newborn, it is wise to make mothers aware of techniques and medications that have the fewest observable effects [3].

ABDOMINAL DECOMPRESSION
In the middle 1950s abdominal decompression as a form of analgesia during labor was initiated by Heyns [7]; it entails the application of negative pressure around the abdomen of the mother in labor. A device is used to draw her abdominal wall anteriorly during a contraction in order to remove the resistance of the anterior and posterior abdominal wall muscles and allow free movement of her uterus. Theoretically this will shorten labor. The negative pressure is in the range of 35 to 77 milliliters of mercury, the higher levels being necessary for analgesia as the strength of contractions increases. After proper instruction, the mother is able to

operate the apparatus herself with each contraction.

Sufficient analgesia is reported to occur in a high percentage of women, with favorable effects on labor and the newborn. However, claims of shortened labor, improved fetal oxygenation, and prevention of fetal hypoxia have not been verified by objective studies. The method has not gained widespread favor [1].

ACUPUNCTURE

Acupuncture has been practiced in China for more than 1000 years. Recently it has been the object of some interest as an alternative to conventional anesthesia for labor and delivery. Unfortunately, no traditional acupuncture points have been developed for vaginal delivery since Chinese women have delivered without anesthesia for many years. To date efforts to use acupuncture in obstetrics have been neither very extensive nor very successful [5].

HYPNOSIS

Hypnosis, one of the oldest medical arts, was first used to produce obstetric pain relief in the 1830s. Isolated reports of its use in obstetrics were published between 1900 and 1940, and since that time interest in its use has grown. It has been accepted by both the American and British Medical Associations as an ethical part of medical practice.

Depending on the skill of the practitioner, about 40 to 50 percent of the women who are prepared antepartally can be successfully hypnotized. While maintaining the active experience of childbirth, these women show reduced levels of fear and apprehension. They are able to relax their perineal muscles effectively, resulting in less trauma to the birth canal, perineum, and fetal presenting part. It is reported that hypnosis shortens the first stage of labor by about 3 hours in primigravidas and by more than 2 hours in multigravidas [6]. Hypnosis precludes the risk of asphyxia in the newborn from chemical analgesics or anesthetics, although the use of posthypnotic suggestion may cause maternal respiratory depression.

Vadurro and Butts [13] report that childbirth under hypnosis can be a very gratifying emotional experience for a couple. In order for it to be successful, the woman must be willing to be hypnotized, and she must have the ability to concentrate, have average intelligence, be unafraid about hypnosis, and have absolute confidence in the practitioner. Hypnotic rapport can be transferred (during the first stage of labor) to other personnel who can, without previous training, induce and maintain the hypnotic state using a prearranged cue. However, it is necessary for the practitioner who has conditioned the woman to be present during the second stage of labor, and particularly during the actual delivery [1].

Many women who have been conditioned for childbirth are unable to remain relaxed in the distracting conditions of a hospital. It is helpful if they are placed in a quiet room and are spoken to as softly and as little as possible, avoiding any word that is suggestive of discomfort. Elements of surprise should be controlled as much as possible. If medication is necessary at any time, the amount given should be no more than enough to maintain the mother's relaxation.

According to Johnson, mothers and their partners who have successfully used this type of analgesia/anesthesia have reported that they saw themselves as active participants in the labor and delivery process. They also have reported the development of feelings of increased closeness as a couple who had control over what was happening to them [8].

REFERENCES

1. Bonica, J. J. *Principles and Practice of Obstetric Analgesia and Anesthesia*, Vols. 1, 2. Philadelphia: Davis, 1972.
2. Brazelton, T. Psychophysiologic reactions in the neonate. II: Effect of maternal medication on the neonate and his behavior. *Journal of Pediatrics* 58:513, 1961.
3. Cohen, S. Evaluation of the Neonate. In S. Shnider and G. Levinson, *Anesthesia for Obstetrics*. Baltimore: Williams & Wilkins, 1979.
4. Cohen, S. Inhalation Analgesia and Anesthesia for Vaginal Delivery. In S. Shnider and G. Levinson, *Anesthesia for Obstetrics*. Baltimore: Williams & Wilkins, 1979.
5. Devore, J. Psychological Anesthesia for Obstetrics. In S. Shnider and G. Levinson, *Anesthesia for Obstetrics*. Baltimore: Williams & Wilkins, 1979.
6. Flowers, C. E., Littlejohn, T. W., and Wells, H. B. Pharmacologic and hypnoid analgesia. *Obstetrics and Gynecology* 16:210, 1960.
7. Heyns, O. S. Abdominal decompression of labour. *Journal of Obstetrics and Gynecology of the British Commonwealth* 66:220, 1959.
8. Johnson, J. Teaching self hypnosis in pregnancy, labor and delivery. *American Journal of Maternal-Child Nursing* 5:98, 1980.
9. Kron, R., Stein, M., and Goddard, K. Newborn sucking behavior affected by obstetric sedation. *Pediatrics* 37:1012, 1966.
10. Levinson, S., and Shnider, S. Systemic Medication for Labor and Delivery. In S. Shnider and G. Levinson, *Anesthesia for Obstetrics*. Baltimore: Williams & Wilkins, 1979.
11. Shnider, S., Levinson, G., and Ralston, D. Regional Anesthesia for Labor and Delivery. In S. Shnider and G. Levinson, *Anesthesia for Obstetrics*. Baltimore: Williams & Wilkins, 1979.
12. Stechler, G. Newborn attention as affected by medication during labor. *Science* 144:315, 1964.
13. Vadurro, J., and Butts, P. Reducing the anxiety and pain of childbirth through hypnosis. *American Journal of Nursing* 82:620, 1982.

FURTHER READING

Anderson, J. A clarification of the Lamaze method. *Journal of Obstetric, Gynecologic and Neonatal Nursing* 6(2):53, 1977.

Blackwell, J. Labor pains. *Nursing Mirror* 11:28, 1978.

Cogan, R. Practice time in prepared childbirth. *Journal of Obstetric, Gynecologic and Neonatal Nursing* 7(1):33, 1978.

Ericson, A. *Medications Used During Labor and Birth*. Rochester, N.Y.: International Childbirth Association, 1977.

Grad, R., and Woodside, J. Obstetrical analgesics and anesthesia: Methods of relief for the patient in labor. *American Journal of Nursing* 77:242, 1977.

Gutsche, B. Maternal analgesia and anesthesia for vaginal delivery. *Journal of the American Society of Anesthesiologists* 24:68, 1978.

Hodgkinson, R., Bhatt, M., Kim, S., et al. Neonatal neurobehavioral tests following cesarean section under general and spinal anaesthesia. *American Journal of Obstetrics and Gynecology* 132:670, 1978.

Larkins, F. The influence of one patient's culture on pain response. *Nursing Clinics of North America* 12:663, 1977.

Mallov, S. Drug interactions. *Clinical Obstetrics and Gynecology* 20:483, 1977.

McDonald, J. Proanesthetic and intrapartal medications. *Clinical Obstetrics and Gynecology* 20:447, 1977.

Nicolls, E., Corke, B., and Ostheimer, G. Epidural anesthesia for the woman in labor. *American Journal of Nursing* 81:1826, 1981.

Ryan, D. Pain of labour. *Nursing Mirror* 40:33, 1978.

Shnider, S. Choice of anesthesia for labor and delivery. *Obstetrics and Gynecology* 58:25 (Suppl.), 1981.

Smith, D. Group process and childbirth education. *Journal of Obstetric, Gynecologic and Neonatal Nursing* 7(4):51, 1978.

Stevens, R. Psychological strategies for management of pain in prepared childbirth. II: a study of psychoanalgesia in prepared childbirth. *Birth and the Family Journal* 4:4, 1977.

Vaterlaus, E. A holistic approach to nursing the patient in pain. *The Canadian Nurse* 23:22, 1979.

PART 4 POSTDELIVERY PERIOD

Chapter 14 Normal Puerperium

The period following birth (puerperium) is generally an exciting and exhilarating time for the couple. However, it is also a time when much work begins for them and it is a time in which they need considerable support. Following the exhausting effort of labor and delivery, the mother faces the task of making many readjustments, physiologic as well as psychologic. During labor she has concentrated her energy on coping with that experience; during the postpartum period, she begins to regain her prepregnancy physical state. The couple are faced with the work of realizing that the baby has actually been born. They must begin the tasks of parenting and assume new roles. In providing care for the woman and the family during this period, you need to assess the physical and behavioral changes occurring in the woman and the needs identified by the new mother and father prior to developing a plan and interventions for their care.

ASSESSMENT OF PHYSICAL CHANGES AND NURSING INTERVENTIONS

Major physical changes occur during the puerperium. In fact, the puerperium is defined as the period beginning immediately after delivery and ending when the woman's body has returned as nearly as possible to its prepregnant state. This readjustment period takes approximately 6 weeks. Assessment of the physical changes occurring during this time is a major nursing function.

Vital Signs

The mother's temperature, pulse rate, and blood pressure are taken frequently in the postpartum period. In normal postpartum mothers, the temperature should not rise about 37.2°C (99.0°F). The transient rise often seen after labor usually falls to normal in 12 hours. While the criteria for febrile temperature elevations vary, those established by the U.S. Joint Committee on Maternal Welfare are generally accepted; they define morbidity as a temperature of 38.0°C (100.4°F) or higher in any two consecutive 24-hour periods during the first 10 days post partum, excluding the first 24 hours.

Temperature elevations due to dehydration occur early after labor, generally within the first 24 hours after delivery. The mother is usually not aware of her elevated temperature, even though she may have warm dry skin, flushed face, and dry mucous membranes. You can easily check the mucous membrane between her gum and her cheek. While the mother's mouth may appear very dry, perhaps due to mouth-breathing, the area between her gum and her cheek will remain moist unless she is dehydrated. With increased fluid intake, her temperature usually returns to normal.

Temperature elevations after the first day post partum are usually due to endometritis or infections of the urinary tract. With both types of infection the mother may initially complain of chills and general discomfort.

Temperature elevations appearing about the third postpartum day were once attributed to milk production or "milk fever." Today it is believed that these elevations are probably due to genital infections, although extreme lymphatic and vascular engorgement may cause a temperature spike for a few hours. With even slight elevations, check the mother's temperature every 2 to 4 hours until it becomes normal for a minimum of two readings.

Bradycardia sometimes found in the postpartum mother may be in the range of

60 to 70, but heart rate may drop to 40 within 2 days after delivery (by the seventh to tenth day, heart rate has returned to normal). This lowered heart rate is considered a good sign, whereas an elevated rate may indicate pain, nervousness, blood loss, infection, or cardiac disease. Although the cause is controversial [6], low heart rate may result from a reduction in cardiac output without a reduction in stroke volume; therefore, the decrease in cardiac output is accomplished by a fall in heart rate.

It is important to take the mother's blood pressure, especially during the first 12 to 48 hours postpartum. Hypertensive disorders related to pregnancy may develop during this time (see Chap. 18).

Changes in the Breast   During pregnancy, large quantities of estrogens secreted by the placenta cause the ductal system of the breasts to grow and to branch. Simultaneously, the stromata of the breasts also increase in quantity, and large quantities of fat are laid down. Equally important to growth of the ductal system are at least four other hormones: growth hormone, prolactin, the adrenal glucocorticoids, and insulin. Each is known to play at least some role in protein metabolism, which presumably explains their use for development of the breasts. Once the ductal system has developed, progesterone acting synergistically with the hormones mentioned previously causes growth of the lobules, budding of alveoli, and development of secretory characteristics in the cells of the alveoli.

Though estrogen and progesterone are essential for the physical development of the breasts during pregnancy, both these hormones also have a specific effect on inhibiting the actual secretion of milk. The hormone prolactin promotes secretion of milk. This hormone, secreted by the woman's pituitary, increases its concentration in her blood steadily from the fifth week of pregnancy until birth of the baby, at which time it has risen to very high levels, usually about 10 times the normal nonpregnant level. In addition to the effects of estrogen, progesterone, and prolactin, the placenta secretes large quantities of human chorionic somatomammotropin, which also has mild lactogenic properties [8].

Lactation suppression during pregnancy is due to the overriding suppressive effects of progesterone and estrogen, which are secreted in tremendous quantities as long as the placenta is still in the uterus. Progesterone and estrogen completely subdue the lactogenic effects of both prolactin and human chorionic somatomammotropin. In the postpartum period, however, the sudden loss of both estrogen and progesterone secretion by the placenta now allows the lactogenic effect of the prolactin from the woman's pituitary gland to function. Within 2 or 3 days the breasts begin to secrete copious quantities of milk. Milk production requires an adequate secretion of other hormones including growth hormone, the adrenal glucocorticoids, and parathyroid hormone, all necessary to provide the amino acids, fatty acids, glucose, and calcium required for milk formation.

The base level of prolactin secretion returns to the nonpregnant level during the first few weeks following birth. However, each time the mother nurses, signals from the nipples to the hypothalamus induce an approximately tenfold surge in prolactin secretion lasting about 1 hour. This prolactin acts on the breasts to provide the milk for the next nursing period. If this prolactin surge is absent, if it is blocked as a result of hypothalamic or pituitary damage, or if nursing does not continue, the breasts lose their ability to produce milk within a few days [8, 9].

The hypothalamus plays an essential role in controlling prolactin secretion. While it stimulates the production of all the other anterior pituitary hormones, it inhibits prolactin production. Consequently, damage to the hypothalamus or blockage of the hypothalamic-hypophysial portal system increases prolactin secretion while it depresses secretion of the other anterior pituitary hormones. Under special conditions, however, such as when the baby nurses, a different type of signal from the hypothalamus can increase the secretion of prolactin.

It is believed that two different hormones formed in the hypothalamus are transported to the anterior pituitary through the hypothalamic-hypophysial portal system to control prolactin release by the anterior pituitary gland. These are called prolactin inhibitory hormone (PIH), which is the dominant hormone under most normal conditions, and prolactin-releasing hormone (PRH), which can intermittently increase prolactin secretion. PIH might be dopamine, which is known to be secreted in the hypothalamus and which also can decrease prolactin secretion as much as tenfold.

Breast Structure   It will be recalled that the breasts are made up of 15 to 24 lobes arranged radially and separated from each other by fat. Each lobe includes several lobules; in each lobule there are smaller alveoli containing many acini cells. These specialized cells form a single layer of epithelium, beneath which lies a layer of connective tissue rich in capillaries. The epithelial layer produces the various constituents of milk. The lobules have ducts that join to form a single larger lactiferous duct for each lobe. These large ducts widen to form milk reservoirs behind the nipple; they narrow and open separately on its surface (Fig. 14-1).

There is little change in the condition of the breasts during the first 2 days post partum. While they do not contain milk, they do produce approximately 150 to 300 milliliters of colostrum per day. *Colostrum*, which often has a laxative effect on the newborn, is a yellowish fluid containing more minerals and protein (especially globulin) but less sugar and fat than mature milk. The production of mature milk generally begins on the fourth day post partum; however, if a newborn nurses within the hour after delivery and frequently thereafter, milk is produced earlier. The breasts are producing mature milk only by the second week post partum.

The intensity and duration of lactation are believed to be dependent on the stimulus of nursing and on the regular withdrawal of milk as well as on the mother's state of mind, health, and nutrition. Through a complex neural mechanism, suckling by the infant not only promotes an adequate supply of milk, but also has a beneficial effect on uterine involution by stimulating oxytocin release from the posterior pituitary. For a discussion of breast-feeding as a method of newborn nutrition, see Chapter 16.

LACTATION SUPPRESSION
While breast-feeding has numerous recognized advantages, some mothers choose to bottle-feed their infants. If this is the case, their natural milk supply needs to be suppressed in some way. Suppression of lactation in non-nursing mothers has been approached through the use of pharmacologic and nonpharmacologic treat-

Figure 14-1. The lactating breast, with nursing infant.

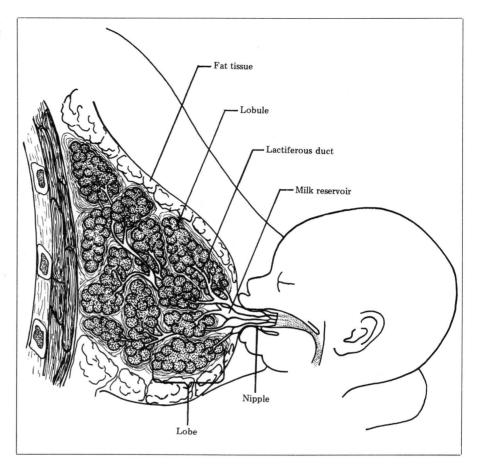

Fat tissue

Lobule

Lactiferous duct

Milk reservoir

Nipple

Lobe

ments. The major pharmacologic agents used to suppress lactation have included estrogen preparations alone or in combination with androgens and, most recently, prolactin inhibitors (Table 14-1). In India, folk medicine prescribes garlic for the newly lactating mother, since it contains plant estrogens and may prevent overfilling.

Estrogens used alone to suppress lactation have been reported to cause nausea, withdrawal bleeding, and rebound breast engorgement. Turnbull [29] reported a rebound lactation in 70 percent of the women he studied. More recently, Niebyl [18], in a prospective double blind study of 99 patients, obtained results that support previous evidence that estrogens delay rather than prevent breast engorgement. Additionally, researchers have focused on a well-established association between estrogens and thromboembolic disease. Studies indicate that the incidence of thromboembolism is significantly increased in the postpartum period, especially in women over 35 years of age and in those having an operative delivery [14, 18]. When estrogen is administered in the days following delivery, it has been reported to cause a significant decrease in antithrombin level III, thus enhancing physiologic changes that predispose to thrombi formation. In 1978, the federal Food and Drug Administration severely criticized the use of diethylstil-

Table 14-1.
Lactation
Suppressants

Preparations	Administered	Side Effects
Synthetic estrogens Chlorotrianisene (TACE)	By mouth. First dose should be given within 8 hours after delivery. Dose: 12 mg qid for 7 days or 50 mg every 6 hours for 6 doses	Nausea, heavier lochial discharge, greater proportion of bright red blood

Estrogen-androgen combination
    Testosterone enanthate and
    estradiol valerate
    (Deladumone OB)
	Intramuscular injection. Administered during the second stage of labor or immediately after delivery. Dose: One 2-cc dose containing testosterone enanthate 360 mg and estradiol valerate 16 mg	Virilizing effects: Hoarse voice, acne

Prolactin inhibitor
    Bromocriptine mesylate
    (Parlodel)
	By mouth. Dose: Usual dose 2.5 mg bid with meals for 14 days beginning the first day following delivery. Dose range: One 2.5 mg tablet daily to three 2.5 mg tablets daily with meals	Nausea, headache, dizziness

bestrol in the treatment of breast engorgement because of its association with uterine, cervical, and breast cancer. The FDA mandated that all women receiving the drug be given information regarding its use, side effects, and risks.

Estrogen-androgen preparations carry all of the previously mentioned side effects plus those associated with androgen therapy. Undesirable side effects of these preparations include rebound lactation, breast engorgement, local pain at the injection site, and manifestations of virilization [30].

Most recently, prolactin inhibitors have been used for suppressing lactation. One of the most commonly used, bromocriptine, inhibits prolactin secretion at the hypothalamic level and also acts directly at the dopamine receptors on the anterior pituitary cells [4, 5, 10, 28]. Pyridoxine (vitamin B_6) promotes the natural conversion of dopa to dopamine, thereby acting to suppress prolactin secretion [15]. Thus far, few undesirable effects of these drugs have been reported other than rebound engorgement in up to 70 percent of the women treated, depending upon the dose of the drug used in the studies.

There has been limited research comparing the effectiveness of nonpharmacologic measures in suppressing lactation. Decreased breast stimulation, binding of the breasts, limiting fluid intake, ice compresses, and analgesics are the most commonly practiced nonpharmacologic measures used to relieve the symptoms of breast engorgement. In one major study, Bristol [2] compared the effectiveness of a compression binder and a supportive brassiere; she found that there was significantly less breast tenderness among those women wearing the supporting brassiere. However, to date, there is little research comparing the effectiveness of these various nonpharmacologic measures against each other.

If the mother is untreated and no effort is made to withdraw the milk after it "comes in," the pressure produced by milk remaining in the ducts and alveoli, as well as the pressure produced by the engorged blood vessels and lymphatics, results in the cessation of secretory activity. The engorgement subsides, usually within 24 hours, and lactation ceases. Nursing mothers may also experience engorgement when the milk initially comes in; engorgement may occur later if the breasts are not adequately emptied when the baby nurses.

DISCOMFORTS DUE TO BREAST CHANGES

Engorged breasts are typically hard, full, tender, shiny, and perhaps reddened. The mother may be made more comfortable with a well-fitting supportive brassiere or binder, applications of warm or cold compresses, or mild analgesics. In addition, the nursing mother may relieve some of the tension within her breasts by manually expressing her milk (Fig. 14-2) by placing her fingers on the periphery of her breast and gradually massaging centrally toward the nipple. With this action the milk is worked down into the reservoirs from which it is expressed by massaging the areola. The mother places her thumb and forefinger at the areolar margin, pressing back in toward her chest and bringing her fingers together rhythmically, approximating the action of a baby's jaws. A lotion or ointment on the peripheral portion of her breast will lubricate the skin and reduce friction. The manual expression of milk is more effective if warmth has been applied; for this reason, many mothers express their milk during or after their shower. This procedure may be done several times each day if necessary.

Figure 14-2. Manual expression of milk.
1. The mother massages her breast, starting from the periphery and working toward the nipple.
2. She then places her thumb and forefinger at the alveolar margin and presses in toward her chest.
3. She then brings her fingers together rhythmically.

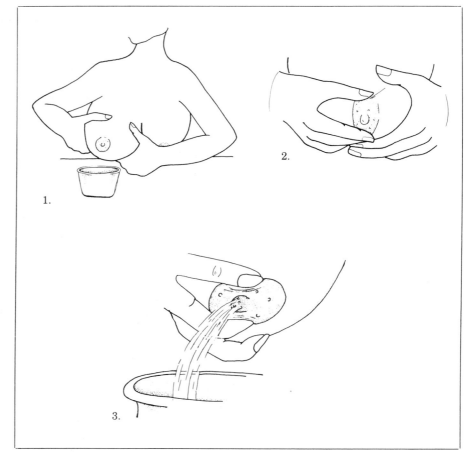

Engorgement is usually resolved in 1 to 2 days. Many authorities discourage the use of a breast pump in the treatment of engorgement, since they feel that its forceful pull traumatizes the tissues. Manual expression of milk is not used to relieve engorgement in the non-nursing mother since the breast stimulation would only help to maintain rather than suppress lactation.

Nipples usually require little extra attention in the postpartum period other than cleanliness and attention to fissures. Since dried milk may accumulate and irritate the nipples, the area should be cleaned with warm water and a soft cloth. Soap should not be used since it removes sebum, which keeps the nipple soft and protected against infection.

Cracked nipples may be caused by a number of factors including an incorrect grasp by the baby. The nipples should be examined under a good light to see whether there is actual cracking or the subepithelial petechiae that are precursors to cracking. Healing measures include exposure to air and light for 20 minutes following nursing. Feeding may have to be discontinued from the involved breast for 24 to 48 hours, then begun again for periods as short as 3 to 5 minutes. A healing ointment such as A and D Ointment may be used. Nipple shields may be used, although these may cause the mother's nipples to be drawn out considerably, which may delay healing or cause additional trauma.

Some nursing mothers have trouble with leaking milk. This problem diminishes as nursing is established and the internal reservoirs have stretched enough to hold the milk [17, 20, 21].

Changes in the Cardiovascular System

In the immediate postpartum period, the woman's blood volume remains high, reflecting the increased blood volume of pregnancy. Within a week it returns to normal, as does the leukocytosis that has been accentuated during labor and immediately after delivery (the leukocytosis will be greater following long labors). During this same period, plasma fibrinogen and sedimentation rate remain elevated. After labor and delivery hemoglobin and hematocrit are also elevated as a result of hemoconcentration, but these values should return to normal levels within 3 to 4 days post partum, as the mother becomes more hydrated. If the hemoglobin and hematocrit are low, additional iron therapy, rest, and possibly transfusions may be necessary. Iron preparations are often routinely given in the postpartum period to compensate for blood loss during delivery and possible depletion of iron stores during pregnancy. In any case, counsel the mother to emphasize foods high in iron in her diet.

As blood volume decreases, women with superficial varicose veins may notice improvement. However, they should continue to wear elastic stockings and to avoid practices that hinder circulation, since the deeper, larger veins may show less improvement.

Changes in the Abdomen, Skin, and Gastrointestinal System

Involution of the woman's abdominal muscles and fascia may require 6 to 7 weeks. In some women the abdominal musculature never regains good tone; the abdominal wall remains flabby and the skin loose. This is most likely to occur when pregnancies follow each other in rapid succession or when the woman's abdomen has been excessively distended and the elastic fibers of the skin ruptured, as in multiple pregnancies or in women with hydramnios.

The woman's abdominal wall generally resumes its normal appearance after 6 weeks. There may be marked separation or *diastasis* of the rectus muscles; if this occurs, that portion of the abdominal wall is formed just by peritoneum, thinned-out fascia, subcutaneous fat, and skin. If the mother raises her head and looks toward her feet as she lies flat in bed, the diastasis becomes accentuated (Fig. 14-3). Take advantage of this opportunity to draw the mother's attention to the condition of her muscles and to interest her in exercises to improve their tone (Table 14-2). One such exercise, which she may begin on the first postpartum day as she lies in bed, involves taking a deep breath, raising only her abdomen, and slowly exhaling. As she exhales, instruct her to pull her abdominal muscles in toward her back, hold them contracted for 5 to 10 seconds, and then relax. She may do this about five times daily.

Although it was formerly thought that an abdominal binder improved muscle tone and hastened involution, it is now known that it has neither effect. A girdle, which may make some women feel more comfortable, is not helpful in this respect either, since the abdominal musculature, not having been exercised, remains as lax as ever when the girdle is removed.

During involution when the abdominal muscles lack tone, they are unable to respond to noxious stimulation by spasm, as is normally the case. Consequently, abdominal rigidity is absent post partum in women who develop a visceral disease such as peritonitis.

For the first few days post partum, mothers perspire profusely, especially at night. This normal reversal of the water retention of pregnancy may add to the increased thirst that is characteristic of the postpartum period. Diaphoresis gradually subsides and becomes normal by the end of a week. Since mothers' perspiration sometimes has a strong odor, daily showers are important, not only for good hygiene but also for personal comfort. Because perspiration is profuse at night, you might advise the mother to wear a hospital gown then and to save her fancy nightgowns for daytime wear.

Pigmentary changes that occur during pregnancy tend to regress during the postpartum period. However, some may never fade completely. Striae gravidarum fade to a silvery color.

Figure 14-3. Postpartum diastasis.

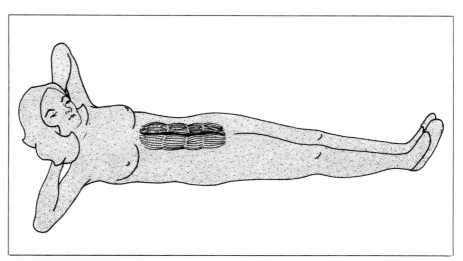

Exercises for the Immediate Postpartum Period (can be performed in bed)

Toe Stretch (tightens calf muscles)
While lying on your back keep your legs straight and point your toes away from you, followed by pulling them toward you and pointing them toward your chest. Repeat 10 times.

Ankle Circle (tightens ankle muscles)
Move your foot only and make a circle as large as possible with your toes. Repeat 10 times.

Pelvic Floor Exercise (tightens perineal muscles)
Contract your buttocks for a count of 5 and relax. Contract your buttocks and press thighs together for a count of 7 and relax. Contract buttocks, press thighs together, and draw in anus for a count of 10 and relax.

Exercises for Later Recovery Period (after first postpartum visit)

Bicycle (tightens thighs, stomach, waist)
Lie on your back on the floor, arms at sides, palms down. Begin rotating your legs as if you were riding a bicycle, bringing the knees all the way in toward the chest and stretching the legs out as long and straight as possible. Breathe deeply and evenly. Do the exercises at a moderate speed and do not tire yourself.

Abdominal Exercise (tightens stomach and thighs)
Raise your upper body to a half-sitting position with palms and elbows on floor. Bring your right knee toward your chest while lifting your left leg about 3–4 inches off the floor. Reverse, drawing the left knee toward the chest and raising the right leg off the floor. Complete 2 sets of 6, relaxing between sets.

Buttocks Exercise (tightens buttocks)
Lie on your stomach and keep your legs straight. Raise your left leg in the air, then repeat with your right leg (feel the contraction in your buttocks). Keep your hips on the floor. Repeat 10 times.

Twist (tightens waist)
Stand with legs wide apart. Hold your arms at your sides, shoulder level, palms down. Twist your body from side to front and back again. Feel the twist in your waist.

While some mothers may have a poor appetite for the first few days post partum, many more have voracious appetites and begin requesting food while they are still in the recovery room. This seems only natural considering the work of labor and delivery and the length of time without solid food. However, the time without solid food may lead to difficulty in having a spontaneous bowel movement.

Constipation may be a problem for other reasons also. The woman's overstretched abdominal and perineal muscles are less effective in aiding defecation, and intestinal peristalsis is still decreased. Other sources of difficulty in having a bowel movement include perineal pain from an episiotomy, fear of rupturing the sutures, hemorrhoidal pain, and the cleansing enema that the mother may have had before delivery. Even if intravenous fluids have been given during labor, there may still be an imbalance between the fluids taken in and those lost during this period, which may leave intestinal contents drier than normal.

Prior to offering suggestions to alleviate constipation, determine the mother's normal bowel habits and what she usually does to relieve constipation. She may be helped by increasing her fluid intake, some of it perhaps in the form of prune juice, or by including fresh fruits and roughage in her diet. In addition, mothers who are ambulatory appear to have fewer problems with constipation. The relaxation that follows perineal tightening exercises may be of use when the mother is about to have a bowel movement.

If all else fails, a mild cathartic such as milk of magnesia may be ordered for the evening of the second day following delivery. If there has been no bowel movement by the morning of the third day, a small enema or a suppository may be effective.

Changes in the Genital Tract   In the immediate postdelivery period, the woman's uterus becomes firm and globular, with its anterior and posterior walls in close apposition. Compared to its condition during pregnancy, it appears blanched because the contracted myometrium has markedly compressed the uterine blood vessels. During the following 6-week period of involution, the woman's uterus decreases in size, mainly because of the autolysis of cellular protein material, particularly actomyosin. As a result there is a tenfold decrease in the size of the hypertrophied myometrial cells, while the actual number of such cells decreases only slightly. The whole process leads to an increase in the nitrogen content of the woman's urine for several days. Just after delivery, the woman's uterus weighs about 1,000 grams (2.2 pounds); by the end of the sixth week the woman's uterus has returned to its normal 50 to 70 grams (1.8–2.5 ounces).

Measure the progress of uterine involution daily by determining the height of the fundus. Following delivery and for the first 2 days thereafter, you will find the fundus usually midline in the abdomen, about 12 centimeters (5 inches) above the symphysis pubis or around the level of the woman's umbilicus. After that, it descends about 1 centimeter (0.4 inch) or one fingerbreadth a day, until by the tenth day it has descended into the cavity of the true pelvis and can no longer be palpated above the symphysis pubis (Fig. 14-4).

The stretched uterine ligaments become shorter as they regain their tone. Until the ligaments, pelvic floor, and abdominal wall are restored to normal tonicity, the uterus is not supported well and may easily be displaced.

After delivery of the placenta and during the postpartum period, uterine contractions continue but occur less frequently than they did during labor. Their pattern becomes incoordinate, a phenomenon that may be due to a decrease in the amount of oxytocin being secreted after delivery or to a decrease in uterine sensitivity to oxytocin stimulation, or both. A primipara's uterus tends to remain tonically contracted, so that she generally has fewer complaints of painful uterine contractions after delivery than a multipara. In about 75 percent of multiparas, the uterus contracts and relaxes at intervals, causing "afterpains" that may on occasion be severe enough to require analgesics. The release of natural oxytocin that accompanies breast-feeding may magnify the intensity of afterpains, as will the administration of oxytocics when they are indicated. In addition, blood clots or retained placental fragments will cause the woman's uterus to contract more vigorously in an effort to expel them. Usually afterpains begin to decrease in intensity after 48 hours. Some mothers find that measures such as assuming a prone position, applying a hot-water bottle to the abdomen, voiding often and keeping the bladder empty, and drinking hot liquids help them to relax and provide some measure of relief.

Since a pregnant woman's uterus requires a more abundant blood supply than a nonpregnant woman's, a readjustment of its vasculature is necessary. Current

Figure 14-4. Involution of the uterus during the puerperium.

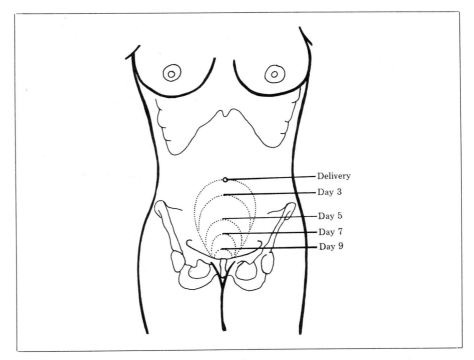

theory suggests that the larger vessels become completely obliterated by hyaline changes and that new and smaller vessels develop in their place. Following delivery, the blood vessels and sinuses of the placental site rapidly become thrombosed. This area, which was originally the size of the palm of the hand, becomes progressively smaller and is replaced by new endometrium. No scar remains when the healing is complete.

Postdelivery decidua consists of the inner portion of the spongy decidual layer in varying thicknesses; within 2 days after delivery it has separated into two layers. The layer next to the myometrium contains the remnants of the uterine glands and is the source of new endometrium. During the first 3 weeks post partum, the epithelium arising from proliferation of these glands covers the uterine cavity, with the exception of the placental site, which is usually covered by the sixth week. When this process is defective, late puerperal hemorrhage may occur. The other layer that lines the uterine cavity is infiltrated by leukocytes, becomes necrotic, and is cast off in the *lochia* (vaginal discharge) within 5 or 6 days after delivery.

The total amount of lochia after delivery is in the range of 150 to 400 milliliters. For the first 2 or 3 days, the red discharge (*lochia rubra*) contains bacteria, fatty epithelial cells, shreds of membrane, decidua, and blood. Later the amount of blood decreases, and the discharge becomes paler or sometimes brownish (*lochia serosa*). After the seventh to tenth day, the lochia becomes whitish or yellowish (*lochia alba*) because of the presence of leukocytes and serum. At about 3 weeks, the amount of lochia decreases; the flow finally stops when the placental site is healed completely. Lochia normally has the odor of fresh blood.

If the woman's lochia remains red after 2 weeks, involution may be delayed or placental fragments may have been retained. If lochia is excessive in amount, has an offensive odor, and contains solid particles, this may be a sign of bits of retained placenta and membranes. Infection should be considered if the woman's lochia is scanty in amount and has an offensive odor. If lochia is scanty but otherwise normal in characteristics, drainage may be poor, possibly because a small clot is obstructing the flow; such an obstruction is usually associated with an elevation in the woman's temperature, which subsides when the obstruction is removed and good drainage is established.

Inform mothers that ambulation usually increases drainage. Women may be needlessly alarmed by the different appearance of blood or an increased amount of blood in the lochia after thay have returned home unless they realize that it may be a sign that their activity level has been too great. With increased rest periods, lochia will usually return to a normal color and amount; however, all lochial changes should be reported.

Lochia may be more profuse in multiparas, and it may be greater when the mother is getting up for the first time. It is observed to be less profuse in nursing mothers, although there may be a temporary increase in the amount of blood in the lochia while the infant nurses.

Immediately after delivery the woman's cervix and her lower uterine segment are flabby collapsed structures. During involution new cervical muscle fibers form and the cervical osses contract, so that by the end of the first 10 days her cervix and lower uterine segment are so narrow that it is difficult to introduce one finger into her external os. A finger will not pass through the internal os at all. The woman's external os does not resume its prepregnant appearance, since lateral depressions from lacerations make it look more slitlike than circular.

After delivery the woman's vagina decreases in size. Mucosal swelling disappears, tone increases, and rugae begin to reappear by the third week. The vagina rarely returns to its nulliparous condition, however. What remains of the hymen are several tags of tissue, the *carunculae hymenales*. The woman's external genitalia lose their fatty cushion and appear more flabby.

The muscles and fascia of the woman's pelvic floor have been overstretched during pregnancy and may have been torn or incised for an episiotomy during delivery. By the sixth postpartum week, their muscular function has returned to normal, and there is little or no gaping of the introitus.

Observe the woman's perineum daily for signs of proper healing, or evidence of infection, swelling, or hemorrhoids. Take special care to prevent infection and irritation of external genitalia from vaginal discharge. Teach the mother to do this for herself, and explain the importance of doing the perineal care correctly. You may choose to do perineal care once a day for the mother in order to observe the condition of her perineum, while carefully noting her facial expressions, which may indicate particularly sore spots.

Perineal care may be done in a variety of ways. Cleansing solution may be poured over the woman's perineum without separating her labia, to prevent the fluid from entering her vagina. The woman's perineum is always cleaned from the vulva to the anal region, wiping with a downward stroke from front to back and using a clean tissue or clean side of the wipe for each stroke. Instruct the mother to do her perineal care with her morning shower and after each voiding and bowel movement. Instruct her to wash her hands well before and after doing this.

Instruct the mother to change her perineal pads (sanitary napkins) as often as necessary and after trips to the bathroom. Teach her to apply the pad with a sanitary belt, sanitary panties, or pins in such a manner that it remains close to her body—not moving back and forth with her activity, which would increase the likelihood of the transfer of organisms from her rectum to her vagina. The pad should not be applied so tightly as to cause discomfort.

Pads are applied and removed from front to back. They should be handled only on the side that will be away from the mother's body. The number of pads required in 24 hours varies according to the amount of lochial discharge; this number provides you with a means of estimating that quantity (if bleeding is heavy or excessive, a pad might be saturated every 30 to 60 minutes). If you suspect excessive bleeding, place the woman on a "pad count" for a certain period of time.

A mother who had an episiotomy or lacerations at the time of delivery will experience varying degrees of perineal discomfort; you may use a variety of measures to provide some relief. Immediately after delivery, the application of ice will decrease swelling and pain. After 24 hours, sitz baths in warm water or a heat lamp directed at her perineum provides improved circulation and relaxation. She may be helped by witch-hazel compresses, analgesic sprays, sitting on rubber rings or pillows, or the application of warm compresses or ice packs (ice in a rubber glove). Exercising perineal floor muscles not only improves circulation of blood in the area but also improves the muscle tone. Instruct the mother to contract her gluteal muscles for 5 seconds and relax; contract gluteal muscles and press thighs together for 7 seconds and relax; and contract gluteal muscles, press thighs together, and draw the anus as though trying to stop a bowel movement for 10 seconds and relax slowly. If the gluteal muscles are held contracted during the process of sitting and moving in bed, this will keep her buttocks together, so that the mother sits on them rather than placing pressure on the suture line.

Sometimes the woman's perineal body does not heal well. Scar formation may distort the base of her bladder and contribute to the development of stress urinary incontinence. Incontinence may also result from lack of good sphincter tone; the mother can improve and maintain this tone by periodically stopping urination midstream for a few seconds.

Changes in the
Urinary System

Soon after delivery there may be an increase in the woman's urinary output, possibly because of increased muscular contractions of the kidney pelves and ureters and release of pressure on her ureters from the presenting part. Increased urinary output may also occur if the mother received intravenous fluid during labor or if she was unable to void because of pressure from the presenting part. Diuresis appearing between days 2 and 5 represents loss of extracellular water accumulated during pregnancy due to hyperestrogenism and elevated venous pressure in the lower half of the body [19].

Voiding after delivery may be difficult for the woman. Her bladder walls, trigone, and urethra may be edematous and hyperemic, with areas of bleeding in the submucosal layers. The woman's bladder capacity post partum is increased, and her bladder may be less sensitive to fluid pressure as a result of trauma by the presenting part or due to the effect of anesthesia. Her vulva may also be edematous, which contributes to the problem.

Mothers should void within the first 8 hours after delivery and should be checked carefully during this time for evidence of bladder distention. A full bladder may appear as a rounded area above the symphysis and may displace the uterus to one side, preventing it from remaining firmly contracted.

When the mother has a full bladder, offer her the bedpan and allow her to concentrate on voiding in private. If she is unable to void, getting her out of bed to the bathroom may be all that is needed. Other helpful measures you might use include turning on the faucet and having her listen to the sound of running water, pouring warm water over her vulva, and having her take a warm sitz bath. Relaxation following perineal tightening may be conducive to starting the flow of urine. When the mother does void, the amount of urine should measure over 100 to 150 milliliters. Amounts less than this usually indicate incomplete emptying; the residual urine remaining in her bladder serves as a medium for the growth of organisms responsible for urinary tract infections.

If the mother is unable to void or if she voids in small amounts, you may need to catheterize her. If this is the case catheterize her after she voids small amounts to check the amount of residual urine remaining in her bladder. If there is more than 135 milliliters of residual urine, you may need to catheterize her after each voiding until the amount of residual urine is approximately 50 to 60 milliliters. As an alternative to frequent catheterizations, you may use an indwelling catheter for 24 hours, until the edema in her urethra, bladder base, and vulva has subsided. When you remove the indwelling catheter, take a culture from the catheter tip or bladder urine to check for possible contamination and infection. After you have removed the catheter, encourage the mother to drink fluids; she should void within the next 6 to 8 hours. When she does void, record the time, the amount that she voids, any other significant characteristics of the urine, and the presence or absence of pain with voiding.

Within 2 to 5 days after delivery, another period of diuresis may occur as the extra fluids retained during pregnancy are excreted. Mothers may void up to 3,000 milliliters per day, as compared to the 1,000 to 1,800 milliliters normally excreted. Their urine may contain lactose secreted from the breasts as they begin milk production. In tests of the urine for glucose, the lactose will yield false positive results. Protein may also appear in the urine, as cells break down during the process of involution. This is usually gone by the third day, but may last for weeks in trace amounts. Acetone may also appear in the urine after prolonged or difficult labor but usually disappears within the next 3 days. Within 2 to 3 weeks the dilatation of the kidneys and ureters is significantly decreased; however, complete return to normal size requires 6 to 8 weeks.

Table 14-3 summarizes some nursing assessments, interventions, and patient teaching topics during the puerperium. For a complete guide, see the Assessment Form at the end of the chapter.

ASSESSMENT OF BEHAVIORAL CHANGES AND NURSING INTERVENTIONS
Taking-in

Reva Rubin [22, 23, 24, 25, 26], one of the most widely quoted authors on the subject of maternal behavior in the postpartum period, has identified the specific phases through which the mother passes. The first, or *taking-in*, phase usually begins with a deep refreshing sleep following delivery. At first the mother may not perceive how exhausted she is because of initial feelings of exhilaration brought about by giving birth or because of emotional tension generated by her

Table 14-3. Assessment,
Interventions, and
Teaching During the
Puerperium

	Assessment	Possible Significance	Interventions/Teaching
Breasts			
Contour	Fullness, firmness, tenderness Tingling with or without pain Venous distention; warm skin; shiny skin; nodular	Milk may be coming in; possible engorgement; possible infection	Proper breast care; process of milk production; breast massage and expression; breast-feeding and diet history and counseling; breast self-examination
Areolae	Soft, compressible, taut; presence of Montgomery's follicles	Areolar engorgement	
Nipples	Prominent, erect, flat, inverted, clean, caked, reddened, sore, fissured, cracked	Grasp of baby may be incorrect	Nipple eversion Proper nursing techniques
Colostrum or milk	Expressed, clear, bluish-white, cream-colored, yellow		
Brassiere	Proper fit and adequate support	Proper alignment of blood and lymph vessels; may prevent engorgement from becoming exaggerated and minimize discomfort	Importance of adequate support
Uterus	Firmness; position with regard to umbilicus and abdominal midline; afterpains; tenderness	Firmness shows proper involution; subinvolution possibly a result of infection, retained placental fragments, atonia; incomplete bladder emptying; fibroids	Process of involution; uterine palpation; activity level after discharge and when to return to work
Bladder	Amount and frequency of voiding; distention; pain or burning on urination; flank tenderness	Normal postpartum diuresis; urinary retention; infection	Proper perineal care to prevent urinary tract infections; adequate fluid intake
Lochia	Amount and type; odor; presence of large clots	Normal involution; possible infection; retained placental fragments; obstructed flow	Changes in lochial appearance; when discharge should cease; proper application of perineal pad; resumption of menstrual periods; resumption of sexual relations; family planning
Perineum	Integrity of suture line; skin temperature and color; amount of discomfort; hemorrhoids	Normal healing; infection; inflammation; hematoma	Perineal care; sitz baths; suture removal; perineal tightening
Bowels	Constipation	Dehydration; inadequate roughage or fluid; discomfort; fear of rupturing episiotomy sutures	Diet history and counseling; assurance of strength of suture line
Abdominal wall	Diastasis	Poor muscle tone	Abdominal tightening; appropriate exercises
Homan's sign	Pain in calf upon flexion of foot with leg extended flat on bed	Possible thrombophlebitis	Inadvisability of leg massage and positions that impede circulation
Emotional status	Dependent, independent; elated, despondent; anorexic	Taking-in or taking-hold; postpartum "blues," possibly more severe depression; inadequate support systems; infant of wrong sex or not as fantasized	"Listening ear"; assurance that mood swings are normal and temporary; referral to proper resource agencies in the community

feelings of anticlimax and emptiness caused by separation from the baby. It has been reported that the mother may have sleep hunger for several days if this initial sleep is interrupted. This should be considered when you plan her nursing care in the immediate postpartum period.

Rubin describes the mother's behavior during this phase as passive and dependent. She accepts what she is given, tries to follow directions, and makes few decisions on her own. Almost all mothers wish to discuss what they recall of their labor and delivery. It is as if a reconstruction of their experience confirms the reality of the postdelivery period. You can be a very supportive listener, and your interaction may be even more meaningful to the mother if you have been with her during labor and delivery. Because of the importance of this reconstruction process, if you have cared for a mother during labor and delivery you should make a special effort to visit her post partum.

During the taking-in phase, sleep and food take on added physiologic as well as psychologic importance in the mother's life. She may often state that she is hungry and require extra snacks throughout the day to become satisfied. This is a good example of how food plays an important part in the asking for and giving of care. She may also express concern about the oral intake of her baby. It is important that you take time to listen to the mother and satisfy her needs and concerns as much as possible, which will help to reinforce her feeling that she and the baby are very important people.

The father, at this time, may find that he must assume the companionship and supportive roles for the family. At the same time he may also be experiencing conflicting feelings and may feel exhausted by the emotional strain of the baby's delivery. He may be concerned about the mother and about her passivity and dependency. If you help him to realize that this is to be expected, it will be easier for him to assume responsibilities for making decisions and for maintaining the routine of home and family, responsibilities that have been previously shared. Give him support by maintaining open lines of communication with him, and providing him with the information and assistance he needs to cope with the changing needs of his new family (Fig. 14-5).

Taking-hold   As the mother's inner resources become replenished during the first few days post partum, she begins to become impatient with her dependency. Rubin describes this as the *taking-hold* phase, during which the mother expresses concerns about the present, particularly regaining control over her own bodily functions. Her anxieties may be increased by doubts about her ability to care adequately for her new baby. Insignificant difficulties she has in handling him may become monumental reinforcements of the concerns she is beginning to feel. Special privileges that were hers alone during pregnancy must now be shared with the baby.

One mother [27] has written of her conflicting feelings during this time; her recollections of old childhood experiences and strange dreams, both pleasant and terrifying, exemplify postpartum introspection. The feelings that she recalls disappeared within a week, as she met success in caring for her baby and became reinvolved with her career.

During the taking-hold phase, the mother becomes more involved with her baby, which facilitates both the development of maternal concern and the tasks of

Figure 14-5. The proud new father also needs support in assuming a new role.

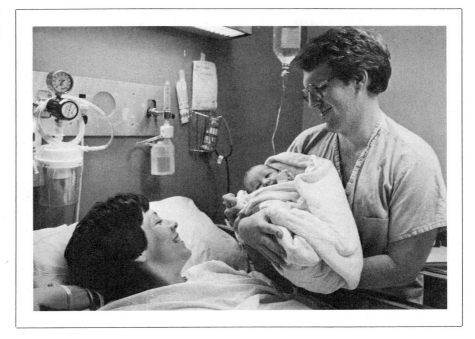

mothering. As she meets success in caring for her newborn, her concern extends to other family members at home and their activities during her absence.

With early discharge of new mothers, most of the period of transition to mothering occurs after the woman has gone home. From a teaching viewpoint, it is unfortunate that the stage of her maximal readiness for learning occurs when supportive nursing staff are not immediately available to her. Therefore, the time you spend with her in the hospital or birth center becomes even more valuable, since your accurate assessment of her needs paves the way for the health teaching, anticipatory guidance, and appropriate referral and follow-up necessary for her smooth transition to motherhood.

It is not uncommon for mothers at some time during the postpartum period to experience frequent temporary mood swings and to feel very vulnerable. Many factors may contribute to this disequilibrium, including the hormonal changes of childbearing, ego regression accompanying increased dependency needs, and discomfort, fatigue, and exhaustion following labor and delivery. In addition, the mother may be overwhelmed by her responsibilities when she goes home or by those responsibilities inherent in her new role. Therefore it is important that you build up the mother's confidence in herself. Such reassurance is rarely solicited by the mother but is gratefully accepted whenever it is offered, particularly in the case of primigravidas.

During this period, the mother may cry for no apparent reason, be irritable, or have a poor appetite or insomnia. These "postpartum blues" often appear about the third day after delivery. A mother may feel guilty about such unaccustomed behavior, especially when she can assign no reason to it; reassure her that it is normal and acceptable. Severe or prolonged depression is usually a sign of a more serious condition.

During the time of the mother's taking-hold, her anxieties may be increased if the father becomes, as Anderson and colleagues [1] note, "totally involved with the baby and does not evaluate and respond to the mother's feelings and reactions . . . Proud and elated over the prospect of parenthood, he may not be sufficiently in tune with the unspoken doubts and questions the mother may have." His behavior may be reinforced by her mood swings and, at times, unpredictable behavior. Your interactions with the parents should focus on encouraging the couple to share ideas and feelings to strengthen the family bonds. Encouragement and praise, along with constant reinforcement and careful teaching, are essential components of your nursing care of the new family.

ASSESSMENT OF NEEDS IDENTIFIED BY MOTHERS

The needs and priorities of new mothers as identified by health personnel are often not the same as the needs, priorities, and concerns identified by new parents themselves. In a study done to determine the postpartum concerns of mothers, Gruis [7] found that both primiparas and multiparas expressed many needs in the first month post partum and, in general, a lack of resources to meet those needs. The concern that predominated in both groups of mothers was coping with the change in their figures. This is not surprising since physical restoration is one of the major tasks of the postpartum period, along with meeting the infant's needs, establishing a relationship with him, and changing life-styles and relationships to accommodate a new family member.

Physical changes and discomforts can present major problems for women and their families. Immediately after delivery women are often pleased to think that they will now have a flat abdomen once again, only to be dismayed if they stand and see a protruding abdomen which may appear almost as large as it did during pregnancy. They may then find that their prepregnant clothes do not fit and that all the weight they hoped to lose with delivery has not been lost. This is only intensified if a woman's partner expresses disappointment that she is not as slim as he thought she would be, an understandable reaction in a culture that values slimness and attractiveness.

Post partum is also a time of physical discomfort, fatigue, and emotional stress. This may be caused in part by the continual demands of the infant. If the woman feels awkward in providing infant care, deficient in supplying breast milk, or unable to quiet her restless, crying infant, she can easily see herself as a failure in the mothering role. The attention required by the new infant may engender feelings of jealousy in the siblings or in the woman's partner. Difficulties in the marital relationship are not unusual during this period. The major concerns of multiparas in Moss's [16a] study centered around the changing relationships within the family and meeting the needs of family members. It is not surprising, then, that the demands of husband, housework, and children constituted the second major concern of postpartum women in Gruis's study. A majority of the 40 women studied mentioned fatigue, emotional tension, feelings of isolation and being tied down, and lack of time for personal needs and interests. Many of these concerns were reiterated by Bull [3a] in a more recent study. The women in Gruis's study did not express concern about the specific details of infant care, obviously a topic well covered during postpartum teaching.

The vast majority of women sought help for these problems from their partners, perhaps because of their easy accessibility. This may, of course, have placed an additional burden on the men who might have been unprepared to accept it. Unfortunately, none of the women in Gruis's study used the nurse as a resource person.

In an additional study by Henning et al. [11], many of the same needs were identified. Most frequently mentioned were more help in the home to allow time for recovery, more time for rest and sleep at home, and guidance in reestablishing family relationships.

In an earlier study by Lesser and Keane [13], the researchers outlined three main physical needs expressed by mothers: sleep and rest, relief of discomfort, and bodily care. Emotional needs identified by mothers in their study were more encompassing; these mothers wanted freedom from responsibility at home, freedom from anxiety, and a choice in whether or not they had to care for the baby initially. Lesser and Keane also reported that nurses generally recognized all the needs that the women themselves revealed; however, their emphasis was different from that of the mothers. Many nurses believed that mothers have very little need for physical care and that they are an independent, happy group. The nurses identified their chief function as teaching the mother care of herself and of her baby. They rarely mentioned the mother's need for a period of dependence and did not emphasize their possible role in meeting these dependency needs.

In keeping with the findings of these studies, the following areas in addition to needs identified by your clients are ones that must be considered in developing an effective care plan and interventions with the mother and family during the puerperium.

Rest, Assistance, and Ambulation

Prior to World War II, women rested longer and remained in bed for 7 to 10 days after delivery. However, during the war, it was often necessary to evacuate the hospital wards in England, and postpartum women were forced to ambulate early. This experience demonstrated the advantages of earlier ambulation. It improves lochial drainage, circulation (with fewer complications of embolism and thrombophlebitis), bowel and bladder functioning, and muscle tone. Mothers generally state that they feel better and stronger when they have been out of bed and walking about. It is now well accepted that mothers may ambulate in 8 to 12 hours or less after delivery. Early ambulation does not, however, negate the mother's need for increased sleep and rest and a period in which her dependency needs should be met.

When attempting to have the mother ambulate for the first time, have her sit on the side of the bed for 5 to 10 minutes before getting up. Place her feet flat on a chair rather than having them hang over the edge of the bed, in order to promote better circulation in her legs. Strongly encourage mothers to wait for assistance before getting out of bed for the first time, since they often become dizzy or faint. The mother may shower once she is ambulating, unless she has had a cesarean delivery or tubal ligation and the incisional area needs to be kept dry.

In anticipating the woman's need for rest and assistance at home, you need to help both the woman individually and the couple understand their need for rest and assistance once the woman and infant return home. The couple have been through an exciting yet emotionally and physically draining experience following the birth of their infant. As the mother and infant return home new adjustments become necessary to meet the demands of the infant. Most couples readily recognize the new demands placed on them but are reluctant to admit their need for additional rest and perhaps outside assistance. In many other cultures, a *doula* (a Greek word for female assistant) spends the immediate postpartum period and often the period of pregnancy and labor and delivery with the mother [3]. Her main purpose is to help the mother learn her mothering tasks. The additional support she provides the family affords them the rest and assistance they need during this transitional period. For many American families the woman's own mother or a member of the family or a friend often serves this function during the new mother's first weeks at home. Help the family with the planning necessary to meet the needs of their own situation (Table 14-4).

Share with the couple that the mother should resume her normal activities gradually once she is discharged. She should rest for at least 30 minutes when she gets home and several times during the day. If possible, she should avoid climbing stairs, especially for the first 3 or 4 days. If this is not realistic, advise her to limit her stair climbing as much as possible. Most importantly, encourage her not to overtire herself.

Coping with Physical Changes
Once allowed out of bed, mothers invariably want to be weighed. Unfortunately, they are often disappointed to find that they have not lost as much weight as they had hoped. They need to be reminded that approximately 5.4 kilograms (12 pounds) are lost after delivery of the baby and the placenta and from fluid and blood loss. Approximately 2.3 kilograms (5 pounds) will also be lost during the postpartum period due to fluid loss. By the end of the postpartum period, any weight above pregnancy weight represents fat or an increase in breast tissue in those mothers who are breast-feeding.

Help the woman understand the other changes that will occur in her physical condition after delivery. The woman has usually been able to anticipate many of the gradual changes occurring during pregnancy. However, changes in the postpartum period occur abruptly. Often the woman and her partner are not expecting her to experience hemorrhoids, a painful episiotomy, voiding and bowel problems, engorged breasts, a flabby abdomen, and less than her expected weight loss. They both need information about these changes, and the woman especially needs an opportunity to discuss her feelings and reactions to them and reassurance that this situation is usual and temporary.

New parents are always interested in knowing when the woman will resume ovulation and normal menstruation. In women who are not breast-feeding, menstruation generally occurs in 4 to 8 weeks. In nursing mothers, menstruation occurs between 2 and 18 months post partum, although it most commonly returns in 4 months. Many women experience a very heavy menstrual flow during their first period after delivery; they should be forewarned of this possibility. The first menstrual period may be anovulatory. Research [12, 19] on nursing mothers indicates that during lactation the ovaries fail to respond to gonadotropins.

For whatever cause, it appears that in the majority of women lactation results in a temporary infertility. This is especially true in those nursing mothers who also experience amenorrhea during lactation. However, infertility during lactation does not occur in all women, and pregnancy is possible during this period. Nursing mothers should be made aware of this so that they may use contraception if they choose. Oral contraceptive agents should be avoided if possible, since the

Table 14-4. Cultural Practices Following Childbirth

Ethnic Group	Cultural Practices
Arab	Much energy is given to fears of the "evil eye" and aspersions of jealous, envious women. Traditional Arab women may interpret expressions of congratulations from female health professionals as indications of envy; the nurse may be casting an evil eye on the newborn. Focus comments on the mother and her labor. If complimenting the baby, touch wood or mention God's blessings
American Indian	Practices differ among tribes
Seminole	The infant sleeps in a hammock suspended from the rafters
Crow	Name for the infant is chosen on the fourth day of life; infant sleeps on a cradle board provided by the father's aunt
Laguna Pueblo	Mother rests for 4 days after birth. Baby sleeps on a cradle board provided by an uncle. Sexual relations are taboo for 9 months after birth
Navajo	Mother drinks hot tea following delivery. The newborn is given an emetic (cedar sap in warm water and a pinch of corn pollen); infant sleeps on a cradle board constructed by the father or an uncle
Mexican	Mother stays in bed for at least 3 days. Before getting up, a wide girdle (*faja*) of coarse cotton cloth is applied. Women remain in the house for 15 days. Afterpains are treated with a teaspoon of olive oil and warm manzanilla tea. Postpartum diet is restricted. For the first 2 days toasted tortillas and boiled milk or *atole* (corn gruel) are served. No vegetables or fruits are allowed. Pork, chili, and tomatoes are avoided for 40 days because they are believed to harm breast milk. Currents of air are thought to be dangerous. *Pasmo* (sudden infection) is believed to result from careless chilling of the body. Chloasma (*pano*) is bleached by applying the infant's wet diapers to the mother's face
Filipino	Depending upon the province and sex of the baby, women may be confined to bed for 10 to 40 days after delivery. Efforts to encourage early ambulation may be interpreted as dislike of the woman. Sponge baths and oil massage are acceptable for cleansing the body after birth rather than showers or tub baths. Spices are restricted for the lactating mother but chicken soup is touted as a milk producer. Parents may spend months with in-laws following birth. In-laws care for the infant and teach the parents infant care
Vietnamese	Postpartum women eat only salty and dry foods. Hot foods are believed to counteract heat loss; cold foods are avoided. Fresh fruits and citrus juices are avoided. Sour or acid foods are believed to cause urinary incontinence. Beef and seafood are avoided for 6 months to avoid itching of the episiotomy site. Soups and water are restricted to avoid stretching the stomach and delaying return of the woman's prepregnancy figure. Early ambulation is avoided for fear that it will cause the organs to move too far down in the body. Intercourse is avoided for 2 to 3 months post delivery. Bathing and showering are avoided for the first month postpartum. Only the hands, face, and perineal area are cleansed. When the mother has been weakened by blood loss, water is believed to cause illness. The room in which the mother stays may be heated with a charcoal fire and kept warm for 1 month postpartum. Vietnamese women believe all babies look similar and fear being given the wrong baby. For this reason, the baby is expected to remain with the mother

Sources: A. Clark, *Culture Childbearing Health Professionals.* Philadelphia: Davis, 1978; A. Hollingsworth, L. Brown, and D. Brooten, The refugees and childbearing: What to expect. *RN* 43:44, 1980; A. Meleis and L. Sorrell, Arab American women and their birth experiences. *American Journal of Maternal-Child Nursing* 6:171, 1981; P. Stern, Solving problems of cross-cultural health teaching: The Filipino childbearing family. *Image* 13:47, 1981; and L. Todd, Indochinese refugees bring rich heritages to childbearing. *International Childbirth Education Association News* 21:1, 1982.

increased estrogen and progesterone tend to interfere with the peripheral action of prolactin, thus decreasing the supply of milk. This is particularly true in the early stages of lactation. The hormones from the pill are present in the mother's milk, but they are not thought to affect the baby, although there have been few long-range studies on this subject.

Nursing mothers also need to know that when the baby is given early supplementary bottle feedings or solid food, the decreased nursing stimulation will result in a decreased prolactin level. This will increase the mother's ability to conceive as she resumes menstruation and ovulation.

Couples are commonly concerned about the question of when they will be able to resume intercourse. Perineal and uterine wounds should be healed before intercourse is resumed. Masters and Johnson [16] report that this occurs within 2 to 4 weeks; most midwives and physicians, however, ask couples to abstain until the first postpartum check-up, when it can be determined if healing has taken place. If a couple does not wish to wait this long, it is important that the man use a condom to prevent introduction of infectious organisms into the woman's genital tract.

Some couples report a change in sexual desire after childbirth, and Masters and Johnson [16] have found in a limited sample of women that their physiologic responses were reduced in rapidity and intensity. By 3 months after delivery these responses were normal again; the mothers who were not nursing recovered faster than the nursing mothers. If sexual response is decreased in the postpartum period, some factors that may contribute to the problem include fatigue, pain, fear, vaginal discharge, poor health, and anxiety about another pregnancy.

Maternal Feelings

While many women feel an immediate fondness for and close relationship with their newborns, others do not. Often physical discomforts and fatigue, an unfamiliar environment without continuous contact and support of family, lack of previous experience caring for newborns, an infant of a different sex or appearance from that expected, and feelings of inadequacy in a mothering role can inhibit the development of maternal feelings. New mothers and fathers need to be reassured that it is not unusual to feel a lack of immediate fondness and intimate relationship with their newborn. Given time, rest, and support this relationship will form in the weeks and months ahead. If obvious signs of total lack of interest and concern for the infant are evident, documentation of parental behaviors and follow-up of the family are most appropriate.

Special Time for Mother and Father

In your postpartum planning and intervention, help the mother and father to identify the need for and help them plan for time they can spend both by themselves and together without the newborn or siblings. Help them identify a need for periods such as these when they may relax alone and resume some of their own special activities. Help them realize these periods together without the children are also necessary for them to resume their relationship together and that they provide a time for them to discuss and share their feelings regarding the new baby, their new roles, and the accompanying new demands. The time in which feelings such as these are shared and worked through is critical for the long-term functioning of the family unit. Helping parents recognize this time as an investment in their future together often helps them provide adequate time for themselves and each other.

Using the "empty bucket" analogy often helps in this instance. Unless parents provide time and opportunity to replenish their own reserves or to fill their own "bucket," it becomes very difficult if not impossible to give of themselves to each other or to their newborn. One cannot pour something from an "empty bucket."

Discharge   Most new mothers and babies are discharged from the hospital in 3 days; however, in some areas they may be discharged in 2 days or even 24 hours after delivery. The earlier discharge reflects the belief that healthy mothers and babies should not remain in institutions where they may come in contact with organisms resistant to antibiotics. Earlier discharge also reduces the cost of hospitalization.

In preparation for discharge, instruct mothers to report any unusual signs or symptoms, such as heavy or foul-smelling lochia or bright bleeding, breast pain (which may indicate mastitis when it occurs around the ninth or tenth day), leg pain (which may indicate venous thrombosis), persistent headache, backache (which may indicate pyelitis), and elevated temperature once they are home. Also review or teach the mother the technique and emphasize the importance of monthly breast self-examination as described in Chapter 7. Providing her upon discharge with learning aids regarding breast self-examination and a list of reportable unusual signs and symptoms is most helpful.

In planning for discharge give the mother your card if you have been her primary nurse, or if not, make sure she has the telephone number of the unit from which she is being discharged so that she has a nursing contact when she leaves the institution. If she has delivered at a birthing center, she will most likely already have established a close relationship with a midwife. After helping the couple assess their needs postpartally, help them make initial contact with additional community resources they or the woman might use such as LaLeche League, nursing mothers groups, parent groups, or the local visiting nursing service. Provide them with information about other resources they may use in the future.

Telephone the woman a short time after she is discharged. Be alert for underlying concerns which she may not verbalize. You might begin by asking her, "What has been happening to you in the last few days?"

Schedule return visits for 2 or 3 weeks instead of 6 weeks so that the woman will have earlier and continued access to professional services. New-parent discussion groups, which meet informally during newborn return visits, provide opportunities to have parents' concerns answered, to share approaches and solutions to problems, and to meet other new parents and form new friendships. Parent discussion groups may be inter- or intradisciplinary and may include such topics as adjusting to parenthood, new roles, relationships, sibling rivalry, and infant care and feeding. If your institution or community does not have such a support group, you might form one.

Case Study   Susan Wilcox

As Susan Wilcox's primary nurse, develop a plan of care for her including both interventions aimed at providing care for her each day and interventions directed toward helping her make the transitional postpartum period at home successful. Each of you will develop your own approach and style in providing care to newly delivered women. Applying the nursing process to the outline following the case study will serve as a guide in organizing your approach to this group of clients while they are in the hospital and in your subsequent follow-up care.

DELIVERY DAY   Susan Wilcox delivered her first baby 1½ hours ago and is now being transferred to the postpartum floor where you are working. You will be the primary nurse.

Susan is a 19-year-old woman whose husband Tom is in the Navy and currently on an "alert" in waters near the Persian Gulf. She is not sure when he will be able to get home. Susan has been working as a secretary in an office in town and would like to return to work if possible. Both her family and Tom's family live approximately 100 miles away. Susan's two closest friends, Jane and Cheryl, work as secretaries in the office where Susan worked and live in the same apartment building as Susan.

Susan's pregnancy was uneventful; with the exception of nausea and vomiting in the first trimester, she felt wonderful the entire time. She attended childbirth education classes at the hospital and appeared very involved in her pregnancy. Tom was able to attend two of the classes with her and also appeared pleased and involved. Susan's physical condition was fine, her pelvic dimensions were adequate, the fetus grew appropriately, her hemoglobin was 11.5, hematocrit 34.5, and she had no complicating illness during pregnancy. Her past health history indicated nothing untoward.

Jane Kennedy, the nurse who was with Susan during labor and delivery, reports that Susan did very well during the experience. She delivered a 7½-pound boy via spontaneous vaginal delivery. His Apgar scores were 8 and 10 at 1 and 5 minutes after birth. Susan received only local anesthesia and had a median episiotomy. Nurse Kennedy reports that Susan had minimal blood loss; her uterus is nicely contracted, at the level of her umbilicus; her vital signs are: temperature 97.6, blood pressure 110/70, pulse 76, respirations 18; her vaginal bleeding is moderate; and she has not voided since delivery but her bladder does not appear distended. Nurse Kennedy again congratulates Susan, tells her what a wonderful job she did during the labor and delivery experiences, and leaves, telling Susan she will be by to see her tomorrow.

Susan complains of a chill, of feeling very fatigued but not sleepy, and of aching in the area of her episiotomy. She asks to use the bedpan and voids 400 cc. Approximately 25 minutes later she voids 350 cc.

DAY 1   The following day, as Susan's roommate gets out of bed to bathe and dress, Susan does likewise. Once out of bed, however, Susan becomes dizzy and sits down quickly on the nearest chair. When you arrive, Susan tells you that she became dizzy and that she still feels very tired. For the remainder of the day, Susan does as you ask and seems content just to follow orders. Her appetite seems enormous even though she remains in bed, and she seems quite thirsty. She is somewhat concerned over her feeling of being fatigued even though she spends so much of the day resting. Despite her fatigue, her beginning attempts to breast-feed her son have been successful, and she appears to enjoy interacting with him although she is awkward in handling him.

DAY 2   On Susan's second postpartum day her vital signs are: temperature 99, blood pressure 112/68, pulse 56, and respirations 20. Her fundus is found two fingerbreadths below her umbilicus, and her uterus is firm. Susan is full of questions: She feels her uterus and wants to know when it will "go away." She also wants to know how long she has to put up with "this period business." In addition, she wants to know if perineal care really does anything for her, but she does admit it feels good when it's done. In the morning she walks down to the treatment room and weighs herself on the scale. She becomes very upset when she finds out that she has lost only 11 pounds of the 27 she gained during pregnancy. She tells you she is sure that she has not lost more because she is constipated, but she "can't go because of the stitches." "What will Tom think of me when he sees me this fat and out of shape?" she asks. She appears rather upset.

DAY 3   Susan has been very interested in breast-feeding but is a little worried since her milk looks very watery: "Will my milk get thicker? This looks like a poor grade of skim milk." When her son is brought to her she still seems ill at ease with him and doesn't appear to know how to hold him. She is also concerned because last evening he "spit up mucus quite a lot. He also doesn't seem to be too interested in drinking." Susan wants to know if she is feeding the baby properly and if he should be so uninterested in drinking. She also notices crampy pains after breastfeeding.

DAY 4   Tomorrow morning Susan will be discharged. She is better at handling the baby now and appears to be more confident in providing his care. Realizing that she will soon be discharged, she wants to known what she should eat or add to her diet in order to have "good milk" for the baby. She also wants to know if she has to continue the perineal care and heat treatments at home, and what the spray is that her roommate puts on her stitches. In addition she wants to know what activities she will be allowed and when she will have to return for a checkup. This afternoon Susan develops breast engorgement and sits in her bed crying.

Assessment Form

Assessment	Plan	Intervention	Evaluation

I. Significant Factors from Pregnancy
  A. Problems during pregnancy
  B. Previous or existing health problems
II. Significant Factors from Delivery
  A. Type
  B. Duration of labor
  C. Infant's condition and Apgar scores
  D. Complications
III. Physical Changes
  A. Breasts
    1. Contour
    2. Areolae
    3. Nipples
    4. Colostrum or milk
    5. Brassiere
  B. Cardiovascular
    1. HB, Hct
    2. Varicosities
  C. Abdomen
    1. Diastasis
  D. Skin
    1. Perspiration
    2. Pigmentation
  E. GI system
    1. Appetite
    2. Bowel movements
  F. Genital Tract
    1. Uterus
      (a) Firmness
      (b) Location
    2. Lochia
      (a) Character
      (b) Amount
      (c) Clots
    3. Cervix
    4. Perineum
      (a) Episiotomy
      (b) Hematomas
      (c) Discomfort
  G. Urinary system
    1. Voiding

Assessment Form			
Assessment	Plan	Intervention	Evaluation

        (a) Character
        (b) Frequency
        (c) Pain
    H. Specific learning needs to cope with
       physical changes
IV. Behavioral Changes
    A. Taking-in
       1. Dependency needs
    B. Taking-hold
       1. Reaching out to others
       2. Increased independence
    C. Mood swings
       1. Elation
       2. Blues
       3. Tearfulness
       4. Severe depression
 V. Needs Identified by
    A. Mother
    B. Father
VI. Needs Identified for Successful Incorpo-
    ration of Newborn into Family and
    the Resumption of Normal Family
    Functioning
    A. Rest and assistance
    B. Special time
       1. For mother alone
       2. For father alone
       3. For couple
    C. Reestablishment of sexual relations
       and contraceptive method chosen
    D. Interaction with newborn
       1. Comfort and expertise in feeding
         and bathing, dressing, cord care,
         circumcision care
       2. Comfort and character of interac-
         tion with newborn—holding, cud-
         dling, talking to, ability to soothe
    E. Sibling interaction with newborn
       1. Sibling rivalry
    F. Resumption of employment by
       father and mother

Assessment Form			
Assessment	Plan	Intervention	Evaluation

      G. Reestablishment of social relationships
VII. Specific Discharge Information
    A. Nurse and physician who can be contacted regarding further questions or concerns
    B. Date of return visit for checkup
    C. Information reinforcing activity level at home
      1. Regarding child care
      2. Regarding breast self-exam
      3. Regarding untoward signs and symptoms to be reported
    D. Community resources available
      1. Parent groups
      2. Nursing mothers groups
      3. Visiting nurse service

REFERENCES

1. Anderson, B., Camacho, M., and Stark, J. *Pregnancy and Family Health*. New York: McGraw-Hill, 1974.
2. Bristol, W. Comparative effectiveness of compressional and supporting breast binders in suppressing lactation. *Nursing Research* 15:203, 1966.
3. Brown, M., and Hurlock, J. Mothering the mother. *American Journal of Nursing* 77:439, 1977.
3a. Bull, M. Change in concerns of first time mothers after one week at home. *Journal of Obstetric, Gynecologic and Neonatal Nursing* 10:391, 1981.
4. Cooke, I., Foley, M., Lenton, E., Preston, E., Millar, D., Jenkins, A., Oblekwe, B., McNeilly, A., Parsons, J., and Kennedy, G. The treatment of puerperal lactation with bromocriptine. *Postgraduate Medicine* 52:75, 1976.
5. Crosignani, P., Lombrosa, G., Caccamo, A., Reschini, E., and Peracchi, M. Suppression of puerperal lactation by metergoline. *Obstetrics and Gynecology* 51:113, 1978.
6. Greenhill, J. P., and Friedman, E. A. *Biological Principles and Modern Practice of Obstetrics*. Philadelphia: Saunders, 1974.
7. Gruis, M. Beyond maternity: Postpartum concerns of mothers. *American Journal of Maternal-Child Nursing* 2:182, 1977.
8. Guyton, A. *Textbook of Medical Physiology*. Philadelphia: Saunders, 1981.
9. Hahn, M., and Hurst, J. Hormonal influences in lactation. *Nursing Times* 64:28, 1980.
10. Harrison, R. Suppression of lactation. *Seminars in Perinatology* 3:287, 1979.
11. Henning, E., Martoglio, G., Quita, M., Reinbrecht, J., and Strickland, M. A Dynamic Nursing Appraisal of the Puerperium. In N. Lytle (Ed.), *Maternal Health Nursing*. Dubuque, Iowa: W. C. Brown, 1967.
12. Keettel, W. C., and Bradbury, J. T. Endocrine studies of lactation amenorrhea. *American Journal of Obstetrics and Gynecology* 82:995, 1961.
13. Lesser, M., and Keane, V. *Nurse-Patient Relationships in a Hospital Maternity Service*. St. Louis: Mosby, 1956.
14. Llewellyn-Jones, D. Inhibition of lactation. *Drugs* 10:121, 1975.
15. Marcus, R. G. Suppression of lactation with high doses of pyridoxine. *South Africa Medical Journal* 49:2155, 1975.
16. Masters, W. H., and Johnson, V. E. *Human Sexual Response*. Boston: Little, Brown, 1966.
16a. Moss, J. Concerns of multiparas on the third postpartum day. *Journal of Obstetric, Gynecologic and Neonatal Nursing* 10:421, 1981.
17. Nichols, M. Effective help for the nursing mother. *Journal of Obstetric, Gynecologic and Neonatal Nursing* 7(2):22, 1978.
18. Niebyl, J., Bell, W., Schaaf, M., Blake, D., Dubin, N., and King, T. The effect of chlorotrianisene as postpartum lactation suppression on blood coagulation factors. *American Journal of Obstetrics and Gynecology* 134:518, 1979.
19. Pritchard, J., and MacDonald, P. *Williams Obstetrics* (16th ed.). New York: Appleton-Century-Crofts, 1980.
20. Riordan, J., and Countryman, B. Anatomy and psychophysiology of lactation. *Journal of Obstetric, Gynecologic and Neonatal Nursing* 00:210, 1980.
21. Riordan, J., and Countryman, B. Some breastfeeding problems and solutions. *Journal of Obstetric, Gynecologic and Neonatal Nursing* 00:361, 1980.
22. Rubin, R. Basic maternal behavior. *Nursing Outlook* 9:683, 1961.
23. Rubin, R. Puerperal change. *Nursing Outlook* 9:753, 1961.
24. Rubin, R. Maternal touch. *Nursing Outlook* 11:828, 1963.
25. Rubin, R. Attainment of the maternal role. 1. Processes. *Nursing Research* 16:237, 1967.
26. Rubin, R. Attainment of the maternal role. 2. Models and Referents. *Nursing Research* 16:342, 1967.
27. Rudolph, S. H. Notes from a maternity ward. *The Atlantic Monthly* 211:122, 1963.
28. Suppressing lactation. *British Medical Journal* 22:18, 1977.
29. Turnbull, A. Puerperal thromboembolism and suppression of lactation. *Obstetrics and Gynecology of the British Commonwealth* 75:1321, 1968.
30. Vorherr, H. Suppression of Postpartum Lactation. *Postgraduate Medicine* 52:145, 1972.

FURTHER READING

Anderson, C. Enhancing reciprocity between mother and neonate. *Nursing Research* 30:89, 1981.
Atkinson, L. Prenatal nipple conditioning for breastfeeding. *Nursing Research* 28:267, 1979.

Berlin, C. Pharmacologic considerations of drug use in the lactating mother. *Obstetrics and Gynecology* 58:17s, 1981.

Beske, E., and Gravis, M. Research-important factors in breastfeeding success. *American Journal of Maternal-Child Nursing* 7:174, 1982.

Brown, B. Maternity-patient teaching—a nursing priority. *Journal of Obstetric, Gynecologic and Neonatal Nursing* 11:11, 1982.

Campbell, S., and Smith, J. Postpartum assessment guide. *American Journal of Nursing* 77:1179, 1977.

Candy, M. Birth of a comprehensive family-centered maternity program. *Journal of Obstetric, Gynecologic and Neonatal Nursing* 8:80, 1979.

Carlson, S. E. The irreality of postpartum observations on the subjective experience. *Journal of Obstetric, Gynecologic and Neonatal Nursing* 5:28, 1976.

Carr, K., and Walton, V. Early postpartum discharge. *Journal of Obstetric, Gynecologic and Neonatal Nursing* 11:29, 1982.

Clark, A. L., and Affonso, D. D. Mother-child relations—infant behavior and maternal attachment: Two sides to the coin. *American Journal of Maternal-Child Nursing* 1:94, 1976.

Donaldson, N. E. Follow-up at home. *American Journal of Nursing* 77:1176, 1977.

Donaldson, N. E. The postpartum follow-up nurse clinician. *Journal of Obstetric, Gynecologic and Neonatal Nursing* 10:249, 1981.

Dungy, C., et al. The nurse clinician: A teaching model for postpartum units. *Journal of Medical Education* 54:507, 1979.

Dutton, M. A. A breastfeeding protocol. *Journal of Obstetric, Gynecologic and Neonatal Nursing* 8:151, 1979.

Erickson, M. P. Trends in assessing the newborn and his parents. *American Journal of Maternal-Child Nursing* 3:99, 1978.

Fawcett, J. Body image and the pregnant couple. *American Journal of Maternal-Child Nursing* 3:227, 1978.

Gardner, S. The mother as incubator—after delivery. *Journal of Obstetric, Gynecologic and Neonatal Nursing* 8:174, 1979.

Giovanti, A. Impact of the firstborn. *Issues in Comprehensive Pediatric Nursing* 2:182, 1977.

Gorrie, T. Postpartum evaluation tool. *Journal of Obstetric, Gynecologic and Neonatal Nursing* 8:41, 1979.

Haight, J. Steadying parents as they go—by phone. *American Journal of Maternal-Child Nursing* 2:311, 1977.

Hall, L. Effect of teaching on primiparas' perceptions of their newborn. *Nursing Research* 29:317, 1980.

Hill, S., and Shronk, L. The effect of early parent-infant contact on newborn body temperature. *Journal of Obstetric, Gynecologic and Neonatal Nursing* 8:287, 1979.

Hoag, L. M., and Cohen, G. D. Family-infant bonding. *Issues in Health Care of Women* 1:3, 1979.

Horn, B. Cultural concepts and postpartal care. *Nursing and Health Care* 11:516, 1981.

Ingalls, A. J., and Salerno, M. C. *Maternal and Child Health Nursing* (4th ed.). St. Louis: Mosby, 1979.

Johnson, N. W. Breast-feeding at one hour of age. *American Journal of Maternal-Child Nursing* 1:12, 1976.

Kindley, K. The sexuality of women in pregnancy and postpartum: A review. *Journal of Obstetric, Gynecologic and Neonatal Nursing* 7:28, 1978.

Kraus, N. Postpartum hospital visits for children. *Issues in Health Care of Women* 1:29, 1979.

Ledger, W. J. The new face of puerperal sepsis. *Journal of Obstetric, Gynecologic and Neonatal Nursing* 3:26, 1974.

Livingston, J. E., MacLeod, P. M., and Applegarth, D. A. Vitamin B_6 status in women with postpartum depression. *American Journal of Clinical Nutrition* 31:886, 1978.

Lotas, M. B., and Willging, J. M. Mothers, babies, perception. *Image* 11:45, 1979.

Luakaran, V., and van den Berg, B. The relationship of maternal attitude to pregnancy outcomes and obstretic complications. *American Journal of Obstetrics and Gynecology* 136:374, 1980.

Ludding-Hoe, S. M. Postpartum: Development of maternicity. *American Journal of Nursing* 77:1171, 1977.

McGowan, M. N. Postpartum disturbance: A review of the literature in terms of stress response. *Journal of Nurse-Midwifery* 12:27, 1977.

McLendon, M., Fulk, C., and Starnes, D. Effectiveness of self breast examination teaching to women of low socioeconomic class. *Journal of Obstetric, Gynecologic and Neonatal Nursing* 11:7, 1982.

Mercer, R. A theoretical framework for studying factors that impact on the maternal role. *Nursing Research* 30:73, 1981.

————. The nurse and maternal tasks of early postpartum. *American Journal of Maternal-Child Nursing* 6:341, 1981.

Miller, D. L., and Baird, S. F. Helping parents to be parents—a special center. *American Journal of Maternal-Child Nursing* 3:117, 1978.

Mynick, A. Instituting a postpartum self medication program. *American Journal of Maternal-Child Nursing* 6:422, 1981.

Norr, K., Block, C., Charles, A., and Meyering, S. The second time around: Parity and birth experience. *Journal of Obstetric, Gynecologic and Neonatal Nursing* 9:30, 1980.

Paukert, S. E. One hospital's experience with implementing family centered maternity care. *Journal of Obstetric, Gynecologic and Neonatal Nursing* 8:351, 1979.

Petrowski, D. Effectiveness of prenatal and postnatal instruction in postpartum care. *Journal of Obstetric, Gynecologic and Neonatal Nursing* 10:386, 1981.

Ritchie, C. A. Depression following childbirth. *Nurse Practitioner* 2:14, 1977.

Schmidt, J. Using a teaching guide for better postpartum and infant care. *Journal of Obstetric, Gynecologic and Neonatal Nursing* 7:23, 1978.

Schroeder, M. A. Is the immediate postpartum period crucial to the mother-child relationship? A pilot study comparing primiparas with rooming-in and those in a maternity ward. *Journal of Obstetric, Gynecologic and Neonatal Nursing* 6:37, 1977.

Senie, R. Possible related risks to breastfeeding. *Journal of Obstetric, Gynecologic and Neonatal Nursing* 11:34, 1982.

Stamps, D. C. and Stamps, I. E. The costs of children: Parenting has a price. *Issues in Health Care of Women* 1:43, 1979.

Strelnick, E. Postpartum care: An opportunity to reinforce breast self-examination. *American Journal of Maternal-Child Nursing* 7:249, 1982.

Sugarman, M. Paranatal influences in maternal-infant attachment. *American Journal of Orthopsychiatry* 47:407, 1977.

Sumner, G., and Fritsch, J. Postnatal parental concerns: The first six weeks of life. *Journal of Obstetric, Gynecologic and Neonatal Nursing* 6:27, 1977.

Sweeney, S. I., and Davis, F. B. Transition to parenthood: A group experience. *Maternal-Child Nursing Journal* 8:59, 1979.

Swenden, L. A., et al. Role supplementation for new parents—a role mastery plan. *American Journal of Maternal-Child Nursing* 3:84, 1978.

Williams, J. K. Learning needs of new parents. *American Journal of Nursing* 77:1173, 1977.

Willson, J. R., and Carrington, E. R. *Obstetrics and Gynecology* (6th ed.). St. Louis: Mosby, 1979.

Chapter 15 Adapting to Parenthood

Following the exhausting effort of labor and delivery, the mother faces the task of making many readjustments, physiological as well as psychological. During labor she has concentrated her energy on coping with that experience. The mother, as well as the father, faces the postpartum period with the work of realizing that the baby has actually been born, beginning the tasks of parenting, and assuming new roles.

PARENTING TASKS Nurses may provide crucial support to parents as they assume their new roles and establish initial relationships with their newborns. One of the parents' first tasks is identifying the infant as theirs, recognizing the separate identity of their baby, and establishing his individuality [27], a process which begins with their initial inspection of him after delivery. This is the time when parents first notice his specific features, and make such comments as "He has his mother's eyes" or "his father's chin." This association with others illustrates their initial steps in seeing him as a separate individual, with characteristics of his own. At the first opportunity encourage parents to unwrap their baby and do a more thorough inspection. You may use this occasion to explain some of the variations in newborns that may seem unusual to the parents, such as the cord stump, milia, and molding of the head. Now is a good time to observe relationships between the parents, and between them and their infant, for clues about family interaction and cohesiveness (Fig. 15-1).

At this time parents are confronted with the reality of their newborn and they must reconcile this with their fantasies of the child they had expected, who may have been of the opposite sex. Sex is probably the major basis for the initial identification process [27]. It can have a strong influence on parents' reactions to the baby, on their handling of him, and on their emotional response of acceptance or rejection. If the differences between the characteristics of the idealized child and the real child are never resolved in the parents' minds, the effects on their relationship with the child may be long lasting. One example known to the authors is a woman who had desperately wanted a girl but had a boy, now 8 years old. She has consistently chosen feminine styles of boys' clothing (and sometimes girls' coats) for him to wear, and she has also painted his fingernails red when he was not in school.

Another important task parents face is determining their relationship to their infant. They must identify his obvious needs, assume responsibility for him, and in some way accommodate their life-style in order to care for him. This becomes readily apparent once the family goes home and assumes total responsibility for the baby. The mother, for instance, may realize she is in need of milk for the baby; she prepares to leave for the grocery store, only to realize that the baby cannot be left unattended. A couple may decide to go to the movies and then realize they must find a babysitter who is able to take care of a newborn. Their fantasy of what having a baby would be like often does not include realities such as these.

Parents are also faced with the tasks of reorganizing the family grouping to include the new member and establishing mutually satisfying roles for themselves. This includes regulating the demands of the infant and of the home

415

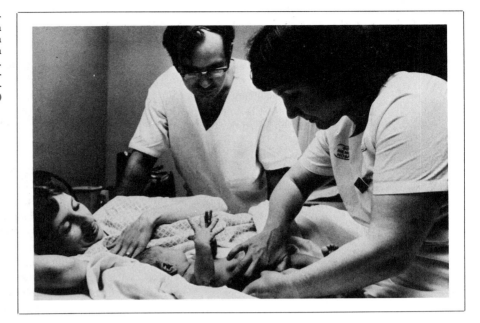

environment and modifying those demands that parents impose upon themselves. What frustrations are now generated in a compulsive house cleaner!

Siblings likewise may become frustrated. Young children often experience anger, guilt, and feelings of desertion when their mother disappears to bring back a new baby. After the new baby comes home, they may show jealousy and resentment and may act out these feelings in a variety of ways. Young children particularly may hesitate to approach their mother on her return, which can be very upsetting to her, especially if she is unaware that this is a common and very temporary reaction. Siblings are often more accepting of the new baby if they are able to attend the birth, visit the mother while she is in the hospital, and see the new baby (Fig. 15-2). If children are made to feel that they are very special people by being given extra love and attention and perhaps a small gift, especially if it is from the new baby, they feel more secure and better able to relate to the baby.

While all parents are faced with basically the same tasks, the quality of their performance differs. A child's normal development is fostered in the atmosphere that is created when parents have warm loving relationships with each other, with their children, and with members of the extended family (Fig. 15-3). It is further enhanced when the infant is able to develop long-lasting relationships with one or more people who are attuned to his needs. The strongest attachment, however, may not always be with the mother. The amount of warm adult-child interaction is an important stimulus in the development of intelligence and language [30], as well as in the development of his innate personality characteristics.

FATHER'S ROLE   In today's society, the new role of father may bring with it many conflicts. One of these conflicts may exist between the traditional role of breadwinner and head of

Figure 15-2. Children meeting their new brother. (Courtesy of Pennsylvania Hospital, Philadelphia, Pa.)

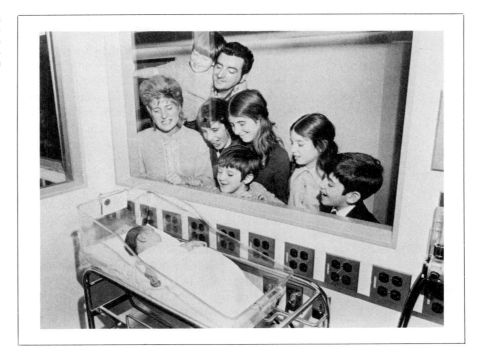

Figure 15-3. The infant develops warm supporting relationships with grandparents who are attuned to his needs. (Courtesy of Pennsylvania Hospital, Philadelphia, Pa.)

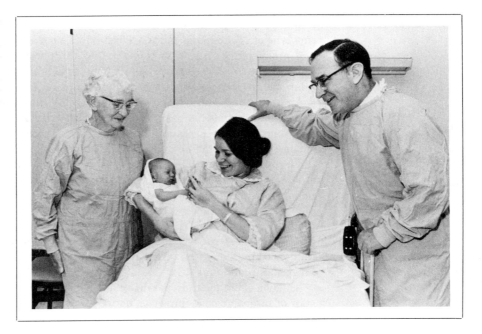

the household and a more recent tendency for parental authority to be shifted to the mother, with fathers assuming some of the nurturant and affectional functions traditionally associated with mothering. With this trend toward greater homogeneity in parental roles, it is generally accepted that fathers may express tender feelings toward their children, but many must still cope with the old concepts of masculine ruggedness and aggressiveness.

Hines [17] notes that "in an environment where the feelings of the father are allowed to be expressed without censure, without fear of embarrassment, and without anyone accusing him of being unmanly, the father shows evidence of deep feelings for his baby right after birth." Today more of these feelings are being openly expressed. A father's investment in the birth of his child is increased by active participation during the prenatal period and during labor and delivery with the support of the members of the health team. In our zeal to involve fathers in the childbearing process, however, we must be careful to meet their needs and not our own, and recognize that some fathers have no desire to participate. Participation may increase the father's feelings of adequacy as a new father, a mate, and possibly a man; in addition, it reinforces his feelings that the children are also his responsibility, not simply that of the mother.

Encouraging the father to have physical contact with his newborn from the time of birth aids in the transition to fathering (Fig. 15-4). In some families where the mother-infant relationship is inadequate, the father-child relationship serves as a balance to support the child. The father, as well as the mother, should benefit from the support and guidance of the health team in adjusting to and caring for their newborn.

DEVELOPING PARENT-CHILD RELATIONSHIPS
Research on Bonding and Attachment

By some definitions a bond is a tie from parent to infant and an attachment refers to the tie from infant to parent. (Today the two terms are often used interchangeably.) A bond is further defined by some as a unique relationship between two people that is specific and endures through time [18]. General indications that this type of relationship exists are behaviors such as fondling, kissing, cuddling, and prolonged gazing. It is thought that the parent-infant tie is the primary source of all of the infant's subsequent attachments, and it is through this relationship over time that the child develops his sense of himself.

A number of factors are important in the formation of the mother's bond to her infant; they include her past experiences with caretaking; whether the pregnancy was planned; her acceptance of its reality once it occurred; having a mate who is supportive of her and accepting of the pregnancy; and her acknowledgement of the fetus as a separate individual. The events of labor and delivery, such as the environment in which they occurred and the length of the process, are also important influences on the woman's interactions with her baby. Peterson and Mehl [25] found the woman's birth experience to be the second most significant predictor of maternal attachment; the first was length of separation of mother and infant after birth. After birth the woman's relationship with her baby is influenced by seeing the infant, touching him, giving care to him, and accepting him as an individual [18].

A major effort to study parent-infant bonding began 15 to 20 years ago when staff of intensive care nurseries noticed that an unusual number of the infants who were discharged in good health were subsequently seen in the emergency

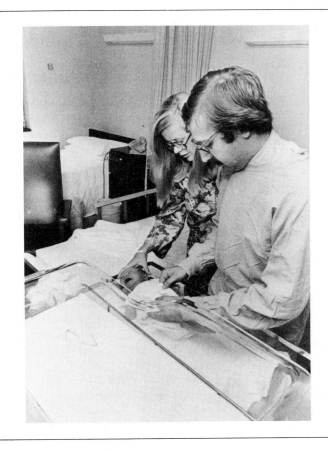

Figure 15-4. Father caring for his newborn. (Courtesy of Pennsylvania Hospital, Philadelphia, Pa.)

room, failing to thrive or victims of child abuse. Subsequent research findings seemed to confirm an increase in the incidence of child abuse and failure to thrive in children who had been separated for long periods from their parents at birth, although it was recognized that many other contributory factors were involved, including the parents' genetic endowments, the parenting each of them received from their own parents, their cultural backgrounds, their relationships with their families, and events surrounding the present as well as past pregnancies [18].

Researchers undertook to investigate further the possibility of the presence of a sensitive period in the human when parent-infant contact might favorably alter parents' later behavior with that infant. Data from several clinical observations and controlled studies performed around the world lend some support to the existence of such a period in the human shortly after birth, whether it be in the first minutes, hours, or days of life. In one group of these studies, some mothers had contact with their infants soon after birth and then at extra extended-time intervals throughout the hospital stay. A year or two later, when they were compared with mothers who had no early or extra contact with their infants, a difference was noted in the mother-infant interactions: The mothers with more contact tended to demonstrate more attachment behaviors, such as soothing, fondling, eye-to-eye contact with their infants [18]. Unfortunately some of the studies have methodological flaws, such as groups that are not comparable because of the influence of a variety of uncontrolled variables. Researchers have also questioned the validity of certain variables used to measure the attachment process.

In one of the most recent of such studies involving 202 mothers, Siegel and associates [31] found that between 2½ and 3.2 percent of the variance in attachment behaviors could be explained by the extra contact; another 10 to 22 percent of the variance was explained by the mothers' background variables such as race, socioeconomic status, age, and education.

Other researchers, using a variety of research designs and subject populations, have studied the effect of additional mother-infant contact in the first hour of life, with contact following this period being similar in experimental and control groups. Results of the research have been varied, with some studies showing significant differences in attachment behaviors between the groups of mothers and other studies showing no differences [11a]. Klaus and Kennell [18] conclude that "at present there are no appropriate studies to tell us the length of time (of contact) required in the first hours and days after birth to produce an effect on the behavior of the mother or child in the subsequent days and weeks of life." One might argue that the lack of early contact does not preclude the later development of attachment between mother and child or parents and child, as in the case of adopted children [34]. It is still unclear whether there is a sensitive period in humans during which contact is essential for the subsequent development of optimal parent-infant attachment.

Facilitating the Relationship

Ainsworth [1] found three maternal behaviors to be highly correlated with strong infant attachments: a positive attitude toward breast-feeding, the amount of care given to the infant, and the mother's knowledge about her infant's behavior. Important maternal and infant behaviors noted by others include eye-to-eye contact, touching, clinging, crying, smiling, and vocalizing. Klaus and Kennell [18] report that touch, eye-to-eye contact, high-pitched voice, movements by the baby in rhythm to the interaction with the parent (entrainment), crying, and odor facilitate attachment.

Brazelton [6, 7], from years of observations of these kinds of behaviors in newborns and parents, has postulated that the infant is an active participant in the interactional process with his parents; according to Brazelton, how the parents respond to the infant depends on the signals he sends them.

During the early postpartum period both parents and baby are involved with each other on many sensory levels. Their behaviors complement each other and serve to bind them together. The infant elicits behaviors from the parents that are satisfying to him; likewise, the parents elicit behaviors in the infant that they find rewarding. The reciprocity acts to ensure the proximity of the parents and child.

For example, when the mother holds her baby close to her, she feels his skin, his motor movements, his clinging to her body. She may be aware of his odor; she may pay attention to his gaze and grimacing (Fig. 15-5). She may move him about in space as she talks, smiles, and makes other facial movements. The infant, on the other hand, may receive tactile and kinesthetic stimulation from her movements. He may have the sensation of being moved in space, the image of his mother's

Figure 15-5. Baby's facial expressions are an important stimulus for parental response.

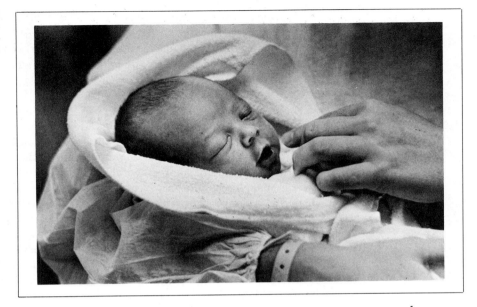

face, and auditory stimulation from her vocalization. He may smell her and feel her body warmth. Both individuals are involved in this communication with each other. You may assess their communication patterns in a number of ways. Observe the amount of time the mother holds the infant (especially face to face), how and when she talks to him, and how she handles him. Is she responsive to the clues he is presenting? Does she call him by name? Does she speak about him with affection? Does she hold him close to her body? Does she change his position gently, in a confident manner?

G. Anderson [3] theorized that the physiologic needs of the mother and infant provide a feedback mechanism to control the type, timing, and amount of interaction that occurs. Subsequent research by C. Anderson [2] indicates that informing mothers about the behavioral characteristics of their infants is an effective means of enhancing the interactional reciprocity. This is supported by several other nurse researchers [12, 32a] who propose the following ways that you might encourage the acquaintance process between parents and their newborns.

1. Have the parents inspect the infant from head to toe.
2. Point out the identifying characteristics of their individual newborn, such as weight, length, hair, skull suture lines, eye color, skin variations, activity level. Identify how the characteristics might change over time.
3. Emphasize the uniqueness of their infant by referring to him by name.
4. Observe and point out the parent-infant reciprocal behaviors. Demonstrate how the parents might elicit responses from their infant: by smiling, cooing, talking, establishing eye-to-eye contact, touching, stimulating reflexes.
5. Instruct the parents in infant care techniques.
6. Compliment the parents on the things that they are doing well.
7. Instruct the parents in infant growth and development patterns so that they might have realistic expectations of their infant.

8. Provide a printed reminder sheet containing information parents may wish to refer to in the future.
9. Plan follow-up care to include home referrals, early clinic appointments, and a 24-hour telephone number for parents to call when they need advice and support.

Klaus and Kennell [18] point out that the human has great powers of adaptation and there are many routes to attachment. Not all parents develop close ties with their babies within the first hour after birth or within a few minutes after the first contact. Mothers and fathers have different ways of reacting to the many environmental influences that occur during this period. If we can make it possible for parents to be with their baby, in privacy, for the first hour and as much as possible during their hospital stay, we may be establishing the most supportive environment in which a relationship can begin. On the other hand, for other parents, such as the mother who is exhausted and prefers to rest, contact with the baby during the first hour post partum may be very stressful. The important point is, as Curry comments, that the needs of individual mothers and fathers should be considered when postdelivery experiences are offered to them [11a]. Since the concept of early bonding has become fairly well publicized in the lay literature, many parents become very disturbed when circumstances (such as an emergency cesarean birth) prevent them from having early contact with their babies, and they fear that their future relationship with the child will be in jeopardy as a result. Many times talking with these families after the birth and reassuring them that nothing irreversible has happened can help to reduce their anxieties [11].

Consumer and professional interest in the bonding/attachment process has stimulated change in health care agencies in the delivery of care to families during the postpartum period. As Tulman comments, as more significant research findings are generated and are subject to critical review, the theoretical base for our practice in this area will grow stronger [34].

Infant-Parent Interaction

INFANT TEMPERAMENT

Parents are well aware that each infant communicates his individuality from the time of birth. Each infant's level of activity may differ, as well as the intensity of his responses to stimuli. Likewise the amount of stimuli needed to evoke a response in a particular infant may vary. It is possible to find in the same family one baby who is friendly and pleasant and who adapts easily to changes in his environment and another who responds in just the opposite manner.

Infants vary in their methods of coping with an overload of stimulation: active physical withdrawal, rejection, decreased sensitivity, and distress signals. They may choose to ignore the stimulus, go to sleep, push the stimulus away, or begin to cry. Some are a joy to be around, placid, easy to care for. Others seem to be fussy, overly active, and difficult to soothe, and may not sleep for long periods of time. The latter baby can be exhausting for the parents.

You can assess infant temperament in a variety of ways. Observe the infant when you are caring for him or when he is being cared for by his parents. This provides an excellent opportunity to determine how he integrates a number of sensory stimuli into appropriate activity. For example, the infant may cry or fuss until he is picked up and fed. As he is moved toward his mother's breast or the bottle, and the nipple is offered, he scans the caregiver's face. As he recognizes the caregiver, there are changes in his respiratory pattern, heart rate, and muscle tone as he cuddles into the caregiver's arms. His reflexes stimulate him to turn in the direction of the nipple and he begins sucking. With appropriate sensations of taste and smell he continues to feed until he is satisfied. Once this happens, he usually drifts into a deep sleep with accompanying changes in autonomic activity, general response level, and muscle tone [28].

Each individual infant will react to stimuli in his environment in his own behavioral style. Health care workers are becoming increasingly interested in this as an area for investigation. For example, Medoff-Cooper and Schraeder [23] have observed behavioral styles of low birth weight infants. Their research indicates that very low birth weight infants may have difficult temperaments in infancy. The 26 infants in their study were described as difficult to soothe, less adaptable, negative in mood, and withdrawing. A low ability to be soothed and negative mood were associated with less maternal responsiveness and involvement.

Whatever the behavioral style of their newborn, parents need help in planning for some time away from their caregiving responsibilities each week. Support systems such as friends or relatives need to be tapped in order that the parents will be able to get their needed rest. Many times parents feel guilty about leaving their baby in the care of someone else. Reassure them that this does not represent neglect of their responsibilities. As Bishop and Brown note, sometimes a little anticipatory guidance in this area will help them to identify the problem before they get to the point of exhaustion and will help to make their decision to seek help easier [4, 8].

INFANT STIMULATION

In the not too distant past, the infant, especially during the neonatal period, was seen as helpless and passive, dependent at first on genetically programmed maturation and after that on the influence of the caretaker who provided the model for him to imitate as he learned adult ways of thinking and behaving [33]. However, in recent years experimental laboratory studies have demonstrated that the infant is not only responsive to patterns of sound but is selectively sensitive to varieties of human speech and to patterns of visual stimuli, especially those characteristic of the human face. Cairns and Butterfield [9] have shown that 2-day-old infants can express an auditory preference for vocal or instrumental music by changing their sucking patterns. Lipsitt [22] describes modifications in sucking patterns as a function of tastes that please or annoy the newborn. Eisenberg [13] has reported infant smiling as a response to sounds characteristic of human speech. Microanalysis of filmed sequences demonstrates that the rhythm of an adult's spoken words in English or another language is reflected in synchronous movements by the infant [32]. Condon and Sander [10] report that by 2 weeks of age, if the infant is exposed to a language that is different from the one heard in the first 2 weeks, he shows some signs of distress.

DeCasper and Fifer [12a] have shown that by 3 days of life newborns are able to discriminate between speakers and demonstrate a preference for higher voices and the mother's voice in particular. In 1976 Lang [21] observed that mothers usually speak to their infants in voices pitched at a higher level than that used in normal conversation.

In 1961 Fantz [15] reported that infants can see at birth, and it has been subsequently demonstrated that newborns have a preference for certain configurations of lines and shapes. Goren and co-workers [16] have speculated that the human face may be the innate form preference of newborns, minutes after birth. Mothers tend to look at their infants in a way that increases the chance that their babies will pay attention and smile back. Since smiling is a strong reinforcer, the visual interaction helps the mother and child to grow closer together. In one study, mothers stated that once their infants looked at them, they felt much closer to their babies [19] (Fig. 15-6).

From a very early age infants have the ability to shut out stimuli in their environment. Stern [32] has noted that infants can sense it when their mothers are staring intensively at them. From a very early age, infants respond to such intrusiveness by averting the mother's gaze or other intense stimulation. Another form of intrusion by the caregiver is that of looming over the infant's face. Bower [5] and others have shown that the infant has an aversive response to objects that move toward his face, stemming from reflexes to protect his eyes and face. Usually, mothers, adults, and older children do not give a second thought to moving in closely to talk, kiss, or otherwise touch the infant. Emde and Robinson

Figure 15-6. Eye-to-eye contact between parents and infants appears to be important during the development of affectional ties. (Courtesy of Pennsylvania Hospital, Philadelphia, Pa.)

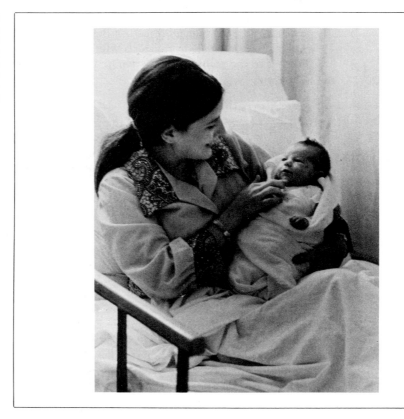

[14] have observed that the infant is usually in the quiet alert state (eyes open, responsive to environment) for a period of 45 to 60 minutes during the first hour after birth. During this time he can see, has visual preferences, and turns his head to the spoken word. After this hour, he usually goes into a deep sleep for the next 3 or 4 hours. The first hour after birth seems to be the ideal time for the newborn to begin interacting with his parents.

Thus, researchers studying the behavioral capacities of the newborn have shown that he sees, hears, reacts to his environment, and moves in rhythm to his mother's voice within minutes and hours after he is born.

It is interesting to note that the tactile contact mothers first have with their infants proceeds in an orderly fashion [19, 28]. The mother begins touching with her fingertips on the baby's extremities, and then proceeds to stroke the baby's trunk with her palm. Still later the mother brings the baby closer to her own body and enfolds him. The activity changes from an exploratory kind of touching to a warm acceptance. Rodholm and Larsson [26] have noted a similar touching sequence in fathers.

Stimulation of the infant's behavioral capacities is an essential element in the development of a parent-infant relationship. Ruffing [29] has presented broad guidelines for nursing practice to facilitate the process of infant stimulation and thus infant response.

1. Help the parents gain confidence in their ability to respond effectively to the baby's crying signals during the first weeks of his life. Crying is the predominant means of infant vocal communication. If they are able to soothe him effectively, he is free to respond to other stimuli in his environment.
2. Explain that sights, sounds, smells, sensations of motion, position, and temperature all provide important opportunities for the infant to learn. His emotional, social, and cognitive potential develops through his sensory experiences. Korner [20] has demonstrated that vestibular stimulation, the experience of being picked up and moved, has a greater effect than body contact both in soothing the infant and in making him more alert.
3. Whenever possible, call the parents' attention to their infant's behaviors that point to his developmental responsiveness. An example might be his gazing at them or at a mobile.
4. Emphasize skills that are necessary to develop social stimulation. This includes visual and hearing stimulation, eye contact, and gaze aversion.
5. Encourage mutual eye contact between parent and infant. As the amount increases, more complex social responses such as smiling and vocalization will emerge from the infant.
6. Reinforce all infant efforts to vocalize. These will emerge at about 6 weeks of age.
7. Encourage regular periods of affectionate play particularly when the infant is alert and responsive. This may follow a daytime feeding session.
8. Teach the new family about the level of the infant's capacity to respond. Infants operate at much higher levels of alertness and responsiveness than is generally realized.

You may also suggest to parents that they can stimulate their infant's senses in a variety of ways:

Change the things he sees.
Change his position.
Hang colored mobiles about 10 to 12 inches from his eyes.
Talk to the baby; use different pitches of voice.
Play music for a short time each day.
Wear perfume.
Move him to the kitchen when meals are being prepared.
Cuddle the baby.
Pat, rock, massage him.
Comfort him when he is upset.
Let other people into his environment.

Although the cumulative effects of early stimulation have yet to be conclusively established, research findings continue to show the infant's great range of responsiveness and discrimination. The finding that infants differ significantly from each other from the beginning suggests that there is more than one way of providing good child care and probably the best way to do so is to respond flexibly to the individual needs of each child.

PARENTING
EDUCATION

Preparation for parenthood begins long before the birth of the baby. It is part of the developmental process that begins with one's own infancy and relationship with one's parents. Pregnancy and childbirth serve to intensify the process.

Almost all couples engage in some preparation for childbirth and child care. For some it will involve only the purchasing of essential clothing and supplies. Others may include discussions of the childbirth experience with their friends and family. Prospective parents may read pamphlets from the doctor's office but what they share with their peers often has much more reality than the contents of an impersonal booklet.

Many communities offer a variety of classes on preparation for parenthood. Some include siblings and grandparents. Topics include promoting self-esteem, understanding, and mutual respect and using reflective listening. Recently more public school systems have been including parenting courses as a part of their health education classes [35]. Some parenting programs are designed to help pre-teenagers learn about normal and handicapped infants and preschoolers through classroom instruction and supervised work in child care centers, hospitals, and health care facilities. Other programs incorporate parenting into classes other than home economics, especially English and social studies. The goal is to increase student ability to resolve conflict, to use social services available to parents, and to care for infants and young children.

Parenting education has been enthusiastically viewed as a solution to many difficulties between parents and children, since it is theorized that if parents knew more about parenting, many problems would cease to exist. Perceiving parent education in this way can be misleading since the notion simplifies the complexity of parenting and ignores the significance of assessing individual needs of mothers and fathers. Wilson [36] conceptualizes the essentials of parenting as a combination of experience, knowledge, and skills. It includes the parent's own

Table 15-1. Family Interactions with Newborn

Assessment	Intervention
Parents' interactions Are the parents interacting comfortably with each other? How are they reacting to their new responsibility?	Provide an environment in which parents can openly express feelings. Acknowledge that becoming parents requires new roles and responsibilities and that this adjustment often takes time
Parent-infant interactions Are the parents comfortable holding him?	Encourage and support both parents in holding him
Are the parents familiar with newborn care? Do the parents know what their newborn's capabilities are?	Teach *both* parents bathing, feeding, dressing, general hygiene of the newborn, how to cope with his behavior; have them care for their baby before discharge to increase their expertise and confidence in caring for him
Do the parents refer to him by name; make eye contact with him; talk to him; touch him; move him?	Provide a role model by talking to the baby, making eye contact and calling him by name; explain the importance of infant stimulation
Do they refer to features that make him unique?	Encourage both parents to examine the baby closely and emphasize features that make him unique; perform newborn physical examination with parents present. Explain his capabilities
What was their "fantasized child"?	Emphasize the positive and unique features of their real child
Sibling reactions What are the reactions of other siblings?	Maintain contact between mother and other siblings by phone or visit. Small gift from mother or baby to other children. Emphasis on the uniqueness of each child: brother's ability to talk when baby can only cry; later other siblings will be able to teach new baby how to do the things they can do

experience of having been nurtured as a child and the parent's skills in establishing and maintaining interpersonal relationships. Parents need external supports, both personal and material, to fulfill their role. (See Appendix II for a list of resources for parents.) They also require an understanding of children's behavior. Awareness of the "whys" of behavior generates a better sense of how to provide care that is appropriate. It is in this respect that parent education can be very helpful [24]. Parents can also learn the mechanics of child care such as feeding and bathing. Understanding the essentials of parenting makes it possible to assess areas in which a parent may need assistance and to intervene appropriately (Table 15-1).

Problem Situation

Adapting to Parenthood

Sally and John Babcock have been married for 12 years. During this time they have enjoyed success in their professional work. (Sally is a chemist and John is the editor of a city newspaper.) They decided to begin a family of two children after much deliberation. After Sally became pregnant, they were careful to choose an obstetrician who was highly recommended by their friends and who would pay attention to their wishes regarding the conduct of their labor and delivery. They wanted their experience to be as "perfect" as possible.

Since neither Sally nor John had brothers or sisters, or much contact with other children while they were growing up, they were concerned about their ability to be good parents. As a result they read as many parenting manuals as they could during the pregnancy.

After a long and difficult labor, their baby girl was born vaginally. Sally and John were glad that she was healthy, but they were just a little disappointed because they had really wanted a boy. On the second postpartum day, when you are caring for Sally and the baby, she has difficulty soothing the infant. She begins crying and says, "I know I will never be a good mother. I can't even make her stop crying." John does not offer much support.

What would be your initial response? What elements would you be sure to include in your nursing care to enhance the couple's development of parenting skills?

REFERENCES

1. Ainsworth, M. Object relations, dependency, and attachment. *Child Development* 40:969, 1969.
2. Anderson, C. Enhancing reciprocity between mother and neonate. *Nursing Research* 30:89, 1981.
3. Anderson, G. The mother and her newborn: Mutual caregivers. *Journal of Obstetric, Gynecologic and Neonatal Nursing* 6(5):50, 1977.
4. Bishop, B. *The Maternity Cycle: One Nurse's Reflections.* Philadelphia: Davis, 1980.
5. Bower, T. Stimulus variables determining space perception in infants. *Science* 149:88, 1965.
6. Brazelton, T. Observations of the neonate. *Journal of Child Psychiatry* 1:38, 1962.
7. Brazelton, T., Koslowski, B., and Moin, M. Origins of Reciprocity: The Early Mother Infant Interaction. In M. Lewis and L. Rosenblum (Eds.), *Origins of Behavior.* New York: Wiley, 1973.
8. Brown, J. Infant temperament: A clue to childbearing for parents and nurses. *American Journal of Maternal-Child Nursing* 2:228, 1977.
9. Cairns, G., and Butterfield, E. Assessing Infants' Auditory Function. In B. Brieflander, G. Sterritt, and G. Kirk (Eds.), *The Exceptional Infant,* Vol. 3. New York: Brunner-Mazel, 1975.
10. Condon, W., and Sander, L. Neonate movement is synchronized with adult speech. *Science* 3:99, 1974.
11. Curry, M. In M. Klaus and J. Kennell (Eds.), *Parent-Infant Bonding* (2nd ed.). St. Louis: Mosby, 1982.
11a. Curry, M. Maternal attachment behavior and the mother's self-concept: The effect of early skin-to-skin contact. *Nursing Research* 31:73, 1982.
12. Dean, P., Morgan, P., and Towle, J. Making baby's acquaintance: A unique attachment strategy. *American Journal of Maternal-Child Nursing* 7:37, 1982.
12a. DeCasper, A., and Fifer, W. The fetal sound environment. *Science* 208:1173, 1980.
13. Eisenberg, R. *Auditory Competence in Early Life.* Baltimore: University Park Press, 1976.
14. Emde, R., and Robinson, J. The First Two Months. In J. Noshpitz and J. Call (Eds.), *Basic Handbook of Child Psychiatry.* New York: Basic Books, 1982.
15. Fantz, R. The origin of form perception. *Scientific American* 204:66, 1961.
16. Goren, C., Sorty, M., and Wu, P. Visual following and pattern discrimination of face-like stimuli by newborn infants. *Pediatrics* 56:544, 1975.
17. Hines, J. Father, the forgotten man. *Nursing Forum* 10:176, 1971.
18. Klaus, M., and Kennell, J. *Parent-Infant Bonding* (2nd ed.). St. Louis: Mosby, 1982.
19. Klaus, M., Kennell, J., Plumbo, N., Zuehlke, S. Human maternal behavior at the first contact with her young. *Pediatrics* 46:187, 1970.
20. Korner, A. Individual differences at birth. *American Journal of Orthopsychiatry* 41(4):608, 1971.
21. Lang, R. *Birth Book.* Ben Lomond, Cal.: Genesis Press, 1972.
22. Lipsitt, L. The Pleasures and Annoyances of Infants: Approach and Avoidance Behavior of Babies. In E. Thoman and S. Trotter (Eds.), *Origins of the Infant's Social Responsiveness.* Hillsdale, N.J.: Lawrence Erlbaum Associates, 1978.

23. Medoff-Cooper, B., and Schraeder, B. Developmental trends and behavioral styles in very low birth weight infants. *Nursing Research* 31:68, 1982.
24. Meier, P., and Peterson, M. A nurse's guide to "how-to-parent" manuals. *American Journal of Obstetric, Gynecologic and Neonatal Nursing* 7(1):46, 1978.
25. Peterson, G., and Mehl, L. Some determinants of maternal attachment. *American Journal of Psychiatry* 135:1168, 1978.
26. Rodholm, M., and Larsson, K. Father-infant interaction at first contact after delivery. *Early Human Development* 3:21, 1979.
27. Rubin, R. Basic maternal behavior. *Nursing Outlook* 9:683, 1961.
28. Rubin, R. Maternal touch. *Nursing Outlook* 11:828, 1963.
29. Ruffing, M. Mothering and early infant stimulation. *Nursing Forum* 18(1):69, 1979.
30. Rutter, M. *Maternal Deprivation Reassessed.* Baltimore: Penguin, 1972.
31. Siegel, E., Bauman, K., Schaefer, E., Saunders, M., and Ingram, D. Hospital and home support during infancy: Impact on maternal attachment. *Pediatrics* 66:183, 1980.
32. Stern, D. A micro-analysis of mother-infant interaction. *Journal of American Academy of Child Psychiatry* 10:501, 1971.
32a. Swanson, J. Nursing intervention to facilitate maternal-infant attachment. *Journal of Obstetric, Gynecologic and Neonatal Nursing* 7(2):35, 1978.
33. Thoman, E. Infant Development Viewed in the Mother-Infant Relationship. In E. Quilligan and N. Kretchmer (Eds.), *Fetal and Maternal Medicine.* New York: Wiley, 1980.
34. Tulman, L. Theories of maternal attachment. *Advances in Nursing Science* 2:7, 1981.
35. Turner, C. Resources for help in parenting. *Child Welfare* 59:179, 1980.
36. Wilson, A. Parenting in perspective. *Family and Community Health* 1(3):65, 1978.

FURTHER READING

Affonso, D. The newborn's potential for interaction. *Journal of Obstetric, Gynecologic and Neonatal Nursing* 5(6):9, 1976.

Avant, K. Nursing diagnosis: Maternal attachment. *Advances in Nursing Science* 2(1):45, 1979.

Benedek, T. Psychobiological aspects of mothering. *American Journal of Orthopsychiatry* 26:272, 1956.

Boudreaux, M. Maternal attachment of high risk mothers with well newborns: A pilot study. *Journal of Obstetric, Gynecologic and Neonatal Nursing* 10:366, 1981.

Bowen, S., and Miller, B. Paternal attachment behavior. *Nursing Research* 29:307, 1980.

Bowlby, J. *Maternal Care and Mental Health.* New York: Schocken, 1966.

Brenton, B. *The Male in Crisis.* New York: Coward-McCann, 1966.

Briggs, E. Transition to parenthood. *Maternal-Child Nursing Journal* 8(2):69, 1979.

Cannon, B. The development of maternal touch during early mother-infant interaction. *Journal of Obstetric, Gynecologic and Neonatal Nursing* 6(2):28, 1977.

Carter-Jessop, L. Promoting maternal attachment through prenatal intervention. *American Journal of Maternal-Child Nursing* 6:107, 1981.

Clark, A. L. The adaptation problems and patterns of an expanding family: The neonatal period. *Nursing Forum* 5:92, 1966.

Clark, A. L. The beginning family. *American Journal of Nursing* 66:802, 1966.

Clark, A., and Affonso, D. Infant behavior and maternal attachment: Two sides to the coin. *American Journal of Maternal-Child Nursing* 1:94, 1976.

Cranley, M. Development of a tool for the measurement of maternal attachment during pregnancy. *Nursing Research* 30:281, 1981.

Donnelly, A., and Conroy, N. Parent-neonate communication in the care-giving system. *Topics in Clinical Nursing* 1(3):1, 1979.

Eckes, S. The significance of increased early contact between mother and newborn infant. *Journal of Obstetric, Gynecologic and Neonatal Nursing* 3:42, 1974.

Friedman, A., and Friedman, D. Parenting: A developmental process. *Pediatric Annals* 6(9):12, 1977.

Funke, J., and Irby, M. An instrument to assess the quality of maternal behavior. *Journal of Obstetric, Gynecologic and Neonatal Nursing* 7(5):19, 1978.

Gay, J. A conceptual framework of bonding. *Journal of Obstetric, Gynecologic and Neonatal Nursing* 10:440, 1981.

Giefer, M., and Nelson, C. A new method to help new fathers develop parenting skills. *Journal of Obstetric, Gynecologic and Neonatal Nursing* 10:455, 1981.

Gordon, R., Kapostins, E., and Gordon, K. Factors in postpartum emotional adjustment. *Obstetrics and Gynecology* 25:158, 1965.

Gordon, V. Teaching concepts of good parenting. *International Nursing Review* 26:137, 1979.

Gottlieb, J. Maternal attachment in primiparas. *Journal of Obstetric, Gynecologic and Neonatal Nursing* 7(1):39, 1978.

Gromada, K. Maternal-infants attachment: The first step toward individualizing twins. *American Journal of Maternal-Child Nursing* 6:129, 1981.

Hall, L. Effect of teaching on primiparas' perceptions of their newborn. *Nursing Research* 29:317, 1980.

Hurd, K. Assessing maternal attachment: First step toward the prevention of child abuse. *Journal of Obstetric, Gynecologic and Neonatal Nursing* 4(4):25, 1975.

Jarrett, G. Childrearing patterns of young mothers: Expectations, knowledge, and practices. *American Journal of Maternal-Child Nursing* 7:119, 1982.

Jenkins, R., and Westhus, N. The nurse role in parent-infant bonding. *Journal of Obstetric, Gynecologic and Neonatal Nursing* 10:114, 1981.

Johnson, C., and Johnson, F. Attitudes toward parenting in dual-career families. *American Journal of Psychiatry* 134:391, 1977.

Johnston, M. Cultural variations in professional and parenting patterns. *Journal of Obstetric, Gynecologic and Neonatal Nursing* 9:9, 1980.

Jones, C. Father-to-infant attachment: Effects on early contact and characteristics of the infant. *Research in Nursing and Health* 4:193, 1981.

Josselyn, I. Cultural forces, motherliness and fatherliness. *American Journal of Orthopsychiatry* 26:264, 1956.

Josten, L. Prenatal assessment guide for illuminating possible problems with parenting. *American Journal of Maternal-Child Nursing* 6:113, 1981.

Kagan, J. The child: His struggle for identity. *Saturday Review* 51:80, 1968.

Kormer, A. Visual alertness in neonates as evoked by maternal care. *Journal of Experimental Child Psychology* 10:67, 1970.

Kunst-Wilson, W., and Cronenwett, L. Nursing care for the emerging family: Promoting paternal behavior. *Research in Nursing and Health* 4:201, 1981.

Lee, G. Relationship of self-concept during late pregnancy to neonatal perception and parenting profile. *Journal of Obstetric, Gynecologic and Neonatal Nursing* 11:186, 1982.

Lidz, T. *The Person.* New York: Basic Books, 1968.

Mercer, R. A theoretical framework for studying factors that impact on the maternal role. *Nursing Research* 30:73, 1981.

Newton, N., and Newton, M. Mothers' reactions to their newborn babies. *Journal of the American Medical Association* 181:206, 1962.

Olson, M. Fitting grandparents into new families. *American Journal of Maternal-Child Nursing* 6:419, 1981.

Palisin, H. The neonatal perception inventory: A review. *Nursing Research* 30:285, 1981.

Paukert, S. Maternal-infant attachment in a traditional hospital setting. *Journal of Obstetric, Gynecologic and Neonatal Nursing* 11:23, 1982.

Reiser, S. A tool to facilitate mother-infant attachment. *Journal of Obstetric, Gynecologic and Neonatal Nursing* 10:294, 1981.

Rising, S. The fourth stage of labor: Family integration. *American Journal of Nursing* 74:870, 1974.

Robson, R. Patterns and determinants of maternal attachment. *Journal of Pediatrics* 77:976, 1970.

Snyder, C., Eyres, S., and Barnard, K. New findings about mothers' antenatal expectations and their relationship to human development. *American Journal of Maternal-Child Nursing* 4:354, 1979.

Sosa, M. Maternal-infant interaction during the immediate postpartum period. *Advances in Pediatrics* 25:451, 1978.

Strauss, S. Abuse and neglect of parents by professionals. *American Journal of Maternal-Child Nursing* 6:157, 1981.

Taubenheim, A. Paternal-infant bonding in the first-time father. *Journal of Obstetric, Gynecologic and Neonatal Nursing* 10:261, 1981.

Thomas, A., Chess, S., and Birch, H. The origin of personality. *Scientific American* 223:102, 1970.

Trevathan, W. Maternal lateral preference at first contact with her newborn infant. *Birth* 9:85, 1982.

Warrick, L. Femininity, sexuality, and mothering. *Nursing Forum* 8:212, 1969.

Wolff, T. Mother-infant interaction in the first year. *New England Journal of Medicine* 295:999, 1976.

Wuerger, M. The young adult: Stepping into parenthood. *American Journal of Nursing* 76:1283, 1976.

Chapter 16 The Normal Newborn

You should examine all newborns immediately after birth, while the newborn is in the delivery room, and more thoroughly once he is taken to the nursery. On each of these occasions you should share the results of the examination with the parents, especially if they cannot be present, so that they do not experience undue anxiety about the condition of their infant.

If you are responsible for providing care to the newborn and the family, you should be able to do a competent physical examination of the newborn, whether it is done in the hospital (when he is admitted to the nursery and prior to his discharge) or on follow-up visits in the home, clinic, or doctor's office. In addition to assessing the physical and behavioral status of the baby, the data establish an initial baseline for the evaluation of future changes in the infant.

Since the newborn's history at this point is that of his parents before conception and, in particular, that of his mother during pregnancy, before performing the physical examination take time to review medical and nursing histories and the nursing care plan on the mother's chart. Review the estimated date of confinement, duration of labor, and type of delivery, as well as any problems such as maternal diabetes, rubella, hemolytic conditions, and addiction that would place the infant at risk. Your physical examination should be systematic and thorough. Remember that just as newborns vary in temperament, so do they exhibit a variety of physical variations that are within normal ranges. When beginning the newborn examination, first make those observations that can be done with minimal disturbance to the newborn such as quality and rate of respirations, auscultation of his chest, color of his skin, motor activity, eye examination, and general appearance.

Gestational Age Assessment

Assessment of whether a newborn is premature, full-term, or postmature is one of the most important considerations in planning his care, since premature and postmature infants may have serious problems adjusting to extrauterine life (see Chap. 21). Neonatal weight, length, and head circumference relationships are important indicators of intrauterine growth and development, but to be of maximal value, these relationships should be based on an accurate and precise measure of gestational age [28].

Several methods have been developed to assess newborn maturity. They are based on external physical characteristics and/or neuromuscular function. (For a detailed discussion of gestational age assessment see Chap. 21.)

Posture, Length, and Weight

Most normal newborns assume a characteristic symmetrical posture. When placed on his abdomen, the infant turns his face to one side, flexes his arms, and holds them close to his trunk. His hands are tightly fisted with his thumb covered by his fingers. His back is bent and his lips are partially flexed, with his knees flexed and drawn up on his abdomen and his pelvis raised off the examining table or mattress (Fig. 16-1). Infants born in a breech position have a tendency to keep their knees and legs straightened rather than flexed, or they may maintain a frog-leg position, depending on the type of breech presentation. Infants born with a face presentation have a tendency to assume an arched posture (opisthotonus).

Figure 16-1. Normal posture of the full-term newborn.

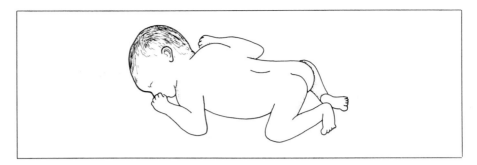

Posture that is not symmetrical may be caused by fractures, commonly of the clavicle or humerus, or by nerve injuries, commonly to the brachial plexus.

The average length of the full-term infant is 51 centimeters (20 inches). Ninety-five percent of all full-term newborns measure in the range of 46 to 56 centimeters (18–22 inches).

In most hospital nurseries, the baby's weight is checked at a fixed time each day. The average birth weight of white male infants in the United States is 3,400 grams (7½ pounds); white female infants weigh approximately 3,200 grams (7 pounds). The weight of 80 percent of full-term newborns falls within the range of 2,900 to 4,100 grams (6 pounds 5 ounces to 9 pounds 2 ounces). Black and Asian infants are generally smaller at birth, while those of northern European ancestry tend to be larger.

Newborns lose from 5 to 10 percent of their birth weight in the first 3 to 5 days after birth but generally regain it in another week. The weight loss is attributed to a loss of fluid from body tissues and to a relatively low food and fluid intake.

Skin   Examine the newborn's skin (under strong natural light) for hair distribution, color, edema, ecchymoses, pigmentary changes, scaliness and desquamation, and hemangiomas. Palpate the consistency of the underlying dermis by lifting a skin fold between your thumb and forefinger. This will give you an estimate of the degree of development of the underlying fatty tissue. During the first 24 hours after birth, the newborn's skin is generally smooth and reddish and may be covered with vernix caseosa, which disappears in about a day if it is not removed. The redness of his skin is due to a high concentration of red cells in the blood vessels, which are closer to the skin's surface because of the lack of subcutaneous fat [3]. The red skin blush changes to a pink hue in the following day or so, and the skin becomes more flaky. Marked scaliness and desquamation are a sign of postmaturity. Slight desquamation is normal over palms and soles and in the groin.

The infant's extremities may appear cyanotic after birth (acrocyanosis) due to immature peripheral circulation, with the feet usually showing more cyanosis than the hands. This is common in newborns less than 3 days old. In addition to being cyanotic, the baby's feet may be cold to touch. Peripheral cyanosis, mottling, cool extremities, and increased activity may indicate cold stress. The infant who becomes cyanotic when crying may be showing signs of some forms of congenital heart disease; if he is cyanotic at rest with relief upon crying, he may be exhibiting signs of pulmonary dysfunction. An infant who has been previously well and suddenly becomes cyanotic and apneic may have thick mucus obstructing his upper respiratory tract. Any generalized pallor in the infant may be due to poor cardiac function, anemia from hemorrhagic disease, or acute blood loss. Pale conjunctiva and mucous membrane of his mouth may also indicate anemia.

Inspect his skin, his creases, fingernails, and umbilical cord for a green staining caused by meconium in the amniotic fluid. In other than babies delivered in the breech position, this may indicate a period of anoxic stress in utero before birth.

Physiologic jaundice is noticeable in less than one-half of all newborns. It generally appears on the second or third day, peaks at about a week, and has disappeared in 2 weeks. It first appears in the skin over the face or upper body and then progresses to encompass a larger area. The initial faint yellow may deepen into orange and become noticeable in the conjunctivae of the eyes. Jaundice may be difficult to observe in infants of low birth weight; because of their decreased subcutaneous fat, the capillaries are close to the surface of the skin, and the color of hemoglobin obscures the jaundice.

Jaundice in the newborn is caused by immaturity of the liver. As red blood cells are broken down, low levels of liver enzymes (mainly glucuronyl transferase) are not able to conjugate bilirubin, and its excretion from the bowel may be delayed. In the newborn, jaundice becomes noticeable when total serum bilirubin rises from a normal level of approximately 1 milligram per 100 milliliters to 6 milligrams per 100 milliliters. Unless there is a pathologic hemolytic condition, the levels do not usually exceed 10 to 12 milligrams per 100 milliliters during the newborn period. The bilirubin levels in breast-fed infants are often higher and the jaundice is more prolonged than in infants who are bottle-fed. One line of research into breast milk jaundice holds that pregnanediol in breast milk inhibits the action of glucuronyl transferase; another links high milk lipase activity with the jaundice. Some research indicates that if breast-feeding is discontinued for 24 hours, presumably allowing glucuronyl transferase to become operative, resumption of breast-feeding no longer has the inhibitory effect [2, 16, 18, 24a].

The presence of edema in the newborn is another important observation for you to make. If the infant has been supine for a period of time, he may have some dependent edema over his buttocks, back, and occiput. The subcutaneous tissues around his eyes, legs, hands, and feet may occasionally be edematous for several days. The fine wrinkles over the dorsal aspect of the hands and feet of the normal newborn are not discernible in an edematous infant. Severe pitting edema may be due to heart failure, congenital heart disease, erythroblastosis, or electrolyte imbalance.

In the immediate period after birth, there may be marked edema and ecchymoses over his presenting part. In a vertex presentation there may be significant edema of his scalp (*caput succedaneum*), which regresses in about 2 days without treatment. This extravasation of serum into the soft tissues of the scalp occurs over the area that was encircled by the cervix; it is particularly evident when labor has been prolonged, causing membranes to rupture and the cervix to fail to dilate fully (Fig. 16-2).

In breech presentations, there may be edema and ecchymoses of the newborn's buttocks or feet, while in shoulder presentations, his shoulder and arm may be affected. Ecchymoses may appear on other parts of his body following a difficult

Figure 16-2. Caput succedaneum, a diffuse edematous swelling of the soft tissues of the scalp overlying the presenting part, which may cross the suture lines. It is caused by pressure of the cervix on the fetus's head during labor.

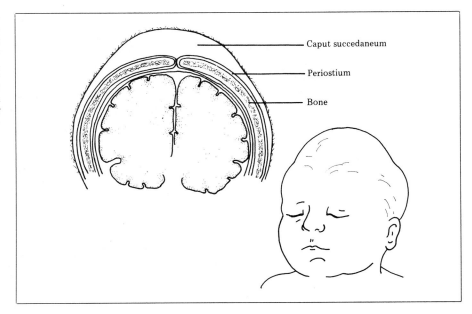

delivery, or they may indicate an infection or bleeding problem. The serum bilirubin may increase when ecchymoses are extensive [19].

Pinpoint hemorrhages (petechiae) may also be seen on the newborn's skin due to increased intravascular pressure, infection, or thrombocytopenia. These hemorrhages generally regress in 24 to 48 hours.

Test for petechiae, jaundice, and ecchymoses by applying direct pressure to the skin, either with your fingers or with a microscope slide. When both index fingers or both thumbs are placed on the baby's skin and then drawn apart while maintaining pressure, petechiae, jaundice, and ecchymoses will remain upon blanching, while red rashes caused by local vascular engorgement will disappear. You may also check for jaundice by examining the mucous membrane of the newborn's mouth.

The most common red rash found on the newborn is called *newborn rash* or *erythema toxicum*; it usually appears on the trunk and diaper area. The rash consists of pinkish-red macules, which frequently contain a central papule (Fig. 16-3) which may be yellow or white, depending on the infant's serum bilirubin level. Since the vesicles contain eosinophils, they give the appearance of being pathologic and are often confused with staphylococcal infections. In order to differentiate between erythema toxicum and a staphylococcal infection, several of the lesions might be circled with a pen. Usually the lesions of erythema toxicum disappear in a few hours, whereas septic lesions will not. The entire rash usually regresses in 48 hours. The rash usually appears around the second day, but new lesions may appear for the first week or more.

Hemangiomas are vascular lesions that are usually present at birth. Port-wine stain (nevus flammeus) appears at birth as a flat, purple or dark-red lesion, appearing most commonly around the scalp and face. Those found over the bridge of the nose may fade, but the others usually do not and require cosmetics for concealment (Fig. 16-4).

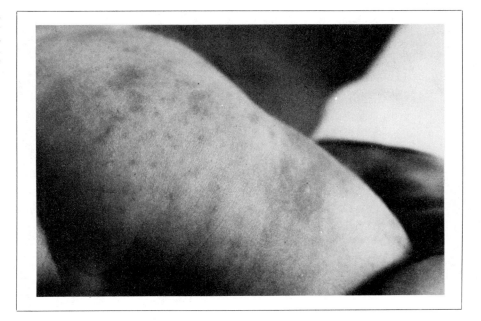

Strawberry hemangiomas may be present at birth, but most often they appear 2 or 3 weeks after birth. They are elevated bright-red lesions containing a collection of small immature blood vessels. They usually regress before the age of 4, but it may take as long as 10 years.

Stork bites (telangiectatic nevi) are flat red or purple lesions with irregular edges, found most often on the back of the neck, lower occiput, upper eyelid, and bridge of the nose. The lesions are areas of capillary dilatation that enlarge and fill when the infant cries. They are very common and disappear in approximately 2 years.

A rather rare nonpathologic condition is *harlequin color change*. When the infant is placed on his side, the dependent half of his body turns red, while the upper half becomes pale. The color changes from the head to the pubic area and stops laterally, abruptly at the midline. Vasomotor instability and the effects of gravity are suggested as causes [23].

In black and Asian infants and those of southern European heritage, areas of blue pigmentation are commonly found over the lower back, sacrum, and buttocks. These *mongolian spots*, which parents often confuse with bruises, are nonpathologic and usually regress by 4 years of age (Fig. 16-5).

Another very common finding is *milia neonatorum* (Fig. 16-6), which consists of enlarged sebaceous glands usually found about the nose but also on the chin, cheeks, and forehead. They usually regress in several days to a week or two. Because they resemble whiteheads, mothers are often tempted to squeeze them; they should be told of the risk of infection from squeezing and cautioned not to do so.

Café-au-lait spots are brown macules usually less than 3 centimeters in diameter. These spots, which are occasionally seen in newborns, are not usually significant, but children with large spots or a large number of spots have been known to develop an underlying neurofibromatosis [31].

Figure 16-4. A. Port-wine stain (nevus flammeus). B. Strawberry hemangioma. C. Stork bites (telangiectatic nevi). (Courtesy of Mead Johnson Laboratories, Evansville, Ind.)

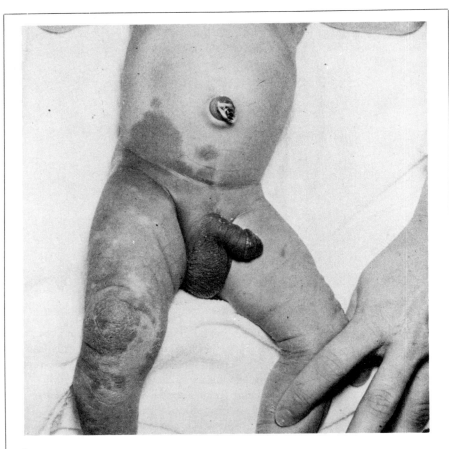

A

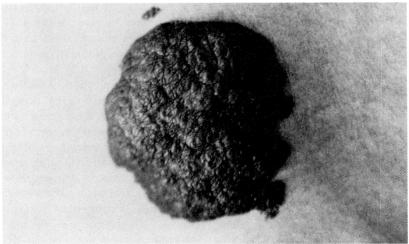

B

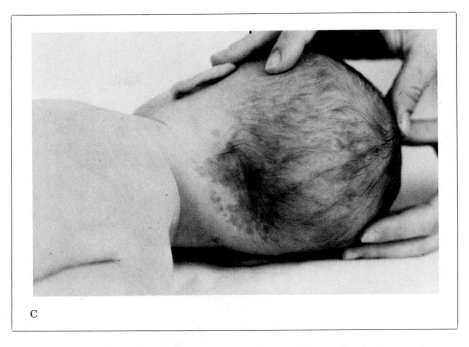

C

Nails   Nails of the full-term infant usually extend beyond the nailbed whereas in preterm infants they are shorter. Spoon-shaped, dysplastic, or absent nails may be indicative of disorders such as fetal alcohol and anticonvulsant syndromes [31].

Head   Examine the newborn's head and face for symmetry, paralysis, weakness, shape, swelling, and movement. The infant's head generally has a biparietal circumference of 33 to 35 centimeters (13–14 inches), approximately 2 centimeters (1 inch) larger than the chest. This measurement is made around the greatest circumference, over the occipital protuberance, and ending in the middle of the forehead (Fig. 16-7).

During the first 24 hours after birth, the infant's head may be equal to or smaller than his chest because of the molding or overriding of the skull bones as the head attempted to accommodate itself to the birth canal (Fig. 16-8). There is generally more molding when the infant's head is engaged for prolonged periods and in first-born infants. There is relatively little or no molding with a breech presentation or in babies delivered by elective cesarean delivery. The molding generally regresses in 24 to 28 hours after birth.

If the newborn's head is over 4 centimeters (1.6 inches) larger than the chest, and this is true of successive measurements over several days, increased intracranial pressure is suspected. Malnourished infants may have significantly larger heads in relation to their chests than normal newborns; the smaller chest measurements may be due to depleted subcutaneous tissue [19].

In addition to measuring the newborn's head circumference, palpate his fontanelles and suture lines. The anterior fontanelle should be open; the posterior may be closed. The size of the fontanelles may be decreased as a result of molding, but this disappears as molding regresses. Check the tension of the fontanelle.

Figure 16-5. Mongolian spots. (Courtesy of Mead Johnson Laboratories, Evansville, Ind.)

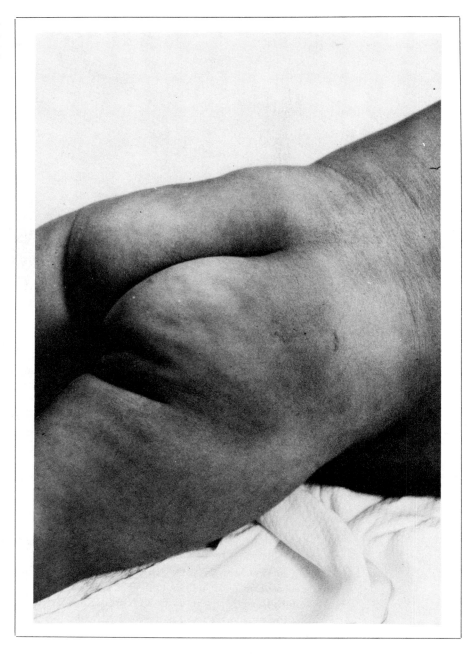

Normally the anterior fontanelle is soft and concave or flat, but with increased intracranial pressure it becomes firm, convex, or bulging; with dehydration it may appear depressed. Since parents are often concerned about touching the infant's "soft spot," inform them that the fontanelle is covered with several layers of protective tissues, so that it can be touched and washed. Explain to them that it will remain open for about the next year and a half to allow for brain growth.

Figure 16-6. Milia neonatorum. (Courtesy of Mead Johnson Laboratories, Evansville, Ind.)

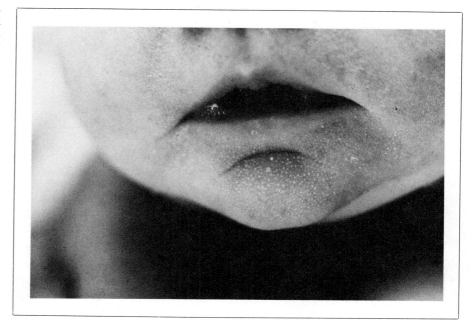

Figure 16-7. Measuring head circumference.

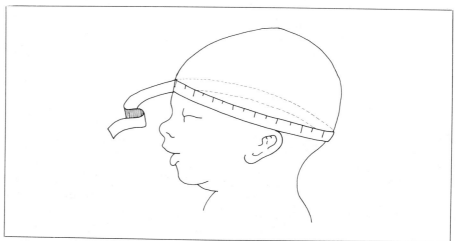

Palpate the suture lines to assess their degree of separation, which may be greater in malnourished infants, whose cranial bones may not have developed sufficiently. The separation may also be greater in infants with increased intracranial pressure due to hydrocephalus, subdural hematomas, cerebral edema, or meningitis. Sometimes due to molding during the birth process, the infant's cranial bones will override each other. This can usually be palpated during the first 24 to 48 hours.

Check the infant's head for *caput succedaneum* and for *cephalohematomas*, the latter of which are collections of blood between the bones and the periosteum (Fig. 16-9). These lesions are found most commonly in the parietal area and in infants who experienced prolonged head compression during labor or rapid traumatic

Figure 16-8. Newborn molding, or overriding of the skull bones.

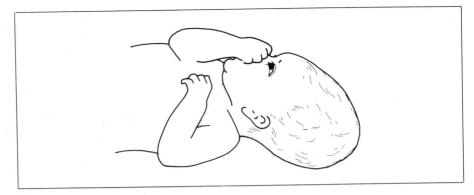

Figure 16-9. Cephalohematoma, a collection of blood between the bones and the periosteum. The swelling does not cross the suture lines and usually feels firm around the periphery and has a soft center.

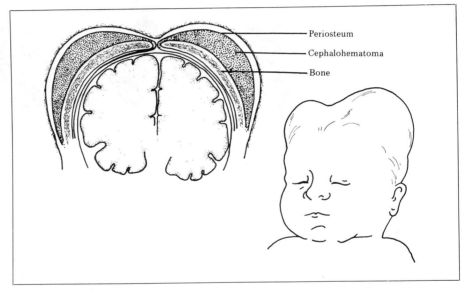

passage through the birth canal. The incidence is also higher in first-born infants.

A cephalohematoma, which is rarely present at birth, may enlarge during the first 3 days. Unlike caput succedaneum, it does not extend across the suture lines, although more than one cranial bone may show a swelling. If the hematoma crosses suture lines, it may indicate a skull fracture [3]. Upon palpation, a cephalohematoma usually is firm around the periphery, with a softer center.

These lesions are absorbed over variable periods of time, depending on their size. While smaller hematomas are rapidly absorbed, the larger ones calcify and are gradually incorporated into the enlarging skull.

The skull may also contain localized areas of softening (craniotabes), commonly along the suture lines in the flat cranial bones, especially the parietal bones. Upon fingertip pressure these areas become indented but resume their shape when the pressure is removed. Craniotabes may be caused by an increase in intracranial pressure or by disturbances of the mother's calcium metabolism [28]. The areas of softening generally calcify rapidly after birth and seldom can be identified later.

Figure 16-10. Facial paralysis.

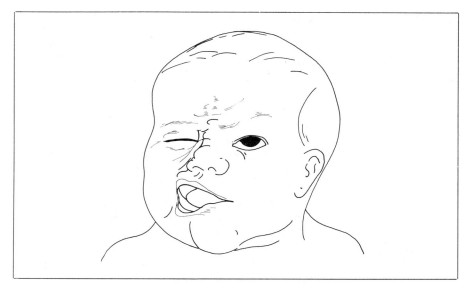

Check the infant's facial movements for symmetry. If there is injury to a facial nerve from trauma at delivery, the affected side of the mouth will fail to retract backward and upward when the infant cries (Fig. 16-10). The majority of these paralyses resolve spontaneously within several days, although total recovery may require several weeks or months [9]; the paralysis may rarely be permanent.

Facial asymmetry may also be due to the position assumed in utero, for example, when the fetus's shoulder has been firmly pressed into his neck. This distortion generally regresses in a few weeks or months, depending on its severity.

Eyes   The newborn has a tendency to keep his eyes closed, making examination of them difficult. He also has a moderate photophobia and will promptly close his eyes on exposure to direct bright light. He will likewise close his eyes in response to loud noises or when his lashes are touched. However, a fully mature protective blink reflex is absent in the newborn. When attempting to examine the infant's eyes, you will find that trying to force his eyelids open meets with resistance. Shading his eyes by placing your hand on the side of his face may induce the infant to open them spontaneously. Slowly raising him from a supine to a sitting position may also be effective (baby-doll reflex).

Begin your examination of the newborn's eyes by noting the external features of the eyes in relation to the face and to each other. Check the size of the eye as well as the angle of an imaginary line between the inner and outer canthus. Normally the outer canthus is slightly higher than the inner canthus in black and white babies. When the slant is pronounced, Down's syndrome may be suspected. Note an epicanthal fold if it is present and the presence and distribution of eyebrows.

While the newborn is quietly alert or semi-dozing, examine his eyelids for any signs of trauma, edema, or ptosis. Sometimes you will see capillary hemangiomas over the eyelids. When the newborn's eyes are open, inspect his conjunctivae for discharge, vasodilation, jaundice, erythema, edema, and hemorrhages.

The sclerae of most full-term newborns are white. Preterm infants have thin sclerae which look bluish. A *distinctly* blue sclera is abnormal in a full-term newborn and suggests possible connective tissue disorders, such as osteogenesis imperfecta [31].

The newborn's pupils should be equal and should constrict in bright light. A small pupil in one eye accompanied by ptosis of the same eye suggests a lesion of the cervical sympathetic chain. In that case there will also be absence of sweating on that side of the face. Since the pupillary light reflex is subcortical, its presence does not rule out cortical blindness [31].

Inspect the newborn's cornea using a point source of bright light (otoscope head) cast tangentially across his eye from the temporal side. Note any cloudiness. The normal newborn's cornea should be shiny and glassy, but the preterm infant may have some haziness in the corneal area during the first week. An unusually large cornea may indicate congenital glaucoma.

Eye color is usually grayish-blue in white infants and brown in dark-skinned infants. Final deposition of pigment and final eye color do not appear for 6 to 12 months, although changes may be seen at 3 months. Likewise, the lacrimal apparatus is not mature at birth, and tears do not accompany crying for approximately 1 month.

Parents often inquire about the baby's ability to see in the immediate newborn period. They are often surprised to learn that their infant can perceive and differentiate between objects with different patterns, colors, and brightness. (For further discussion of this point see Chap. 15.) They are also often concerned with their newborn's transient "crossed-eyes" (strabismus) or jerky uneven eye movements (nystagmus). The parents need to be assured that these immature and uncoordinated eye movements are normal in the newborn and are the result of poor control of the eye muscles; the eye movements should become more coordinated by the third or fourth month. Infants exhibiting strabismus after the age of 6 months should generally be referred for treatment.

For approximately 48 hours after delivery the newborn's eyelids may be swollen, generally due to pressure on his head during delivery. The pressure may also cause rupture of capillaries in the sclera, resulting in subconjunctival hemorrhages, which appear as a red crescent band, either on the side of the iris or completely surrounding it. These hemorrhages are common; they appear in approximately 40 percent of all newborns and regress in about 2 weeks.

Another common finding is chemical conjunctivitis due to the instillation of silver nitrate drops at birth. The eyelids are edematous, the conjunctiva is red, and a purulent discharge may be present. The infant is usually treated with a warm saline eye irrigation several times a day, and the discharge usually disappears in a day or two. Similar discharges may be due to infections caused by staphylococcus, gonococcus, or a variety of gram-negative rods [19]. Generally these are not evident as soon after birth as chemical conjunctivitis.

Nose   The newborn's nose should look symmetrical and relatively flat. Since the infant breathes through his nose and not through his mouth, obstructions such as mucus, choanal atresia, or stenosis will cause varying degrees of respiratory distress. Examine the infant for adequate air flowing through his nose by holding a wisp of cotton close to each nostril. As the baby exhales, the cotton will move away if there is adequate exchange. If there is not, you may have to open his mouth to establish an efficient airway. Ordinarily his nose does not move with normal respiration. Unilateral choanal atresia sometimes remains undiscovered until much later when the child begins to have persistent nasal discharge from the affected side or unequal noisy nasal breathing, commonly during upper respiratory infections.

Ears   In examining the infant's ears, check their formation, position, and amount of cartilage present. Cartilage that gives the pinna a firm feeling is indicative of a full-term infant. The ears of a preterm baby are softer because they have less cartilage.

With the ear in a normal position, the helix is on the same plane as the angle of the eye (Fig. 16-11). Ears that are twisted or rotated often appear to be low set but actually are not. Genuinely low-set ears may indicate Potter's syndrome (bilateral renal agenesis) or one of several other chromosomal abnormalities.

Examine closely the formation as well as the position of the external ear. Significant flattening of the superior helix and large flabby ears that slant forward are often found in infants with unilateral absence of the kidney and congenital obstruction of the urinary tract [20]. Urogenital anomalies are often associated with malformations of the ear, since the embryonic development of both occurs during the same period.

Occasionally, accessory auricles are found around the ear in the form of small skin tags. They are usually treated by tying them off with a ligature.

Since the auditory nerve tracts are mature at birth, infants are able to hear well within a few days. By this time their eustachian tubes are clear of fluid and mucus. Testing of a newborn's hearing can be done by observing his responses to loud noises such as a hand clap or a shout.

Figure 16-11. Normal position of the ears, with the helix on the same plane as the angle of the eye.

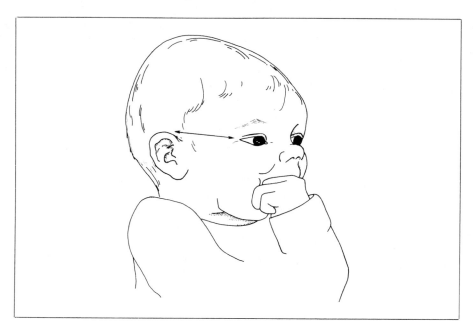

Mouth   Inspect the newborn's lips, gums, tongue, palate, and oropharynx. Check his mouth for palate closure, size of tongue, presence of teeth, and signs of infection. When you examine the newborn's mouth, it is best to have the baby cry rather than to try to visualize his mouth and pharynx by depressing his tongue.

A small mouth (microstomia) occurs in a few generalized syndromes (trisomies 18 and 21). Microstomia is seen in mucopolysaccharidosis but is otherwise rare. Corners of the mouth that turn down ("fish mouth") are uncommon but may be seen in fetal alcohol syndrome [31].

Cleft lip and palate are obvious abnormalities. Cleft lip is an abnormality that may occur alone or with cleft palate. It can vary in degree from a small opening in the lip (most commonly on the left side) to a complete separation (usually bilateral), which extends into the nasal floor. It is possible that infants with large defects may also have midline brain defects and need further evaluation. Check for cleft palate by placing a gloved finger in the infant's mouth. (This also can be used to check the sucking reflex.)

About one infant in 2,000 will be born with teeth (predeciduous), usually the lower central incisors. As a rule the roots are poorly formed or absent, and only the crowns are calcified. If the teeth become loose or interfere with feeding, they should be removed. Occasionally true deciduous teeth erupt shortly after birth; these can be differentiated from the predeciduous teeth by x-ray and should not be removed.

Epstein's pearls, which are small white nodules (accumulations of epithelial cells) usually found on either side of the hard palate, are often mistaken for teeth by parents. They are of no significance and usually disappear a few weeks after birth.

The newborn's tongue may appear to be large but true macroglossia is rare. An excessively large tongue may be indicative of cretinism, Down's syndrome, or other abnormalities. Occasionally the frenulum of the tongue gives the appearance of what parents call "tongue tie" (frenulum linguae). This sharp thin ridge of tissue begins at the base of the tongue, runs along its undersurface, and extends far forward to the tip of the tongue. Previously it was clipped because it was thought to interfere with speech and eating; however, it is now known that this is not the case. In addition, because of the close proximity of a large vein which may be severed when it is clipped, there is danger to the infant from bleeding and infection if the procedure is performed.

Sometimes sucking blisters, which appear as rounded thickened areas, may be found in the midline of the upper lip. Sucking calluses may also be seen, appearing as dried crusts or plaques, which run horizontally along the middle of the lips. During the first few weeks, the older ones are shed and new ones form.

The mouth should also be carefully inspected for signs of infection. A fungal infection (thrush), caused by *Candida albicans*, is occasionally found in the newborn; it is transmitted from the mother's vaginal secretions during birth. It appears as white or gray-white plaques on the tongue and mucous membrane and can easily be mistaken for curdled milk (Fig. 16-12), but the plaques cannot be wiped off or brushed away as milk curds can. Thrush is treated with a solution of aqueous gentian violet or nystatin suspension (100,000 units/ml) swabbed over the mucous membranes 3 or 4 times a day.

Figure 16-12. Newborn thrush caused by *Candida albicans*. (Courtesy of Mead Johnson Laboratories, Evansville, Ind.)

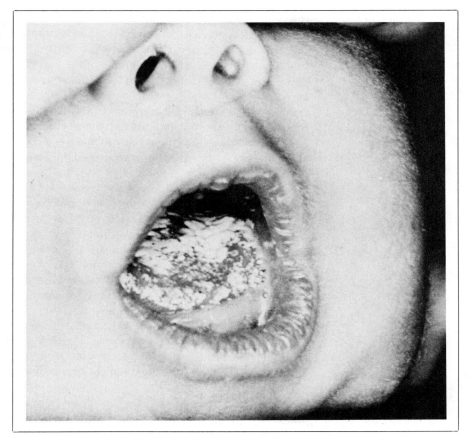

Neck Inspect and palpate the newborn's neck. You will notice that it appears short, especially in infants who have more fat deposits. An extra thickening of skin in female infants at the posterolateral area may be indicative of the "web neck" commonly found in Turner's syndrome [31].

Palpate the newborn's neck along his cervical spine, over his sternocleidomastoid and trapezius muscles, and anteriorly to locate the larynx, cricoid area, and thyroid gland. While you palpate his neck, palpate each clavicle for possible fractures, especially if he has a history of difficult or breech delivery.

Sometimes a newborn will have torticollis, a spasmodic, one-sided contraction of neck muscles, so that his head tilts toward the affected side and his chin turns away from that side. Usually this results from a hematoma of the sternocleidomastoid muscle, occurring either in utero or during a traumatic delivery. Usually no treatment is required.

Thyroid enlargement is rare except in endemic goiter areas and in newborns whose mothers have taken either medication containing iodine or antithyroid drugs. Such goiters are usually easily palpable and may also be visible. Rarely would they be large enough to cause respiratory distress.

The presence of palpable lymph nodes in the newborn's neck area is unusual and suggests the possibility of congenital infection.

Chest and Lungs   In evaluating the soft and bony thoracic tissues, the lungs, and the heart, you will use inspection, percussion, palpation, and auscultation. First inspect the size and shape of the thoracic cage. Measure the chest circumference across the nipple line. The average chest circumference of the normal full-term newborn is 33 ± 3 centimeters (12–13 inches), about 2 centimeters smaller than the head circumference.

Palpate the newborn's sternum and ribs to determine any asymmetry in contour or number and to locate any masses that might be present. At the lower end of the newborn's sternum you will find a small, sharp, cartilaginous mass, the xiphoid process. Parents sometimes need to be reassured that this finding is normal [31].

Inspect the newborn's breasts and nipples for number, symmetry, size, color, turgor, and discharge. Extra nipples (small pigmented areas) are sometimes present in a line vertical to the main nipple on the right or left side. The full-term newborn's areola is stippled, has a raised edge, and a diameter of at least 0.75 centimeter. Nipple and areola size are less pronounced in preterm babies and serve as an aid in estimating gestational age.

Frequently newborns experience breast enlargement at around the third day of life due to the withdrawal of maternal hormones, particularly estrogen, which have crossed the placental membrane during pregnancy. The engorged breasts may also secrete a thin white fluid known as *witch's milk*, probably related to the presence of prolactin in the newborn. Caution parents against massaging or squeezing their infant's engorged breasts, to prevent the occurrence of breast abscesses or mastitis. The enlargement generally regresses in about 2 weeks.

Pulmonary Status   There is a wide range of what are considered "normal findings" for the newborn's pulmonary examination. Pulmonary evaluations are influenced by the time that the examination is done after birth, the sleep-awake status of the baby, when he was fed, the drugs his mother took prior to and during delivery, and his physical environment.

Observe the infant's respiratory pattern before he is disturbed. Count his respirations for a full minute. Normal newborns breathe at a rate of between 40 and 60 breaths per minute. Rapid rates are usual for a few hours after birth; the respirations also tend to be shallow, with an irregular rhythm.

Note the environmental temperature. Extremes in temperature can either slow or accelerate the newborn's respiratory rate. In the case of a cesarean birth his respiratory rate may be higher for the first 4 to 6 hours after birth than that of the infant born vaginally; presumably this is related to the delay in disappearance of fluid from the pulmonary tree of the infant born by cesarean.

Many newborns exhibit periodic breathing (resumption of respiration after a 5–15 second period without respiration), especially those at higher altitudes and those who are preterm. Periodic breathing episodes decrease over time.

Observe the symmetry of the newborn's chest expansion. If it is not symmetrical, there may be problems such as diaphragmatic hernia and pneumothorax. Observe the newborn's use of his respiratory muscles.

The infant's respiratory movements are mainly diaphragmatic, since his thoracic muscles are weak. His intercostal muscles remain relatively still, as his abdomen expands with inspiration and falls with expiration. Frequently on inspiration his soft lower ribs tend to be drawn in as his abdomen protrudes, which is often apparent when the infant cries. Under abnormal conditions the newborn will use his abdominal muscles to accomplish respiration. You will see a "see-saw" breathing pattern since his abdomen and chest will move asynchronously up and down.

Abnormal respiratory signs include [19]:

1. Generalized cyanosis (most obvious and most serious).
2. Sustained respiratory rate in excess of 60 respirations per minute (tachypnea) when measured for 30 seconds or more on several occasions.
3. Irregular respirations associated with repeated apneic episodes often caused by central nervous system depression from hypoxia or intracranial hemorrhage. These may also signal sepsis, hypoglycemia, or cold stress.
4. Retractions, which indicate obstruction to the air flow through the respiratory tract. Upon inspiration the thoracic wall retracts between the ribs, above the clavicles, and below the inferior costal margins.
5. Respiratory grunt, in which the infant attempts to retain air and increase PO_2; an audible sigh during each expiration is equivalent.
6. Flaring of the nostrils (seen with air hunger).

Breath sounds may be difficult to evaluate. The newborn's chest is small, and breath sounds are transmitted freely throughout. Use a warm stethoscope with a small diaphragm and bell not more than 2 centimeters in diameter. With practice, you will be able to detect the exchange of air in the lungs, particularly if there is a difference in exchange between the two lungs. Decreased breath sounds or delayed air entry is heard with shallow respirations, hyaline membrane disease, atelectasis, and emphysema. The newborn's posture may also influence your findings since infants who lie in one position aerate certain portions of their lungs better than others.

You may also hear rales, which are caused as air rushes through fluid in the terminal bronchioles and alveoli. The sound is crackling in nature and may be heard in infants in the first minutes of life or in infants with hyaline membrane disease, pneumonia, and pulmonary edema. Occasionally rales are heard in normal babies. Rhonchi, which are coarse sounds that resemble snoring, are caused as air rushes through fluid contained in the large bronchi. They can be heard after aspiration of fluid or feedings [19].

Cardiac Status   An examination of the newborn's heart is complex because of many factors that cause findings to change during the first hours and days of his life: changing cardiac function and changing systemic and pulmonary vascular capacity and resistance, gestational age, amount of time after birth, behavioral state, environmental temperature, and maternal or neonatal medications to which he has been exposed. For purposes of collecting the greatest data base, ideally you should examine the newborn's heart at birth and again at 6, 24, and 72 hours after birth. Of these times, 24 and 72 hours after birth are the most important.

Begin your assessment of cardiac status by checking the color of the newborn's skin and mucous membranes for cyanosis (blue), pallor (white), plethora (purple), or normal coloration (pink). In darkly pigmented infants, check those areas that are likely to be less pigmented such as the tongue, gingivae, and nailbeds. Note the intensity and quality of light in the room since it will influence your findings. Use natural light whenever possible.

If you detect cyanosis, record the location, the effect of crying on the cyanosis, and the change in color over time. As mentioned previously, acrocyanosis (distal extremities) or cyanosis of the face or scalp may be normal in the first hours of the newborn's life. Cyanosis of mucous membranes during crying may also be normal in the immediate newborn period but should not persist beyond that time.

If you detect pallor, note its distribution over the newborn's body. Generalized pallor is suggestive of peripheral vasoconstriction, infection, cardiac failure, and very low hemoglobin. Plethora, on the other hand, may stem from a combination of saturated and unsaturated hemoglobin and may be associated with cardiopulmonary and neurologic abnormalities [31].

If you notice sweating in the newborn despite a normal environmental temperature, it may be a sign of congestive heart failure or drug withdrawal if it is accompanied by other pertinent signs and symptoms.

Assess the infant's capillary filling time by depressing his skin over one central and one peripheral area. Note the time it takes for the blanched skin to return to its normal color. If it takes longer than 3 seconds, it is probably an abnormal finding [31].

Using your index fingers, examine the newborn's pulses when he is resting quietly. Note their presence or absence, their amplitude, and symmetry. Check the pedal pulses on both sides. Since the newborn's pedal pulses are not always detectable, their absence is not necessarily abnormal. Palpate both femoral areas. If the femoral pulses are absent, it is indicative of inadequate aortic blood flow (coarctation of the aorta), and if they are significantly bounding, it may indicate congenital heart disease [14]. You should find it easy to palpate both brachial and radial pulses as well.

Scanlon et al. [31] recommend that blood pressure be taken in every newborn using a cuff with a width of about one-third or one-half the circumference of the extremity being examined. The best method of routine indirect systolic and diastolic blood pressure determination in the newborn seems to be artery wall motion detection using a pulse sensor attached to a Doppler ultrasonic transducer. Most newborns weighing more than 3 kilograms will have a systolic blood pressure between 60 and 80 millimeters of mercury and a diastolic reading between 35 and 55 millimeters of mercury.

Using a single finger on the newborn's chest, begin to palpate the precordium by locating the point of maximal impulse (PMI). You will usually find the PMI on his left side in the fourth to fifth intercostal space, medial to the midclavicular line; in the immediate newborn period it may be found farther to the right. Palpate across the infant's entire anterior chest since the PMI can be shifted by either congenital or acquired intrathoracic problems such as pneumothorax, diaphragmatic hernia, or dextrocardia [31].

Next, auscultate the newborn's heart. Count the heart rate for one full minute. The heart rate in the newborn ranges between 100 and 160 beats per minute. At birth the rate tends to be at the higher end of the scale, but it then falls; however, during crying it may reach 200.

It may be difficult to detect abnormalities in the rhythm of the newborn's heart. It is normal for brief periods of deceleration to be followed by periods of acceleration. Because his heart rate is so rapid, at first you may find it difficult to evaluate his heart sounds. They are usually loud and clear, the second sound being higher in pitch and sharper than the first. Third and fourth sounds are rarely heard in the newborn. Murmurs are common, although the great majority of those detected in this period are transitory and not associated with anomalies. Most are systolic ejection murmurs of a vibrating quality heard in the second left intercostal space. Some may be explained by decreasing pulmonary vascular resistance and/or changing blood flow through the ductus arteriosus [31].

Abdomen and Back The newborn's abdomen is cylindrical, appears to protrude slightly, and moves synchronously with the chest in respiration. If his abdomen is distended, the skin appears tightly drawn and the subcutaneous vessels can easily be seen. Distention may be due to the enlargement of a solid abdominal organ, to bowel obstruction (especially if peristalsis is visible), or to infection. If the newborn's abdomen appears flat and flabby, abdominal muscle tone may be decreased due to drug or neurologic depression. Auscultate bowel sounds for presence, quality, and intensity.

Palpate the newborn's abdomen when he appears quiet and relaxed. Giving him a pacifier will help. After locating the margin of his liver below his ribs on the right side, place the palmar surface of your right index figure just above the groin parallel to the right costal margin. Apply gentle pressure and gradually move your finger upward until the liver edge slips below it, usually about 1 to 2 centimeters below the costal margin. The normal newborn liver edge is sharp; a rounded edge may be suggestive of congestive heart failure, especially when accompanied by other relevant signs. When you palpate the anterior liver surface, you should find that it is firm, not hard or nodular [31].

You should use a similar technique to palpate the newborn's spleen on the left side. Most of the time you will be able to feel only its tip. If the spleen itself is palpable, it is probably enlarged.

Palpate the rest of the newborn's abdomen for any masses. You will probably find a gap between the two rectus muscles, which is especially visible when the baby cries. You may feel an umbilical hernia, which is a defect in his anterior abdominal wall.

Palpate the newborn's kidneys for size, shape, and texture. This may be done most easily within 6 hours after birth, before the intestines fill with air. With the newborn supine, support his upper trunk and occiput and flex his hip to relax his abdominal musculature. On the same side as the flexed hip, place the fingers of your free hand posteriorly on his flank. Place your thumb on his abdomen and press posteriorly to meet your fingers, moving it up, down, and laterally. Another technique which may be helpful involves placing your hand in the posterior flank for upward pressure, then using the fingers of the other hand to apply gentle downward pressure toward the posterior (Fig. 16-13). Enlargement of the kidneys usually suggests hydronephrosis.

The ability of the kidney to concentrate urine and to excrete a solute load is considerably less in a newborn than in an older child or adult. Urine may contain uric acid crystals, which appear on the diaper as reddish blotches that may be mistaken for blood. Uric acid crystals may yield false positive results if you test the infant's urine for albumin [33].

Figure 16-13. Palpating the kidney in the newborn.

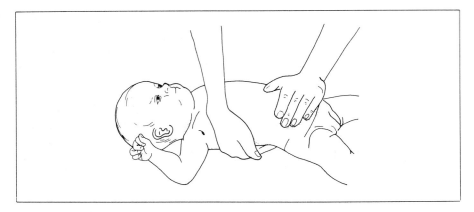

In addition to palpating the kidneys, you should check for bladder distention, which appears as a firm globular mass that can be felt in the suprapubic region. Usually the infant voids within the first 24 hours; a record is kept of the number of voidings as well as any unusual characteristics. After the first few days, the infant voids from 10 to 15 times a day.

On the admission examination, check the umbilical cord for the normal number of blood vessels. A single artery is often associated with congenital problems, especially renal abnormalities. Occasionally a newborn may have an *umbilical hernia*, which is a defect in the anterior abdominal wall. All but the larger ones close spontaneously by approximately 2 to 3 years of age, as the child's abdominal muscles strengthen. The *cutis navel* (skin navel) is often confused with an umbilical hernia (Fig. 16-14). In the cutis navel the cord stump protrudes from the abdominal wall and is covered by abdominal skin; it cannot be returned to the abdomen as an umbilical hernia can, and it becomes flatter with time.

Examine the infant's anal area for fistulas, presence of anus, and tone of anal

Figure 16-14. Umbilical hernia and cutis navel.

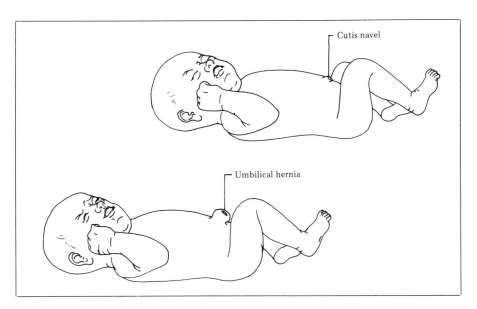

sphincter. Meconium is usually passed in the first 24 hours, but its appearance may be delayed. However, if there is no stool by the end of the first day, check the patency of the anus by passing a small tube into the anus no further than 1 centimeter (½ inch) [19]. The passage of meconium persists for about 48 hours, followed by transitional stools and milk stools. Transitional stools are a combination of the tarry black color of meconium and the yellow of milk stools. The stool gradually changes to a golden yellow of soft consistency if the infant is breast-fed or a light yellow of pasty consistency if the infant is bottle-fed. The number of stools decreases from six daily to two daily as the infant grows older. After several weeks a breast-fed infant may have one to three bowel movements per week. As long as the baby is healthy and alert and his abdomen is soft, it matters little if he has several stools a day or only one or two a week.

While the infant is in a prone position, check to see that the spinal column is of normal curvature. Lateral curvature on the first examination may be due to positioning in utero. Sometimes you may find a sacrococcygeal cleft or pilonidal dimple; this is generally benign provided that it does not connect with an underlying sinus or deeper structure. Palpate the spine for the presence of any masses that may be meningomyeloceles. They may be covered by skin, subcutaneous tissue, or meninges. If you find decreased anal sphincter tone or neurologic deficits in the lower extremities, a spinal cord defect may be present.

Genitalia   In examining a full-term male infant, you should be able to palpate the testes in the scrotal sac, which is wrinkled and, provided that he is warm, hangs loosely from the infant's body. During the examination close off the inguinal canal with the thumb and index finger to prevent the testes from slipping back into it (Fig. 16-15). When the infant is chilled, the dartos muscle layer within the scrotum contracts, making the sac appear rather small and very close to his body. Parents are often concerned when this happens and should be informed that the scrotum will appear larger and hang more loosely when their baby is warm. In preterm infants the testes may still be in the inguinal canal; the scrotal sac is smaller and less wrinkled and is held more closely to the body.

Examine the glans penis of the newborn male to locate the urethral opening.

Figure 16-15. Examining the genitalia of a male infant, using the thumb and forefinger to block the inguinal canal to prevent the testes from slipping back into it.

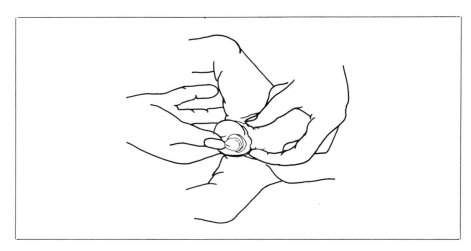

When the opening is ventral rather than central, it is known as *hypospadias*; when the urethra opens dorsally it is known as *epispadias*. If either of these congenital deformities are present, surgical repair is generally carried out by 2 years of age to prevent future embarrassment to the child. Since the foreskin is often used in making these repairs, these children are usually not circumcised. Hypospadias and epispadias are generally easily observed, so that there is no need to forcibly retract the tightly adherent prepuce covering the glans. The prepuce is usually retractable by 4 to 6 months of age [26]. If the urethral orifice is located far back on the penis and close to the perineum, adrenogenital syndrome should be considered. In this abnormality there is both failure to secrete cortisol and excessive androgen production by the adrenal glands. In female infants with the adrenogenital syndrome, the clitoris is enlarged.

Edema of the scrotal sac or a *hydrocele* may also be noted in a newborn male. Edema is more prevalent in babies born in breech presentations and regresses within a few days. A hydrocele, a collection of fluid in the scrotal sac, usually regresses within 1 to 3 months.

In full-term female infants, the labia majora are generally larger than the labia minora, while the reverse is true for premature infants. Occasionally you may see a piece of hymenal tissue protruding from the vagina; this hymenal tag regresses in several weeks. You may see white mucoid discharge and sometimes small amounts of blood (pseudomenstruation) on the infant's diaper or in her vagina. Both are due to a drop in maternal hormones, especially estrogen. While the bloody discharge appears for only a brief period, the white mucoid discharge may be present for a week or two. Virilization of the female fetus may result in an enlarged clitoris.

Extremities   A general inspection of the infant's skeletal system will give you a picture of his general posture (which usually reflects his intrauterine posture), the tone of his musculature, and his ability to move spontaneously in a well-coordinated, if sporadic, fashion. If you cannot change an unusual posture by passive manipulation, then an abnormality may be present. If you are aware of the infant's history, you can make a more meaningful assessment. For example, infants who were born breech frequently lie with their hips abducted and knees flexed [31].

Assess the upper extremities by examining the newborn's clavicle, scapula and humerus, elbow, forearm, and hand. Palpate the clavicles over their entire length. Suspect a fractured clavicle if the infant has a history of a difficult birth and if you note some irregularity on palpation, decreased movement, or odd position of the extremity.

Palpate the scapula and humerus for contour and symmetry. Observe movement of the newborn's shoulder. Check his elbow, forearm, and wrist for range of motion and contour of the bones. You will be able to detect an absence of the radius or ulna, which is often associated with other congenital anomalies.

Examine the infant's hands and feet for *polydactyly* (extra digits), a disorder more commonly found in black newborns. The most frequent form of polydactyly is an extra digit attached to the small finger of the hand. Usually the extra digit contains only soft tissue without bone and is treated by tying it off with a silk suture. In a few days it becomes gangrenous, dries, and falls off. If the extra digit contains bone, it must be surgically removed. *Syndactyly* (the fusing of two digits) is found infrequently and most commonly involves the toes; separation requires surgery.

Check the shape, size, and posture of the infant's hands and fingers, and inspect his palms for the configuration of creases.

Examine the newborn's lower extremities by palpating his legs for fractures or masses. Put his hips through range of motion and check carefully for hip dislocation, which is more common in girls, especially after breech deliveries. There is a high incidence in some families; Brown and Valman [12] also report a racial predisposition, noting that the disorder is more common in Italians. Examine the infant by placing him in a supine position, flexing his knees, and abducting his hips out to the side and down toward the table's surface (Fig. 16-16A); suspect hip dislocation if there is resistance to the abduction or if a click is heard, which signifies that the femur has slipped from the acetabulum. Another method is to flex the infant's knees, keeping his feet flat on the table (Fig. 16-16B). The knee on the affected side will be lower (Allis' sign). A dislocated hip may also be indicated by unequal, higher, or extra gluteal or thigh folds on the affected side (Fig. 16-16C).

Neurologic
Examination
Abnormal neurologic signs in the newborn may be transient phenomena but must nevertheless be evaluated. As Korones [19] notes, predictions of later brain dysfunction cannot be made with consistent accuracy on the basis of neurologic abnormalities during the newborn period. It is usually best to do the neurologic examination after 24 hours, when the effects of the birth process (edema, medication) have decreased.

In doing a neurologic examination on a newborn, first check those reflexes that cause the least disturbance to the baby. Your observation should begin with his general level of activity, noting his spontaneous movements to see if he moves both sides equally well, and his lower extremities as well as his upper extremities.

Observe the *tonic neck reflex* when the infant is at rest or asleep (Fig. 16-17). When lying on his back, the newborn turns his head toward one side, with the arm and leg of that side extended while the opposite arm and leg are flexed. This has been described as the "fencing position." If the baby's head is gently turned toward the other side, often the position of the extremities can be reversed.

The *grasp reflex* is usually strong in full-term infants and weaker in premature or depressed newborns. Test this reflex by placing your finger across the infant's palm; the normal newborn will grasp your finger so tightly that he can be pulled up almost to a sitting position (Fig. 16-18).

Check the *rooting reflex* by lightly stroking the corner of the infant's mouth or cheek; his response is to turn his head toward the stimulated side in search of a nipple. Touching his upper lip causes him to open his mouth and turn his head slightly upward.

Test *sucking* ability by placing a nipple in the infant's mouth. The response of the normal newborn is an immediate forceful and coordinated suck, while preterm and depressed babies respond less, as do babies who have recently been fed. A coordinated suck-swallow pattern is not evident before 33 to 34 weeks' gestation.

Test the Moro reflex and the stepping reflex after an evaluation of muscle tone,

Figure 16-16. Examining for hip dislocation (see text for details).

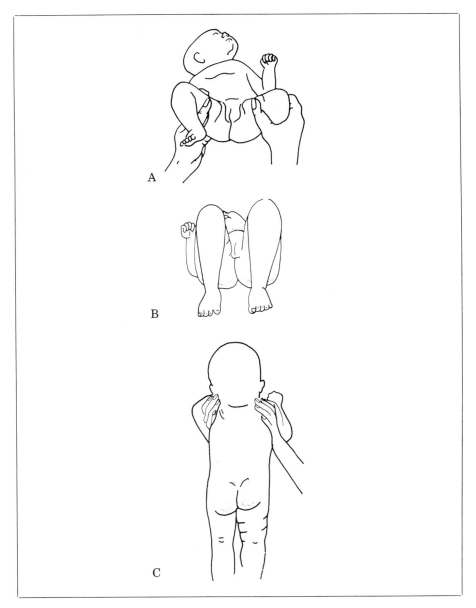

A

B

C

since eliciting the Moro reflex, in particular, does disturb the infant. In evaluating muscle tone remember that normal newborns maintain some flexion in all extremities. When you extend the infant's arm or leg, he normally responds by flexing it again when the extremity is released. Preterm infants and those who have suffered intrauterine hypoxia show less flexion at rest and little or no flexion in response to testing.

Always check head control. This can be done by lifting the infant and holding him by the wrists. If the baby has good head control, he contracts his shoulder and arm muscles and flexes his neck as he is pulled to a sitting position (Fig. 16-19).

Figure 16-17. Tonic neck reflex.

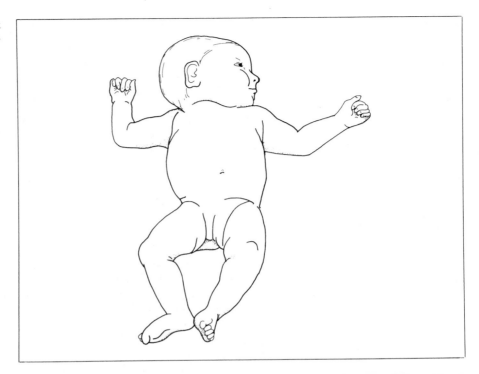

Figure 16-18. Grasp reflex.

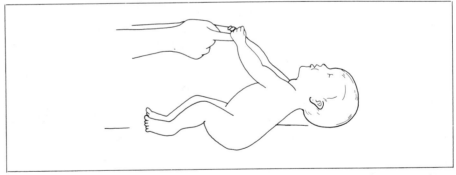

When the infant reaches a sitting position, he should use his neck muscles to prevent his head from falling on his chest. Infants with Down's syndrome or intrauterine hypoxia show little head control or ability to contract their arm, shoulder, or neck muscles.

Check muscle tone by holding the infant horizontally in the prone position (ventral suspension), with your hand under the infant's chest (Fig. 16-20). A full-term infant may momentarily hold his head in line with his trunk (3 seconds), but, for the most part, his head will remain at an angle of 45 degrees or less from the horizontal line. The maneuver allows you to see the infant's control of his head, trunk, arms, and legs.

The *Moro reflex* (startle reflex) may be elicited by jarring the crib or by the preferred method of holding the newborn in a supine position with one hand

Figure 16-19. Evaluating head control in the newborn.

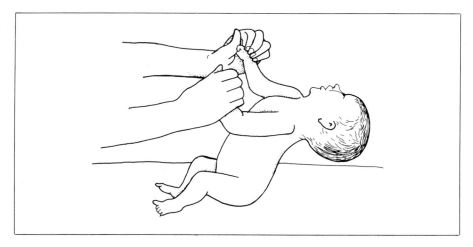

under his head and one under his buttocks. When the hand under his head is moved to his back, allowing his head to drop slightly, the reflex is activated. The infant's arms, wrists, and fingers quickly extend and abduct, followed by flexion of his arms and legs in an embracing motion and usually a cry (Fig. 16-21). It is important to check the response for symmetry. If one extremity does not respond it may indicate neurologic damage or a fracture.

Check the *stepping reflex* by holding the infant in a standing position with his feet on the examining table. The normal baby's response will be to straighten his trunk and make alternate stepping movements with his legs.

Normal newborns also have a positive Babinski reflex. The presence of the previously discussed reflexes in the normal newborn indicates appropriate neurologic response. Many reflexes, such as rooting, sucking, blinking, sneezing, coughing, gagging, and grasping, have an obvious functional value. Other reflexes, such as the Moro and the tonic neck reflexes, are thought to be vestigial reflexes handed down from the ancient past and still seen in lower animals. These primitive reflexes normally disappear in approximately 3 months (Table 16-1).

Elicit *tendon reflexes* by sharp percussion with your finger over the appropriate

Figure 16-20. Evaluating muscle tone in the newborn by holding him in the prone position.

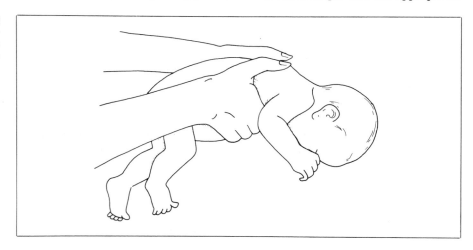

Figure 16-21. Moro or startle reflex (see text for details).

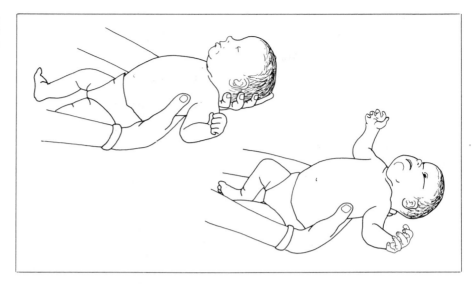

structure. These reflexes may be more brisk in the newborn than in the older child and are influenced by the awake or sleep state of the infant. The biceps, knee, and ankle reflexes should be symmetrical; these reflexes test the C5–6, L2–4, and S1–2 spinal cord segments, respectively.

The integrity of other segments of the spinal cord can be tested using a firm stroke with a cotton swab. These include *truncal incurvation* (T2 to S1), in which a firm stroke to one side or the other of the infant's spine from the neck to the coccyx will cause it to curve in that direction. Segments S4 and S5 can be tested by the *anal wink reflex* in which the anus will constrict when you stroke the lateral anal margin [31].

CRANIAL NERVES

As part of the neurologic exam you may want to test the newborn's cranial nerves. The olfactory nerve (I) may be tested by his response to some aromatic substance. While doing his examination you will already have tested his optic nerve (II); you will have noted whether his pupils constrict, whether he blinks in response to a bright light, and whether he follows the movement of a brightly colored object. In testing the oculomotor (III), trochlear (IV), and abducens (VI) nerves, you should check for pupillary constriction to light and lack of eyelid ptosis. In addition, you might check for doll's eyes; turning the supine newborn's head to the left and then to the right causes his eyes to move in the opposite direction. When you have elicited his rooting reflex, you have checked the trigeminal nerve (V). Check the facial nerve (VII) by observing his facial tone when he cries. The angles of his mouth should not droop. Assess his auditory nerve (VIII) by observing his response to a loud noise. Glossopharyngeal nerve (IX) is intact if he has a strong gag reflex during which his uvula does not deviate to one side. Listen to his cry; if it is not hoarse then his vagus nerve (X) is intact. You might check the accessory nerve (XI) in the newborn by turning his head to the side and observing his efforts to return it to its original position. Test his tongue strength (hypoglossal nerve—XII) by inserting your gloved finger in his mouth and feeling the force of his suck [31].

Table 16-1. Examination
of the Newborn

Body Part	Examination Procedures
Head	Measure circumference Palpate suture lines and fontanelles Observe for indication of molding, caput succedaneum, cephalohematoma
Eyes	Observe for evidence of edema, discharge, conjunctivitis, subconjunctival hemorrhage, pupil capacity
Ears	Observe position, size, and formation; note presence of cartilage
Nose	Observe for patent nasal passages, nose breathing, nasal flaring, discharge
Mouth	Check for palate closure, presence of teeth, Epstein's pearls, evidence of infection (thrush), size of tongue; note character of cry
Chest	Measure circumference Examine heart and lung sounds; observe respirations Observe breasts for enlargement, discharge, development, supernumerary nipples
Abdomen	Observe for symmetry Palpate liver and kidneys Observe condition of umbilical cord
Genitalia Female	Observe labia for development and protection provided by majora clitoris for size; check for vaginal bleeding or discharge, presence of hymenal tag
Male	Observe penis for evidence of epispadias or hypospadias; scrotum for rugae and presence of testes, evidence of swelling
Back	Observe for straight spinal column, evidence of dimpling of skin over sacral vertebrae, patency of anus
Extremities	Examine for fractures, polydactyly, syndactyly, club feet, posture, and symmetrical use of extremities Observe creasing on hands and feet Examine for hip dislocation
Skin	Observe color and thickness Check for indication of cyanosis, edema, ecchymoses, jaundice, lanugo, vernix caseosa, petechiae, desquamation, turgor Check for evidence of milia, mongolian spots, erythema toxicum, hemangiomas, infection
Neurologic system	Check Moro's, grasp, suck, rooting, and tonic neck reflexes Observe muscle tone, head control, posture, and movements

Behavioral Assessment

The newborn can respond in a relatively sophisticated manner to the stimulation of all five of his senses. When you assess the newborn, you should simultaneously record his state of wakefulness or sleep since it will influence his actions for a variety of reflex and behavioral responses. In addition, be aware of drugs that have been administered to his mother (such as analgesics, hypnotics, and anesthetics) which may still be having an effect on the infant's ability to respond to stimuli. Brazelton [10] and others have identified "states" of a newborn's behavior as follows: "quiet deep sleep"—no spontaneous activity, eyes closed, respirations regular; "light active sleep"—random startles, respirations irregular, eyes closed, rapid eye movements observable, frequent change of state with response to stimulation; "drowsy awake"—eyes open or closed, eyelids fluttering, variable activity level, mild startles from time to time, delayed response to stimulation, frequent change of state; "quite alert"—eyes open, little motor activity, focuses attention on source of stimulation; "alert active"—eyes open, much motor activity with thrusting of extremities, increase in startles in response to stimulation, some fussiness; "crying"—intense crying which is difficult to interrupt with stimulation. Although each state is fairly distinct, the newborn may make very smooth transitions between the awake-alert states and between these states and the sleep states.

GENERAL HYGIENE
Assessment and Intervention

When you work with newborns and their parents you will have numerous opportunities to incorporate many of the pertinent observations previously described into their care, teaching, and follow-up. Remember that parents are extremely critical of minute anatomic and physiologic variations in their babies. Anatomic asymmetries, such as one eye being open more than the other (especially on the side farther away from the source of light in the room), molding of the head, irregular breathing, engorged breasts (especially in the male), and variations in external genitalia, become magnified. One of the many times you can discuss such variations with the parents is during the baby's bath.

BATHING THE NEWBORN

Babies can be cleansed in a variety of ways without violating basic underlying principles of safe care. At one time, daily soap and water and/or oil baths were the rule, but today complete baths are often not given. Blood, meconium, and excess vernix caseosa are wiped off with dry or water-moistened cotton balls and thereafter the diaper area is cleaned as necessary.

During the 1960s, in response to an increase in staphylococcal infections in newborn nurseries, the American Academy of Pediatrics recommended that infants be bathed in a liquid detergent containing 3% hexachlorophene after birth and then every other day. Subsequent research [5] has indicated that although the rate of staphylococcal colonization and staphylococcal skin diseases is indeed reduced, there is no documented proof that the use of 3% hexachlorophene ever arrested a serious nursery epidemic. In addition, its use has increased the colonization of gram-negative organisms and the incidence of gram-negative disease.

In recent years the actual safety of daily bathing of infants with a solution containing 3% hexachlorophene has been questioned, since it leaves protective residue that reaches a peak effectiveness after three baths and is absorbed through intact skin. When it was disclosed that blood levels found in newborns bathed daily in 3% hexachlorophene have been shown to approach levels known to be neurotoxic in experimental animals, the Food and Drug Administration ruled that hexachlorophene could be distributed only by prescription. Therefore, the routine prophylactic use of hexachlorophene for total body bathing of newborns in hospital nurseries or in the home is no longer recommended. The most actively promoted alternative, povidone-iodine (Betadine), can cause local and systemic reactions in hypersensitive infants, and there is no proof that it is safer [17].

The Committee on the Fetus and Newborn of the American Academy of Pediatrics [5] recommends dry skin care for newborns, which involves the use of plain nonmedicated soap and tap water, or tap water alone, on the baby's skin in the areas that need attention: face, neck, axillae, and groin, and the buttocks with each diaper change. If a nursery infection is present, once-daily prophylactic bathing of the newborn with 3% hexachlorophene, followed by prompt and thorough rinsing, may be given on a short-term basis.

The committee emphasizes that the two most important factors in the transmission of infection from infant to infant are hand contact and lapses in hygienic technique. Scrupulous handwashing with an iodine preparation, a 3% hexachlorophene emulsion, or any other cleansing agent before and between handling babies is essential.

It is important for the parents to have the opportunity to observe a bath being given to their baby and for one or both of them to give him a bath themselves before the family leaves the hospital or birth center. Take this opportunity to explore with the parents their plans for caring for the baby, the methods they have considered using, and the facilities they have at home, so that, as a part of the dialogue, modifications can be suggested if necessary.

Parents who have other children are not necessarily uninterested in being taught to bathe their new infant. Many times they are anxious to learn new techniques or to review their own, especially if some time has elapsed since their last child was born. In addition, encourage them to share what they have learned from their past experiences, so that their "tips" might be passed on to new parents.

The baby's bath may be given at any time of the day but is usually given before a feeding. If the day is particularly warm, a sponge bath may be repeated two or three times during the day, taking care to rinse and dry all skin folds and creases thoroughly. Parents may not realize how active newborns really are; stress the importance of never leaving the baby alone on an elevated surface where he could roll off; it is best for them to get into the habit of keeping one hand on him at all times.

Whether you demonstrate the bath for the parents or they do it themselves, certain principles are basic. If all necessary supplies are organized before beginning the bath, the parent will be less likely to leave the baby alone or unduly exposed once the bath is begun. Safety pins should always be closed and put well out of the baby's reach. It is also preferable to have an area where dirty linen and soiled items can be placed. The room should be warm (75°–80°F) and free from drafts, and the bath water should feel warm to the elbow (98°–100°F).

The baby should be cleaned starting from the cleanest area and proceeding to the most soiled, in the following order: eyes, face, ears, scalp, neck, upper extremities, trunk, lower extremities, and finally genitalia and buttocks. The infant's eyes receive special care, and are gently cleaned with sterile water or tap water from the inner canthus to the outer canthus, to avoid contaminating the lacrimal ducts. A clean surface of the washcloth or a clean cotton ball is used for each stroke.

Throughout the procedure, various parts of the baby are washed, rinsed well, and dried thoroughly, with particular attention paid to the creases and body folds. Usually only one area of the infant is exposed at a time in order to avoid chilling, since the newborn's temperature-regulating mechanism may not be fully developed at birth and his heat production is low. During the first few days his temperature is unstable, responding to slight stimuli with considerable fluctuation above or below the normal level [13]. For this reason in many nurseries where a soap and water bath is routine, the baby's initial bath after birth is often delayed for several hours to allow his body temperature to stabilize.

Researchers [21] have demonstrated that the temperature of the newborn may fall precipitously following delivery, to levels lower than are generally recognized. They suggest that temperature fluctuation and a decreased temperature may be desirable or even essential for a rapid and satisfactory adjustment to extrauterine life. Due to the extreme sensitivity of skin thermal receptors, a peripheral thermal stimulus, such as bathing, might be an important factor in heat production. Nursing research by Whitner and Thompson [34] has demonstrated that bathing the newborn did produce a greater initial drop (0.5°C, or 1°F) in body temperature than was seen in unbathed babies. However, subsequent to this initial drop, the body temperature of the bathed newborn showed a significant increase (approximately 0.2°C, or 0.5°F), which was not seen in the unbathed control group of babies. This would seem to indicate that the bathing tended to produce a more rapid return toward the desired level of body temperature (36.1°–37.2°C, or 97°–99°F), although the researchers question whether or not the same effect might have been achieved through stimulation by a light friction rub with a warm towel.

At the other end of the spectrum are those nurseries where no attempt is made to clean the baby, except for removing blood on his face and scalp. The vernix caseosa is not removed since most of it either rubs into his skin or rubs off onto his clothes within 12 to 24 hours. Sometimes it tends to remain longer in body creases and skin folds, such as the neck, axillae, and between the labia. This may encourage infection or irritation of these areas; therefore, the vernix caseosa is wiped away after 24 to 48 hours.

The baby is not given a tub bath until after the cord has dropped off, usually within 2 weeks. However, most parents are interested in learning how to support the baby's body during his tub bath. Usually this is done by placing the left arm under the baby's head and shoulders, grasping his left arm firmly. The right hand is used to grasp his ankles, and may be used to wash him after he is lowered into the tub. If a small towel is placed in the bottom of the tub, its surface will not be as slippery.

The so-called football carry is a useful hold for washing the baby's hair or to free one hand to arrange bath items. One arm is placed under the baby's body, with his head on that hand and his buttocks held securely between the adult's hip and elbow, leaving the other hand free.

SKIN CARE

The newborn's skin becomes irritated easily because the dermis and epidermis are very loosely connected. During the first 2 or 3 days after birth, the skin becomes increasingly dry; often cracks will appear, particularly around his wrists and ankles. Usually these are not significant and disappear spontaneously.

Because the newborn's skin is so easily irritated, the use of strong soap and excessive amounts of baby oil or baby powder should be avoided. Most of these products contain perfume, which, while it makes the baby smell nice, may actually have an irritating effect on his skin. Excessive use of powder, especially by shaking it on the baby, may leave large amounts of it to collect and become caked in his skin creases, and there is also the danger that he may inhale it.

Advise parents to shake the powder on their own hands and smooth it on the baby. Many parents are interested to learn that cornstarch, a much less expensive substitute, provides the same effect as the commercially prepared baby powders. Baby oil is also perfumed and may be an irritant; it is also a good medium for bacterial growth if left on the skin in large amounts and should therefore be used sparingly.

CORD CARE

The baby's daily care involves not only bathing but also inspection and observation. One area that is routinely inspected is his umbilical cord, and parents are often concerned about its proper care.

Within 24 hours after birth, the evaporation of Wharton's jelly has caused the umbilical cord to lose its bluish-white moist appearance, and within a few days it becomes shriveled and almost black. Several days later the stump sloughs, leaving a small granulating wound, which after healing forms the umbilicus. Separation of the cord from the body most frequently occurs around the tenth day but occasionally takes several weeks; no attempt should be made to dislodge it before it separates naturally.

Formerly care of the cord was not given too much attention, and neglect of asepsis resulted in the transmission of infections through the umbilical vessels, with the eventual death of many infants. Sometimes even today serious umbilical infections are found, most frequently caused by *Staphylococcus aureus, Escherichia coli,* or *Pseudomonas aeruginosa.*

The blood vessels at the base of the cord are initially sealed off by formation of thrombi. Final obliteration does not occur until the end of the first month, when the vessels become fibrous cords. Until this anatomic closure occurs, the blood vessels may be portals of entry to pathogenic organisms. Signs of infection include any unusual or foul odors of the cord, red inflamed areas around the stump, and drainage from the cord, but the baby may have a serious umbilical cord infection without any local signs.

Observe the newborn's cord for bleeding as well as infection, particularly during the first 24 hours. Bleeding seems to occur most often between the second and sixth hours of life, sometimes in association with crying or the passage of meconium. The danger appears to be greatest with a bleeding disorder or when the cord initially contains a large amount of Wharton's jelly; in the latter case, the cord shrinks, and the previously tight tie or clamp becomes loose. Usually a blood clot at the end of the cord stump prevents such bleeding, but if bleeding should occur, a hemostat should be placed on the cord as far away from the abdominal wall as possible, to allow for the application of another tie or clamp. As a rule, cord ties remain in place until the cord separates. Clamps are usually removed in 24 hours if the cord appears dry (Fig. 16-22).

Since infants' cords dry more quickly and separate more readily when exposed to air, dressings are usually not applied. Diapers are usually placed below the cord for this reason and also to prevent urine from keeping the cord area moist. Cord care commonly involves wiping the cord stump with a cotton ball saturated with antiseptic solution or with a 70% solution of alcohol to further encourage drying until healing is complete. If the cord seems unusually moist, applying the alcohol several times a day enhances drying.

Figure 16-22. A. Hollister cord clamp. B. Clamp closed on cord stump.

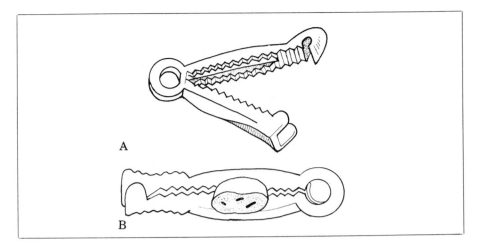

GENITALIA

Advise parents to clean the genitalia of baby girls gently and carefully with moistened cotton balls or a soft cloth, wiping from front to back. A clean portion of the cloth or a new cotton ball is used for each stroke. Smegma, a thick cheesy secretion of the sebaceous glands, is removed from between the folds of the labia.

If a baby boy is not to be circumcised, parents are instructed to ease the foreskin back very gently during the daily bath in order to clean the smegma from around the glans. No force should be applied in attempting to retract the foreskin, since, as mentioned previously, it may be several months before it is easily retractable.

Circumcision, a sterile surgical procedure in which the foreskin (prepuce) of the penis is removed, traditionally has been done for religious or cultural reasons. In the United States it has been believed to be of medical value as well and has been almost routinely performed on all male newborns. This is not the case in many other areas, including Europe, South America, and Japan. Consumers as well as physicians are questioning the routine circumcision of newborns, and some physicians are advising it only when a specific reason exists for the procedure [25].

In the past, circumcision has been routinely recommended to prevent the occurrence of disorders such as phimosis, cancer of the penis, and cancer of the cervix, and to save the "different" uncircumcised male "locker room embarrassment." It is also argued that the circumcised penis is cleaner and more aesthetic, and that it provides greater pleasure during sexual intercourse, although this latter fact is controversial.

Some physicians view circumcision as a basically unnecessary body mutilation, while others who argue against routine circumcision feel that circumcision, like any surgery, is associated with occasional hazards and complications. Primarily these complications involve infection, surgical trauma, and hemorrhage; the danger of hemorrhage seems particularly pertinent in light of the newborn's hypoprothrombinemia. It is generally felt, however, that the vitamin K injection given the newborn lessens the danger of hemorrhage.

Research [26] indicates that the increased incidence of genitourinary cancers in populations that do not practice circumcision appears to be related to poor genital hygiene, inadequate hygienic facilities, and venereal disease. The conclusion is that in groups where a high standard of cleanliness could presumably be expected, circumcision at birth would not seem to be justified.

At this time in the United States, circumcision of the newborn is still frequently performed, either in the delivery room shortly after birth, or on the second or third postnatal day, unless it is a religious ritual circumcision. The operation is usually performed without anesthesia, and the baby will cry probably as much from being restrained as from discomfort from the procedure. Sometimes he may be comforted by a sterile nipple pacifier or by a warm blanket.

The raw incision is usually covered with sterile petrolatum-saturated gauze. The main principle in circumcision care is to keep the wound clean and observe it for bleeding. In most instances, the circumcision dressing is carefully removed postoperatively when the infant voids for the first time and is then replaced. Dressings are usually not reapplied after 24 hours; the wound is cleaned with warm water following diaper changes, and the penis is sometimes coated with petrolatum until healing is complete, usually within a few days.

Because the newborn does have a transitory hypoprothrombinemia, the circumcision is particularly observed for bleeding every hour during the first 24 postoperative hours. Usually the baby's crib is tagged with a special sign, so that nursery personnel are alerted to the fact that he is newly circumcised. Only one layer of diaper should cover his penis, so that any bleeding will be evident; usually undue irritation is avoided by not placing the baby on his stomach. If bleeding does occur, it is usually stopped with very gentle pressure. Sometimes a 1:1000 solution of epinephrine is applied locally to the bleeding point. Of course, if the bleeding persists, notify the physician.

The parents are usually anxious when their baby is to be circumcised and want to see him immediately following the procedure. This is a good time to show them the wound and begin the explanation of its care. After the circumcision, the baby finds comfort from being held, cuddled, and fed, since feedings are usually withheld prior to the procedure.

DIAPER RASH

Another source of concern for parents is the diaper rash that babies often get, caused by a reaction of bacteria with the urea in the urine, resulting in an ammonia dermatitis. The best treatment consists of keeping the area clean and dry, with exposure to air and light several times a day. Additional warmth is provided by the use of a lamp (with a bulb no brighter than 40 watts) placed 30 centimeters (12 inches) or more from the buttocks for 30 minutes at a time. When the baby is being fed and has his diaper on, the area can be protected by ointments, such as petrolatum jelly, zinc oxide, or A and D Ointment. This helps keep stool off the raw area and aids in the healing process. A frequent cause of diaper rashes at home is inadequate rinsing of the infant's diapers. Diaper rashes may also be associated with a thrush infection. Persistent rashes should be reported to a health professional.

PARENTS' CONCERNS
Assessment and Intervention

You can alleviate many of the concerns that parents have and will encounter in caring for their baby at home. This can only be done if you spend time with the parents, participating in the baby's care with them and giving them encouragement and positive reinforcement. Review such topics as taking the baby's temperature, signs of hunger, normal occurrence of regurgitation, sneezing, hiccupping, and characteristics of normal stools. You may also use this time to observe and evaluate the parents' comfort and ability in holding, dressing, feeding, bubbling, and positioning the baby.

In a hospital it is conceivable that if the baby is in a central nursery and is brought to the mother every 4 hours for feeding, the parents may take him home without ever having heard him cry. Sometimes they voice a concern about what his cry means or what to do if the baby does not stop crying when he is picked up. Tell them that the crying is his way of telling them that his diaper is dirty or that he is about to have a bowel movement, that he is hungry or has a gas bubble, or that he is being stuck by a pin. Sometimes a sudden noise will startle a baby; in this case cuddling usually quiets his crying. Often a warm bath will soothe and calm him. Parents need to be made aware of the fact that a certain amount of crying is normal and aerates the lungs.

Parents often ask when they can take the baby outside. Usually when the mother feels like going out for the first time, the baby may go along. This, of course, depends on the weather. The baby should be well protected from temperature extremes and from direct exposure to sun or wind. The amount of clothing the baby needs is generally comparable to that which the parent is wearing.

If the parents will be travelling in a car, they should be reminded to use a car seat for the baby and not to put the baby on the floor, where exhaust fumes tend to collect. Some physicians feel that flying should be postponed for the first several weeks, because the baby's middle ear is not developed enough to adapt to changes in pressure. It is important at take-off and landing that the baby be sucking on his bottle or nipple to assist in adjustment to changes in pressure.

NEONATAL
IMMUNOLOGY
*Assessment and
Intervention*

Before birth the infant is protected by the surrounding membranes, the uterus, and the biologic defense mechanisms of the mother. At birth he leaves this sterile environment and enters one contaminated by infectious organisms. His own protective mechanisms, aided by antibodies passed across the placenta from the mother, should successfully defend him against the common infectious agents. However, since his general resistance remains low, he should be exposed to as few of these organisms as possible.

Several natural portals of entry exist in the newborn, for example, vessels of the umbilical cord, circumcision, and breaks in his skin. Opportunities for infection are inherent in certain anomalies, such as omphalocele and exstrophy of the bladder; in babies who receive repeated exchange transfusions or fluids or who have frequent blood sampling through the umbilical vein; in babies who require resuscitation; and in babies who are placed in isolettes that have not been thoroughly cleaned. Special precautions should be taken if the mother's membranes were ruptured more than 24 hours before delivery, or if she had a fever or infection during the last week of pregnancy, prolonged labor, foul-smelling or purulent amniotic fluid, traumatic delivery, or an infectious disease, such as syphilis or tuberculosis.

The relative immune deficiency of the newborn makes him unusually able to develop serious infections, such as meningitis and septicemia, which are significant causes of severe disease or death in the neonate. He is also susceptible to the common viruses, such as cytomegalovirus and rubella.

The newborn's first line of defense is the surface protection provided by his intact skin and mucous membrane; there are also several basic host response mechanisms that operate in varying degrees [15,19]. The initial inflammatory response of the newborn is delayed, and he cannot concentrate inflammatory cells at the site of infection as well as adults can, so it is less likely that his infection will remain localized.

The newborn's serum is deficient in its capacity to opsonize organisms (prepare organisms for phagocytosis by polymorphonuclear leukocytes). The part played by lymphocytes and macrophages in the newborn's defense is probably also decreased.

Serum immunoglobulins (IgG, IgM, and IgA) are important in the immunologic defenses of the newborn because of their role in opsonizing bacteria for phagocytosis, in killing bacteria in specific systems, and in neutralizing viruses. IgG globulins contain antibodies to a majority of bacterial and viral organisms to which the mother has previously been exposed. These are the only globulins to cross the placental membrane, first appearing in the fetus around the third gestational month. They accumulate progressively, until they equal the mother's level at term. Therefore, the length of gestation as well as the mother's antibody complement is the determinant of the IgG level at birth; the average concentration in serum is 1,000 milligrams per 100 milliliters at term, but lower levels are found in the premature infant. Most of these globulins are catabolized over the first 3 months of life; however, the infant's own synthesis of IgG increases gradually after the age of 3 months to cover the loss.

The fetus can produce IgM globulins at about the twentieth week of gestation. Since intrauterine infections may produce this immunologic response in the fetus, the measurement of this globulin is used to establish the presence of such an infection. Some specific antibodies can be identified within the IgM fraction, including syphilis, toxoplasmosis, cytomegalovirus, rubella, and herpesvirus. Usually the IgM level at birth is below 20 milligrams per 100 milliliters of serum.

IgA globulins do not usually cross the placenta and are not detectable in most normal infants at birth. The fetus and neonate are slower to manufacture IgA than IgM globulins, so they are found less regularly in the serum of infected infants at birth.

PROTECTION FROM INFECTION

Nothing administered to the newborn, including commercial gamma globulin, will improve the functioning of his immune defense system; consequently, it is important to protect him from undue exposure to organisms in the environment and to be alert for rapid diagnosis and treatment of infections when they develop. This is achieved by maintaining aseptic and clean technique in his care and by preventing his contact with persons who are themselves infected.

To further ensure protection from infection, the American Academy of Pediatrics sets certain standards and recommendations for hospital care of newborns [4]. Ideally the nursery itself should be enclosed and have some system of ventilation or air conditioning in which there is an adequate filtering device. The floor is always considered contaminated, and dropped objects must be discarded or sterilized before they are used again. All linen, clothing, formulas, and solutions used in infant care must be clean, and each infant should have his own set of supplies. When the baby is moved to a common facility (scale or treatment table), a clean paper or sheet should be used for his protection. If he is in an incubator, he should be placed in a clean one every 4 days or every week.

Access to the nursery should be through a scrub room where personnel change clothes and thoroughly scrub their hands and arms, paying special attention to their nails. Handwashing is repeated when personnel move from one infant to another. These policies apply to each member of the nursing staff and to everyone else who enters the nursery, including cleaning personnel, aides, medical students, and physicians. Since exposure to agents most likely to make the newborn ill comes from persons in his environment, anyone who has infections of the skin or upper respiratory tract, diarrhea, or fever of unknown origin is automatically excluded from the nursery. This ban includes parents and visitors as well as nursery staff. At home such hazards are fewer because of the relatively small number of individuals in contact with the baby.

In order to minimize the risk of infection when the baby is taken to his mother, some hospitals do not allow visitors on the unit during that time. The mother washes her hands before her baby is brought to her; if she has an infection, her baby can be taken to the door of her room so that she can see him, and she can be given reports of his progress.

Infection in the newborn is not always indicated by fever; hypothermia or marked temperature variations may be present, indicating the infant's inability to control his temperature. Infection may be suspected when the baby is inactive and/or does not eat well. Other indications of infection include jaundice beginning after the third day, a mottled appearance to his skin, abdominal distention, diarrhea, vomiting, changes in respiratory patterns, and skin lesions. A full fontanelle, a high-pitched cry, and irritability indicate an infection of the central nervous system.

Well before the family leaves the hospital or birth center explore with the parents their plans for follow-up health care for the infant and the mother. Make them aware of community agencies nearby and the services they provide for continued health supervision and guidance. If the postpartum stay is short, follow-up by a community health nurse may be welcome, especially in the absence of helpful relatives nearby. Parents should be helped to arrange for some form of continued health supervision, through a midwife, a private physician, a hospital, or a community health center. Here the baby can be assessed for normal patterns of growth and development and given necessary regular immunizations when his immunologic system is producing antibodies in good fashion, by the age of 2 or 3 months. In general, parents and their new infant make the first of many visits for continued health supervision within 4 to 6 weeks post delivery.

NEWBORN NUTRITION
Assessment and Intervention

FLUID

Normal nutrition for newborns includes providing water, electrolytes, and nutrients in adequate but not excessive amounts. Moore [22] outlines the main reasons why fluid balance is more precarious in the newborn than in older children and adults. Since metabolic rates of the newborn are higher, he utilizes a greater quantity of water. (The newborn produces 45–50 calories per kilogram of body weight per day, while adults produce 25–30 calories per kilogram per day.)

The newborn has a larger surface area in proportion to his body mass. Therefore he has a higher ratio of water loss through evaporation, about twice that of the adult. Because of this, his fluid balance is more susceptible to environmental temperature and humidity variations.

In the newborn the proportion of water in relation to total body mass is 70 to 75 percent, greater than at any other life period. Extracellular water comprises 30 to 35 percent of his total body weight, compared to 25 percent in an older infant and 20 percent in an adult. In a 24-hour period he excretes 50 percent of his extracellular water, compared to the 14 percent an adult excretes; therefore, he has less reserve.

The kidneys of premature and full-term infants have about half the concentration power of the normal adult, and they function satisfactorily under usual conditions but not during times of stress. Since the newborn is not able to conserve water by concentrating urine, even in dehydration his output may not decrease. The normally higher levels of phosphate and potassium in his urine are also related to kidney immaturity.

The newborn's water requirement is 80 to 100 millimeters per kilogram of body weight per day during the first 10 days and 125 to 200 milliliters per kilogram per day thereafter. Babies must have at least 75 to 90 milliliters per kilogram of body weight per day. Otherwise they may exhibit the characteristic signs of dehydration: dry skin, loss of skin turgor, depressed fontanelle, weight loss, rapid and weak pulse, increased temperature, and soft eyeballs. When dehydration occurs, fluids are given intravenously and are carefully calculated to replace lost electrolytes. An infant's electrolyte balance is relatively unstable, especially sodium and potassium levels, because of the rapid exchange of water and the ease with which the balance is upset.

NUTRIENTS

Calories. By the tenth day the infant needs 110 to 130 calories per kilogram of body weight per day (50–60 calories per pound) in order to provide energy for his relatively high basal metabolic rate, increasing activity, and rapid growth. However, needs will vary within the given range even for babies of the same age and size. The newborn should have 9 grams of protein daily (7–16 percent of calories) to provide for growth and to make up for losses from his skin and in his urine. (At 1 month he needs 14 grams of protein per day; at 2 months, 15 grams per day; and from 3 months to 1 year, 16 grams per day.)

About 40 percent of the newborn's calories should be in the form of carbohydrates. When carbohydrates comprise less than 20 percent of the calories, the baby will not be able to tolerate the high percentage of protein and fat in the formula. If over 50 percent of the calories are provided by carbohydrates, the baby will probably have loose stools due to his inability to hydrolize disaccharides, which will eventually result in impaired growth and development.

About 55 percent of the calories should be provided by fat. If fat content is too low, then either the protein intake will be so high that the renal solute load will be excessive, or the high level of carbohydrate will lead to diarrhea.

Vitamins. Most babies in the United States receive supplementary vitamins, and as a result, vitamin deficiencies are relatively rare. In addition, in many hospitals babies are given vitamin K (0.5–1.0 milligrams) routinely at birth, since it is only after birth that normal intestinal flora are established and begin to synthesize vitamin K. Because formulas and breast milk contain B-group vitamins, it is felt that their deficiency would be unlikely in the newborn. Since the optimal amounts of B-group vitamins are not fully determined, however, many physicians believe that a supplement is desirable, if not essential. Folic acid deficiencies may be overlooked because they can be masked by a common iron deficiency anemia.

On the other hand, with vitamin A the danger is overdosage. Healthy infants receiving human milk, cows' milk, and most commercial formulas do not need any extra vitamin A; 600 I.U. per day is adequate (most formulas have 1,500–2,700 I.U. per liter). If a milk-free or skim-milk formula is used, vitamin A must be supplemented since much of it is removed with the fat. However, a good concentration of vitamin A exists in the fish liver oils used to supply additional vitamin D.

With vitamin D there is a possibility of toxicity. In the United States, evaporated milk, most commercial formulas, and most fresh whole milk are fortified at least to the level of 400 I.U. per liter. Skim milk, some commercial milk, and human milk contain less than the 400 I.U. daily requirement; infants fed with these need supplemental vitamin D. The premature infant needs more vitamin D than does the full-term infant.

The minimum daily requirement of vitamin C is 25 milligrams; if the infant is breast-fed, his supply of this vitamin will be adequate if his mother has a sufficient quantity in her diet. Heated cows' milk has little or no vitamin C, but orange juice and other citrus juices supply it in good quantity. One ounce of fresh orange juice or 2 ounces of reconstituted frozen orange juice per day will satisfy the infant's requirement. However, the most common and easiest method of satisfying all his vitamin needs is through administration of a vitamin supplement in pill or liquid form. It should be emphasized that this is not really necessary for every infant but depends on the quantity and quality of his intake.

Minerals. The need for minerals is met with little difficulty, with the exception of iron. Over 75 percent of the total iron content in the newborn's body at birth is in erythrocytes, but a small amount is stored in other tissues. The iron from the erythrocytes is retained in the body when the red blood cells break down and is reclaimed later for hemoglobin synthesis. The amount of iron available depends on the initial hemoglobin mass and may be inadequate to meet the infant's needs in later months if the initial hemoglobin level was low or if the infant was of a low birth weight. After birth the hemoglobin drops steadily until it reaches a low of 11 grams per 100 milliliters with a hematocrit of 33 percent at about 3 months. A combination of factors accounts for this change, including lack of or slow hematopoiesis, breakdown of red blood cells, and growth and expansion of the circulatory system. In the full-term infant, the recovery of erythrocytes and hemoglobin levels begins at 2 months when the hematopoietic process resumes. In the premature baby, this physiologic anemia persists for a longer period, up to 4 months, since he has a smaller hemoglobin mass initially and a rapid growth rate.

Iron deficiency (hemoglobin below 10 grams per 100 milliliters) may be found in 25 to 76 percent of infants over 6 months of age from economically deprived areas and in 1 to 2 percent of babies from more affluent families. Formulas fortified with iron are frequently used for babies who have a high risk of developing iron deficiency anemia. The use of iron-fortified cereals is also recommended.

FEEDING

The newborn faces the task of adjusting to the change from fetal nutrition to that of taking in food, digesting it, and assimilating its nutrients on his own. His gastrointestinal tract previously has not been required to utilize much muscle, chemical, or absorptive activity in handling food. Now he must do this for himself with the help of his sucking, swallowing, and gagging reflexes.

As soon as the infant cries, he swallows a large amount of air into his stomach. Once he ingests liquid as well, his stomach may easily increase to a size four or five times that of its empty contracted state. Its capacity at birth is about 30 to 35 milliliters, about 75 milliliters by the second week, and 100 milliliters by the end of the first month (the average adult capacity is 1,000 milliliters). The newborn has 2 million gastric glands (the adult has 25 million), which begin to secrete acid before birth. The proteolytic activity of these glands in the newborn is less than 20 percent of that in the 2- or 3-month-old baby. The stomach musculature, including the pyloric sphincter, is moderately developed at birth, but the elastic tissue is poorly developed. Peristaltic activity in the newborn does not occur in a progressive wave but rather in a simultaneous contraction of most of the stomach musculature.

The supporting musculature of the newborn's intestinal tract is poorly developed; since his abdominal wall is weak, his abdomen often appears distended. His intestinal tract does have well-developed secretory and absorbing surfaces, but peristalsis is weak and discontinuous.

The digestive system of the normal full-term infant has the functional capacity to propel, digest, and absorb every type of food in liquid form except complex carbohydrates. The major portion of the feeding leaves his stomach in 3 to 4 hours, most in 1½ to 2 hours after the meal, but there are wide variations. Human milk leaves the stomach more rapidly than cows' milk, and formula made from unboiled cows' milk stays in the stomach longer than formula made from boiled cows' milk.

Feeding Schedule. It seems best to begin feeding each baby according to his individual need, which usually occurs within 4 to 12 hours after birth, instead of adhering to an established routine. Plain water may be given first, followed by glucose water. First feedings test the infant's ability to suck and swallow adequately. If he aspirates the feeding, water will be less damaging to his lung tissue than milk. If the baby is in good condition and his mother is ready, he may nurse in the delivery room. How often and how much he is fed depends on the baby, and this is a somewhat unknown quantity in the beginning.

Many infants are placed on a demand schedule by their mothers and are fed when they show signs of hunger: waking up, crying, refusing water with disgust, seizing the nipple, and nursing vigorously. The baby usually takes what he wishes and stops when he has had enough. Most babies eat six or eight times a day, with a time lapse of from 2 to 8 hours between feedings, which may vary from day to day. After 3 or 4 days, the infant may have several days on which he may want to eat very frequently. After a week or two, he establishes a fairly regular schedule.

It is not unusual for babies to dawdle over their feedings during the first few days. Parents must be patient then, and they will find that it is easier to feed their baby when he appears hungry. This is particularly true if the baby is breast-feeding since if he is not hungry, he is less likely to grasp the nipple well. This will be unpleasant for him and cause unnecessary concern for the mother. Help the parents in the process of getting to know their newborn's eating patterns; this support can consist of help in holding the baby while he eats, adjusting his position, placing the nipple in the baby's mouth, or bubbling him.

Choice of Method.   The choice of infant feeding methods is sensitive to cultural and social changes. In ancient times, from the moment of birth a mother and her newborn were together. Breast-feeding occurred early and often, about 8 to 12 times per day during the early weeks, whenever the infant searched for his mother's breast and cried with hunger. Swaddled to the mother, the baby was carried and rocked by the swaying movements of her body as she spent her day gathering food. At nightfall, they lay down to sleep together, and her infant's needs for the breast were easily met at the mother's side. When a mother died in childbirth, a lactating relative took the baby to nurse. This was the precursor of the hired wet nurse in later societies [27].

Although breast-feeding was practically the universal method of infant feeding until recent times, there is evidence that artificial feedings were attempted. Feeding vessels have been found in Egyptian graves dating back to 2500 B.C.; others found in Europe appear to have been in use about 500 years later. Spouted feeding cups from the grave of premature twins circa 600 B.C. were found in Sudan. Milk from goats, donkeys, and other animals is believed to have been used in the vessels. Direct suckling of animals was also used according to Egyptian etchings and Greek myths.

Pap gruels, forerunners of modern baby foods, were first used in the 1600s. Pap was a liquid, usually milk, combined with bread, rice, or flour. Its use generally led to underfeeding since it had to be diluted to pass through the opening in the container.

Artificial feeding was associated with high infant mortality from infection, especially diarrhea. During the 1800s in Europe, seven of eight artificially fed infants perished. Foundling hospitals in the late 1700s reported mortality of 80 percent or more. To avoid the dangers of artificial feeding during this era, affluent mothers hired wet nurses. Wet nursing became so widespread and profitable in the cities that in order to obtain easy employment as a wet nurse, girls contrived to initiate lactation by having illegitimate babies whom they sent to "baby farms" in the country where the infants, more often than not, perished [27].

As a result of scientific and technological advances infant mortality and morbidity due to artificial feeding decreased dramatically. Most significantly, discoveries in bacteriology and the emerging science of biochemistry resulted in the boiling, modifying, and canning of cows' milk. As a result of these and numerous social changes, the incidence of breast-feeding decreased dramatically.

Today mothers usually request information on which to base their decision of whether to breast-feed or bottle-feed; this is a cultural decision rather than one based on health in most instances. Personal attitudes, social pressures, and psychologic needs all play a part. The cultural values of some nurses are strongly in favor of one or the other method of feeding, and such an opinion can interfere with good nursing care if the mother is made to feel guilty or inadequate because of her choice. Prenatal counselors can do much to reassure the mother and to solve practical problems in advance; this may lead some hesitant mothers to give breast-feeding a trial. The danger of excessive persuasion does exist, however, and may result in the creation of a sense of guilt, defeat, or frustration in the mother who does her best to breast-feed but fails. If the mother has a chronic disease (heart, kidney, tuberculosis), breast-feeding can be an additional strain. If the infant is premature and if active breast-feeding is delayed beyond 3 or 4 weeks, the likelihood of maintaining lactation is diminished.

Anthropologists in some countries measure the level of acculturation by the incidence of artificial feeding—the less breast-feeding, the higher the sophistication level. In developing countries where the water supply is often unsafe, sanitary facilities are not well established, education levels are low, and money is not available to buy bottles and nipples, breast-feeding is decreasing. This is especially unfortunate since gastrointestinal disease, a result of contaminated water and formula, is still a major cause of infant mortality. The *Lactobacillus* flora in the gastrointestinal tract of the breast-fed baby creates an environment unfavorable to *E. coli* growth and discourages this source of infant morbidity.

Protein-calorie malnutrition (PCM) is a common and unfortunate result when poor families try to stretch expensive formula by diluting it with contaminated water. In the Caribbean, it may cost up to 30 percent of the family's weekly income to purchase a week's supply of canned milk [27].

The potential contraceptive value of total breast-feeding is especially important in developing countries where women have difficulty obtaining alternative methods of birth control. It is estimated that total breast-feeding may decrease the incidence of pregnancy in the first 9 months after delivery by as much as 90 percent [27].

World health leaders are concerned about the trend away from breast-feeding in developing countries. They attribute it to the advertising and economic pressures of commercial food companies. In poor countries breast-feeding often becomes a lifesaving necessity, so they feel that the activities of multinational food manufacturers deserve some scrutiny and criticism. To counteract the influence of these companies, governments of some developing countries and many international agencies are beginning to appropriate money for education about breast-feeding [27].

FORMULA FEEDING

Bottle-feeding may be easier for some mothers than breast-feeding since the position of the bottle can be more readily adjusted than that of the breast. The nipple of the bottle is usually of adequate length and size to fit the baby's mouth, and the flow is even and easily maintained. In addition, bottle-feeding more readily allows someone other than the mother to participate in the infant's feeding, and thus is one way to permit the father an earlier and more active role in infant care.

Most hospitals purchase commercially prepared formula; served moderately cold or at room temperature, it is tolerated well by most babies. As mentioned previously, babies are best fed when they are hungry, dry, and comfortable. Whether it is the parents or the nurse who does the feeding, it is important that the baby be *held* throughout. This provides another opportunity to foster development of a feeling of closeness and security. Babies are usually held in a semireclining position, with the bottle tilted enough so that the nipple is constantly filled with milk (Fig. 16-23). Since sucking is ineffective when the baby's tongue is raised, it is important to make sure that the nipple is placed over the tongue. If the baby is obtaining formula, there will be air bubbles in the bottle; sometimes a clogged nipple prevents this. Needless to say, the nipple is considered sterile and should not be handled when the baby is being fed. Normally the infant consumes his feeding in about 15 to 20 minutes.

The common practice of propping the bottle by the baby's side is potentially dangerous, since the baby may choke or suck in considerable air. Research [8] has also indicated that propping the bottle with the baby supine may predispose him to recurrent middle-ear infections. His eustachian tube is shorter and wider than in the adult, and it lies at such an angle that milk may be propelled to the middle ear through it following the tremendous amount of suction that the infant exerts when feeding.

Figure 16-23. Proper position for feeding. The infant is in a semireclining position and able to make eye contact with the nurse. (Courtesy of Thomas Jefferson University, Philadelphia, Pa.)

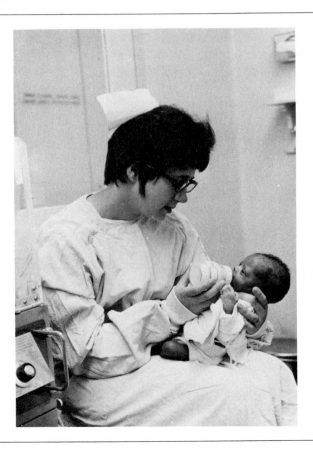

When the baby goes home, his parents may choose to continue feeding him the particular formula he received in the hospital or birth center or they may use one of a number of different preparations (Tables 16-2, 16-3, 16-4). A formula made with *evaporated milk* is still popular, low cost, generally available, sterile in the can, and convenient to store and handle; most brands of evaporated milk are equivalent in composition. For the newborn, evaporated milk is usually diluted with water in the ratio of 1:2 or 2:3, and the dilution for older infants is 1:1. The purpose of the dilution is to lessen the fat component of the milk; since the carbohydrate content is also diluted, additional sugar or corn syrup must be added. Nearly all brands are fortified with vitamin D (400 I.U. in a 13-ounce can). The amount of calories provided depends on dilution and on the amount of carbohydrate added. A dilution of 1:2 yields 14 calories per ounce; the 1:1 dilution yields 22 calories per ounce. Each 1 percent of carbohydrate added increases the energy value by 1.2 calories per ounce; the added carbohydrate allows normal metabolism of fats, permits protein to be used to build new tissues instead of to provide calories, and encourages normal water balance.

Table 16-2. Comparison of Components of Types of Milk

Type of Milk	Ratio	Calories/Ounce	Grams per 100 Milliliters			
			Protein	Fat	Carbohydrate	Minerals
Human milk	Undiluted	20	1.1	4.5	6.8	0.2
Whole milk	Undiluted	20	3.3	3.5	4.8	0.72
Evaporated milk	1:1	22	3.6	4.2	5.3	0.75
Commercial preparations						
Enfamil	1:1	20	1.5	3.7	7.0	0.35
Similac	1:1	20	1.7	3.4	6.6	0.38

Table 16-3. Formula Preparation for Newborn

Basic Component	Daily Requirement
Calories	55 calories per pound of body weight (approximate)
Fluid	3 ounces per pound of body weight
Carbohydrates	40 percent of caloric daily requirement: cane sugar (48 calories per tablespoon) or corn syrup (60 calories per tablespoon)

Table 16-4. Formula for 6-Pound Baby, Using Undiluted Evaporated Milk, Corn Syrup, and Water

Basic Component	Daily Requirement
Calories	330 calories (approximate)
Fluid	18 ounces
Carbohydrates	132 calories*

6 ounces of evaporated milk*	=	264 calories
1 tablespoon of corn syrup*	=	60 calories
12 ounces of water		324 calories
18 ounces of fluid		

* 1 ounce of evaporated milk contains approximately 3.1 grams of carbohydrate, so 6 ounces contain about 18 grams of carbohydrate. Each gram of carbohydrate represents 4 calories (18 × 4 = 72 calories [in evaporated milk]). Corn syrup is all carbohydrate (1 tablespoon = 60 calories of carbohydrate). 60 + 72 = 132 calories of carbohydrate.

Fresh milk is usually boiled to modify the curd and to complete sterilization. Ordinarily water in amounts not exceeding half the volume of milk is used to dilute it for young infants. The added water is mixed with 5 to 8 percent carbohydrate (sugar or corn syrup). Fresh milk, likely to be fortified with vitamin D, is more expensive and cumbersome than evaporated milk, and it also requires refrigeration and a constant fresh supply. When fresh cows' milk is not modified, it yields 20 calories per ounce.

If *dried milk* is used, boiled water is used to reconstitute it to its original strength. Low-fat or nonfat dried milk will have a lower caloric value and will need a vitamin D supplement. The advantages of dried milk include low cost and the ability to be stored in bulk.

Hypoallergenic formulas are available when it becomes necessary to alter or avoid the protein fraction; these formulas use processes involving evaporating, drying, or boiling the milk, or consist of a nonmilk product, such as soybeans or almonds. These formulas have an unpalatable taste and are somewhat lower in nutritional value.

Preparation of Formula in the Home. Artificial formula is usually made either by dilution of commercially prepared concentrated formula or by mixing an evaporated milk formula. If the baby is breast-fed, with only an occasional bottle, the commercial powdered formula is often used. It may be stored without refrigeration after opening.

The choice of preparation method depends on the kind of formula, the safety of the water and milk supply, the mother's ability to use the method, the presence of refrigeration in the home, and the number of bottles used each day. If safe milk and a pure municipal water supply are used, sterilization of the formula is usually unnecessary after the first few weeks.

With the *aseptic* method, the bottles, nipples, nipple-caps, and equipment used in making formula are sterilized (boiled for 10 minutes) or washed in a dishwasher before the formula is prepared. The formula is made according to directions, put into each bottle, nippled, capped, and refrigerated.

Terminal sterilization involves formula preparation under clean but not aseptic conditions. The equipment is washed thoroughly, the prepared formula is poured into the bottles, and the nipples and caps are applied loosely. They are placed in a sterilizer or large pot with a tight-fitting lid and boiled in water for 25 minutes. Prepared formula should not be left standing at room temperature but should be refrigerated as soon as it has cooled. Before refrigeration the screw caps are tightened.

When the baby does not take all of the formula from the bottle, what is left should either be discarded or used immediately in preparing cooked food, such as pudding. Generally this formula is considered unsafe for use for another feeding, even if it is refrigerated. Formula prepared for a single feeding should be used immediately.

BREAST-FEEDING

Reports indicate that approximately 50 percent of mothers in the United States breast-feed their infants. A recent report by Arafat and colleagues of breast-feeding practices and attitudes of over 400 mothers in New York City found that mothers in the lowest income bracket and those in the four top income brackets were much more likely to breast-feed than mothers in the middle income brackets [6]. The study also found that while religious affiliation did not make a significant difference in the method of infant feeding, ethnicity was a significant factor. Thirty-three percent of the black mothers reported breast-feeding at least one child compared to 55 percent of the white mothers and 67 percent of the Hispanic mothers. Other factors related to positive choices to breast-feed are the mother having been breast-fed herself, encouragement and support of breast-feeding from family, friends, and health professionals, and educational programs about breast-feeding.

In our own culture perhaps the number of breast-feeding mothers would increase if a woman's breasts were associated more with feeding babies than with sexual pleasure. As Nichols [24] notes, even though the

sexual display of breasts on any public beach, or in evening dress where the breasts are emphasized, or even see-through blouses with the no-bra look are circumstances we are fairly comfortable with, or at least not unduly shocked by, the sight of a nursing baby is somehow embarrassing. If we were to see a mother openly nursing a baby in a public place, our reaction would likely be discomfort or embarrassment.

Mothers, too, are affected by this cultural attitude, and because of it may choose not to breast-feed.

Advantages of Breast Milk. Many advantages are customarily attributed to breast milk: It is of correct chemical composition, it is constantly fresh and available at an even temperature, it is free from bacteria, it involves no preparation, and it is associated with a lower incidence of allergy, most notably eczema. In addition it is readily digested and assimilated, has a laxative effect on the baby, and results in less frequent and less severe feeding upsets. The flow of milk is well regulated, and the baby can suck until he is satisfied. Occasionally it is claimed that breast-feeding is cheaper, but in reality the recommended nutritional intake of the lactating mother makes breast-feeding a more expensive method of infant nutrition than some others. Poor maternal nutrition does not usually affect the quality of the milk, since the mother draws on the resources of her own tissues in its manufacture. Only the vitamin content is directly related to daily maternal intake. However, the quantity of milk can be affected; as a result, the malnourished mother probably will not have a sufficient amount of milk to adequately feed her infant.

Whether or not breast milk contains antibodies that are absorbed by the infant is a matter of controversy. Differences in the incidence of respiratory and enteric infections in breast-fed and bottle-fed babies are documented, although some research [1] indicates that these differences fade in middle-class families with good hygiene. In populations where these differences do exist, it is hard to judge whether they are due to the beneficial effects of breast milk or to increased contamination during bottle-feeding.

There are certain components of breast milk that may provide protective properties [11]. It is suggested that IgA, the predominant immunoglobulin in milk, effects an antimicrobial protection of mucous membranes and probably acts locally on the gastrointestinal tract. Breast milk containing polio antibodies prevents successful oral immunization of the newborn with live polio virus vaccine by neutralizing the virus in the gut; therefore, the vaccine is given later. The content of IgA in early colostrum may be as high as 20 to 40 milligrams per milliliter; after the first 2 to 4 days, the IgA content of breast milk drops to 1 milligram per milliliter. It is postulated that an increase in milk production compensates for the drop. In addition to antibodies, breast milk is also thought to contain lymphoid cells, neutrophils, and macrophages with phagocytic activity. These may play a part in protecting the maternal lactiferous glands as well as the infant's gastrointestinal tract from infection. Breast milk contains a large amount of lactoferrin, which has a strong bacteriostatic effect on *E. coli.*

Colostrum, the first milk produced after the baby's birth, is a yellow substance with more protein (in the form of globulins) and salts than mature milk, and less fat and sugar. During this initial period of lactation the baby gets no more than ½ ounce of colostrum at nursing, so that it is of minimal nourishment. Its beneficial effects, other than the transfer of globulins, include the early establishment of the milk supply with a decreased possibility of subsequent breast engorgement. For these reasons many authorities advocate allowing the baby to start sucking as soon as possible after birth.

Mature milk, which appears about the third day, is a bluish-white liquid with an alkaline or possibly neutral reaction; colostrum cells are usually absent after the twelfth day. Fat globules are small, numerous, and of uniform size. For the first 2 weeks mothers' milk is higher in protein and lower in fat, but in the following weeks the protein decreases while the fat and carbohydrate content increases. The last milk the baby gets from the breast at each feeding is richest in fat.

Breast milk can be stored, usually by pasteurizing and freezing or canning it for future use. Throughout the country there are breast milk centers or banks for the collection of surplus breast milk, which is made available for premature infants or for those babies with special nutritional problems.

If the mother has decided to breast-feed her infant, she should understand the physiology of lactation, breast-feeding routines, length of nursing, positioning for breast-feeding, and solutions to common problems encountered during nursing.

Physiology of Lactation. In order to successfully breast-feed, the mother should have an understanding of the basic anatomy and physiology of lactation. Following birth, the loss of estrogen and progesterone secretion through loss of the placenta allows the lactogenic effect of prolactin from the mother's pituitary to function. Within 2 to 3 days the breasts begin to secrete copious amounts of milk. During the next few weeks postdelivery the base level of prolactin secretion returns. However, each time the mother nurses, signals from the nipples to the hypothalamus cause approximately a tenfold surge in prolactin secretion lasting about 1 hour. This prolactin acts on the breasts to provide the milk for the next nursing period. If this prolactin surge is absent, if it is blocked as a result of hypothalamic or pituitary damage, or if breast-feeding does not continue, the breasts lose their ability to produce milk within a few days [28].

LET-DOWN REFLEX.   Whether or not the milk in the breasts is readily available to the baby depends on the milk ejection reflex, generally called "let-down." Some milk collects in the milk reservoirs, or sinuses, which lie under the areola. As the baby first sucks, he compresses the sinuses and thus the fore-milk is the milk he gets. The stimulation of his sucking on the sensitive nipple nerve endings causes the hypothalamus to direct the pituitary to secrete oxytocin. Oxytocin released into the bloodstream results in immediate and dramatic action in the alveoli, i.e., the myoepithelial cells banding the secretory cells contract, milk is ejected into the ductules and ducts, and the milk sinuses refill. With the let-down, the baby receives the hind-milk, the part of the milk that contains the fat content. The fat particles are sticky and adhere to the walls of the alveoli. They are forced out only when the milk ejection reflex functions. It is easy to see how important let-down is for the proper nourishment of the baby; in order to get enough calories he must receive the hind-milk as well as the fore-milk.

In the early weeks of nursing, let-down may not function reliably and automatically. The reflex is affected by the mother's emotional state, anxiety, and discomfort. Subjectively, let-down is felt as a tingling sensation or as a filling sensation. Nichols [24] suggests when assessing mothers to determine if they are experiencing let-down, ask the mother if she has any leaking or spraying of milk from one breast while nursing on the opposite one. If she does, you can reassure her that when let-down becomes well conditioned, this leaking will no longer occur. The sphincter muscles around the nipple will hold back the milk until it is actually taken by the baby.

Beginning Breast-feeding. Ideally, nursing should start as soon as possible after birth. Some researchers indicate that the newborn has a heightened sucking reflex shortly after birth. Other advantages frequently cited are that early nursing stimulates early milk production, it gives the infant full benefit of the colostrum, and stimulation of oxytocin production in the mother helps contract her uterus.

The breast-fed infant nurses more frequently in the early weeks—often 8 to 12 times a day—with only one or two periods when he sleeps for 4 to 5 hours between feedings. The infant's stomach is small and breast milk is so readily digestible that he can rarely be expected to go more than a couple of hours between feedings. While on some days he will seem less interested in feeding, during future growth spurts his demands will increase. These occur generally 2 weeks, 6 weeks, between 2½ and 3 months, and between 4½ and 6 months after birth. At these times he may fret and cry more easily and will require increased feedings.

Positioning. The mother may assume one of several positions during breast-feeding (Fig. 16-24). Changing nursing positions is helpful for the comfort of the mother, for complete emptying of her breasts, and for the prevention and treatment of nipple tenderness and plugged ducts [24]. The mother may choose to nurse the infant while she is lying on her side, or sitting upright, or the baby may be nursed placed on the mother's chest. This latter position is helpful if the mother has had spinal anesthesia and is to remain flat in bed. Tailor sitting is another comfortable position for breast-feeding.

Feeding Technique. To successfully breast-feed, the infant must have both the areola and nipple in his mouth. To help the baby get a firm grasp on the nipple and areola, the mother may "point up" the nipple by gently pressing the areola between two fingers. As the baby begins to nurse, he should be prevented from pressing his nose against the breast and obstructing his nasal pathway. If this

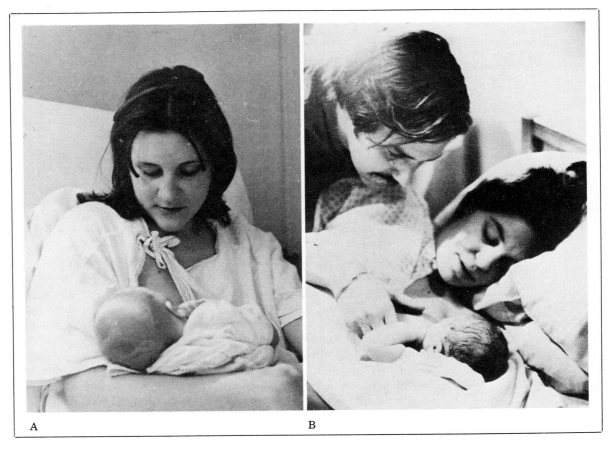

A   B

Figure 16-24. A. Breast-
feeding in sitting posi-
tion. B. Lying on side
while breast-feeding.
(Courtesy of Booth Ma-
ternity Center, Philadel-
phia, Pa.)

occurs, the mother should place her finger against her breast, pressing it back from the baby's nose. When the baby's jaws close, his gums compress the areola over the lacteal sinuses, squeezing the milk out. Air is sealed off by the baby's lips and flat cheek muscles. Breaking the infant's suction may be accomplished by placing a finger at the corner of the baby's mouth before pulling him away (Fig. 16-25). This will prevent the nipple from becoming sore.

The initial nursing time should be 5 to 7 minutes on each breast for the first day or two, gradually increasing to 10 to 15 minutes on the first breast as long as the baby nurses well on the second breast. Nursing time varies considerably from baby to baby according to how hungry he is and how much he desires to suck. The baby may close his lips tightly around the nipple only and suck vigorously. With this method he obtains very little milk, and the nipple is likely to be injured by his vigorous sucking. If nipples become sore, nursing time can be restricted to 5 to 10 minutes on each breast, just enough time to empty them through the period of soreness. Both breasts should be offered at each feeding, and the woman should alternate the breast she starts with. This ensures that each breast will get adequate stimulation. Pinning a safety pin on one side of her bra will help the mother remember on which side to start the next feeding.

Figure 16-25. When the infant is finished eating, suction can be broken by placing a finger in one corner of the infant's mouth.

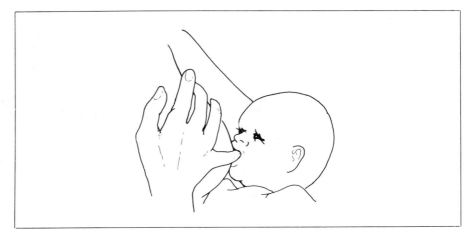

It is important that the mother be prepared for the initial grasp pain when the baby latches onto her breast. This will decrease as lactation becomes well established. She should also be aware of how to use the baby's rooting reflex to best advantage, since he will turn toward her breast and nipple when it touches his cheek. Refrain from trying to stimulate the rooting reflex manually, since the baby is likely to turn toward your hand rather than the mother's breast.

Many babies begin nursing easily and suck immediately, but occasionally a baby needs to experiment before he begins. Sometimes moistening the mother's nipple with a few drops of expressed colostrum or a few drops of formula or sugar water will prompt the baby to take the nipple more eagerly. If he does not nurse after approximately 10 minutes of trying, it is best to stop and try again at the next feeding or when he seems hungry.

It is difficult to determine the amount of milk a breast-feeding baby has taken. In some nurseries the baby is weighed before and after feeding to determine this, but most of the time other factors are used as indications that he is getting enough: his satisfaction, sleeping patterns, time between feedings, weight gain, and number of wet diapers.

Sometimes it is necessary for the mother to empty her breasts in order to relieve engorgement, to maintain milk supply when the baby cannot empty her breasts in the early days of nursing, or to allow fissures to heal.

A hand pump may be used; with this, suction may be obtained by collapsing the rubber bulb at one end, placing the other, widened end over the nipple and areola, and releasing the bulb. The process is repeated until the desired amount of milk is emptied. This method is often used to soften the breast before the baby nurses. There are a variety of types of hand pumps. Tibbetts and Cadwell [29] give a detailed comparison of them (see Table 16-5).

Breast-feeding Problems. PAIN. During the first few weeks the mother may experience some pain in her breasts at each nursing. She may be assured that this is common and is often related to a let-down that is not yet functioning smoothly. Within a few weeks, as she learns to relax and becomes more self-confident in feeding, she will find that the pain will disappear. In the meantime, a mild analgesic may be helpful.

*Table 16-5. Breast
        Pumps*

Pump	Availability	Sterility	Capacity	Power Source	Cost	Portable	Instructions	Equipment
Loyd B. Pump	By mail	Yes	4 oz (baby food jars can be used)	Woman	$35–$37	Yes	Limited	All glass parts; good for working mothers
Egnell	Rental depots	Yes	8 oz	Electricity	Rental $17.50 for first 5 days, $1.70 for each additional day	No	In booklet and on pump	All plastic parts; good for long-term use
Kaneson Expressing and Feeding Bottle	By mail	Yes	3 oz	Woman	$23.95 plus $1.25 shipping	Yes	Booklet	Plastic parts; good for situations where milk can be directly fed to baby
Evenflo Natural Mother Breast Pump Kit	Available in pharmacies, Sears, Penney's	Yes	4 oz	Woman	Less than $3	Yes	Booklet	Plastic parts good for working mothers
Hand pump	Pharmacies	Poor	Less than ½ oz	Woman	Less than $3	Yes	No	Plastic container; rubber bulb
Hand expression	To anyone who learns the skill	Yes	No limit	Woman	Free	Yes	See Chapter 14	Natural; good for woman with occasional need to collect milk

Source: E. Tibbetts and K. Caldwell. Selecting the right breast pump. *American Journal of Maternal-Child Nursing* 5:262, 1980.

ENGORGEMENT.   The initial filling of the mother's breasts may be accompanied by engorgement, but this varies considerably from mother to mother. The engorgement is due partly to increased vascularity and partly to the increased accumulation of milk. There may be secondary lymphatic and venous stasis if milk cannot be removed. Sometimes the ducts become occluded by congested tissues and/or blockage with earlier secretions that have become thickened. The mother needs reassurance that the discomfort of engorgement will subside in a day or two.

Engorgement may be prevented through frequent nursing. When it does occur, hand expression or use of a breast pump to release some of the milk to reduce the pressure and expose the nipple further is helpful prior to feeding the infant. If the areola is engorged and firm, the baby cannot compress the milk reservoirs underneath with his jaws. As a result, he may grasp the nipple alone, which will lead to tenderness, soreness, and cracking. Areolar massage will soften the area prior to nursing. A hot shower or hot compresses to the breasts before nursing should also relieve the discomfort.

SORE NIPPLES. Soreness can be prevented by proper nipple care, avoiding engorgement by frequent nursing, and proper positioning of the infant. Simply washing the nipples daily with plain water should be sufficient to keep them clean. Washing the nipples with plain water before and/or after nursing washes off the emollient sebum of the skin and the natural antiseptic lysozyme contained in human milk. It is far more important that the mother wash her hands carefully. Avoiding engorgement by frequent feedings is very important in nipple care. When an infant nurses every 2 to 3 hours he is less ravenous than when he waits 4 to 5 hours and tends to exert less trauma on the mother's nipples.

Proper positioning of the infant on the breast as well as nursing in different positions is also important. Changing positions for nursing ensures that the most tender areas of the nipple are not continuously exposed to the same pressures of the baby's mouth. Sore nipples usually reach a peak of discomfort, then improve rapidly if the infant is correctly positioned and breast-fed frequently.

Further aids for sore, cracked, or fissured nipples include exposing the nipples to air, application of lanolin, or brief exposure to an ultraviolet sunlamp. After each nursing the woman should air-dry her nipples and let the flaps of her bra down for 15 to 30 minutes two or three times a day. No plastic liners should be in the bra or on disposable nursing pads, for these trap moisture and impede air circulation. A wire tea strainer may be placed inside the mother's bra to keep clothing away from the sore nipple. It allows circulation of air and encourages more rapid healing [30]. A very light application of hydrous lanolin after air drying is soothing on sore nipples, but lanolin can cause difficulties if either the mother or infant is sensitive to wool. Some mothers find A & D Ointment also soothing on sore nipples. Whatever substance is used should be safe for mother and baby and should not have to be washed off before nursing, since the less washing or scrubbing of the nipples, the better.

If nipple soreness is severe, cracked ice wrapped in a clean white cloth and applied to the nipple area only has been very helpful to some mothers. Nipple healing in severe cases may also be speeded by using an ultraviolet sunlamp. At a distance of 4 feet, initial exposure should be ½ minute the first day, 1 minute the second and third days, 2 minutes the fourth and fifth days, and 3 minutes the sixth day and thereafter, unless the skin becomes red. The mother's eyes should be protected when the lamp is being used, and if used at home it should be kept away from other children to prevent accidents.

INFECTIONS. Mastitis and breast abscesses generally require medical intervention. Some clinicians recommend that the mother should be strongly urged to continue to breast-feed the baby on both breasts, and even to increase the frequency of nursing. Breast infections will not harm the baby. Usually the infection is interstitial, not intraductal, and even in the rare case of some infective material reaching the baby, the anti-infective properties of mothers' milk seem to prevent harm to the baby. The best treatment for mastitis, to prevent abscess development and hasten recovery, includes the application of moist heat, forcing of fluids, administration of antibiotics to which staphylococcus is not resistant, bed rest, and continued frequent breast-feeding. (See Chap. 20 for a discussion of the issues surrounding continuation or discontinuation of breast-feeding during mastitis.)

If the mother has been nursing without discomfort and then rapidly develops extremely sore nipples thrush should be suspected. Check the mother's breasts for inflammation of the nipples and areola and the infant's mouth for white patches indicative of the infection. Treatment may consist of nystatin or 1 to 2% gentian violet swabbed in the infant's mouth.

LACK OF REST.   Among the most common problems for breast-feeding mothers are the frequency with which the baby nurses and lack of rest. Mothers should be told that breast-fed infants nurse frequently in the early weeks, usually 8 to 12 times a day. Discussions with the mother about putting her baby's needs first and minimizing the care of her house should also be a part of discharge planning for self-care. Help the nursing mother do advance planning to meet her increased need for rest. Encourage her to relax, nap when the baby is asleep, and let others who are available to help take care of house, laundry, and cooking while she devotes herself to her baby's and her own well-being [29].

Weaning.   Addition of solid foods to the baby's diet around the middle of the first year is the first step in weaning for most babies. As time goes by, the outside world becomes more and more interesting to him, and the the baby wants to nurse less and less. Some babies give up breast-feeding on their own even before a year, others around 12 to 15 months of age; still others seem to need to continue for a little or much longer.

As Riordan and Countryman note, ideally, weaning will occur in response to the baby's needs, whatever his age. Some mothers, however, feel a need to wean the baby before the baby is fully ready. When this is necessary, the mother should be encouraged to wean very gradually. Eliminating one feeding a day for a few days, omitting a second for several more days, and likewise slowly eliminating additional feedings will enable the baby to adjust with minimal trauma. Mothers who undertake weaning should endeavor to give the baby a great deal of additional holding, cuddling, and attention to replace the loss that the baby is experiencing [29].

Transfer of Drugs and Other Substances in Breast Milk.   Nearly all drugs that the mother takes may be found to some extent in her breast milk but not all of them appear in significant amounts. It is important, therefore, to consider not only what she is taking but how much. Unless the mother is taking large doses, alcohol, barbiturates, antibiotics, narcotics, salicylates, caffeine, and psychotherapeutic drugs appear in insignificant amounts in breast milk [7]. Mineral oil, milk of magnesia, and aspirin in the normal recommended doses may be safely taken. Atropine may decrease milk production and may cause intoxication in the baby. Ergot may cause vomiting, diarrhea, and weak pulse in the baby. If the mother is taking oral anticoagulants, her baby should be watched for bleeding tendencies. Steroids, bromides, cascara, and metronidazole (Flagyl) may cause symptoms in the baby. Radioactive iodine may be transmitted in the milk and may have a suppressive effect on the infant's developing thyroid; if the mother has had studies using it in the recent antepartal period, it is felt that it is wise to stop breast-feeding for a time. Smoking may decrease the mother's excretion of milk, but if she smokes only moderately, she should not be made to feel that she should give it up solely for the baby's sake. However, she should avoid smoking near the baby, since smoke inhaled by the baby increases the incidence and severity of respiratory diseases. As mentioned previously, oral contraceptives may inhibit lactation, particularly if they are begun before the fifth or sixth postpartum week. Long-range effects of marijuana on the infant have not been documented. The fact that breast milk contains more DDT than cows' milk is known; its importance depends on the amount received by the baby, who appears to be in no danger from present levels of DDT in breast milk (see Table 16-6).

Table 16-6. Transfer of Substances in Breast Milk

Drugs Contraindicated in Breast-feeding Mothers

Chloramphenicol	Hematologic suppression of bone marrow in high serum concentrations
^{131}Iodine (half-life 10 days) ^{125}Iodine (half-life 30 days) ^{67}Gallium (half-life 14 days) ^{99m}Technetium (half-life 2 days)	Transported in milk in high concentrations. If the woman needs diagnostic tests with one of these radioactive substances, she should not nurse her infant for the number of days indicated according to the agent
Mercury	Concentrated in breast milk. Can cause severe toxicity in the infant
Anticancer agents	May be mutagenic or carcinogenic. Should be avoided until more data are available
Environmental pollutants	Should be avoided as much as possible
Lipid-soluble sulfonilamides	Potential risk in the presence of neonatal hyperbilirubinemia when the potential for displacement of bilirubin from protein binding sites exists. Sulfisoxazole recently reported *not* to be contraindicated
Lithium	Concentrations in infants can reach therapeutic levels

Drugs Which May Be Contraindicated in Breast-feeding Mothers
(due to lack of data or equivocal findings)

Oral contraceptives	Ethylbiscoumacetate
Diazepam (large doses)	Cimetidine
Metronidazole	Loperamide
THC (9-tetrahydrocannabinol)	Senna
Cascara	

Drugs Not Contraindicated in Breast-feeding Mothers

Warfarin	Phenothiazines	Digoxin
Most antibiotics	Anticholinergics	Antacids
Antihistamines	Metroprolol	Acetaminophen
Decongestants	Carbamazepine	Aspirin
Epinephrine	Captopril	Narcotics
Corticosteroids	Non-lipid soluble sulfas	Butorphanol
Ethanol	Tricyclic antidepressants	Methenamine
Propranolol	Haloperidol	Sprionolactone
Heparin	Phenytoin	Thiazide diuretics
Propylthiouracil	Theophylline, caffeine	

Source: Adapted from J. Bertino. The pharmacology of human milk. *Birth and the Family Journal* 8:237, 1981.

BUBBLING THE BABY

When the baby's stomach is full, his sucking becomes slow and intermittent and he gradually falls asleep. Since he normally swallows air as he nurses, it is important to raise the air bubbles from his stomach. It is good practice to stop once or twice during each feeding to attempt to raise the bubble. If this is not done, the baby will burp when he is put back in bed and milk will be likely to come with it, increasing the danger of aspiration. Sometimes a baby stops sucking because a large air bubble has made his stomach feel full; after he is burped, he begins to suck with renewed interest.

Most babies are easily bubbled. If the infant is held in an upright position, the air will rise to the top of his stomach. If his body is supported against the nurse's or the mother's body or shoulder and he is gently patted or stroked on the back, the air comes up with a definite belch. Sometimes a change in position alone, from reclining to upright, is all that is needed. If the baby has not burped in 2 or 3 minutes, it probably would be wise to put him down and try again later. If this is still not successful in raising a bubble, he is put to bed and positioned either on his right side or on his abdomen. Hiccuping is common and is generally not significant.

Some babies, characterized as "spitters," regurgitate more than the usual amount; such a baby should be handled as gently as possible, fed in a calm relaxed atmosphere, and bubbled frequently, in a sitting position. When he is placed in his crib, he should be put on his right side or abdomen in a reverse Trendelenburg position. It should be remembered that regurgitation relates to an overflow of milk, not to be confused with actual vomiting. The amount regurgitated is frequently less than it appears, and the baby is usually retaining an adequate amount unless he fails to gain weight.

Case Study Baby Smith*

As Baby Smith's nurse, develop a plan of care for him, including short- and long-range goals. Each of you will develop your own approach to newborn care. Applying the nursing process to the outline following the brief case study will help to organize your approach to the care of newborns and their families while they are in the health care agency and when they return home.

Baby boy Smith was born at 6:32 A.M. on Wednesday, September 18. He was delivered with low forceps and epidural anesthesia after 10 hours of an uneventful labor. His Apgar scores were 8 at 1 minute and 10 at 5 minutes. He received routine newborn care in the delivery room and was later transferred to the newborn nursery. His mother, Susan Smith, a 28-year-old primigravida, is married to Henry Smith, a 30-year-old manager of a shoe store.

Upon admission to the nursery, Baby Smith's vital signs are assessed; his weight is 3,200 grams; his length is 51 centimeters. He is estimated to be a full-term baby by dates and appearance, AGA. His head circumference is 33 centimeters; chest, 31 centimeters; and abdomen, 31 centimeters. He is placed in a warming bed. Susan plans to breast-feed the baby. From the verbal report you

* Case study developed by Andrea Hollingsworth.

learn that his mother was too tired to nurse him in the recovery room, even though she has been very enthusiastic about the prospect of breast-feeding him. As you prepare to do the admission nursing assessment on Baby Smith, you notice that he appears somewhat listless.

Around 10 A.M. the same day Baby Smith's temperature is 98.6°F, taken rectally. After being bathed and dressed he is placed in a bassinet crib. At 10:30 A.M. he receives a feeding of sterile water. He takes 1 ounce well and regurgitates a small amount of mucus. When he is taken out to his mother, she smiles and reaches out to hold the baby. "Is he OK?" she asks. After an explanation that everything appears normal, she unwraps the baby. "You can take him back now," Susan states, "I'm tired."

That evening, when Baby Smith is brought out to his mother for the 10 P.M. feeding, Susan begins to feed the baby and she does not appear to need help. She handles the baby with confidence. When the nursery nurse returns, Susan is watching television and the baby is lying at the foot of the bed on his abdomen, sleeping.

The next morning, a class is to be held on baby care. A nurse invites Susan to come and join the other mothers. Susan states, "Oh, my stitches hurt too much and, besides, my mother knows all about taking care of babies—she had eight of her own." She then turns her attention back to the television.

On September 20, the baby appears jaundiced and the serum bilirubin is 13 mg/100 ml. The doctor orders phototherapy for Baby Smith. As Susan walks by the nursery window, she notices her baby under the hyperbilirubinemia lamp with his eyes covered. She stops at the nursery nurses' station and asks about her baby. The nurse invites her in and explains the baby's treatment. Susan listens and says, "But he's OK? Right?" The nurse assures her and she leaves.

Assessment Form

Assessment	Plan	Intervention	Evaluation

I. Pertinent History
  A. Mother's age, socioeconomic level, ethnic cultural group, education, marital status
  B. Mother's/family's past medical history
  C. Mother's past obstetric history
  D. Mother's present prenatal history
  E. Labor and delivery
II. Physical Findings
  A. Posture, length, weight
  B. Gestational age
  C. Skin
    1. Hair distribution
    2. Turgor
    3. Color
      (a) Cyanosis
      (b) Pallor
      (c) Plethora
      (d) Jaundice
      (e) Pink
      (f) Meconium staining
    4. Vernix
    5. Dryness or peeling
    6. Other
      (a) Edema
      (b) Ecchymoses
      (c) Petechiae
      (d) Erythema toxicum
      (e) Hemangiomas
      (f) Telangiectatic nevi
      (g) Milia
      (h) Harlequin color change
      (i) Mongolian spots
      (j) Café-au-lait spots
      (k) Nails
  D. Head
    1. Biparietal circumference
    2. Symmetry, shape, swelling
      (a) Caput succedaneum			

Assessment Form			
Assessment	Plan	Intervention	Evaluation

      (b) Cephalohematoma
      (c) Molding
      (d) Facial movements, asymmetry
    3. Fontanelles—anterior, posterior
      (a) Enlarged
      (b) Bulging
      (c) Sunken
      (d) Size
    4. Sutures
      (a) Overriding
      (b) Separation
  E. Face
    1. Eyes
      (a) Color
      (b) Hemorrhagic areas
      (c) Edema
      (d) Discharge
      (e) Conjunctivitis
      (f) Jaundice
      (g) Pupils
      (h) Size
    2. Nose
      (a) Patency
      (b) Nasal flaring
      (c) Discharge
    3. Ears
      (a) Formation
      (b) Position in relation to eye
      (c) Cartilage
      (d) Hearing
    4. Mouth
      (a) Size
      (b) Palate lip
      (c) Size of tongue in relation to mouth
      (d) Predeciduous teeth
      (e) Epstein's pearls
      (f) Frenulum linguae
      (g) Sucking blisters

Assessment Form			
Assessment	Plan	Intervention	Evaluation

      (h) Infections (thrush)

      (i) Gums

F. Neck

  1. Mobility

  2. Torticollis

  3. Length

  4. Goiter

G. Chest

  1. Circumference

  2. Symmetry

  3. Breast

    (a) Engorgement

    (b) Nipples

    (c) Areola

    (d) Accessory nipples

  4. Respiratory system

    (a) Rate

    (b) Rhythm

    (c) Type of respiration

    (d) Grunting

    (e) Retraction

    (f) Lungs

      (1) Rhonchi

      (2) Rales

  5. Cardiovascular

    (a) Rate

    (b) Rhythm

    (c) Murmurs

    (d) Capillary filling time

    (e) Pulses

      (1) Radial

      (2) Brachial

      (3) Femoral

    (f) Blood pressure

H. Abdomen and back

  1. Appearance

    (a) Shape

    (b) Distention

      (1) Abdominal

      (2) Bladder

Assessment Form

Assessment	Plan	Intervention	Evaluation

2. Liver, kidney, spleen
   (a) Size
   (b) Shape
3. Umbilicus
   (a) Infection
   (b) Hernia
   (c) Cutis navel
   (d) Vein and arteries
   (e) Bleeding
4. Bowel sounds
5. Spinal column
   (a) Curvature
   (b) Pilonidal cyst
   (c) Masses

I. Genital-anal
   1. Appearance
      (a) Male
         (1) Testicles
         (2) Scrotum
             a. Rugae
             b. Edema
         (3) Urethral patency
         (4) Hypo- or epispadias
         (5) Foreskin
         (6) Ambiguities
      (b) Female
         (1) Prominence of labia majora/minora
         (2) Vaginal discharge
         (3) Hymenal tag
         (4) Urethral patency
         (5) Ambiguities
   2. Anus
      (a) Patency
      (b) Stool transition

J. Musculoskeletal
   1. Posture, muscle tone
   2. Extremities
      (a) Contour
      (b) Symmetry

Assessment Form			
Assessment	Plan	Intervention	Evaluation

      (c) Fractures (clavicle, scapula, humerus, femur)

      (d) Range of motion

      (e) Paralysis

      (f) Irregular position

      (g) Polydactyly, syndactyly

   3. Hip

      (a) Hip click

      (b) Gluteal folds

  K. Neurologic

   1. Muscle tone

   2. Head control

   3. Cranial nerves

   4. Reflexes

      (a) Tonic neck

      (b) Grasp

      (c) Rooting

      (d) Sucking

      (e) Moro

      (f) Stepping

      (g) Babinski

      (h) Baby doll

      (i) Tendon

      (j) Truncal incurvation

      (k) Anal wink

III. Behavioral Assessment

  A. Response to stimulation

  B. State

   1. Quiet deep sleep

   2. Light active sleep

   3. Drowsy awake

   4. Quiet alert

   5. Active alert

   6. Crying

  C. Sleeping pattern

  D. Feeding pattern

   1. Type of feeding

   2. Intake

  E. Voiding pattern

  F. Stool pattern

Assessment Form

Assessment	Plan	Intervention	Evaluation

G. Temperature regulation
H. Relationship with parents
   1. Parental interest
   2. Eye-to-eye contact
   3. Refusal to handle baby
   4. How refer to baby
   5. Support systems at home
   6. Need for referral to clinical or community resources
   7. Date for return visit to pediatrician or pediatric nurse practitioner			

REFERENCES

1. Adebonojo, F. Artificial vs. breast feeding. *Clinical Pediatrics* 11:25, 1972.
2. Adlard, B. P. F., and Lathe, G. G. Breast milk jaundice: Effect of pregnanediol on bilirubin conjugation by human liver. *Archives of Diseases in Childhood* 45:186, 1970.
3. Alexander, M., and Brown, M. *Pediatric Physical Diagnosis for Nurses.* New York: McGraw-Hill, 1974.
4. American Academy of Pediatrics. *Standards and Recommendations for Hospital Care of Newborn Infants.* Evanston, Ill., 1976.
5. American Academy of Pediatrics, Committee on Fetus and Newborn. Hexachlorophene and skin care of newborn infants. *Pediatrics* 49:625, 1972.
6. Arafat, I., Allen, D., and Fox, J. Maternal attitude and practice toward breastfeeding. *Journal of Obstetric, Gynecologic and Neonatal Nursing* 10:91, 1981.
7. Arena, J. Contamination of the ideal food. *Nutrition Today* 5:2, 1970.
8. Beauregard, W. Positional otitis media. *Journal of Pediatrics* 70:294, 1971.
9. Behrman, R., and Mangurten, H. Birth Injuries. In R. Behrman (Ed.), *Neonatology.* St. Louis: Mosby, 1973.
10. Brazelton, T. Neonatal Behavioral Assessment Scale. In *Clinics in Developmental Medicine,* No. 50. London: Heineman, 1973.
11. Breast milk and defence against infection in the newborn. *Archives of Diseases in Childhood* 47:845, 1972.
12. Brown, R. J. K., and Valman, H. B. *Practical Neonatal Pediatrics.* Oxford: Blackwell, 1973.
13. Davis, V. The structure and function of brown adipose tissue in the neonate. *Journal of Obstetric, Gynecologic and Neonatal Nursing* 9:368, 1980.
14. Driscoll, J. M. Physical Examination. In R. Behrman (Ed.), *Neonatology.* St. Louis: Mosby, 1973.
15. Gordon, R. Neonatal immunology: A review of host response to infection. *Michigan Medicine* 72:219, 1973.
16. Hargreaves, T., and Piper, R. F. Breast-milk jaundice. *Archives of Diseases in Childhood* 46:195, 1971.
17. Hexachlorophene in the nursery. *Medical Letter on Drugs and Therapeutics* 15:1, 1973.
18. Jaundice. *LaLeche League News* 13(4): July–August, 1971.
19. Korones, S. *High-Risk Newborn Infants.* St. Louis: Mosby, 1981.
20. Longenecker, C. G., Ryan, R. F., and Vincent, R. W. Malformation of ear as clue to urogenital anomalies. *Plastic and Reconstructive Surgery* 35:303, 1965.
21. McClure, J. H., and Caton, W. L. Newborn temperature: Temperature of term normal infants. *Journal of Pediatrics* 47:583, 1955.
22. Moore, M. L. *Newborn Family and Nurse.* Philadelphia: Saunders, 1981.
23. Neonatologists and the critical first hours. *Journal of the American Medical Association* 202:41, 1967.
24. Nichols, M. Effective help for the nursing mother. *Journal of Obstetric, Gynecologic and Neonatal Nursing* 7:22, 1978.
24a. Poland, R., Schultz, G., and Garg, G. High milk lipase activity associated with breast milk jaundice. *Pediatric Research* 14:1328, 1980.
25. Poole, C. Neonatal circumcision. *Journal of Obstetric, Gynecologic and Neonatal Nursing* 8:207, 1979.
26. Preston, E. N. Whither the foreskin. *Journal of the American Medical Association* 213:1853, 1970.
27. Riordan, J., and Countryman, B. Part I: Infant feeding patterns past and present. *Journal of Obstetric, Gynecologic and Neonatal Nursing* 9:207, 1980.
28. Riordan, J., and Countryman, B. Part II: Anatomy and psychophysiology of lactation. *Journal of Obstetric, Gynecologic and Neonatal Nursing* 9:210, 1980.
29. Riordan, J., and Countryman, B. Part V: Self-care for continued breastfeeding. *Journal of Obstetric, Gynecologic and Neonatal Nursing* 9:357, 1980.
30. Riordan, J., and Countryman, B. Part VI: Some breastfeeding problems and solutions. *Journal of Obstetric, Gynecologic and Neonatal Nursing* 9:361, 1980.
31. Scanlon, J., Nelson, T., Grylack, L., and Smith, Y. *A System of Newborn Physical Examination.* Baltimore: University Park Press, 1979.
32. Tibbetts, E., and Cadwell, K. Selecting the right breast pump. *American Journal of Maternal-Child Nursing* 5:262, 1980.
33. Vulliamy, D. *The Newborn Child.* Baltimore: Williams & Wilkins, 1972.
34. Whitner, W., and Thompson, M. The influence of bathing on the newborn infant's body temperature. *Nursing Research* 19:30, 1970.

FURTHER READING   Applebaum, R. M. The modern management of successful breast feeding. *Pediatric Clinics of North America* 17:203, 1970.

Atkinson, L. Prenatal nipple conditioning for breastfeeding. *Nursing Research* 28:267, 1979.

Ballard, J. A simplified score for assessment of fetal maturation of newly born infants. *Journal of Pediatrics* 95:769, 1979.

Berlin, C. Pharmacologic considerations of drug use in the lactating mother. *Obstetrics and Gynecology* 58:17s, 1981.

Beske, E., and Garvis, M. Research—Important factors in breastfeeding success. *American Journal of Maternal-Child Nursing* 7:174, 1982.

Bornstein, M., Kessen, W., and Weiskopf, S. The categories of hue in infancy. *Science* 191:201, 1976.

Brazelton, T. Behavioral competence of the newborn infant. *Seminars in Perinatology* 3:35, 1979.

Britten, G. Early mother-infant contact and infant temperature stabilization. *Journal of Obstetric, Gynecologic and Neonatal Nursing* 9:84, 1980.

Brodish, M. Perinatal assessment. *Journal of Obstetric, Gynecologic and Neonatal Nursing* 10:42, 1981.

Broome, M. Breastfeeding and the working mother. *Journal of Obstetric, Gynecologic and Neonatal Nursing* 10:201, 1981.

Browne, M. Controversial questions about breastfeeding. *Journal of Obstetric, Gynecologic and Neonatal Nursing* 4:15, 1975.

Burd, B. Nurses' messages about breastfeeding. *American Journal of Nursing* 81:1491, 1981.

Cadwell, K. Improving nipple graspability for success at breastfeeding. *Journal of Obstetric, Gynecologic and Neonatal Nursing* 10:277, 1981.

Cash, J., and Giacoia, G. Organization and operation of a human breast milk bank. *Journal of Obstetric, Gynecologic and Neonatal Nursing* 10:434, 1981.

Crelin, E. *Functional Anatomy of the Newborn.* New Haven, Conn.: Yale University Press, 1973.

Eiger, M., and Olds, S. *The Complete Book of Breastfeeding.* New York: Workman, 1973.

Foley, K. Caring for the parents of twins. *American Journal of Maternal-Child Nursing* 4:221, 1979.

Fomon, S. Nutrition in Infancy. In D. Lauler (Ed.), *Infant Nutrition.* New York: Medcom, 1972.

Giefer, M., and Nelson, C. A new method to help fathers develop parenting skills. *Journal of Obstetric, Gynecologic and Neonatal Nursing* 10:455, 1981.

Grimes, D. Routine circumcision reconsidered. *American Journal of Nursing* 80:108, 1980.

Gromada, K. Maternal-infant attachment: The first step toward individualizing twins. *American Journal of Maternal-Child Nursing* 6:129, 1981.

Haddock, N. Blood pressure monitoring in neonates. *American Journal of Maternal-Child Nursing* 5:131, 1980.

Hall, J. Influencing breastfeeding success. *Journal of Obstetric, Gynecologic and Neonatal Nursing* 7:28, 1978.

Hall, L. Effect of teaching on primiparas' perceptions of their newborn. *Nursing Research* 29:317, 1980.

Hayes, B. Inconsistencies among nurses in breastfeeding knowledge and counseling. *Journal of Obstetric, Gynecologic and Neonatal Nursing* 10:430, 1981.

Hill, S., and Shronk, J. The effect of early parent-infant contact on newborn body temperature. *Journal of Obstetric, Gynecologic and Neonatal Nursing* 8:287, 1979.

Iles, J., and McCrary, M. Cuddle bathing can be fun: The rewards of research. *American Journal of Maternal-Child Nursing* 1:350, 1976.

LaLeche League International. *The Womanly Art of Breastfeeding.* Franklin Park, Ill., 1963.

Leonard, L. Breastfeeding twins: Maternal-infant nutrition. *Journal of Obstetric, Gynecologic and Neonatal Nursing* 11:148, 1982.

Livingston, R., Crane, V., and Mims, L. Clinical assessment of gestational age. *Journal of Obstetric, Gynecologic and Neonatal Nursing* 6(6):17, 1976.

Meyer, H. What parents worry about in their newborn infants. *Medical Times* 100:51, 1972.

Nalepka, C. Understanding thermoregulation in newborns. *Journal of Obstetric, Gynecologic and Neonatal Nursing* 5(6):17, 1976.

Oehler, J. *Family Centered Neonatal Nursing Care.* Philadelphia: Lippincott, 1981.

Olson, M. Fitting grandparents into new families. *American Journal of Maternal-Child Nursing* 6:419, 1981.

Peters, D., and Worthington-Roberts, B. Infant feeding practices of middle-class breastfeed-ing and formula feeding mothers. *Birth* 9:91, 1982.

Pryor, K. *Nursing Your Baby.* New York: Harper & Row, 1973.

Reiser, S. A tool to facilitate mother-infant attachment. *Journal of Obstetric, Gynecologic and Neonatal Nursing* 10:294, 1981.

Riordan, J., and Rapp, E. Pleasure and purpose, the sensuousness of breastfeeding. *Journal of Obstetric, Gynecologic and Neonatal Nursing* 9:109, 1980.

Scahill, M. Helping the mother solve problems with feeding her infant. *Journal of Obstetric, Gynecologic and Neonatal Nursing* 4:51, 1975.

Schaffer, A., and Avery, M. E. *Diseases of the Newborn.* Philadelphia: Saunders, 1971.

Senie, R. Possible related risks to breastfeeding. *Journal of Obstetric, Gynecologic and Neonatal Nursing* 11:34, 1982.

Simkin, P. "Physiologic" jaundice of the newborn. *Birth and the Family Journal* 6:23, 1979.

Stern, L. Physiology of the newborn: I. Bilirubin metabolism. *Progress in Pediatric Surgery* 12:1, 1978.

Stevenson, R. *The Fetus and Newly Born Infant.* St. Louis: Mosby, 1973.

Sullivan, R., Foster, J., and Schreiner, R. Determining a newborn's gestational age. *American Journal of Maternal-Child Nursing* 4:38, 1979.

Taubenheim, A. Paternal-infant bonding in the first-time father. *Journal of Obstetric, Gynecologic and Neonatal Nursing* 10:261, 1981.

Whitley, N. Preparation for breastfeeding. *Journal of Obstetric, Gynecologic and Neonatal Nursing* 7:44, 1978.

Williams, J., and Lancaster, J. Thermoregulation of the newborn. *American Journal of Maternal-Child Nursing* 1:355, 1976.

Wood, B. Factors affecting neonatal jaundice. *Archives of Disease in Childhood* 54:111, 1979.

Wood, C. Immunology related to the newborn. *Nurse Practitioner* 1(6):37, 1976.

Yaffe, S. Drugs and chemicals in breast milk. *Professional Pharmacy* 6:1, 1979.

PART 5 COMPLICATIONS OF CHILDBEARING

Chapter 17 Fetal Assessment

In the past, there were relatively few ways of determining fetal maturity or well-being apart from determining estimated date of confinement, carefully observing uterine growth, and listening to fetal heart sounds. Currently a number of diagnostic methods are available to determine fetal maturity and the presence of sex-linked disorders, chromosomal abnormalities, hemolytic disease, and various enzyme deficiencies. The list of disorders that can be diagnosed in utero is growing rapidly as methods of detection become more sophisticated (Table 17-1). This knowledge provides the parents of severely affected fetuses with options not previously available to them; it also gives infants who must be delivered prematurely a much greater chance of being delivered when viable. Much of this testing, as well as counseling on genetic matters, is done in centers located throughout the country. When working with childbearing families, you need to be aware of the nearest counseling center that provides these services in case referral is necessary.

FETAL MATURITY
Amniocentesis

Tests to determine fetal maturity generally involve amniocentesis. In this commonly used procedure, the obstetrician anesthetizes the woman's skin over her lower abdominal wall and inserts a needle through it and through the wall of her uterus into the amniotic cavity. A syringe is attached to the needle, and amniotic fluid is withdrawn. This procedure can be done successfully as early as the twelfth gestational week.

Complications from the procedure are uncommon and are reported at 1 percent or less. They include abortion or premature labor, maternal hemorrhage or infection, fetal puncture wounds, fetal pneumothorax, and damage to the placenta and umbilical vessels. In order to avoid complications, ultrasound visualization may be used prior to or during the procedure to localize the placenta and fetal parts.

NURSING INTERVENTION

In preparing the woman for amniocentesis ask her to void prior to the procedure if she is past the twentieth week of gestation. Before this time, her full bladder will hold the uterus steady and out of the pelvis. Have her lie on her back with her hands and a pillow under her head. Take her vital signs including fetal heart rate (FHR) before the procedure so that a baseline has been established should complications occur. Having explained the procedure to the woman previously, now keep her informed of each step while it is being done. Hogan and Tcheng [11] note that women express discomfort or fear about local infiltration, possible injury to the fetus, and lower abdominal cramping for a few hours after the procedure. They note that by keeping the woman informed during the procedure and reducing her anxiety, physical discomfort and stress perception are minimized. Lower abdominal cramping has not been found to have an adverse effect on pregnancy. Following the procedure, monitor the woman's vital signs including any signs of uterine contractions for 30 minutes to 1 hour.

Amniotic fluid may be tested for lecithin-sphingomyelin (L/S) ratio, creatinine, bilirubin, fat cells, alpha-fetoprotein, and other substances.

Table 17-1. Prenatal Diagnosis by Amniocentesis[a]

Chromosomal Disorders
   Trisomy 21 (Down's syndrome)
   Trisomy 18
   Turner's syndrome
   Mosaicism (two different cell lines)
Neural tube defects (anencephaly, spina bifida)
Rh isoimmunization
Metabolic disorders
   Hurler's syndrome
   Galactosemia
   Pompe's disease (glycogen storage disorder)
   Disorders of lipid metabolism
      Fabry's disease
      Gaucher's disease
      Tay-Sachs disease
      Sandhoff's disease
      Krabbe's disease
      Metachromatic leukodystrophy
      Mucolipidosis II, IV
      Niemann-Pick disease
      Wolman's disease
   Maple syrup urine disease
   Cystinosis
   Methylmalonic acidemia I, II
   Propionic acidemia
   Adenosine deaminase deficiency
   Alpha-thalassemia
   Adrenogenital syndrome
   Acute intermittent porphyria
   Congenital erythropoietic porphyria
   Congenital nephrosis
   Familial hypercholesterolemia
   Hypothyroidism
   Lesch-Nyhan syndrome
   Lysosomal acid phosphatase deficiency
   Menkes' disease
   Sickle cell disease
   Xeroderma pigmentosum

[a] Partial list.

Sources: M. Golbus, and J. Stephens. Prenatal diagnosis of chromosomal abnormalities and neural tube defects. *Clinics in Perinatology* 6:245, 1979; M. Mahoney. Prenatal diagnosis of inborn errors of metabolism. *Clinics in Perinatology* 6:255, 1979; and J. Miles, and M. Kabock. Prenatal diagnosis of hereditary disorders. *Pediatric Clinics of North America* 25:593, 1978.

LECITHIN-SPHINGOMYELIN

As the fetus matures, phospholipids necessary for lung expansion and gas exchange at birth are present in the alveoli of the lung. This material can be detected in amniotic fluid in the later months of gestation. Prior to lung maturity, two important lipoproteins, lecithin and sphingomyelin, are in equal concentrations. Lecithin is produced in two major pathways, the choline and methylation pathways. Until the thirty-fifth week of gestation, methylation is the primary pathway, while after 36 weeks of gestation lecithin is produced through the choline pathway. The choline pathway yields a more stable and effective form of lecithin, whereas lecithin produced by the methylation reaction is easily inhibited by hypothermia, hypoxia, acidosis, and possibly cesarean birth. After 34 to 35 weeks of gestation the concentration of lecithin usually increases in amniotic fluid, while that of sphingomyelin remains the same. When the ratio of lecithin to sphingomyelin in amniotic fluid is 2 : 1, the choline pathway of lecithin synthesis is functional, the fetal lung is considered mature, and the chances that the infant will develop respiratory distress syndrome are low [4, 17].

In normal pregnancies, a mature L/S ratio (2 or greater) predicts absence of respiratory distress syndrome in approximately 98 percent of subjects studied. Alternately, a ratio indicating an immature fetal lung has been associated with respiratory distress syndrome in only 40 to 80 percent of fetuses tested. The lower the ratio, however, the more likely the infant will be affected with the syndrome [12].

While L/S ratios are accurate in normal pregnancies, in higher risk pregnancies the correlation is not so predictive. In the latter, fetuses with advanced gestational ages may have low L/S ratios while younger ones may have ratios indicative of lung maturity. Maternal conditions in which placental blood flow is reduced may stress the fetus increasing fetal corticosteroid which stimulates production of surfactant in type II alveolar cells (Table 17-2). This same phenomenon is believed to occur when the woman's membranes have been ruptured from 48 to 72 hours or longer. Blood or meconium in the amniotic fluid sample yields low L/S ratios.

In some instances fetuses with mature L/S ratios experience respiratory distress after birth. It has been postulated that stress during labor and delivery may have impaired surfactant activity after the specimen was obtained.

Two other phospholipids found in smaller quantities in amniotic fluid, phosphatidyl glycerol (PG) and phosphatidyl inositol (PI) are important in stabilizing lecithin in the surfactant layer that lines the alveoli. The presence of PG may be a more accurate predictor of lung function than the L/S ratio [21].

A rapid foam test is in use that indicates the presence of mature L/S ratios in amniotic fluid. The fluid is mixed with ethanol and shaken vigorously for 15

Table 17-2. Disorders Associated with Alteration from Normal Time of Appearance of Mature L/S ratio

Mature ratio before 35 gestational weeks (accelerated maturation)
Maternal conditions
  Toxemia (early onset)
  Hypertensive renal disease
  Hypertensive cardiovascular disease
  Sickle cell disease
  Narcotic addiction
  Diabetes, class D, F, R
  Chronic retroplacental hemorrhage
  Hyperthyroidism
  Corticosteroids, aminophylline
  Maternal infections
  Placental insufficiency
Fetal disorders
  Prolonged rupture of membranes

Mature ratio after 35 gestational weeks (delayed maturation)
Maternal condition
  Diabetes, class A, B, C
  Chronic glomerulonephritis
Fetal condition
  Rh disease
  Smaller of identical twins

Source: Modified from L. Gluck. *Clinical Obstetrics and Gynecology* 21:547, 1978.

seconds. In 15 minutes a reading is taken. A stable foam ring forms in the presence of adequate amounts of lecithin and remains for 15 minutes while lesser amounts form varying degrees of bubbling. The shake test is a good screening measure for determining mature lungs; however, in the absence of foam an L/S ratio is usually recommended. The foam stability test to detect respiratory distress syndrome may also be used on gastric aspirate taken from the baby within 1 hour after birth.

CREATININE AND URIC ACID

Creatinine levels found in amniotic fluid are considered by some physicians to be reliable measures of gestational age when used in conjunction with other measurements. After 34 weeks' gestation, the concentration in amniotic fluid rises progressively and rapidly. Most amniotic fluid specimens with levels in excess of 1.6 to 1.8 milligrams per 100 milliliters of fluid correlate with gestational ages over 36 weeks in 94 percent of women tested [6, 7]. The concentration, however, depends on fetal muscle mass, kidney excretion, amniotic fluid volume, and maternal serum levels [15]. Misleadingly high levels are found in women with impaired renal function such as hypertensive disorders of pregnancy and often in diabetic women. Lower than expected levels are often found in the amniotic fluid of women with Rh disease.

Uric acid levels were used in the past with creatinine levels to determine fetal age. Uric acid, like creatinine, increases significantly as gestation increases, reflecting an increased urinary output and muscle mass of the maturing fetus [23].

BILIRUBIN

By using spectrophotometric analysis of amniotic fluid, it is possible to measure minute quantities of bilirubin and other breakdown products of hemoglobin. Bilirubin normally appears in the amniotic fluid as early as the twelfth week, peaks between 16 and 30 weeks, and then decreases as gestation advances. In most instances there is no bilirubin in amniotic fluid beyond 36 weeks' gestation, presumably because the liver has matured and is able to conjugate it. This finding is variable, however, and bilirubin determination is not too valuable for estimation of fetal maturity. Bilirubin levels remain high or increase in the presence of hemolytic disease, and determination of levels is valuable in assessing the severity of Rh disease. It is difficult to obtain good test results if there is meconium or blood in the amniotic fluid specimen or if hydramnios is present [6, 15]. In addition, specimens obtained for bilirubin analysis must be protected from light.

FAT CELLS

The number of fat cells in amniotic fluid also indicate fetal maturity. There is a sharp rise in the number of these cells after 36 weeks, possibly due to the functional maturity of fetal sebaceous glands. The fetus is considered mature when a 20 percent fat cell count is found in amniotic fluid. These same fat cells, which stain orange with a 1% Nile blue sulfate stain, can be identified in vaginal smears when the woman's membranes have ruptured [7, 10]. The test is considered valuable by some physicians in both normal and high-risk pregnancies.

Ultrasound Testing   Ultrasound testing involves using reflected sound waves as they travel in tissue; it can be used to produce an echocardiogram. When the ultrasonic pulse beam is directed appropriately through the fetal head, the biparietal diameter may be measured accurately. A cross section can be obtained using an oscilloscopic beam and the ultrasonic beam so that the echo dots yield a cross-sectional anatomic picture (Fig. 17-1).

Ultrasound can detect pregnancy, multiple pregnancy, fetal abnormalities (such as anencephaly and hydrocephalus), hydatidiform mole, fetal death, fetal presentation, fetal soft tissue abnormalities, and hydramnios. It can also be used to determine placental position and fetal weight.

Using ultrasound, pregnancy can be identified as early as 5 weeks when a circle of echoes form the gestational sac. Measurement of the sac provides estimates of gestational age. At 6 to 7 weeks fetal parts can be recognized, and crown rump measurement for estimation of fetal age is possible. When ultrasound testing is performed prior to the 14th week, the estimated date of confinement is predictable within 4 to 5 days in 95 percent of women. At 14 weeks maturity can be determined by measuring the biparietal diameter of the fetal head. After 28 weeks biparietal and thoracic diameters are measured in order to determine maturity and evidence of normal growth. Infants of diabetic mothers, for example, will maintain normal head measurements until after the thirty-seventh week when they may become larger. The macrosomia of these infants, however, can be evaluated by comparing the thoracic diameter with the biparietal diameter. Alternately, women with hypertensive disease may have an infant with normal head size for gestational age but smaller thoracic diameter, reflecting preferential sparing of the brain with curtailed overall body growth. Biparietal and thoracic dimensions should be taken in series in order to evaluate fetal growth over time in women with high-risk pregnancies.

When gestational age is certain and growth has been normal, determinations of fetal weight alone may be needed. Weight can be determined by biparietal

Figure 17-1. Drawing simulating ultrasonic transverse scan of the fetal head.

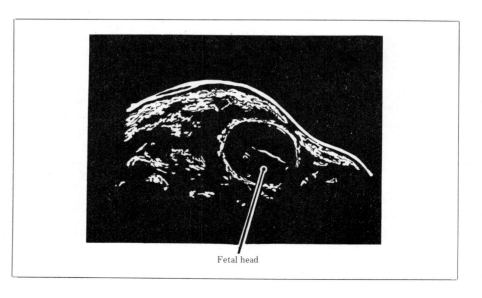

Fetal head

measurements. Thompson [22] found that 91 percent of fetuses with biparietal diameters of 8.5 centimeters (3.3 inches) or greater weighed over 2,500 grams (5.5 pounds), and Stocker et al. [20] found that 90 percent of fetuses weighed over 3,000 grams (6.6 pounds) when the diameter was 9.1 centimeters (3.6 inches). Weight determinations have been inaccurate with fetuses who were small or large for their gestational age, unless serial determinations were performed. Problems measuring the biparietal diameter are also encountered when the fetal head is deep in the pelvis, in breech presentations, and when the mother is obese or has hydramnios.

Currently, portable real-time imaging is used to provide visualization of the fetus in motion. (The image may also be filmed for later evaluation.) Fetal breathing movements, cardiac activity including activity of the heart valves and chambers, swallowing, and motion can be observed. Fetal movement can be seen as early as 7 weeks, cardiac activity between 7 and 8 weeks. This method is also used during amniocentesis so an insertion of the needle does not accidently hit the fetus or placenta.

X-Ray   X-rays have been used to determine fetal maturity based on specific epiphyseal centers of ossification, the size of the fetal skull, fetal length, and calcification of fetal teeth. This method has the inherent problem of exposure to radiation for the fetus and mother as well as intrinsic inaccuracies resulting from variations in growth rate and skeletal maturation. X-rays have also been used to identify multiple pregnancies, hydrocephalus, anencephalus, fetal death, and the edema and "Buddha position" so indicative of severe erythroblastosis with hydrops fetalis.

In general, the distal femoral epiphysis is apparent at 36 weeks, and the proximal tibial epiphysis at 38 weeks; however, female fetuses are more advanced in bony development than males, and the skeletal maturation of black fetuses develops more rapidly than that of white fetuses [5, 10]. The use of x-ray to determine fetal maturity has largely been replaced today by the use of ultrasound measurements.

FETAL WELL-BEING   Tests to determine fetal well-being may require a blood specimen from the mother, a 24-hour urine collection, and an endoscopic examination, amniocentesis, or fetal monitoring.

Estriol   One test of fetal well-being depends upon the determination of estriol levels from samples of maternal urine collected over a 24-hour period. Serial estriol determinations provide information about the fetoplacental unit, since the biosynthesis of estriol within the placenta cannot occur without precursor substances produced in the fetal adrenal gland. Therefore, results of this test reflect placental and fetal adrenal functioning. Since there are marked differences in the amount of estriol produced by individual women, serial estriol levels are important to determine how the placenta is functioning for a period of time; a single estriol level might appear misleadingly high or low.

The level of estriol excretion is influenced by the length of gestation, fetal and placental size, existence of multiple pregnancy, maternal renal function, and adequacy of the urine collection. The levels may also be influenced by ingestion of drugs such as antibiotics and aspirin [17]. As pregnancy advances, the low urinary values found in the first and second trimesters increase, particularly during the last 3 to 4 weeks. Levels above 12 milligrams per day after 34 weeks are considered adequate by some clinicians. Levels that drop 50 percent or more in a week signify danger to the fetus, and at levels of 4 milligrams per day or less fetal death may occur within 48 hours [7]. Urinary estriol is absent when the fetus is dead and in an anencephalic fetus where the fetal adrenal gland is absent.

In women with hypertensive disease and renal disease normal estriol values are reliable indicators that the fetus is well. In women with Rh sensitization, low estriol values are reliable indicators of fetal jeopardy; low values in pregnant women with diabetes are not as reliable.

Estriol levels in amniotic fluid specimens have also been studied, but reports indicate that correlations using this method are not any better than those using specimens from urinary collections [10]. Plasma estriol levels are being investigated, but to date the technique remains complex and is not in widespread use. Total plasma estriol is measured in conjugated and unconjugated forms. The unconjugated form, which demonstrates a sudden increase at 36 weeks' gestation, appears more predictive than other fractions measured [12].

Alpha-Fetoprotein

Alpha-fetoprotein, which is currently receiving much attention in the determination of fetal well-being, is a major plasma protein of early fetuses, synthesized by the fetal liver and yolk sac but not the placenta. Its function is not known but it may bind estrogens. Alpha-fetoprotein levels are highest in fetal serum during the first 13 weeks of gestation. After this period the concentration of alpha-fetoprotein in the fetal serum decreases and that of albumin increases. After 13 weeks, the levels in fetal serum and amniotic fluid decrease rapidly. Greatly increased amniotic fluid levels have been found in fetuses with spina bifida, anencephaly, and other neural tube defects [14, 18] (see Table 17-1).

The concentrations of alpha-fetoprotein levels in maternal serum are only one-hundredth to one-thousandth those of fetal serum. Low maternal levels rise slowly during the second trimester and reach a plateau early in the third trimester. Increased levels in maternal serum are associated with maternal immunization against Rh and ABO blood factors, severe fetoplacental dysfunction, and intrauterine death.

Studies in Great Britain have indicated that testing maternal plasma is a useful tool in identifying neural tube defects in the fetus. When levels in maternal plasma were sufficiently elevated and the possibility of a neural tube defect was present, amniocentesis was performed to determine if elevated levels were present in amniotic fluid. Sonography was also used to visualize any defects. The screening of some 11,600 pregnant women between 16 and 20 weeks' gestation detected 93 percent of afflicted fetuses [9]. While routine screening of alpha-fetoprotein in maternal serum has not been advocated, many physicians recommend that amniotic fluid obtained for other reasons between 15 and 19 weeks' gestation be tested for alpha-fetoprotein also.

Fetoscope

The fetoscope provides direct visualization of the fetus and the placental blood vessels. It has been used to obtain samples of fetal blood for the prenatal diagnosis of some hemoglobinopathies such as sickle cell anemia and beta-thalassemia, to visualize structural anomalies, and to take minute fetal skin biopsies. The position of the fetus and placenta are determined by ultrasound. The woman's abdominal skin is anesthesized, followed by a small skin incision and insertion of a trocar into the amniotic sac. The trocar is then replaced by the fetoscope. The procedure is currently in the research stages.

Amnioscopy   Amnioscopy has limited value in determining fetal well-being. An amnioscope may be passed by aseptic technique into the woman's cervical canal to visualize the amniotic fluid for the presence of blood or meconium. However, the procedure may cause cervical trauma, vaginal bleeding, and possibly premature rupture of membranes or premature induction of labor [1].

Nonstress Test   The nonstress test (NST) is used to evaluate fetal heart rate response to stress caused by fetal movement [16]. It is used for pregnant women who have prolonged pregnancies, diabetes, hypertensive disorders, abnormal estriol levels, a history of stillbirths, or other pregnancy complications. In performing the test, the pregnant woman is monitored externally, and the fetal heart rate is evaluated for accelerations that normally occur in response to fetal activity. Responses are classified as reactive, nonreactive, sinusoidal, and inadequate. The criteria used by Weingold et al. [25] for NST screening are as follows:

Reactive	Accelerations of 15 beats per minute or more above baseline, last 15 seconds or more with 5 fetal movements in 20 minutes
Nonreactive	No accelerations with fetal movements or fewer than 5 accelerations in 20 minutes; test period must be 40 minutes minimum to allow for fetal rest cycle patterns
Sinusoidal	Oscillations of fetal heart rate occurring with a frequency of 2 to 5 cycles per minute with an amplitude of 5 to 15 beats per minute
Inadequate	Unreadable FHR data or no fetal movements recorded

NURSING INTERVENTION

In preparing the woman for a NST, a brief history will indicate the reason for the test if her chart is not available. Take her initial blood pressure with her in a sitting or side-lying position to avoid a baseline reflective of positional hypotension. With the woman sitting in a comfortable recliner or a bed with her head elevated approximately 45 degrees, outline fetal position and attach the fetal monitoring equipment. Ask the mother to mark the tracing paper each time she feels a fetal movement. Take her blood pressure approximately every 10 minutes to detect supine hypotension that might affect fetal heart rate and the outcome of the test. If no fetal movement occurs, rubbing or palpating the mother's abdomen will stimulate the resting fetus. Observe any uterine contractions the mother may have for duration, frequency, and intensity.

Lieber [13] notes that "few women scheduled for a nonstress test view it as a casual procedure, even when they consider it only a safety measure." They express anxiety about the fetus's condition, the concerns of other family members regarding the test, and the cost, and often exhibit a lack of knowledge or misinformation about the test. As the women become more anxious, they become less able to understand what is happening and what is expected of them. She suggests that by understanding the women's anxieties and by offering supportive reassurance through eye contact, gentle handling of the woman's body, and skillful application of equipment, we can provide comfort along with a valid assessment of the unborn baby's health and development.

The NST is as effective as the oxytocin challenge test in evaluating normal intrauterine fetal status. It is also noninvasive and easy to perform, there are no contraindications to its use, and it can be performed in an outpatient setting.

Oxytocin Challenge Test

The oxytocin challenge test (OCT or Stress Test) is generally used when a woman has had an abnormal nonstress test. In order to evaluate the fetus's ability to withstand the stress of labor, the woman undergoes a short period of simulated labor contractions. This test may be carried out any time after the thirty-fourth week of gestation. The fetal heart rate is monitored for 30 minutes to establish a baseline. Contractions are then started and maintained by giving the woman an intravenous infusion of oxytocin. The infusion is maintained until the woman has three adequate contractions within a 10-minute period. The external fetal monitor records the fetal response to each uterine contraction, showing type II dips when placental reserve is insufficient (see Chap. 12). If the FHR shows this intolerance to the stress of the contractions, the test is considered positive and the intravenous infusion is discontinued.

Between 57 and 75 percent of the positive tests yield abnormal fetal outcomes. While negative test results are reliably predictive of good fetal outcomes, positive results are less reliable. With cautious assessment, vaginal delivery is possible when the test is positive. However, cesarean birth is often used to avoid further stress on the fetus. The test is not used in women with vaginal bleeding, incompetent os, ruptured membranes, a uterine scar such as from a previous cesarean delivery, or an overdistended uterus such as occurs with twins.

Placental Polypeptides

Placental function has been monitored by determining levels of human chorionic gonadotropin (HCG) and human placental lactogen (HPL). In early pregnancy, women with threatened abortions excrete decreasing amounts of HCG. In later pregnancy, women with diabetes, Rh immunization, and preeclampsia excrete high levels of HCG, suggesting that near term high levels may signify impending fetal death.

It has been reported that as pregnancy advances there is a linear increase in the production of HPL (chorionic somatomammotropin). Levels falling below 4 micrograms per milliliter after 30 weeks of gestation indicate fetal danger. Rather than a single test, serial determinations (as in estriol studies) are performed to follow the progress of the pregnancy in diabetes, hypertensive disorders, isoimmunization, intrauterine growth retardation, and threatened abortion. Since this test merely indicates placental function, it is used in conjunction with other tests that indicate fetal status or maturity [19]. It has not been used extensively.

Hormonal Cytology

Hormonal cytology has also been used to determine the status of the pregnancy, as reflected in the morphologic appearance of desquamated vaginal cells. When abortion threatens, there is an increase in the number of karyopyknotic cells. Fetal death is associated with a decrease in small cells and the appearance of parabasal cells. Persistent ferning of cervical mucus beyond the first 2 to 3 months of pregnancy confirms a poor prognosis for that pregnancy [10].

Enzyme Studies   Maternal plasma levels of diamine oxidase (histaminase) have been used to evaluate fetal well-being in the first two trimesters. The amount increases normally during the first 20 weeks of pregnancy, while falling levels during this time indicate threatened or missed abortion. Enzyme titers greater than 500 units per milliliter indicate that pregnancy will be maintained into the third trimester [10].

Enzyme studies may also be carried out on cultures of fetal cells obtained from amniocentesis. Results of these studies can establish the presence of enzyme deficiencies in the fetus, such as the deficiencies found in galactosemia and the Lesch-Nyhan syndrome. Other enzyme deficiencies, such as the low levels of hexosaminidase A found in Tay-Sachs disease, may be detected in amniotic fluid cells as well as in the liquor itself.

The karyotyping of cultured cells can demonstrate the presence of various chromosomal abnormalities, including mongolism. Some physicians routinely require karyotype screening on pregnant women who are 40 years of age or older because of the increased incidence of trisomy in this age group. Karyotyping can also establish the fetal sex, which may be helpful for couples who have a history of sex-linked disorders such as hemophilia.

Cortisol   Cortisol has been the subject of much research to determine its role in fetal development and its use as a measure of fetal well-being. Experimental and clinical observations suggest that glucocorticoids have an important role in the normal process of fetal lung maturation [3]. Receptors for glucocorticosteroids have been demonstrated in fetal lung tissue. There is indirect evidence that glucocorticoids stimulate acceleration of pulmonary surfactant and enhance fetal lung maturation. Premature birth, prior to the 24 to 48 hours of increased cortisol levels in utero that is found in full-term births, is associated with respiratory distress syndrome. Although the treatment remains controversial, premature infants reportedly have a lower incidence of respiratory distress syndrome (even though as fetuses in utero they were shown to have low L/S ratios) if the mother receives glucocorticoids 24 hours prior to the birth [2]. One study [8] reported amniotic fluid cortisol levels 2.4 times higher at 35 to 40 weeks of gestation than those found at 20 to 34 weeks. Respiratory distress syndrome did not occur when total amniotic fluid cortisol was greater than 60 milligrams per milliliter. Pregnancies over 40 weeks were reported to have further increases in total cortisol; values over 120 milligrams per milliliter were found in this group.

ASSESSMENT AND
INTERVENTIONS
Assessment   When women require tests of fetal status there is some question of possible complication of the pregnancy. Not only may the woman's anxiety be increased but that of her family as well. You will want to assess the reason for the required test and what the results may mean in relation to this or future pregnancies. Has there been any history of the possible problem with other pregnancies or with other women in the family? What does the woman understand about the test and its possible implications? What is her husband's or family's understanding regarding it? What are their major concerns? How is the test and its implications affecting the woman's, husband's, or other family members' sense of self-esteem and family functioning?

Interventions   You may begin your interventions by attempts to decrease the woman's anxiety after you know her major concerns. Encourage women in this situation to express, correct, modify, and confirm their understanding of the situation. Correct misunderstandings the woman, her husband, or other family members may have. Often not only the woman but her husband and other family members may feel guilt when possible complications arise. The husband may feel guilt for having impregnated his wife. The extended family may feel they have done something or passed something through the family lines to cause the current problem. The woman may feel not only guilt for something she perceives she may have done wrong but also fear for the life of the baby and perhaps for herself as well. In addition to giving information and correcting misinformation, reassure her wherever possible. Praise her for the concern and care she is taking of her fetus and herself by following through on the advice of the health team.

Susan Weil [24], a nurse who herself had several complicated pregnancies, suggests other ways we can help clients with complicated pregnancies. These include referral to a support group, support for husbands, sexual counseling, and childbirth education classes for high-risk couples. If the woman is having difficulties during the pregnancy, ask her what assistance would be most helpful to her during the remainder of her pregnancy. It may be possible to provide her with counseling or to put her in touch with a community agency or other member of the health care team who could meet her most pressing concerns. It may be that simply maintaining continued contact with her on subsequent visits or by telephone is all that is necessary.

REFERENCES

1. Ansari, A. New approach to amnioscopy. *Journal of the American Medical Association* 212:321, 1970.
2. Avery, M. E. Prenatal diagnosis and prevention of hyaline membrane disease. *New England Journal of Medicine* 292:157, 1975.
3. Bishop, E. Acceleration of fetal pulmonary maturity. *Obstetrics and Gynecology* 58:485, 1981.
4. Brown, B., Gabert, H., and Stenchever, M. Respiratory distress syndrome, surfactant biochemistry, and acceleration of fetal lung maturity: A review. *Obstetrical and Gynecological Survey* 30:71, 1975.
5. Cruz, A. C., Buhi, W. C., and Spellary, W. N. Comparison of fetogram and L/S ratio for fetal maturity. *Obstetrics and Gynecology* 45:147, 1975.
6. Droegemueller, W., Jackson, C., Makowski, E. L., and Battaglia, F. C. Amniotic fluid examination as an aid in assessment of gestational age. *American Journal of Obstetrics and Gynecology* 104:424, 1969.
7. Duhring, J. L. The high risk fetus. *Hospital Medicine* 10:77, 1974.
8. Fenci, M., and Tulchinsky, D. Total cortisol in amniotic fluid and fetal lung maturation. *New England Journal of Medicine* 292:133, 1975.
9. Ferguson-Smith, M., May, H., Vince, J., Robinson, H., Rawlinson, H., Tait, H., Gibson, A., and Ratcliffe, J. Avoidance of anencephalic and spina bifida births by maternal serum alphafetoprotein screening. *Lancet* 1:1330, 1978.
10. Greenhill, J. P., and Friedman, E. A. *Biological Principles and Modern Practice of Obstetrics*. Philadelphia: Saunders, 1974.
11. Hogan, K., and Tcheng, D. The role of the nurse during amniocentesis. *Journal of Obstetric, Gynecologic and Neonatal Nursing* 7:24, 1978.
12. Korones, S. *High-Risk Newborn Infants*. St. Louis: Mosby, 1981.
13. Lieber, M. "Nonstress" antepartal monitoring. *American Journal of Maternal-Child Nursing* 5:335, 1980.
14. Milunsky, A., and Alpert, E. The value of alpha fetoprotein in the prenatal diagnosis of neural tube defects. *Journal of Pediatrics* 84:889, 1974.
15. Myers, J., Harrell, M. J., and Hill, F. Fetal maturity: Biochemical analysis of amniotic fluid. *American Journal of Obstetrics and Gynecology* 121:961, 1975.

16. Paul, R., and Petrie, R. *Fetal Intensive Care.* Wallingford: Corometrics Medical Systems, Inc., 1979.
17. Pritchard, J., and MacDonald, P. *Williams Obstetrics* (16th ed.). New York: Appleton-Century-Crofts, 1980.
18. Seppala, M., and Ruoslahti, E. Alpha-fetoprotein in Rh-immunized pregnancies. *Obstetrics and Gynecology* 42:701, 1973.
19. Spellacy, W. N., Buhi, W. C., and Birk, S. A. The effectiveness of human placental lactogen measurements as an adjunct in decreasing perinatal deaths. *American Journal of Obstetrics and Gynecology* 121:835, 1975.
20. Stocker, J., Mawad, R., Deleon, A., and Desjardins, P. Ultrasonic cephalometry. *Obstetrics and Gynecology* 45:275, 1975.
21. Quilligan, E., and Kretchmer, N. *Fetal and Maternal Medicine.* New York: Wiley, 1980.
22. Thompson, H. E. The clinical use of pulsed echo ultrasound in obstetrics and gynecology. *Obstetrical and Gynecological Survey* 23:903, 1968.
23. Tsudaka, T., Bloch, D., and Wolf, P. An automated profile of amniotic fluid. *Laboratory Medicine* 2:32, 1971.
24. Weil, S. The unspoken needs of families during high risk pregnancies. *American Journal of Nursing* 81:2047, 1981.
25. Weingold, A., Yonekura, M., and O'Kieffe, J. Nonstress testing. *American Journal of Obstetrics and Gynecology* 138:195, 1980.

FURTHER READING

Coetzee, E., et al. Using ultrasound for midtrimester and difficult late-third-trimester amniocentesis. *Perinatology/Neonatology* 12:41, 1979.

Cranley, M. Antepartal fetal assessment. *American Journal of Nursing* 78:2098, 1978.

Gal, D., Jacobson, L., Ser, H., Park, S., and Lancer, M. Sinusoidal pattern: An alarming sign of fetal distress. *American Journal of Obstetrics and Gynecology* 132:903, 1978.

Hallman, M., et al. Absence of phosphatidylglycerol (PG) in respiratory distress syndrome in the newborn: Study of the minor surfactant phospholipids in newborns. *Pediatric Resident* 7:714, 1977.

Kopf, R. Nonstress test. *American Journal of Nursing* 78:2115, 1978.

Levine, A., and Imai, P. Intrauterine treatment of fetal hydronephrosis. *Association of Operating Room Nurses* 35:655, 1982.

NIH Consensus Development Conferences. Antenatal diagnosis: Amniocentesis. *Clinical Pediatrics* 18:454, 1979.

NIH Consensus Development Conferences. Antenatal diagnosis: Predictors of fetal malnutrition. *Clinical Pediatrics* 18:533, 1979.

Patterson, P. Fetal therapy: Issues we face. *Association of Operating Room Nurses* 35:663, 1982.

Sethi, S. Oxytocin challenge test. *American Journal of Nursing* 78:2112, 1978.

Shields, D. Maternal reactions to fetal monitoring. *American Journal of Nursing* 78:2110, 1978.

Wladimiroff, J. W., et al. Real-time and M-mode ultrasonic assessment of fetal and neonatal cardiac geometry and function. *Perinatology/Neonatology* 13:15, 1980.

Wheeler, L., Duxbury, M., Raff, B., and Carroll, P. *Fetal Assessment.* White Plains, N.Y.: National Foundation March of Dimes, 1979.

Chapter 18 Complications of Pregnancy

Spontaneous abortion, the loss of a fetus up to 20 weeks of gestation or weighing less than 500 grams (1.1 pounds), accounts for the loss of 1 in every 5 to 7 pregnancies [15]. It is not known what causes most spontaneous abortions; however, it is known that in the early months of pregnancy, spontaneous expulsion of the conceptus is preceded by fetal death.

Spontaneous abortions have been attributed to abnormal uterine environment, defects in germ plasm, and defects in early development, possibly due to teratogens such as chemicals, viruses, radiation, or poisoning from heavy metals or anesthetic or illuminating gases. They have also been attributed to systemic disease in either parent, maternal thyroid dysfunction, and severe maternal anemia. In one study, 76 percent of the spontaneously aborted fetuses were abnormal [16]. Depending on the population studied, chromosomal abnormalities were found in 22 to 60 percent of the aborted fetuses; the earlier the abortion occurred, the more severe the associated anomaly [3,34]. It has also been documented that women over the age of 35 have a higher incidence of spontaneous abortion and of infants born with congenital malformations [15].

One maternal factor believed to favor abortion is decreased amounts of progesterone produced by the corpus luteum early in pregnancy or by the placenta later in pregnancy. Early in pregnancy the deficient progesterone is unfavorable to implantation and development, while deficiency later may increase uterine sensitivity and allow coordinated uterine contractions to expel the pregnancy.

Maternal infection has also been cited as a cause of spontaneous abortion, which may result from a transfer of bacterial toxins and microorganisms that affect the fetus. It is also possible that the infectious process in the mother may increase her temperature and metabolic needs while compromising those of the fetus and placenta. Chronic infections with *Listeria monocytogenes* and *Toxoplasma* have been cited as causes of abortion.

Perhaps surprisingly, a woman may undergo anesthesia and surgery without spontaneous abortion, provided that hypoxia is avoided. Likewise, while abortion may result from trauma, it is an extremely rare occurrence.

ASSESSMENT AND INTERVENTION

Abortions early in pregnancy result in the loss of all the products of conception, while abortions later in pregnancy usually result in the loss of the fetus but retention of the placenta or portions of the membranes. Pregnancy tests may continue to yield positive results as long as portions of the placenta continue to produce HCG.

When *threatened abortion* occurs and the woman complains of pelvic cramping, backache, and possible bleeding, most physicians prescribe bed rest and abstinence from intercourse, although many would agree this treatment has no basis in fact. The pain of an abortion may be anterior and rhythmic, simulating mild labor; it may be a persistent low backache associated with a feeling of pelvic pressure; or it may be a dull pain at the midline accompanied by tenderness over the woman's uterus. Diethylstilbestrol has been used as a treatment for threatened abortion in the past, but vaginal clear-cell carcinoma has been reported among the female children of these pregnancies [9]. Some physicians will give progesterone if a pregnanediol test shows decreased progesterone excretion. Progesterone, however, can cause masculinization of the female fetus if given before the twelfth week or phallic enlargement when given over long periods. Also, a recent study reported that 73 percent of women threatening to abort and given hormonal support aborted on the average 20 days later, while 67 percent of the women in the control group receiving no hormonal support aborted on the average 5 days later. The researchers concluded that progestational agents did not improve the outcome but only delayed the inevitable [33].

If rest does not relieve her symptoms, the woman may be asked to resume some of her activities, in the belief that the pregnancy will be lost and the activity may shorten the time. Many clinicians, citing the high percentage of abnormal fetuses expelled in spontaneous abortion, question whether any attempt should be made to try to retain a pregnancy once an abortion threatens. It should be noted that approximately one out of every five women has some spotting of blood during the early months of pregnancy, and only one-half of these pregnancies are lost [30].

When abortion becomes *inevitable* as the external cervical os dilates and the membranes rupture, pieces of the conceptus may be expelled. When a portion of the conceptus remains in the woman's uterus (*incomplete abortion*), bleeding continues; if it is not removed, infection can ensue. The uterus is evacuated with a curette or a vacuum extractor. If the pregnancy has advanced past the first trimester and the cervix is not open, oxytocin induction may be used.

Habitual abortions (which are said to have occurred when women have lost three or more pregnancies) have been attributed to thyroid dysfunction, uterine abnormalities, pathologic ova, hormonal imbalance, tumors, and an incompetent cervical os. With treatment, 70 to 80 percent of all women who have experienced habitual abortion are able to carry a pregnancy successfully [30].

In habitual abortion caused by an *incompetent cervical os*, the woman loses the pregnancy during the second trimester as the cervix silently dilates, the membranes rupture, and the fetus is expelled. The cervix rarely dilates prior to the sixteenth week, since the products of conception are believed to be too small to cause cervical dilation prior to that time. Therefore, the treatment consists of surgical reinforcement of the weak cervix with a purse-string suture prior to this time or before the cervix has dilated 4 centimeters (Fig. 18-1). Two similar surgical procedures are used, the McDonald and the Shirodkar procedures. With the McDonald procedure, the cervical suture is removed at 38 to 39 weeks, allowing the woman to progress through labor and vaginal delivery. With the Shirodkar procedure, either the suture is snipped prior to or at the beginning of labor, or it may be left in place for the next pregnancy, in which case a cesarean delivery is performed. When working with a laboring woman who has had either of these procedures performed, you may find that progress is slow due to fibrotic changes in the cervix, but this slow progress may be followed by very sudden cervical dilatation and delivery. Cervical lacerations may also occur.

A woman who experiences a *missed abortion* retains her dead fetus in utero without undergoing the uterine contractions that would expel it; the reasons for this are unknown. The fetus becomes macerated, developing flabby skin, soft

Figure 18-1. Shirodkar procedure for reinforcing a weak cervix.

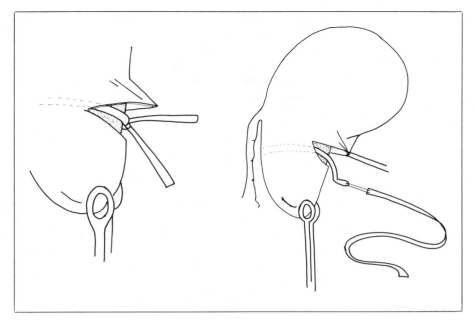

tissues, and loose bones, or more rarely, becomes mummified as it dries and becomes leathery. With fetal death, pregnancy tests may remain positive if chorionic villi are still active. The woman usually experiences a regression in breast and uterine size; after 3 weeks, blood fibrinogen decreases as a result of intravascular coagulation. The woman may notice bleeding from her nose or gums or bleeding from slight trauma. The decreased fibrinogen may be averted by intermittent administration of heparin subcutaneously [13]. If spontaneous abortion does not occur soon after diagnosis, oxytocin induction may be used in an effort to expel the uterine contents and avoid the possibilities of the woman's developing disseminated intravascular coagulation (DIC) or possible infection.

Ectopic Pregnancy

Ectopic pregnancy, or pregnancy outside of the normal uterine environment, is a complication that ranks high among the causes of maternal mortality. Because its symptoms are sometimes vague, it may be confused with other abdominal conditions, resulting in a delay in diagnosis and treatment. In about three or four out of 1,000 cases of ectopic pregnancy, the woman disregards vaginal staining for several days or weeks and then she collapses and dies as a result of hemorrhagic shock before she can be treated surgically.

An ectopic pregnancy occurs once in every 87 to 300 deliveries, and 98 percent of the time implantation takes place in one of the fallopian tubes [32]. Causes of ectopic pregnancy vary, but many such pregnancies result from a congenital anatomic irregularity in the tube or the presence of diverticula, either of which may impede or prevent the progress of the dividing trophoblast through the tube. Other factors that may contribute to the incidence of ectopic pregnancy are endometriosis of the oviduct, previous tuboplasty, previous tubal pregnancy, and the use of an intrauterine contraceptive device. The current increase in cases of venereal disease may result in an increased incidence of ectopic pregnancies, since the accompanying pelvic inflammatory complications and formation of scar tissue result in narrowed tubal lumens. The use of antibiotics in treatment has also probably contributed to the incidence of ectopic pregnancy by preventing tubal occlusion (sterility) but not preventing injured mucosa and scar formation. There is some evidence that postabortion infections may produce a similar result [29].

The trophoblast may implant in the interstitial, isthmic, or ampullary portion of the oviduct. An interstitial or cornual implantation occurs least often and is the most dangerous, since diagnosis is often not made before rupture occurs. Hypertrophy of the cornua allows the conceptus to reach sizable proportions before the trophoblast penetrates the uterine and tubal walls and causes rupture. Sometimes signs and symptoms do not appear before the beginning of the second trimester. The rupture is similar to rupture of the uterus, and the intra-abdominal hemorrhage is sudden, massive, and an immediate threat to life.

Implantation in the tubal isthmus is more common. Hypertrophy of the tubal musculature at the isthmus is insufficient to accommodate the growing ovum, and the wall at the placental site is weakened. Any trauma—straining at stool, coitus, or bimanual examination—may cause slight hemorrhage in this area. Within 2 or 3 weeks after the first missed period, the tube bursts from overdistention of the thinned necrotic wall, and there is bleeding into the peritoneal cavity. Although the rupture is usually on the abdominal surface, occasionally it is into the broad ligament. Sometimes a hematoma will form there, resulting in mild discomfort. Further growth of the pregnancy and hematoma will result in rupture of the broad ligament and its contents into the abdominal cavity.

Ampullary implantations are the most frequent form of tubal pregnancy. When the implantation occurs near the distensible fimbria, the conceptus may grow for 6 to 12 weeks before it is lost. It may be extruded into the abdominal cavity without injury to the tube, and transient pelvic pain for only a few hours may be the only symptom. If bleeding is extensive, signs of intra-abdominal hemorrhage will be present. Sometimes the conceptus may reimplant in the abdominal cavity or in a mass of adhesions and continue to grow as a secondary abdominal or tuboabdominal pregnancy. If the implant is medial to the fimbria, the woman's clinical course is comparable to an isthmic pregnancy.

Ovarian pregnancies, which are very rare, result from the implantation of the egg within the follicle; usually surgery becomes necessary by the end of the first trimester. Very rarely the implantation site is the cervix, and the initial diagnosis is likely to be placenta previa. Cervical implantation usually results in hemorrhage severe enough to necessitate a hysterectomy.

An abdominal ectopic pregnancy, an exceedingly rare event, occurs when the egg implants on the surface of the ovary, on another reproductive structure, or on the pelvic peritoneum. It may be a primary implant or secondary to a tubal abortion. This pregnancy may go to term, but the fetal prognosis is very poor due to hemorrhage or separation of the placenta. The universal symptom is pain, and a soft tissue x-ray is usually diagnostic. The placenta is absorbed if left in place, but it may separate before the vessels completely thrombose. Sometimes the condition may go completely undetected, in which case the fetus becomes a small lithopedion (calcified fetus), only to be identified years later during abdominal surgery or autopsy.

ASSESSMENT

Unfortunately as yet no reliable diagnostic laboratory procedures definitely establish or exclude ectopic pregnancy, and the diagnosis is rarely made before tubal rupture or hemorrhage takes place. The woman with an ectopic pregnancy may have a history of longstanding infertility or pelvic inflammatory disease. She will experience the physical changes of pregnancy, such as increases in uterine and breast size, but may have vaginal bleeding as a result of degeneration and sloughing of uterine decidua. Pregnancy tests may be positive since the chorionic villi are producing HCG, although the total amount produced may be less than normal. She will give a history of irregular vaginal staining, possibly dysuria or dyspareunia, one or more missed or scanty periods, and the sudden onset of abdominal pain and syncope while doing something strenuous. Her other symptoms of lower abdominal and pelvic discomfort may be vague but may be localized to the side of gestation.

If rupture has occurred, her signs and symptoms will be governed by the amount of hemorrhage. She may have abdominal tenderness, rigidity, and generalized sharp, knifelike abdominal pain. Her uterus is likely to be enlarged because of the trophoblastic estrogen and progesterone, and movement of her cervix will elicit a sharp localized pelvic pain because blood has irritated the pelvic peritoneum. This cervical movement may also give her the urge to void, defecate, or vomit. If the blood has irritated the diaphragm, her pain may be referred to her shoulder or chest. Pain in the flank, rectum, or suprapubic region is not uncommon. Blue skin about the umbilicus (Cullen's sign) appears late and is present only if the hemorrhage is extensive. If the rupture occurs gradually, her symptoms will be less characteristic and may vary from hours to weeks in their appearance. Culdoscopy, culdocentesis, and laparoscopy are useful diagnostic procedures for the visualization of the pelvic structures or for detection of blood in the peritoneal cavity.

INTERVENTION

In most cases the treatment is immediate surgery to establish hemostasis and combat shock. Blood replacement is begun. Monitor blood volume by central venous pressure. The affected tube is usually removed, although if one tube has already been lost, there is usually an attempt to save the remaining one by resection. The ultimate prognosis is good for the woman in whom rupture occurs early. Surgical removal of an unruptured ectopic pregnancy carries no more risk than the hazards of anesthesia and laparotomy. Remember that Rh isoimmunization may follow an ectopic pregnancy, so if the woman is Rh negative and not yet sensitized she should receive Rh_o immune globulin.

Care of the woman with an ectopic pregnancy initially revolves around the prevention of a life-threatening hemorrhage. Monitor her very carefully, keep her on bed rest, pad counts, and frequent vital signs. Since this is a completely unexpected event most of the time, many couples are completely overwhelmed once they understand the seriousness of what is happening. They need a chance to discuss their fears and concerns, particularly regarding their chances for a subsequent successful pregnancy.

SECOND-TRIMESTER
COMPLICATIONS
*Gestational
Trophoblastic Disease*

A hydatidiform mole is a hydropic swelling or "degeneration" of the connective tissue of immature chorionic villi resulting in segmental grapelike accumulations of fluid within the villous branches (Fig. 18-2). These grapelike clusters are grossly visible and tend to develop when the villous circulation fails to develop normally. Vesicles become attached by fibrous strands to one another, distending the entire uterus. There may be no fetus (complete mole), or there may be the remains of a degenerating fetus if embryogenesis has proceeded normally for some time (incomplete mole). The karyotype of a complete mole is 46 XX, which is now believed to be derived from a paternal haploid, X-carrying set of chromosomes that reaches the 46 XX status by duplication of its own nucleus. The original nucleus of the ovum is either absent or inactivated [18].

A hydatidiform mole occurs once in 1,500 to 2,000 pregnancies in the United States. The incidence is much greater in the Far East, especially China, the Philippines, and Malaya, where it occurs once in every 145 to 500 pregnancies [15]. Martin reports the incidence of mole as one in 257 deliveries among native Alaskans. Additionally, the incidence of mole after 45 years of age is 10 times more frequent than at ages 20 to 40 [25].

Figure 18-2. Hydatidi-
form mole.

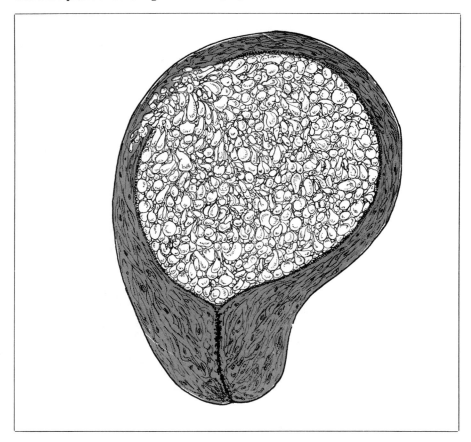

ASSESSMENT

The diagnosis of a benign hydatid mole is often confused with multiple pregnancy or with a threatened abortion accompanied by concealed hemorrhage, both of which cause one of the signs of molar pregnancy: a uterus that is unusually large for the time of gestation. If you are caring for a woman whose uterus is larger than expected for her EDC, which has been established, and you find no fetal heart tones, you will want to ask her a number of additional questions. Ask the woman if she has had vaginal bleeding. Vaginal bleeding, usually the first symptom of a molar pregnancy, commonly occurs at the beginning of the second trimester, but it may not occur until the sixth month. Occasionally the bleeding may be accompanied by the passage of some of the hydropic villi. The bleeding may be slight or profuse, as part of the mole becomes separated from its attachment. Bleeding may be brown (like prune juice) or bright red and will probably result in anemia, so the woman may appear pale and weak. Usually the woman's HCG titer is markedly increased beyond the ninetieth day of gestation, when it would normally be expected to drop. Ask the woman if she has experienced vomiting since about 30 percent of women with molar pregnancies have hyperemesis. About 10 percent have elevated thyroxine levels as the trophoblastic cells produce a molar thyrotropin similar to the hormone isolated from the pituitary gland and placenta, but few women develop signs of hyperthyroidism [26]. About 20 percent of the time these women will experience symptoms of preeclampsia before the twentieth week of gestation.

When you examine the woman, you will find no fetal heart tones by auscultation or amplification techniques; no fetal skeleton will appear on ultrasound or x-ray.

INTERVENTION

Once the diagnosis is made and the woman's blood loss is replaced, the mole is removed by dilatation and curettage, suction curettage, or (if it is more advanced than 14 weeks) hysterotomy. Hysterectomy is considered if the woman is 40 years or older, since the potential for development of subsequent malignancy is high in this group. Development of subsequent malignancy is one of the complications of molar pregnancy, along with the possibility of preeclampsia, recurrent hemorrhage, and perforation of the uterus.

Once the mole is removed, the cure rate is 85 to 90 percent. The antimetabolite drugs, methotrexate or actinomycin-D, may be given both before and after removal of the mole to prevent the development of trophoblastic disease, although many clinicians prefer to use these potent drugs only if evidence of persistent trophoblast remains [30]. This type of prophylaxis may be used when the incidence of malignant disease is high and the chances of follow-up poor. Because of the toxic side effects of these drugs, they are not administered unless the woman is kept under close observation, with appropriate blood and kidney studies.

A woman who has had a molar pregnancy is followed routinely for 1 year for gonadotropin activity; HCG levels should be negative within 6 weeks after evacuation. Chest x-rays are done at intervals to determine if any metastasis of molar tissue has occurred. So that HCG levels are not masked by those of a subsequent pregnancy, counsel the woman to wait for at least 6 months to 1 year before attempting another pregnancy. The incidence of a repeat mole is minimal. As a rule there is no specific follow-up treatment for women whose HCG titers fall quickly and do not rise again.

Chorioadenoma Destruens (Invasive Mole)

If the mole retains the invasive qualities of the trophoblast, it may invade deeply into the myometrium and perforate blood vessels and may also invade the vagina or parametrium. This invasive phenomenon occurs in 1 out of every 6 to 10 women who have a mole and is diagnosed by biopsy. Chemotherapy yields good results, although in some cases hysterectomy may be advocated. Chorioadenoma destruens is more malignant than the benign mole but less malignant than choriocarcinoma.

Choriocarcinoma

Choriocarcinoma is one of the most malignant neoplasms affecting women, but fortunately it is very rare. About 20 percent of the cases of choriocarcinoma develop following pregnancy (intrauterine or ectopic) after the twentieth week of gestation; about 40 percent develop following a molar pregnancy and 40 percent following an abortion [30]. The woman's symptoms are similar to those of a woman who has a mole, but the disease is accompanied by early metastasis to the lung and the vagina. It is diagnosed by an increased HCG titer and by x-ray demonstration of metastatic lung lesions. Treatment includes chemotherapy and hysterectomy.

The current cure rate of women with persistent gestational trophoblastic neoplasia of all severities is 90 percent [23].

Hyperemesis Gravidarum

Hyperemesis gravidarum is pernicious vomiting during pregnancy. A dangerous and abnormal situation exists when a woman's vomiting continues after the first trimester and interferes with fluid balance and other phases of nutrition. Fortunately, hyperemesis gravidarum is rare today.

The specific etiology of hyperemesis is unknown, but it is probably related to trophoblastic activity and gonadotropin production. It may be related to an increased amount of HCG, although the increase is probably a result of the state of dehydration rather than being caused by increased secretion. However, in molar pregnancies, the increased HCG levels are associated with a greater incidence of hyperemesis. No foreign or specific protein substance has been identified as a possible cause of hyperemesis; one suggestion is that it may be a reflex from uterine displacement [32]. Many clinicians believe that there is a psychosomatic component in hyperemesis, resulting from insecurity, anxiety, or a negative attitude toward the pregnancy.

ASSESSMENT

Women with hyperemesis are usually hospitalized for treatment. Nursing care should be supportive and focused on maintaining a quiet relaxed environment, control of vomiting, and restoration of fluid and electrolyte balance and food intake. Your initial assessment includes evaluation of the woman's physical condition and feelings about herself and her pregnancy.

The woman with hyperemesis experiences vomiting, especially when her stomach is empty. She may also have nausea at the mention or sight of food, weight loss, increased pulse, dehydration, signs of vitamin deficiency, thirst, hiccups, heartburn, ptyalism, constipation, and scanty, concentrated urine.

In addition to evaluating her physical condition and symptoms, elicit her feelings about the pregnancy. What are her family's feelings? Was this a planned pregnancy? How has it affected her already and how will it affect her life-style? What are her support systems and have they been effective in supporting her? What does she identify as major problems or concerns and does she see herself being able to solve them?

INTERVENTION

Women with hyperemesis are usually restricted from oral intake and given intravenous fluids for 48 hours. Then, if symptoms have subsided, they are permitted frequent small meals, which they choose themselves but which are predominantly carbohydrate. Small doses of sedatives and tranquilizers and the frequent use of mouthwash will often help.

Hospitalization removes the woman from pressing duties and responsibilities. This is often essential to improvement in her condition. Often no visitors are permitted in this protected environment, occasionally not even the husband. Encourage family members to call for progress reports during this period of separation.

THIRD-TRIMESTER COMPLICATIONS
Placenta Previa

About 5 to 6 percent of pregnant women have vaginal bleeding or staining in the latter half of pregnancy. Sometimes the open blood vessels thrombose and the bleeding ceases, but occasionally the hemorrhage is of such magnitude that the death of the mother and fetus results.

One of the major causes of hemorrhage in the latter half of pregnancy is placenta previa, which occurs when the ovum implants on or near the isthmic portion of the uterus. During the following growth and development, the placenta covers a portion of the lower uterine segment, including the cervix. In total placenta previa, the internal cervical os is completely covered; in partial placenta previa, it is partially covered; and in a low placental implantation (marginal placenta previa), a margin of the internal os is covered by the placenta. As the cervix dilates in later pregnancy or during delivery, the placental attachment tears loose and is followed by hemorrhage from the exposed vessels (Fig. 18-3).

The incidence of placenta previa is approximately one in every 200 to 250 pregnancies in the United States. As parity increases, placenta previa becomes more frequent, presumably due to atrophic changes of the endometrium.

Although the etiology of placenta previa is uncertain, it may develop when the ovum encounters an area of healthy endometrium in the lower portion of the uterus. It could develop following implantation in the upper segment owing to faulty or poorly vascularized endometrium. In the presence of this relative ischemia, the placenta will spread over a large area and extend into the lower uterine segment. The placenta is likely to be thin with a large surface area and additional cotyledons in the form of succenturiate lobe formation. Marginal insertion of the cord commonly occurs. Since the lower uterine segment is covered with significantly less endometrium than the uterine body, the development of placenta accreta (a placenta that is abnormally adherent to the uterine wall) occurs, although rarely. It may be that placenta previa develops from a portion of

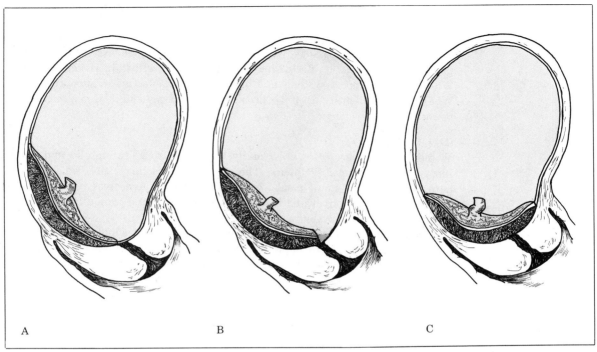

Figure 18-3. Types of placenta previa. A. Marginal placenta previa. B. Partial placenta previa. C. Total placenta previa.

the decidua capsularis located near or in contact with the lower uterine segment, in which case the villi of the chorion laeve beneath the particular area of the capsularis persist [32].

ASSESSMENT

Placenta previa is characterized by painless vaginal bleeding in the latter half of pregnancy, especially in the last trimester. It occurs without warning and in the absence of trauma; very often the woman will awake in a pool of blood of varying amounts, usually about a cupful. In cases of total placenta previa the bleeding is usually greater and appears earlier than in partial placenta previa. Most often the mother contacts the clinic nurse, midwife, or obstetrician by telephone, and she is advised to come to the hospital immediately by ambulance, even though the initial episode of bleeding is rarely fatal. In each subsequent episode the bleeding is greater.

Since she is likely to be taken to the labor floor, the nurse there is the one who usually will give her initial care. The amount of her bleeding is checked (50 milliliters, small amount; 100 milliliters, moderate amount; 500 milliliters, profuse amount). Ask about the bleeding: When did it start? More or less than a menstrual period? Any previous episodes? Pain, cramping, contractions? Was the doctor notified? Did she have any accidents? When is the baby due? Check her vital signs (blood pressure, temperature, pulse, respiration, and fetal heart tone) and palpate her abdomen for tenderness, rigidity, and fetal position. Often the placental souffle can be heard above the symphysis pubis. Evaluate the woman's emotional status.

Initial treatment usually includes blood work (Hb, Hct, WBC, differential), an intravenous infusion, close monitoring, and oxygen if necessary. Ultrasound is used to confirm the diagnosis, although historically a very careful speculum examination was done. After the diagnosis has been made, no further vaginal or rectal exams are permitted to avoid initiating further hemorrhage.

Placental localization can be achieved in a number of ways. X-ray methods include cystography, with a contrast medium in the bladder, and femoral angiography, a test that outlines the intervillous spaces and is 97 percent accurate. Soft tissue x-ray is 90 to 95 percent accurate, and a radioactive isotope scan is also highly accurate. Thermography, another method, depends on the presence of warmth over the highly vascularized placenta. Ultrasound, used to outline the boundaries of the placenta, is used most commonly. Angiography and ultrasound are accurate by the early and middle portions of the third trimester. Isotope scans and soft tissue x-ray are less accurate before the thirty-fourth week [15]. Abnormal fetal presentations are common with placenta previa and can be identified early. They often provide the first clue, before the initial bleeding episode, that tests to localize the placenta should be done.

INTERVENTION

Through the eighth month of pregnancy, delivery is delayed whenever possible to increase fetal maturity and enhance both fetal and maternal prognosis. This may mean a prolonged hospitalization for the woman, or she may be sent home with instructions for decreased activity, if the previa is marginal and the bleeding controlled.

Your role in the continuing care of this woman includes making appropriate referrals to other agencies for homemaking services or financial assistance. In addition, as Kilker and Wilkerson note, telephone contact or home visits will provide an on-going assessment of her condition [22]. This may include planning activities at home, helping to prepare the children for the mother's next hospitalization, preparing the family for a possible premature baby and evaluating the home for his care, beginning preoperative teaching (since the woman may eventually need a cesarean delivery), and possibly drawing blood for hemoglobin and hematocrit. The expectant parents are usually frightened if there is a second episode of bleeding and when delivery is anticipated, but your continuing care will ensure that they are better prepared for what is to come.

If the woman remains hospitalized she will be on bed rest. Monitor her for bleeding. Monitor vital signs including fetal heart rate and hemoglobin and hematocrit levels. No vaginal or rectal examinations are performed. If vaginal examination is necessary, it is carried out under a double setup (the delivery room is set up for both a vaginal and a cesarean delivery). In this situation, should profuse bleeding occur, an emergency cesarean delivery can be undertaken immediately.

After the fetus has reached a gestational age of 37 weeks or more, the neonatal mortality is not greatly improved by further intrauterine development [30]. If the woman is bleeding and the diagnosis is confirmed, she is delivered. Cesarean is the accepted method of delivery in practically all instances of placenta previa [30]. If the placenta lies far enough posterior, a lower uterine segment incision can be made. The classic approach (through the upper uterine segment) is often used to avoid incising the placental site to decrease blood loss (since with placenta previa the lower uterine segment is rather vascular and easily traumatized) and to provide greater access to the fetus who is high in the uterus.

In rare instances a vaginal delivery is performed using artificial rupture of membranes. Theoretically, the release of amniotic fluid will allow the presenting part to enter the pelvis and tamponade the portion of the placenta comprising the previa, thus producing hemostasis. Oxytocin may be given very carefully. The hazard that accompanies vaginal delivery in a woman with placenta previa is the interference with fetal circulation by pressure of the presenting part against the placenta or umbilical cord. Constant monitoring of fetal heart tones is imperative, and preparations should be made for an immediate cesarean delivery in case it becomes necessary. Fetal distress or recurrent bleeding during the course of labor necessitates cesarean delivery in about half of the women who have placenta previa in which vaginal delivery is attempted. Your role in closely monitoring the mother cannot be overemphasized.

Postpartum hemorrhage may occur, since the placental site is in the lower uterine segment, where there are not as many muscle fibers to contract and occlude blood vessels. There is an increased risk of uterine infection from prolonged rupture of membranes, retained placental fragments, and anemia. Rupture of the uterus may occur if the muscle has been weakened by the ingrowth of the placenta and the presence of blood sinuses. Additionally, since there may also be a significant loss of blood from the fetal circulation via placental hemorrhage, it is wise to make routine checks of the infant's hematocrit.

Placenta previa has a 1.5 percent maternal death rate, from hemorrhage, infection, traumatic rupture of the uterus, and air embolism. Overall perinatal mortality is below 15 percent, primarily resulting from prematurity and intrauterine asphyxia due to the placental position and the chance of cord prolapse. When the delivery occurs after the thirty-fifth week of gestation, perinatal mortality does not exceed 5 percent. The relatively low mortality is attributable to overall improvements in anesthesia, adequate blood replacement prior to the termination of the pregnancy, and expert care of the premature infant.

Abruptio Placentae *Abruptio placentae* refers to the premature detachment of a normally implanted placenta during the latter half of pregnancy, particularly during the last trimester. It is one of the most serious complications of pregnancy, occurring in about one of 150 to 200 pregnancies. In about 10 percent of the women, the separation is severe enough to contribute to maternal mortality from hemorrhagic shock. In the other 90 percent of women, only a small area of the placenta is detached and the result is not as serious. Abruptio placentae appears to be more common in women with toxemia and vascular and renal disease. Its incidence increases in women over 30; in women over 40, the frequency is double that in women under 30. The frequency of abruptio placentae is also increased in women with a parity of five or more [14].

Although the etiology is largely unknown, a popular theory attributes it to interference with the afferent flow of blood to the intervillous space. Some degeneration and necrosis of the decidua near its junction with the trophoblast occurs normally in the last trimester. If it becomes pronounced, the vascular channels lose support and collapse, causing bleeding from the placental site. It is also postulated that a folic acid deficiency or tension on a short umbilical cord may be contributory. Although it is possible that the vena cava syndrome (obstruction of vena cava) may increase venous pressure in the intervillous space sufficiently to detach the placenta through the formation of a retroplacental hematoma, most of the time a human adaptive mechanism stabilizes the uterine circulation. Excessive intrauterine pressure, as in marked hydramnios or multiple pregnancy, can produce pressure necrosis of the decidua. A sudden and marked decrease in intrauterine pressure, as in spontaneous rupture of membranes in hydramnios, might also be contributory. In about 33 to 50 percent of women with abruptio placentae, there is some degree of hypertension and proteinuria. Associated constricted arterioles may lead to decidual degeneration.

Placental separation may occur at the periphery, in which case bleeding may be visible as the blood flows from the edge of the placenta under the membranes, through the cervix into the vagina. Sometimes the amniotic fluid is a burgundy red color. Separation may also be initiated centrally by the formation of a blood clot behind the placenta; the clot may sometimes measure as much as 1,000 cubic centimeters. In severe cases the myometrium may be infiltrated with blood (Couvelaire uterus). If the hemorrhage is concealed, the amount of bleeding cannot be estimated and the situation is potentially very serious. If the amount of bleeding is great, it may distend the uterine wall toward the abdominal cavity.

ASSESSMENT AND INTERVENTION

The diagnosis of abruptio placentae is usually not difficult for the physician to make but the extent of the separation is hard to estimate. Usually the woman reports some vaginal bleeding, the sudden onset of severe continuous abdominal pain and/or low back pain, and a rigid, tender, irritable uterus. The woman is hospitalized immediately (Table 18-1).

If the abruption is mild and if the mother is near term, labor may be induced and the mother delivered vaginally as quickly and as atraumatically as possible. Since the placenta may separate during labor, be alert for a significant change in the woman's condition. The first indication of danger may be her complaint of a

Table 18-1.
Characteristics of
Abruptio Placentae and
Placenta Previa

Characteristic	Abruptio Placentae	Placenta Previa
Onset	Third trimester	Third trimester (commonly in eighth month)
Bleeding	May be concealed, external dark hemorrhage, or bloody amniotic fluid	Mostly external, small to profuse in amount, bright red
Pain and uterine tenderness	Usually present; irritable uterus, progresses to board-like consistency	Usually absent; uterus soft
Fetal heart tone	May be irregular or absent	Usually normal
Presenting part	May or may not be engaged	Usually not engaged
Shock	Moderate to severe depending on extent of concealed and external hemorrhage	Usually not present unless bleeding is excessive
Delivery	Immediate delivery, usually by cesarean section	Delivery may be delayed, depending on size of fetus and amount of bleeding

charley-horse type of pain in her abdomen [22], and her uterus may become irritable, rigid, and boardlike. Fetal heart rate may become irregular or absent, and there may be a definite increase in fetal activity. Sometimes the fundal height increases, and active bleeding may or may not be observable. Since maternal apprehension increases greatly, explain everything that is happening to both of the expectant parents. They should be mentally prepared for a possible cesarean delivery. Without giving false reassurances, reinforce the positive aspects of the woman's condition by having the couple listen to the fetal heart tones and telling them when vital signs are stable and when there is no evidence of further bleeding. The seriousness of the situation demands your constant supervision.

Hypofibrinogenemia, a complication associated with abruptio placenta, is the result of consumption of fibrinogen by disseminated intravascular coagulation (DIC), caused by absorption of thromboplastin-like material from the placental site. Fibrinogen levels, ordinarily elevated in pregnancy, may drop to incoagulable amounts (below 100 milligrams per 100 milliliters) within a matter of minutes in rapidly developing premature separation of the placenta. Prompt delivery usually limits the progression of this disorder and eliminates the need for further therapy if uterine tone is maintained. Supportive treatment includes type and crossmatch, blood transfusions, clotting mechanism evaluation, and intravenous fluids.

If the placental separation is moderately severe or severe, a cesarean delivery is done in order to save the fetus and the mother, after hypofibrinogenemia, if present, is corrected. If a Couvelaire uterus has developed, it will not contract sufficiently during labor, making vaginal delivery impossible. If maternal hemorrhage is uncontrollable, a cesarean delivery will be performed to allow an immediate hysterectomy.

Your interventions following cesarean delivery for this woman are much the same as for other women who have had the procedure (Chap. 19). In addition, it is essential that you monitor this mother closely for postpartum hemorrhage and indications of renal failure due to periods of extreme hypovolemia and renal ischemia.

Perinatal mortality accompanying abruptio placentae is approximately 15 percent; fetal complications arise from premature birth, anemia, and hypoxia, but early cesarean increases the chances of fetal survival. The maternal mortality for this disorder is 6 percent. Late postpartum hemorrhage may be a subsequent problem.

Coagulation Defects   The terms used for coagulation defects include the defibrination syndrome, consumptive coagulopathy, and DIC, the last of which is the most common. Coagulation defects are associated with longstanding intrauterine fetal death and severe abruptio placentae. DIC may be a secondary effect of amniotic fluid embolism and is seen in association with some cases of sepsis or endotoxin shock; it involves a decrease in plasma fibrinogen concentration and other clotting factors, with a sharp fall in platelets.

DIC is more common in women with Rh-negative sensitization, hypertension, or preeclampsia; in these women, fetal death in utero and abruptio placentae are fairly common.

The etiology is controversial but definitely involves a reduction in circulating fibrinogen to levels of 100 milligrams per 100 milliliters or less [32]. It is due either to the direct effect of primary fibrinolysis or to intravascular clotting with resultant activation of the fibrinolytic system. In either case, hemorrhage is the end result. The most consistent findings are decreased fibrinogen, decreased plasminogen, and varying degrees of thrombocytopenia. Most cases involve disseminated intravascular clotting, with fibrinolytic activity appearing in response to fibrin deposition (Fig. 18-4).

It is possible that in normal pregnancy some intravascular clotting may occur in undetectable amounts due to the increase in Factors VII, VIII, IX, and X, and fibrinogen (Factor I) [17,32]. The process of fibrin deposition may normally be required to maintain the integrity of the intervillous space, which is constantly being challenged by myometrial contractions. Fibrin deposition may also keep the placental surface intact [32], but occasionally it reaches pathologic proportions and decreases placental transport.

ASSESSMENT

DIC is rarely encountered before the twentieth week of pregnancy. Many intrauterine fetal deaths occur between 5 and 8 months of pregnancy, when the spontaneous onset of labor is less likely. DIC more often occurs when a dead fetus is retained for 5 or more weeks. Fortunately most women deliver within this time, but about 40 percent of women in whom the dead fetus is retained longer will develop DIC. It is often heralded by the appearance of ecchymoses and bleeding from mucous membranes, which may first present during delivery.

A clot observation test is a rapid and practical method of identifying a clotting defect. Normal blood clots in 8 to 12 minutes, and the clot remains intact for 24 hours. If a clotting defect is present, the blood may not clot, or if it does, the clot may undergo partial or complete dissolution within 30 to 60 minutes [32]. This indicates a low fibrinogen level and/or fibrinolytic activity; a fibrinogen level determination confirms the diagnosis.

Figure 18-4. Disseminated intravascular coagulation. (Modified from C. McLennan and E. Sandberg. *Synopsis of Obstetrics*. St. Louis: Mosby, 1974.)

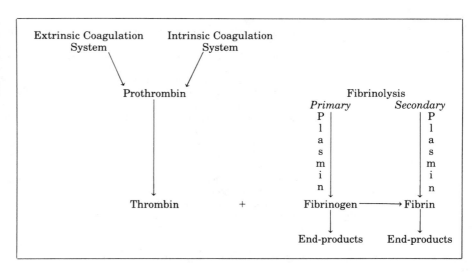

INTERVENTION

With the diagnosis of DIC, the mother is given fibrinogen (Factor I), together with whole fresh blood. Minimal treatment of women with severe cases consists of the administration of 2 to 4 units of blood with 4 to 8 grams of fibrinogen. Heparin, advocated by some clinicians to block the disseminated intravascular coagulation has most recently been condemned by Pritchard and MacDonald as likely to aggravate the hemorrhage [30].

Evacuation of the uterine contents helps to control the loss of blood and removes the stimulus to clotting. However, effective hemostasis at the time of delivery does require a stable clot. Bleeding in severe cases in the past may have been attributed to atony, when it has actually been the result of a defect in the clotting mechanism.

Hypertensive Disorders in Pregnancy

Hypertensive disorders in pregnancy rank among the leading causes of maternal mortality and make a significant contribution to perinatal mortality. Preeclampsia and eclampsia (formerly termed toxemia) are two major hypertensive disorders, which are characterized by the development of hypertension, edema, and proteinuria and are usually relieved by termination of the pregnancy (Table 18-2). Edema is usually the first symptom to appear, generally observed as rapid weight gain. A rise in blood pressure follows, followed by proteinuria.

PREECLAMPSIA AND ECLAMPSIA

Preeclampsia, unique to human gestation, is the development of hypertension with proteinuria, edema, or both, induced by pregnancy after the twentieth week of gestation. It appears most frequently in young primigravidas and in women

Table 18-2.
Classification of
Hypertensive Disorders of
Pregnancy

Gestational edema: The occurrence of a general and excessive accumulation of fluid in the tissues of greater than 1+ pitting edema after 12 hours' rest in bed, or of a weight gain of 5 pounds or more in 1 week due to the influence of pregnancy.

Gestational proteinuria: The presence of proteinuria during or under the influence of pregnancy, in the absence of hypertension, edema, renal infection, or known intrinsic renovascular cause.

Gestational hypertension: Gestational hypertension is the development of hypertension during pregnancy or within the first 24 hours postpartum in a previously normotensive woman.

Preeclampsia: The development of hypertension with proteinuria, edema, or both due to pregnancy or the influence of a recent pregnancy. It occurs after the twentieth week of gestation but may develop before this time in the presence of trophoblastic disease. Preeclampsia is predominantly a disorder of primigravidas.

Eclampsia: The occurrence of one or more convulsions, not attributable to other cerebral disorders such as epilepsy or cerebral hemorrhage, in a patient with preeclampsia.

Superimposed preeclampsia or eclampsia: The development of preeclampsia or eclampsia in a patient with chronic hypertensive, vascular, or renal disease. When the hypertension antedates the pregnancy, as established by previous blood pressure recordings, a rise in the systolic pressure of 30 mm Hg, a rise in the diastolic pressure of 15 mm Hg, and the development of proteinuria, edema, or both are required during pregnancy to establish the diagnosis.

Chronic hypertensive disease: The presence of persistent hypertension, of whatever cause, before pregnancy or prior to the twentieth week of gestation, or persistent hypertension beyond the forty-second day of the postpartum period.

Sources: The American College of Obstetricians and Gynecologists; and D. N. Danforth (Ed.), *Obstetrics and Gynecology* (3rd ed.). Hagerstown, Md.: Harper & Row, 1977.

with molar pregnancies, diabetes, multiple pregnancies, or hydramnios, and in women who are obese or who have a history of previous hypertension in pregnancy.

Assessment.   Preeclampsia varies in severity. Women with preeclampsia may be comparatively symptom-free and may have little or no peripheral edema remaining after bed rest. Their blood pressure is usually near or above 140/90, or about 30 millimeters of mercury above normal systolic and 15 millimeters of mercury above normal diastolic pressures. Young women who normally have blood pressures of 90/60 may have significant problems when their blood pressures approach 120/80, therefore it is essential that a baseline blood pressure reading be recorded early in pregnancy. In women with pregnancy-induced hypertension (PIH), the normal circadian rhythm of blood pressure may be altered or completely eliminated. Instead of the normal morning peaks and nighttime lows, the blood pressure of women with PIH peaks during the night [41]. In the woman with preeclampsia, a 24-hour urine collection contains about 1 gram of albumin. A random, clean, midstream specimen shows +1 or +2 albumin (Table 18-3).

Milder forms of preeclampsia may rapidly progress to severe preeclampsia and possibly eclampsia. In severe preeclampsia generalized edema is apparent, and there may be pitting edema over the lower extremities, abdominal wall, face, hands, and sacral area. Severe preeclampsia is characterized by a sudden and marked weight gain of more than 0.9 kilogram (2 pounds) over a period of a few days or a week. Blood pressure generally is 160/110 or higher and the daily 24-

Table 18-3. Symptoms of Preeclampsia

Symptom	Definition
Mild preeclampsia	
Hypertension	Increase of 30 mm Hg or more systolic, or systolic level of 140 mm Hg or more; increase of 15 mm Hg or more diastolic, or diastolic level of 90 mm Hg or more
Proteinuria	+1 or +2 or 1 gm/liter in midstream or catheterized urine specimen (found in two specimens at least 6 hours apart)
Edema	Generalized, facial, hand and fingers; reflected in a rapid weight gain of over 0.7 kg (1.5 pounds) per week
Severe preeclampsia	
Hypertension	160/110 or above
Proteinuria	5 gm or more in 24-hour urine collection or +3 or +4 reading on turbidometric analysis
Edema	In addition to generalized edema, possibly pitting edema; weight gain may be 0.9 kg (2 pounds) or more over a period of a week or less
Headache	
Blurred vision	
Oliguria (less than 400 ml in 24-hour urine collection)	
Epigastric pain	

hour urine albumin is 5 grams or more, or +3 or +4. The woman may also experience frontal headache, nausea, vomiting, cerebral or visual disturbances, listlessness, hyperreflexia, oliguria (less than 400 ml/24 hr, or less than 30 ml/hr), increased hematocrit, and finally epigastric pain. Eclampsia develops when the woman has convulsions.

A screening test called the supine hypertensive or "roll-over" test is sometimes used between 28 and 32 weeks of pregnancy to predict hypertensive disease developing in later pregnancy. To carry out the test the woman lies in the left lateral recumbent position and her blood pressure is taken 5 and 15 minutes later to establish a baseline diastolic blood pressure. The woman then rolls over to a supine position and her blood pressure is taken immediately and 5 minutes later while she is still in the supine position. If the woman's diastolic blood pressure increases 20 milliliters of mercury or more, the test is considered positive. Results of studies using this test indicate that 90 percent of the women having a negative rollover test remained normotensive, whereas 84 percent of those with a positive rollover test developed pregnancy-induced hypertension in later pregnancy [19, 24]. Some clinicians report less success with the test [20a].

Pritchard and MacDonald note that pregnancy-induced hypertension is much more likely to develop in a woman who is exposed to chorionic villi for the first time, who is exposed to a superabundance of chorionic villi and covering trophoblast as with twins or hydatidiform mole, who has preexisting vascular disease, or who is genetically predisposed to the development of hypertension during pregnancy [30].

Preeclampsia appears in about 5 percent of all pregnancies. Because of improved antepartal care, better general health and nutrition, and early detection and treatment of the disorder, the incidence of preeclampsia has decreased by 25 to 50 percent, and the incidence of eclampsia has decreased by 60 to 95 percent. Unfortunately the cause of these conditions is essentially unknown, but functioning trophoblastic tissue is apparently necessary to their development, and vasospasm is basic to the disease process. Vasospasm occurs with arteriolar vasoconstriction and increased peripheral vascular resistance. The vasospasm is thought to be due to the exquisite sensitivity of the vasculature to vasopressors. Plasma renin activity and circulating angiotensin II levels are lower in women with pregnancy-induced hypertension than the levels of those of normal pregnant women. Other substances implicated in the pathogenesis or maintenance of hypertension of pregnancy include catecholamines, prolactin, vasopressin, prostaglandins, and as yet unidentified pressor agents. Environmental factors (such as climate and socioeconomic status) and personal factors (such as genetic predisposition, diet, activity, and health habits) may be contributory. The exact relationship of good nutrition to the development of preeclampsia is obscure, but the frequency of the disorder appears to be higher in populations in which diets are deficient, particularly in protein (see Chap. 8). Another theory holds that preeclampsia is an autoimmune disease, since the placenta may be considered antigenic [32]. DIC may also be a mechanism involved.

Preeclampsia is also believed to be caused by uterine ischemia, although it is possible that the ischemia is a result, rather than a cause, of the disease. Mechanical factors in or around the uterus fail to allow the blood flow to adapt to the requirements of the uterus and fetus [15]. Decreased uterine blood flow leads to the production by the ischemic placenta (or by ischemia-induced decidual degeneration) of pressor polypeptides, thromboplastin, or thromboplastin-like substances. Ischemia is augmented by mechanical factors, such as increased myometrial tension (resulting from multiple pregnancy or during labor), or excessive amounts of trophoblast (hydatid mole). Primigravidas have decreased vascular hypertrophy. Women with chronic hypertensive vascular disease already have arteriolar sclerosis and increased vascular resistance.

The kidney consistently shows the effects of preeclampsia or eclampsia with decreased renal blood flow and decreased glomerular filtration rate. A "classical" lesion (capillary endotheliosis) develops in the kidney and involves all glomeruli equally. The glomeruli swell and become ischemic, obstructing the capillary lumens. The lesions usually regress by 2 weeks after delivery. Tubular capacity for reabsorption of sodium appears to be increased, and cardiac output is increased. In women with severe preeclampsia, the cardiac load is significantly increased because of increased peripheral vascular resistance and elevated viscosity of the blood, as a result of hemoconcentration. Plasma volume is lost to the interstitial space in PIH and causes a hypovolemia. The decreased plasma volume leads to high serum uric acid, a finding correlated with poor fetal outcome. Decreased volume may also be the mechanism for sodium retention associated with the disorder [41]. Uterine blood flow decreases with hypertension, and the decreased uteroplacental blood flow is a principal cause of fetal death and of the tendency for infants to be small for gestational age. The placenta shows an increased number of infarcts. Pulmonary edema, congestive heart failure, cerebral hemorrhage, and complications of operative obstetrics are major causes of death in women with preeclampsia and eclampsia. Retinal edema and spasm of retinal arteries may result in actual detachment of the retina. Increased cerebrovascular resistance may lead to dulling of the sensorium.

Intervention.   Care of the woman with severe preeclampsia is directed toward the prevention of convulsions by decreasing blood pressure, establishing diuresis, and continuing the pregnancy until the fetus is mature. The woman may be hospitalized or placed on bed rest at home. Sedatives or hypotensive agents may be used. Encourage her to lie on her left side so renal and uterine blood flow increase, which may result in diuresis and the return of her blood pressure to normal levels. During pregnancy, arterial blood pressure has been found to be highest when the woman is sitting, intermediate when she is supine, and lowest in the left lateral recumbent position [36a]. When taking the woman's blood pressure, take it in the same arm with the woman in the same position. Monitor her vital signs every 4 hours; if she is at home a responsible friend or family member may be taught to do so. Record her weight and her intake and output daily. Fluids are not necessarily restricted. Under this regimen her symptoms usually diminish. There is some evidence that the development of preeclampsia or eclampsia may be related to nutrition, specifically protein deficiency [40]. It is no longer regarded as valid to restrict calorie intake to avoid large weight gain (accumulation of fat) in the hope of avoiding preeclampsia. A high protein diet is usually advised. Another common practice, based on rather dubious evidence, has been the routine restriction of salt in the hope of preventing edema. Actually, the restriction of sodium intensifies the normal renin-angiotensin-aldosterone mechanism, which results in a positive sodium balance [28]. Therefore, sodium restriction should probably not be a major part of the routine treatment of preeclampsia, and there are many questions as well, about the routine use of diuretics. However, some preeclamptic women may not handle sodium well, and on this basis the restriction is indicated when hypertension develops [15].

The woman's pregnancy is maintained until at least the thirty-sixth week, if possible. Nonstress tests, urinary estriol determinations, and ultrasound measurements of fetal growth are often used to monitor the condition of the fetus. In the management of severe preeclampsia, blood pressure is usually lowered by a pharmacologic agent. Magnesium sulfate, commonly administered intramuscularly in a 50% solution with 1% procaine, is a popular choice. It has a depressant action on the myoneural junction, decreasing hyperreflexia and resulting in some vasodilatation. It also depresses the central nervous system and may cause osmotic diuresis, secondarily decreasing intracranial pressure.

Magnesium sulfate (usually 5–10 grams in 10–20 milliliters) is injected deep into the gluteal muscle (Fig. 18-5). Because the solution is very irritating to tissues, the needle used to draw it up should be discarded. As the injection is made, the needle is rotated like a wheel, because of the large amount of solution. Usually the dose is divided equally between the two buttocks, and the tissue is massaged well following the injection. Since magnesium sulfate is eliminated chiefly by the kidneys, a high serum concentration may be reached if urine output is low. As a result, respiration or cardiac action may be depressed, although respiratory depression does not occur until after the patellar reflex disappears. If this reflex is absent, if respirations are below 16 per minute, or if urine output is under 30 milliliters per hour, repeat doses of magnesium sulfate are not given. Calcium gluconate is an effective metabolic antagonist and should be kept

Figure 18-5. Technique for injecting magnesium sulfate (see text for details).

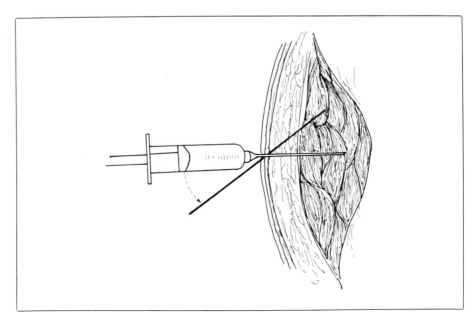

available. Other medications used to decrease hypertension are hydralazine (which decreases arteriolar resistance) and morphine and other sedatives (Table 18-4).

If eclampsia develops (i.e., if convulsions occur), monitor the woman very carefully. She is put on bed rest with padded side rails; intravenous fluids, a central venous pressure line, and a Foley catheter are inserted. Restrict her oral intake. Record her output hourly, and record her vital signs frequently. The foot of the bed may be elevated to facilitate tracheobronchial drainage. Suction to prevent aspiration, oxygen, and padded tongue blades should be readily available. Make every effort to decrease the woman's sensory stimulation. Promote a quiet environment and give her only the care that is absolutely necessary. When her convulsions cease, irritability decreases, blood pressure decreases, and her pulse is below 100, then thought is given to the termination of her pregnancy. If her cervix is favorable for labor, her membranes are ruptured and oxytocin may be given. A cesarean delivery is usually performed if the induction fails, her labor slows, her condition worsens, or fetal distress develops. Monitor her blood loss

Table 18-4.
Medications Used in the Treatment of Hypertensive Disorders of Pregnancy

Drug	Use	Dose	Adverse Reactions
Phenobarbital	Sedative; anticonvulsant (raises threshold for seizures)	Oral: 30–100 mg BID or TID in preeclampsia IM or IV; large doses for eclampsia	Tolerance may develop; rashes; ataxia
Magnesium sulfate	Anticonvulsant; depresses CNS function especially at neuromuscular junction; reduces muscle excitability; peripheral vasodilation; in large doses osmotic diuretic	IM: 10 gm initially as 50% solution followed by 5 gm every 4 hr until reflexes are reduced IV: loading dose of 4 gm given over 10 min. Followed by 1 gm/hr until therapeutic blood levels of 6–7 mEq/liter are reached	Respiratory depression, depression of deep tendon reflexes; IM injections may produce pain and swelling at injection site
Sodium amobarbital (sodium amytal)	Anticonvulsant; used in eclampsia when convulsions persist	IV: up to 0.25 gm injected over a 3-min period	
Diazepam (Valium)	Anticonvulsant; used to control or reduce convulsions	IV: 5 mg IM: 10 mg Dose is administered every 2 hr until convulsions are controlled	Fetal tachycardia and loss of fetal heart rate variability, newborn lethargy, hypotonia, respiratory depression, failure to suck
Hydralazine (Apresoline)	Antihypertensive; dilation of vascular smooth muscle, especially arterioles	IV: when diastolic blood pressure is 110 mm Hg test dose 5 mg followed by 10 mg, repeated until diastolic blood pressure is 90–100 mm Hg (usual dose 5–20 mg)	Chills, fever, depression, headache, palpitations, dizziness, vomiting, tachycardia, sweating
Hydrochlorthiazide	Diuretic; used in treating women with chronic hypertension; not used in prevention of preeclampsia (no documented advantage)	Oral: 50 mg BID	Fatigue, weakness, anorexia, heartburn, nausea, vomiting, decreased fetal birth weight

Sources: E. Dickason, et al. *Maternal and Infant Drugs and Nursing Intervention.* New York: McGraw-Hill, 1978; S. Aladjem. *Obstetrical Practice.* St. Louis: Mosby, 1980; E. Quilligan, and N. Kretchmer. *Fetal and Maternal Medicine.* New York: Wiley, 1980; J. Pritchard, and P. MacDonald. *Williams Obstetrics* (16th ed.). New York: Appleton-Century-Crofts, 1980; and T. King. Maternal and fetal effects of cardiovascular drugs. *Symposia Reporter* 4:15, 1981.

carefully since it has been demonstrated that eclamptic women experience twice the blood loss of women who deliver with noncomplicated pregnancies [13a].

The pathophysiologic changes associated with preeclampsia and eclampsia tend to regress rapidly following delivery, but eclampsia may develop during the first 24 hours after delivery. Diuresis in the first 12 hours following delivery is often a first and valuable sign of recovery. Mothers are supervised carefully for about 10 days post partum. Usually edema and proteinuria decrease progressively and are gone by the fifth postpartum day.

Maternal mortality increases with the severity of the disorder. Chances of reoccurrence in subsequent pregnancies range between 13 and 45 percent. Additionally, the rate of diabetes found in later years in women who have had preeclampsia is 2.5 times greater than that found in the general population [30]. Fetal mortality has ranged from as low as 0.9 percent for women with preeclampsia who are treated to as high as 15 percent, when eclampsia occurred. It is primarily due to prematurity, although some infants are low birth weight and some are stillborn.

It is uncertain whether preeclampsia and eclampsia can be prevented. Antepartal care is given the most credit for alerting health personnel to signs and symptoms that can be treated. Dietary salt restriction and the use of thiazide diuretics have no documented value in prevention, nor is weight control thought to be of any value in this regard. In some research, early manifestations of preeclampsia have actually been relieved by an increased salt intake [15]. Needless to say, pregnant women should be aware of the symptoms that should be reported to the nurse, midwife, or obstetrician so that they can be more carefully monitored.

CHRONIC HYPERTENSIVE VASCULAR DISEASE
Some women who have hypertensive disorders of pregnancy have chronic hypertensive vascular disease (CHVD). In these instances the hypertension precedes the pregnancy and exists prior to the twentieth week of pregnancy.

Women with CHVD are placed on bed rest. The use of sodium restriction, diuretics, sedatives, and hypotensive drugs is controversial, and their use is variable, depending often upon physician preference. Women return for weekly visits. The woman's pregnancy is terminated as soon as possible, but every effort is made to prolong it to 34 weeks or more.

A high fetal loss is associated, especially if preeclampsia is superimposed; many infants are small for their gestational age. CHVD is also associated with abruptio placentae, stillbirth, and late abortion. Most women survive, but there is a tendency for their condition to be more severe with succeeding pregnancies. Therefore a discussion of contraception is an important element of your teaching plan for them.

MULTIPLE PREGNANCY   On the average, multiple pregnancy resulting in twins occurs in 1 of 80 pregnancies; triplets occur in 1 of 6,400 pregnancies; and quadruplets occur in 1 of 512,000 pregnancies. Monozygotic (identical) twinning occurs apparently at random in 1 of about 200 pregnancies. Dizygotic (fraternal) twinning is controlled by various factors, especially ethnic and familial, and is subject to pituitary secretion of follicle-stimulating hormone (FSH), with the ova coming from the same graafian follicle or from separate ones, in the same or opposite ovary. The number of mature ova released from the ovary depends on the balance between the action of the pituitary gonadotropins and the inhibiting action of ripening follicles on the maturation of other follicles. If such inhibition does not occur (due to endocrine imbalance, such as excessive pituitary stimulation), two or more ova can be released.

Twinning is most common among blacks, less common among whites, and least common among Orientals. Dizygotic twinning is familial, and families that have a history of dizygotic twins have a higher incidence of multiple births. The twin-bearing mother probably has a higher FSH secretion rate, leading to polyovulation. The trait may be inherited through the father; however, accurate studies to support that assumption have not been made [32].

Multiple births may also be the result of treatment for infertility with human FSH. Twinning appears to be increased with advancing maternal age up to 39 years, probably due to higher levels of gonadotropin. The incidence is decreased after the age of 39, probably due to a decline in ovarian function. Higher frequency of twinning with increasing parity may be due to permanent changes in the activity of the pituitary gland or ovary during pregnancy.

Dizygotic twins always have two chorions and two amnions. Genetically as dissimilar as any other siblings, fraternal twins are definitely diagnosed as such if one twin is male and one female (Fig. 18-6).

Monozygotic twins have one chorion and two amnions about 70 percent of the time, and two chorions and two amnions about 30 percent of the time. This is dependent on the time of the twinning impetus (splitting of the ovum). If it is on day 3 or after, when the chorion is established, they will be monochorionic. If it is on day 8 or after, they will be monoamnionic, since by then the amnion is established. Once the embryonic axis is formed, after day 14, true twinning is presumably impossible; if it does occur, the twins are likely to be conjoined [32].

The diagnosis of monozygotic twinning can be made with certainty at birth when the placenta is available, or later, using blood groups and skin grafting. A single placenta is usually associated with identical twins, although dizygotic placentas may fuse and appear as one. Triplets may be monozygotic, dizygotic, or trizygotic.

Spontaneous abortion is more likely to occur with multiple fetuses than with a single fetus. Both perinatal mortality and maternal mortality are greater in multiple births than in single ones; in pregnancies lasting over 20 weeks, 14 percent of twins die in the perinatal period, compared to 3 percent of singletons. Since 50 to 80 percent of all twin pregnancies are delivered before term, prematurity is the major cause of the increased mortality. Monoamnionic twins have the highest mortality, often due to entangled umbilical cords and blocked circulation. There may be a significantly greater hazard for the second twin as a result of prolonged exposure to anesthesia, uterine contraction with detached placenta, or the greater likelihood of breech presentation. Abnormal placental insertions of the cord occur in about 7 percent of twin pregnancies, compared to 1

Figure 18-6. A. Monozygotic twins—one chorion, two amnions, and one placenta. B. Dizygotic twins—two chorions, two amnions, and two placentas. C. Dizygotic twins—two chorions, two amnions, and a single fused placenta.

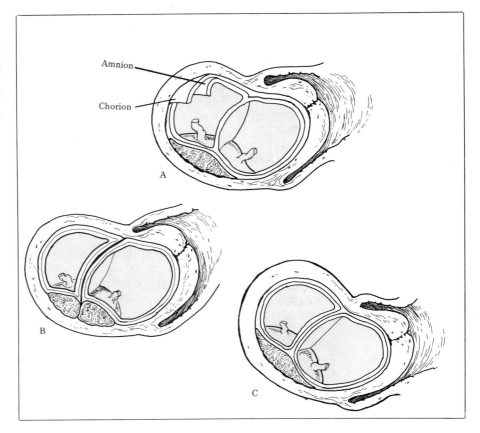

percent in singletons. Congenital anomalies tend to appear more frequently as well. Abortions are common.

Maternal complications of hypertensive disorders, polyhydramnios, anemia, and placenta previa are more common, and overdistention of the uterus may contribute to a greater incidence of postpartum hemorrhage. Labor may be abnormal, since overstretching of the myometrium may cause uterine contractions to be ineffective in dilating the cervix during the active phase. This, plus the resulting increase in operative deliveries, tends to increase the incidence of infection.

Assessment and Intervention

The primary goal in caring for the woman with a multiple pregnancy is to help her bring her pregnancy to the point where the fetuses are viable. If she gets adequate rest, nutrition, and antepartal care, it is likely that she will not develop preeclampsia or have premature dilatation of her cervix. The presence of a skilled pediatrician in the delivery room will benefit the infants.

Multiple pregnancy is diagnosed when the woman's abdomen is larger than expected for the length of gestation. It is often associated with rapid uterine growth, pronounced edema, proteinuria, and fetal motion over her entire abdomen. Two fetal heart tones can be counted simultaneously, but since fetal size may be small, the heart tones are less likely to be audible at a time when the size of the uterus would indicate they should be heard. Abdominal palpation yields many small parts by 6 or 7 months. Ultrasonography or x-ray is used for a positive diagnosis. Twinning may not be suspected or diagnosed until after the birth of the first infant, when the mother's uterus remains almost as large as before.

Women who are carrying twins are seen more frequently for checkups. Good general hygiene and rest at home or preadmission to the hospital for bed rest between the twenty-eighth and thirty-sixth weeks of gestation may prolong pregnancy and prevent premature labor. Since hypertensive disorders may accompany multiple pregnancy, teach these women the pertinent signs and symptoms that they need to report to the nurse, midwife, or obstetrician.

Their excessive abdominal distention because of the oversized uterus often leads to digestion difficulties, constipation, hemorrhoids, backaches, pedal edema, and dyspnea. Varicose veins and urinary stasis (resulting in chronic urinary tract infection) may also develop. Pressure symptoms are relieved if the woman lies on her side whenever she is taking one of her frequent rest periods. Pelvic rocking exercises will help her backache as will sitting frequently with her legs elevated. Small frequent meals will make digestion easier. The woman with twins also needs a diet high in protein, iron, and calcium to meet the needs of the growing fetuses.

As Leonard notes, clinicians differ in their counseling regarding added daily calories for women carrying twins. The added calories suggested range from a daily increase of 300 kcal to 1,000 kcal once pregnancy reaches 20 weeks' gestation [22a].

Complications during labor include uterine dysfunction due to an overstretched myometrium, abnormal fetal presentations, and premature labor. Monitor both fetuses with external monitors or with one internal and one external monitor. After the birth of the first infant, monitor the one remaining in the uterus very carefully.

The interval between the actual delivery of each twin is usually 3 to 15 minutes. Since the uterus contracts to accommodate to the decreased intrauterine volume, there is the danger of placental separation while the second twin is still inside the uterus. In many instances the second twin is in a transverse lie, or his presenting part is above the inlet. In both instances prolapse of the cord or dystocia is more likely to occur. Therefore, an internal podalic version may be done and the second twin delivered breech.

Both twins are vertex about 45 percent of the time; one vertex and one breech, 38 percent; both breech, 9 percent; one transverse, 7 percent [15]. If they happen to be interlocked, the delivery is usually by cesarean; vaginal delivery is very difficult, resulting many times in the loss of one twin. If labor must be stimulated in multiple pregnancy, oxytocin is used with extreme caution.

Since the mother is unlikely to be able to take care of two or more babies at home without some assistance, help her investigate the resources at her disposal, making appropriate referrals or later doing follow-up visits. Since the mother's delivery is likely to be early and complex, prepare her for the possible procedures she will encounter and for the appearance of her babies, should they be premature. Sometimes following a multiple birth parents need to be reminded of the uniqueness of each of their infants.

Transfusion Syndrome and Blood Chimerism Sometimes in monochorionic (monozygotic) twins there is an interfetal anastomotic vascular connection (transfusion syndrome). During the development of a single placenta, some blood vessels almost regularly join, whether artery to artery, vein to vein, or artery to vein. The most significant degree of transfusion syndrome results when a single arteriovenous communication exists. An artery from one fetus supplies a cotyledon, which is drained by a vein from the other fetus. As a result, one fetus (A) continuously loses blood to the other (B). Therefore, B gets hypervolemia and presumably hypertension, cardiac hypertrophy, and occasionally edema, and he generally grows larger. He may urinate excessively, resulting in hydramnios. Nourishment for the two twins is, of course, unequally divided. When the process occurs very early in gestation, one twin (B) will tend to overpower the other, with the weaker heart dilating into a tortuous vessel. This fetus remains undeveloped. At times one of the twins dies before birth. In this instance, the fluid constituents are gradually resorbed, and the twin becomes a shriveled, compressed appendage (fetus papyraceus) of the placenta. If the A twin survives, he is likely to be small and to suffer from microcardia, anemia, dehydration, and perhaps oligohydramnios. Such a different prenatal environment may cause such identical twins to remain different for quite some time.

Postnatally, if the donor twin (A) has a hemoglobin of below 13.3 grams per 100 milliliters in the first 24 hours, a transfusion is usually given [38]; this infant may have an early iron deficiency anemia. The recipient twin (B) has polycythemia, and jaundice and hyperbilirubinemia are postnatal threats. He is prone to dehydration because of frequent urination. Treatment aims to decrease polycythemia and blood viscosity. A hematocrit over 75 percent warrants phlebotomy or partial exchange of plasma for blood, which will also help to correct the hyperbilirubinemia.

Sometimes dizygotic twins who have an anastomoses of their fetal circulations will show a blood group chimerism, which means that they contain a mixture of two distinct types of blood. Blood chimerism has been detected in only a few sets of monozygotic twins.

POLYHYDRAMNIOS (HYDRAMNIOS) AND OLIGOHYDRAMNIOS An excessive amount of amniotic fluid (polyhydramnios) or a very small amount (oligohydramnios) may be associated with maternal disease, such as diabetes mellitus, heart disease, and kidney disease; with multiple gestation; or, as in 25 to 33 percent of the cases, with fetal abnormalities. In about half of the cases of hydramnios and oligohydramnios there is no demonstrable cause.

Instances of hydramnios (Fig. 18-7) in which the amount of amniotic fluid is 2 to 4 liters or more are often associated with particular fetal anomalies including atresias and neural tube defects. In esophageal and duodenal atresia an insignificant amount of fluid may be swallowed, and in anencephaly or hydrocephaly the swallowing reflex may be disturbed through an alteration in brain structure. In spina bifida, it is thought that cerebrospinal fluid may be added to the amniotic cavity through the exposed meninges.

Assessment Chronic polyhydramnios is usually noticed around 28 to 38 weeks of gestation, and the accumulation of fluid is gradual. Acute polyhydramnios, the result of a very rapid process over a few days, is usually noticed around 20 to 24 weeks of

Figure 18-7. Woman with extreme case of hydramnios (5,500 milliliters of amniotic fluid was measured at delivery). (From L. M. Hellman and J. A. Pritchard. *Williams Obstetrics* [14th ed.], 1971. Courtesy of Appleton-Century-Crofts, Publishing Division of Prentice-Hall, Inc.)

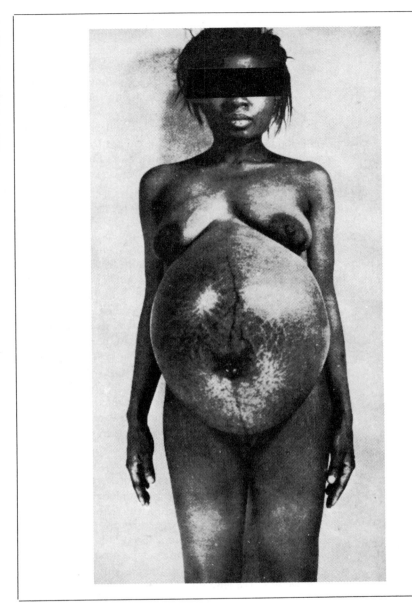

gestation. In the latter instance, spontaneous labor often results before the end of the second trimester as a result of rapid uterine expansion. Premature delivery is common, not only because of uterine enlargement but also because the woman's cervix is often effaced and considerably dilated due to the pressure exerted on it.

Interventions   Two or 3 liters of fluid may be removed by amniocentesis, which may maintain the woman's pregnancy to fetal viability. In extreme situations repeat amniocentesis may have to be done. The main difficulty with removing amniotic fluid is that too much may be removed too rapidly, thus initiating labor. Approximately 500 milliliters are removed per hour until 1,500 to 2,000 milliliters have been removed. Removal takes place in a closed system with the flow of amniotic fluid controlled by a screw clamp. Monitor the mother's vital signs carefully during the procedure. In the past some physicians recommended the use of diuretics. Currently they are regarded as ineffectual and potentially dangerous [15]. It is rarely necessary for the pregnancy to be terminated.

With polyhydramnios of 3 or more liters, the woman often experiences pain in her abdomen, back, and thighs, caused by increased pressure. She may complain of dyspnea, nausea, and vomiting, and she may have edema of her abdominal wall, vulva, and lower extremities. Usually you will find it difficult to hear the fetal heart tones. You will not easily palpate the fetus. The focus of your interventions is to have the mother rest, preferably on her side, semirecumbent, to increase blood flow to her uterus and fetus and to relieve her symptoms. She will also need reassurance regarding her outcome and that of her infant. She may also need help in augmenting her support system through community resources.

The maternal prognosis is usually good, although abruptio placentae, uterine dysfunction, and postpartum hemorrhage may occur. Abnormal fetal presentations are common, and surgical interventions may be required; postpartum hemorrhage in this instance is even more likely. Maternal shock may also result postpartally from the sudden decrease in intra-abdominal pressure. Fetal prognosis is poor, since in many cases the baby will be born prematurely and have anomalies and prolapsed cord, or he may be the victim of abruptio placentae.

Oligohydramnios, a rare condition in which the amount of amniotic fluid may be only 100 to 200 milliliters, is sometimes associated with fetal renal agenesis or postmaturity. If it occurs early in pregnancy, the amnion may adhere to the fetus, or amniotic bands may form around one of his arms or legs, with resulting deformities in either case. The fetal skin may be wrinkled, leathery, and dry. The infant may be born with a club foot or hand or with amputated digits, and shortness of muscles may lead to torticollis (wry neck).

In some instances labor may be premature. As a rule, uterine contractions are ineffectual, and the labor may be prolonged. Fetal hypoxia may occur because the decreased surrounding fluid results in cord compression.

ABNORMALITIES OF THE PLACENTA AND CORD
Placental Abnormalities

It is believed that flat subchorial infarcts form the basis for two placental abnormalities: placenta marginata and placenta circumvallata [15]. If these infarcts occur at the edge of the placenta, they may form a more or less complete white infarcted ring (placenta marginata). In this case the fetal membranes may adhere to the decidua and the placenta may be delivered without them, with postpartum hemorrhage resulting from the retention of the membranes.

If the infarcted ring is raised from the surface, the attached membranes may double back over its edge, resulting in a dense ring of tissue (placenta circumvallata) (Fig. 18-8). The fetal vessels descend from the cord and end at the margin of the ring instead of coursing through the entire surface area of the placenta. Often this condition is asymptomatic, but it may be associated with premature bleeding during the second and third trimesters of pregnancy and premature delivery.

Placenta succenturiata occurs when one or more accessory lobes are attached to the main placenta. Usually it is not symptomatic until the third stage of labor,

Figure 18-8. Placenta circumvallata. (From L. M. Hellman and J. A. Pritchard. *Williams Obstetrics* [14th ed.], 1971. Courtesy of Appleton-Century-Crofts, Publishing Division of Prentice-Hall, Inc.)

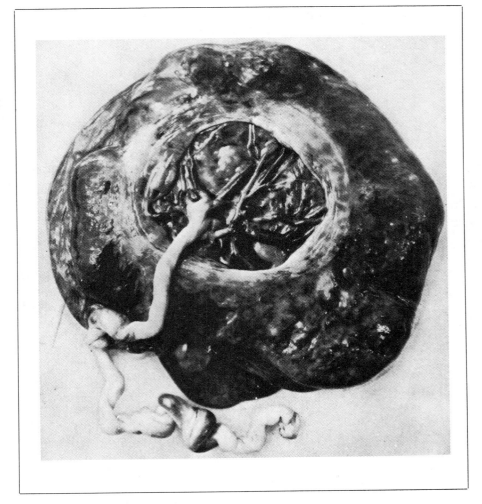

when the lobes may be inadvertently left in the uterus, predisposing the mother to hemorrhage.

If infarcts occur within the placenta itself, they may compromise fetal oxygenation or nutrition; if they involve a substantial portion of tissue, they may even cause fetal death. Calcium deposits on the basalis surface of the placenta are a sign of its normal aging process and are frequently found in term pregnancies, particularly if the gestation has been prolonged. Usually they are of no clinical importance, but extensive calcification is associated with a poor fetal prognosis.

Abnormalities of the Cord

Ordinarily the cord inserts at or near the center of the placenta, although an insertion at a different position is not uncommon. If the cord is inserted at the placental periphery (battledore placenta), there may be slight bleeding, which could be confused with placenta previa.

A velamentous insertion occurs when the cord inserts into the membranes in such a way that the umbilical vessels travel between the amnion and the chorion to the placenta (Fig. 18-9). This is often accompanied by other placental anomalies, such as infarcts, placenta succenturiata, or placenta previa. Its occurrence is nine times more frequent with twins than with single births, and it occurs very frequently with triplets. This type of cord insertion is particularly dangerous to the fetus when the vessels travel along the lower uterine segment and cross over the internal cervical os (vasa praevia). The vessels are usually torn when the membranes are ruptured, and fetal hemorrhage may result.

Since the umbilical vein is longer than the arteries and since the vessels are longer than the cord itself, the vessels become twisted and coiled in an effort to accommodate to the available space. Usually at these points the Wharton's jelly is a little thicker, and false knots or nodes tend to appear in the cord. True knots are very rare, and occur when the fetus passes through loops in the cord. True knots may tighten during fetal descent in the birth canal and compromise his oxygen supply.

About 20 percent of the time, the fetus is so active in utero that the cord becomes coiled around its neck (nuchal cord). This is a potentially serious complication, since it may make the cord functionally short and may interfere with the mechanism of descent. Cord compression during labor and delivery may cause fetal asphyxia. For these reasons the midwife or obstetrician will feel for the cord immediately after delivering the baby's head; if loops are present, they are uncoiled before attempting to deliver the baby's shoulders.

DIABETES   Pregnancy represents an additional physiologic stress to the woman with a chronic illness. Helping this woman and her family through a pregnancy that results in delivery of a healthy infant requires much teaching and support, a knowledge of appropriate community agencies, and a thorough knowledge of the interaction of pregnancy and chronic illness.

The number of women with diabetes who are choosing to have children is increasing each year. Prior to the advent of insulin, pregnancy for these women was rare. Many diabetics never lived to reproductive age, and the women who did were very frequently infertile. Diabetic women who did become pregnant faced a 25 percent chance of dying during childbearing and only a 50 percent chance of having a living child [30]. Today diabetic women are becoming pregnant and, with good health care, are delivering live, healthy infants. Achieving successful pregnancy outcomes, however, requires coordinated and comprehensive care by a health care team, most commonly in a regional high-risk perinatal center.

A diabetic woman who wishes to become pregnant should be counseled about getting ready for pregnancy. Her diabetes should be in good control, and she should be in good nutritional status and know how to avoid infections. If the diabetes does not remain in control, the woman may abort, usually because of ketoacidosis and placental insufficiency. Early in pregnancy the fertilized ovum may not survive or it may not implant at the blastocyst stage. Controlling her diabetes is not always easy, since pregnancy causes increased peripheral resistance to insulin, and a placental insulinase increases the rate of destruction of insulin. In addition, chorionic somatomammotropin mobilizes lipids while sparing carbohydrates for fetal use, thereby antagonizing the action of insulin [1]. The problems with insulin regulation may be compounded by nausea and vomiting in early pregnancy, and further compounded if the woman develops an infection of any kind.

Figure 18-9. Velamentous insertion of umbilical cord. (From K. L. Moore. *The Developing Human: Clinically Oriented Embryology* [3rd ed.]. Philadelphia: Saunders, 1982.)

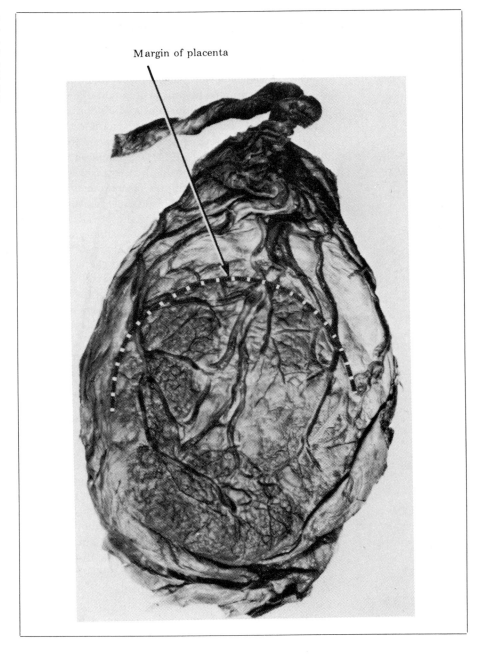

Margin of placenta

Assessment and Intervention

During the course of the pregnancy, the woman, as well as the family, needs much support in coping with the changes in her diabetic state, as well as with the usual changes of pregnancy. The woman who has successfully regulated her blood sugar for a number of years may now find it far harder to control. The effects of progesterone on gastrointestinal motility and the increased pressure of the growing uterus increase the absorption time of food. This effect and the effects on insulin noted above may leave the woman feeling as though she has lost control of the diabetes. Reassure her by explaining the changes in food absorption and insulin that occur during pregnancy and tell her that after delivery her diabetes will most probably respond as it did prior to her pregnancy.

Two recently developed methods to monitor and regulate blood sugar in diabetes are proving helpful to pregnant diabetics. One is the home blood glucose monitoring system, a simple procedure done in the home by the diabetic, using blood samples instead of urine to monitor the degree of control achieved. The procedure involves placing a drop of blood from a self-inflicted finger prick onto either a Chemstrip, which is then compared to a color chart for an estimation of the blood glucose level, or a Dextrostix, which is then inserted into a portable reflectance meter for a digital measurement of the blood glucose level. Advantages of self-monitoring of blood glucose over urine testing are that it improves regulation of glycemia, enables the physician to make treatment adjustments over the phone on the basis of solid information, eliminates the need to admit many diabetic women to the hospital for stabilization, and improves the motivation of diabetics for self-management of the diabetic regimen.

Home blood glucose monitoring may well replace urine testing as a method of determining blood sugar levels of diabetics. While the approach has not been in use long enough to determine if improvement of glycemia will retard such long-term complications as retinopathy, its present effects on the well-being of diabetics have been proven beneficial.

Another method of controlling blood sugar currently being tested is the use of various insulin pumps which deliver intermittent doses of insulin. One such pump weighs approximately 1 pound and is fitted with a 3-milliliter plastic syringe. The syringe (filled with regular insulin) is connected to a plastic tube that ends with a small, 27-gauge needle, inserted under the skin of the abdomen and held in place with tape. Daily changing of the injection site is recommended, but some patients use the same site for as long as 4 days. For the basal (between meal) dose, the pump is programmed to give a small amount of insulin every 8 to 16 minutes. To give a larger, pre-meal dose, the woman turns up the Dosage Selector Dial on the pump and presses the Instant Dose button. After the pump infuses the pre-meal dose, which takes 30 to 90 seconds, the woman resets the pump to the basal rate. The pump is removed during activities such as bathing and swimming, since it is not water-tight. An alternate model automatically returns to the basal rate after the woman turns a screw to infuse the pre-meal dose. Effectiveness of the pumps is currently being investigated [35].

The woman's insulin requirements will change during pregnancy. During this period women often receive a mixture of insulins, intermediate acting (Lente or NPH) and short acting in a ratio of 2 to 1 respectively; they may also require an evening dose in a ratio of 1 to 1 intermediate and short acting. Many women find that their insulin requirements remain the same or even decrease during the first half or two-thirds of pregnancy, only to increase tremendously during the last trimester. In the second half of pregnancy insulin requirements may be as high as 70 to 100 percent above prepregnancy needs [4]. This presumably occurs as the effects of chorionic somatomammotropin increase. Some women find that their insulin requirements gradually increase throughout the pregnancy; others whose diabetes had been controlled by diet alone may require insulin for the course of the pregnancy. Oral hypoglycemics are not as effective during pregnancy, are teratogenic in some species, and may cause hypoglycemia in the newborn [15]; they are not used during pregnancy.

Some women who show no signs or symptoms of diabetes in the nonpregnant state become symptomatic when pregnant, a condition known as gestational diabetes. Research indicates that if these women receive insulin during the last trimester of pregnancy their infants tend not to become macrosomic. In one study women received 20 units of NPH with 10 units of regular insulin daily each morning to maintain their blood sugars between 100 and 200 milligrams per 100 milliliters; they delivered normal sized infants [8]. When not treated, this condition may lead to fetuses who are large for their gestational age and who often die in utero [21]. The diabetic symptoms disappear following the pregnancy, but many of these women become overt diabetics later in life [1] (Table 18-5).

Women who have been diabetic for some time are aware of periods throughout the day when their blood sugar is low. During pregnancy they will find that this pattern has changed and that hypoglycemia may occur at very unexpected times. In addition, much larger amounts of fast-acting carbohydrates, such as fruit, sugar, or glucose, may be required, to raise their blood sugar. Carefully assess the pregnant woman's knowledge of the symptoms of insulin shock and diabetic ketoacidosis, and her awareness of what she should do at the onset of such symptoms. The immediate family members also should be aware of these signs and symptoms, and someone should be able to administer an injection of glucagon to the woman if needed.

The woman's diet during pregnancy is usually 30 to 35 K calories per kilogram of ideal body weight. The usual K calorie range is 1,800 to 2,400 with 125 grams of protein and a carbohydrate spread of 30, 30, 30, and 10 for breakfast, lunch, dinner, and an evening snack [4].

Insulin Shock

ASSESSMENT AND INTERVENTION

Not infrequently, pregnant diabetics will experience insulin shock, which may result from changes in intestinal absorption and insulin action. It may also occur when the woman regulates her insulin dose according to the amount of glucosuria. During pregnancy there is a tremendous increase in glomerular filtration without a concomitant increase in tubular reabsorption of solutes; as a result, some glucose may be lost in the urine. Lactose may also appear in the urine and will yield a positive reaction when glucose testing is done. The diabetic woman who wants to be well controlled during her pregnancy may adjust her insulin dose on her own, or she may not eat as much at her next meal when she tests her urine and finds a positive reaction to glucose. Her blood sugar may already be low, and she may soon be in shock. Many of these episodes can be avoided if the woman is aware of the changes that occur in pregnancy. She should be told that it may be safer for her to have small amounts of sugar in her urine and that she need not be concerned unless she has a large amount (+3 or +4) of sugar or any trace of acetone. If she feels shocky, 2 tablespoons of honey or corn syrup mixed in a glass of fruit juice should help. If she is not at home, cola is usually available and should be effective. The woman who has been having repeated episodes of shock may need to carry a dose of glucagon in her handbag, or keep one at home where a member of the family can administer it. She should also carry a card in her wallet

Table 18-5.
Classification of Diabetes in Pregnancy (Duration of Disease More Important than Age at Onset)

Class A Gestational Diabetic (90% of all patients with diabetes seen by the obstetrician)
1. Normal fasting blood sugar
2. Abnormal glucose tolerance test
3. Usually controlled by diet
4. Infant LGA

Class B
1. Onset after age 20
2. Present less than 10 years
3. No vascular complications
4. May have been controlled by diet; now insulin-dependent
5. Infant LGA

Class C
1. Onset between ages 10–19
2. Present 10–19 years
3. No vascular complications
4. Insulin-dependent before pregnancy; now insulin requirements increase
5. Infant LGA

Class D
1. Onset under age 10
2. Present 20 years or more
3. Peripheral vascular disease
4. Retinal changes
5. Hypertension
6. Insulin-dependent
7. Infant SGA

Class F
1. Includes nephropathy with proteinuria and decreased creatinine clearance
2. Infant SGA

Class R
1. Proliferative retinopathy which may intensify
2. Therapeutic abortion may be a consideration

Class G
1. When many failures have occurred in pregnancy; it is thus possible to have Class A–G

Class H (new)
1. Includes patients with cardiopathy (may be symptomatic)

Classes may change during pregnancy!

Source: Modified from P. White. Diabetes mellitus in pregnancy. *Clinics in Perinatology* 1(2): 331, 1974.

that identifies her as a diabetic and preferably wear a Medic Alert bracelet during pregnancy. If she has been having repeated episodes of shock, her husband, a family member, or a neighbor should phone or visit periodically during the day.

The woman and members of her family are always concerned about the fetal effects of an episode of insulin shock or acidosis. They can be told that the fetus seems not to be as affected by hypoglycemic episodes; however, episodes of ketoacidosis are tolerated poorly by the fetus [15].

Concerns of the Family   One of the most essential components of care for the family is listening to their concerns. In addition to worrying about the status of the baby, the woman may be very concerned about loss of control over her diabetes. Her husband may also be very concerned about this, wondering if this lability will continue after the baby is born and if they will be able to care for the infant in that case. He may also wonder if he can cope with the lability on a continuing basis. The family may also have financial concerns, especially if the woman is hospitalized during the course of pregnancy. If there are other children in the family, arrangements must be made for their care in their mother's absence. Costly tests to determine serial urinary estriol levels, nonstress tests, or ultrasound measurements may be made in the later months of pregnancy. The woman may be hospitalized a week prior to delivery to assess her status as well as that of the fetus and to prepare her for delivery.

Delivery   ASSESSMENT AND INTERVENTION

Delivery of the infant of a diabetic woman is also costly. In the past, all diabetic women were delivered by cesarean prior to their expected date of confinement, since many fetuses died in utero. Fetal death may result from premature placental aging and consequent insufficiency, which is common among diabetic women. Currently many physicians allow a woman to go to term and deliver vaginally, provided the fetal status is not compromised. Labor may begin spontaneously, or it may be induced. Nonstress tests may be done weekly after the thirtieth week, estriol levels and monthly ultrasound scans provide a measure of the functioning of the placenta and fetus, and fetal monitoring during labor allows assessment of fetal response during this period. If these testing methods are not available, or if there is a sudden change in insulin requirements late in the pregnancy, women with overt diabetes are usually delivered between 36 and 38 weeks of gestation, either by induction or by cesarean. If the woman's placenta decreases its functioning, its hormone production and insulin antagonism decrease suddenly. The woman who is receiving considerable insulin may now have hypoglycemic episodes. In this instance she is usually delivered shortly after these episodes. On the day of delivery, long-acting insulin is usually not given. The woman is generally kept hydrated with intravenous fluids of 5% dextrose in water, and regular insulin is used to control blood sugar and ketone levels. The physical exertion of labor decreases her insulin requirements.

During the first few days post partum, the mother's insulin requirements may fluctuate markedly, often dropping abruptly following delivery. This fluctuation stabilizes within a few days. If her diabetes is controlled, there is no contraindication to breast-feeding.

The diabetic woman is more likely than the nondiabetic woman to encounter complications during pregnancy and delivery. Pregnant diabetics have an increased incidence of hypertensive disorders, infection, hydramnios, and postpartum hemorrhage. Pregnancy in some diabetic women results in a progression of retinopathy, which may stop or regress after delivery [5].

Infants born to diabetic mothers may be larger, encounter respiratory difficulties after birth, have an increased tendency to inherit diabetes, and have an increased incidence of congenital anomalies. The incidence of anomalies is greater when the mother's diabetes is of long duration, when she is insulin dependent, and when she has vascular complications. The possible causes of anomalies in the infant include hypo- or hyperglycemia in the mother early in pregnancy, a teratogenic effect of insulin, uterine and placental insufficiency, and chromosomal aberrations. One study of women with malformed infants reported that 30 percent of the women developed overt diabetes 25 years later. Congenital anomalies of infants of diabetic mothers include skeletal, cardiac, and central nervous system defects [12].

It has been reported that children of diabetic mothers who had acetonuria (reflecting ketoacidosis) during pregnancy have lower IQs than the general population and than children of diabetic mothers who did not have this complication [7]. It also has been reported that infants of diabetic mothers tend to be more immature than expected for their gestational age, possibly due to an immature enzyme system [10]; they have delayed development of ossification centers, a high incidence of hyperbilirubinemia and respiratory distress syndrome, and a higher concentration of fetal hemoglobin than other infants of similar gestational age. The perinatal death rate ranges between 10 and 15 percent. The major cause of perinatal death is congenital malformation followed by respiratory distress syndrome.

All of these factors can severely tax the coping ability of the family. They clearly need constant support and comprehensive care during the pregnancy and in the postpartum period.

CARDIAC COMPLICATIONS
Assessment and Intervention

The woman with cardiac disease needs counseling prior to becoming pregnant. She should be aware of the reason for the restrictions that will be placed on her activities and her diet, and she should be aware of the statistical chances of delivering a live infant. However, she also needs to know that there is no evidence to date that normal childbearing causes any permanent deterioration of cardiac status or that giving birth shortens her life expectancy [6]. She and her partner may then thoughtfully consider pregnancy as well as other options in starting their family. If they do decide on pregnancy, they will then begin with a knowledge of what the woman's care will involve.

Pregnancy imposes a significant circulatory burden on the woman, due to increases in her cardiac output, oxygen consumption, and blood volume. The burden begins in the first trimester, increases throughout the second, and persists to term [30]. During labor, cardiac output increases 20 to 30 percent during each uterine contraction. The pulse rate, blood pressure, and left ventricular work also increase. In women receiving saddle block or caudal anesthesia, however, these changes were not seen according to one study, prompting Greenhill and Friedman [15] to comment that this finding suggests that response to pain, anxiety, and muscular activity play a more important role in raising cardiac output than any autotransfusion from the uterine sinuses into the systemic circulation. This reemphasizes the importance of supportive nursing measures to relieve the anxiety and pain of all women in labor.

Following delivery the woman usually has bradycardia as she becomes more relaxed and is relieved of pain and as the venous return is augmented. The first uterine contraction following birth of the infant puts a significant amount of blood into the general circulation and gives a brief rise in plasma volume. Blood loss over the next few hours reduces the plasma volume. However, this reduction is brief, since the fluid that has accumulated in interstitial spaces during pregnancy begins to enter the general circulation, raising the plasma volume to abnormally high levels [15]. This explains the normal diuresis in the first few days post partum. Observe the woman with cardiac disease very carefully during this period of increased cardiac burden. The elevated plasma volume continues for approximately 2 weeks.

Maternal mortality associated with heart disease ranges between 1 and 5 percent, the major cause of death being cardiac decompensation and heart failure. The majority of problems occur in the periods during pregnancy, labor, and puerperium when the cardiac burden is greatest. If the woman is cyanotic during pregnancy, she is likely to deliver an infant who is small for his gestational age or to go into labor prematurely; if the woman is very severely cyanotic, the fetus may die in utero. Whittlemore et al. reported fetal wastage to be 36 percent in women with hypoxic congenital heart disease [39]. The woman who is acyanotic and does not experience cardiac failure generally delivers a healthy infant.

Most heart disease found in pregnant women is the result of rheumatic fever. However, the incidence of congenital heart disease is increasing, as children with congenital heart defects have corrective surgery and reach their reproductive years; women with such defects run the risk of delivering infants who are also congenitally deformed.

The functional classification of the American Heart Association serves as an important guide in caring for the pregnant woman with cardiac disease (Table 18-6). Most women in classes I and II are able to handle the physiologic demands of pregnancy. The cardiac status of women in all of the classifications should be evaluated very early in pregnancy, if not before. This usually includes chest x-rays, an electrocardiogram, and tests for vital capacity. They should continue under close medical supervision throughout pregnancy and for some time following delivery.

Women with cardiac disease must get adequate rest—at least 10 hours of sleep at night as well as rest periods throughout the day—since physical exertion is an important cause of heart failure. Recommend only light housework if any and restrict climbing stairs. One study [30] suggests that even women with classes I and II heart disease have limited blood flow and oxygen supply to the fetus and should substantially restrict physical activity. Recommend that women avoid abdominal compression and the supine position and wear support hose to prevent venous pooling in the legs. All stresses, emotional as well as physical, must be avoided. Infection is one of the more serious stresses, and prophylactic antibiotics may be administered during pregnancy. Pregnant women with cardiac disease

Table 18-6.
Classification of Patients
with Cardiac Disease

Class	Definition
I	No limitation of physical activity; no symptoms of cardiac insufficiency or anginal pain
II	Slight limitation of physical activity; comfortable at rest; excessive fatigue, palpitations, dyspnea, or anginal pain with ordinary physical activity
III	Marked limitation of physical activity; comfortable at rest; excessive fatigue, palpitations, dyspnea, or anginal pain with less than ordinary physical activity
IV	Inability to perform any physical activity without discomfort; symptoms of cardiac insufficiency or anginal syndrome possible at rest; discomfort increased with physical activity

Source: Based on Functional Classifications of the New York Heart Association.

need treatment immediately if they experience infection of any kind. Upper respiratory infections, especially bronchitis and pneumonia, are leading causes of severe heart failure in pregnancy. Dental caries may also become foci of infection. The woman needs a well-balanced diet high in iron, protein, vitamins, and minerals to prevent anemia, which also would severely tax her heart.

Assess the woman for signs of impending cardiac decompensation particularly during the latter months of pregnancy. The first sign of cardiac failure is likely to be persistent rales at the lung bases, frequently with a cough. The rales are present after the woman has taken two to three deep breaths. Additionally, increasing dyspnea on exertion and attacks of smothering with cough and hemoptysis are other signs of impending cardiac failure. How is her color? Does she have rales, palpitations? Is she coughing? Does she have signs of edema in her face, ankles, or hands? Is her respiration labored, her pulse fast? How is she handling restrictions placed on her activities? All of these assessments should be made each time she visits.

Labor and Delivery   Hospitalization of women with classes I and II cardiac disease before delivery is common. Carefully follow these women during labor. The importance of relieving anxiety and pain has already been mentioned. Carefully monitor and record the woman's vital signs every 15 minutes, or more often as labor progresses, noting any signs of beginning cardiac failure. A pulse rate of 100 beats per minute or greater between contractions and in the absence of fever, and respirations greater than 24 with associated dyspnea suggest approaching cardiac failure. Also be alert for rales. Continuous fetal monitoring is most helpful.

When analgesics are needed, give them to the woman promptly. Combinations of a narcotic analgesic and a synergistic tranquilizer are generally used. Regional anesthesia may be used for pain relief during labor and delivery except in those mothers where hypotension may be life-threatening, such as the woman with a cardiac shunt.

Have the woman labor upright in bed or on her side in a semirecumbent position. She may need oxygen during the course of labor. Since bearing down increases the cardiac burden, the woman is delivered as soon as possible after she is fully dilated. Although she may deliver spontaneously, she is usually delivered with low forceps to avoid the stress of pushing and prolonging the second stage. The blood loss associated with cesarean delivery places additional burdens on the woman, making it a less desirable method of delivery that is used only when absolutely necessary.

During and following delivery take special care to prevent excessive blood loss, which would further tax her heart. Postpartum hemorrhage, puerperal infection, and thromboembolism are much more serious complications of pregnancy in the woman with cardiac disease. Use synthetic oxytocin rather than ergonovine to avoid increases in blood pressure. Intravenous therapy is limited; if blood is needed, packed erythrocytes are used to reduce the amount of fluid introduced. Make sure that the mother receives a great deal of rest in the postpartum period. You may need to restrict visitors and manipulate the environment so that rest is possible. The mother may need oxygen and she may need to remain in Fowler's position to ensure adequate oxygenation. Ambulate the woman early to prevent thromboembolic complications. Take precautions to avoid exposing the mother to infection of any kind, particularly upper respiratory infection. Because of the severe complications that result from infection, prophylactic antibiotics are continued during labor and following delivery.

Women with class III cardiac disease may be hospitalized, ideally, for the length of their pregnancy. Any woman with cardiac disease is hospitalized if she begins showing signs of impending or overt heart failure and usually remains hospitalized for the duration of the pregnancy. Heart failure in pregnancy is usually left-sided and is treated in the same way that it would be in the nonpregnant state. The woman receives digitalis, oxygen, sedatives, bed rest, diuretics, a low-sodium diet, and restricted fluids.

Discharge preparation for all women with cardiac disease should include discussion of the necessity for help at home for several weeks or more, limited activity and much rest, good nutritional status, prevention of infection, and contraceptive counseling.

Cardiac surgery may be performed early in the pregnancy and may make childbearing safer for some women. The risk of some types of cardiac surgery is not significantly greater during pregnancy than when the woman is not pregnant. However, even with surgery complications may still arise during pregnancy, and therapeutic abortion is the alternative chosen by some women.

ANEMIA
Assessment and
Intervention

Both in early pregnancy and near term, the hemoglobin level of healthy women is usually 11.0 grams per deciliter or higher. It is generally accepted that during pregnancy or the puerperium, women with hemoglobin levels less than 10.0 grams per deciliter are considered anemic. Also remember that hemoglobin levels decrease slightly during the second trimester as the volume of plasma expands more rapidly than the volume of erythrocytes. Later in pregnancy plasma expansion ceases while erythrocyte production continues and hemoglobin levels increase slightly from those found during the second trimester [30].

The majority of women who develop anemia during their pregnancy do so because of iron deficiency. Often these women had a diet poor in iron prior to becoming pregnant; they may have had excessive menstrual bleeding; and often they have had a number of pregnancies in rapid succession. These women begin their pregnancy already anemic or with low iron reserves, and as pregnancy advances, anemia results from the additional iron demands created by pregnancy and by the needs of the fetus. It will be recalled that the maternal need for iron caused by pregnancy with a single fetus is approximately 800 milligrams. About 300 milligrams are needed by the growing fetus and 500 milligrams are used to expand maternal hemoglobin mass. Anemia at this time is a potentially dangerous condition, since there is some evidence that the fetoplacental function is impaired in pregnancy anemias [2].

Laboratory evaluation of a woman with moderate anemia may include measurements of hemoglobin, hematocrit, smear of peripheral blood, serum iron concentration, and a sickle-cell preparation if the woman is black.

The frequency of anemia during pregnancy varies considerably, depending upon whether supplemental iron is taken or not. One report indicates that hemoglobin levels at delivery among women who took iron supplements averaged 12.4 grams per deciliter whereas levels in women not receiving iron averaged

11.3 grams per deciliter. No one in the group not receiving iron had levels below 10.0 grams [30].

Provide pregnant women with diet counseling as well as iron supplements if they are anemic. Ferrous sulfate (300 milligrams, three times a day) is usually prescribed. Encourage the woman to take the iron with meals to avoid gastric irritation, which is often a problem. Your counseling, emphasizing a well-balanced diet high in iron, should also stress the need for adequate fluids, roughage, and vitamin C foods if the woman is receiving oral iron preparation. Roughage will decrease constipation, which often occurs as a side effect of iron therapy, and vitamin C enhances iron absorption. Iron preparations should be taken throughout pregnancy and for about 6 months after delivery in order to restore normal hemoglobin and hematocrit levels and to replenish iron reserves. Women who are unable to tolerate oral iron preparations may be given intramuscular or parenteral preparations if the anemia must be corrected quickly. This approach may be necessary when a woman is severely anemic and close to term.

Infections and folic acid deficiencies are also causes of anemia during pregnancy. A variety of subacute and chronic infections may produce anemia by altering reticuloendothelial function and iron metabolism. Anemia is often found in women with acute pyelonephritis, chronic renal disease, malignant conditions, and rheumatoid arthritis.

Folic acid deficiency causes a megaloblastic anemia. Women with this type of anemia generally consume low amounts of animal protein and fresh vegetables, especially green leafy vegetables. They sometimes consume large amounts of alcohol and little nourishing food. These women often develop nausea, vomiting, and anorexia during pregnancy. In addition to diet counseling, folic acid supplements are usually required. As little as 1 milligram of folic acid daily produces a striking response.

Less commonly, women experience anemia caused by abnormal hemoglobins. Sickle-cell anemia, which occurs predominantly in blacks, is one example. Pregnancy is a significant stressor to the woman with this disorder. Any situation that triggers hypoxemia will cause the abnormal hemoglobin to assume a sickle shape; the change in the shape of the hemoglobin causes the red blood cells to block small vessels and cause ischemia to tissues resulting in a pain crisis. The erythrocytes then agglutinate and are destroyed.

Women with sickle-cell anemia hemoglobin C have lower maternal and perinatal mortality and morbidity rates than women with sickle-cell anemia hemoglobin S. Women with sickle-cell trait do not tend to have higher maternal or perinatal mortality rates than the general population, but these women tend to have higher rates of asymptomatic bacteriuria than black women without the trait. Women with sickle-cell anemia experience a more intense chronic anemia during pregnancy, frequent infections, and periodic crises marked by abdominal and joint pain. Occasionally a pain crisis is assumed when a woman with sickle-cell anemia is actually experiencing other serious obstetric problems such as ectopic pregnancy, placental abruption, or pyelonephritis.

Women with this disorder usually maintain hemoglobins of 7 grams per deciliter during pregnancy if they have no infection or nutritional deficit. Since erythropoiesis is very active in these women, to compensate for the short life span of their own red blood cells, folic acid supplements of 1 milligram per day are usually given. Good diets, vitamin supplements, rest, and efforts to avoid infection or other situations that would stimulate maternal hypoxemia are essential for these women during pregnancy.

During labor the care of women with sickle-cell anemia is directed toward measures to avoid their becoming upset and taxed physiologically. They are kept comfortable but not oversedated. Packed red blood cells and whole blood are on hand if surgery is necessary or if excessive blood is lost. The medical management for these women is much like that for women with cardiac disease.

Pregnancy loss in women with sickle-cell anemia is high. Loss from abortion or perinatal death approaches 30 to 50 percent [27,30] in women with hemoglobin S. In women with hemoglobin C, the figure is far lower, approximately 15 percent [30]. Because of the large perinatal loss and the great stress that pregnancy imposes on a woman with sickle-cell disease, sterilization or an adequate contraceptive is often advocated following the birth of one living infant. Oral contraceptives are avoided because of the effects of estrogen on blood-forming elements.

Within the last decade, some physicians have routinely used prophylactic transfusions in women with sickle-cell anemia. These women are transfused with packed erythrocytes containing no S hemoglobin. With adequate hemoglobin levels the woman's own bone marrow reduces the production of erythrocytes. By thus maintaining low levels of hemoglobin S, these women have fewer crises and associated problems and much lower maternal and perinatal mortality and morbidity. One study of 40 women so transfused reported no maternal mortality and only one abortion and one stillbirth in the group [30].

INFECTIONS   In general, pregnant women are no more susceptible to acute infectious disease than other women, but the consequences are serious if one is contracted. Frequently abortion results, the acute infection may become worse because of the stress of the pregnancy and labor, and maternal and fetal mortality increases (Table 18-7).

Syphilis   ASSESSMENT AND INTERVENTION
Serologic testing for syphilis is a part of routine early prenatal care, and the test is repeated in the third trimester to detect any infection contracted during pregnancy. If serologic evidence of syphilis is found, the woman is treated with antibiotics with the goal of treatment being the elimination of the spirochete from the fetus. Women with untreated syphilis often experience premature labor.

The 1979 recommendations of the Centers for Disease Control (CDC) for treatment of syphilis during pregnancy are as follows:

1. For women exposed to syphilis within the preceding 3 months or for those having syphilis of less than 1 year's duration, the treatment is benzathine penicillin G, 2.4 million units total, half in each buttock. Aqueous procaine penicillin G, 600,000 units per day for 8 days for a total of 4.8 million units, is also recommended. For women allergic to penicillin, oral erythromycin, 2 grams per day for 15 days, should be administered.
2. For women who have had syphilis for an undetermined length or for more than 1 year, the treatment is benzathine penicillin G, 2.4 million units intramuscu-

Table 18-7. Effects of
Maternal Infection on
Fetus and Neonate

Infection	Effect(s) on Fetus and Neonate	Associated Factors	Prognosis of Infant
Coxsackie virus	? Congenital malformations in first trimester Transplacental meningoenceph-alitis and/or myocarditis Acquired infections	Maternal infection mild	Depends on the extent of the disease
Cytomegalic inclusion body disease	Intrauterine death Premature delivery Severe generalized disease—jaundice, hemolytic anemia, thrombocytopenia, hepato-splenomegaly, central ner-vous system disease (includ-ing cerebral calcification and chorioretinitis), microcephaly, and undergrowth	Half the women in early childbearing years show no immunologic response to this virus; mothers are most often asymptomatic	Early death in majority of severely affected infants; severe mental and motor retardation in some survivors
Hepatitis B	Abortion Neonatal hepatitis	Newborn infection most common in symptomatic mother	
Herpes simplex	Mild infection with a few skin lesions; infant does not ap-pear ill Viremia, severe generalized dis-ease, CNS involvement ? Congenital malformations	Maternal herpetic vulvovag-initis usually present. Transplacental infection of fetus may occur	Mild disease—recovery Severe disease—usually fatal
Influenza	Increased incidence of abortion and premature labor Occasional association of con-genital malformations, espe-cially anencephaly and me-ningomyelocele	Active immunization by an attenuated vaccine should not be given during preg-nancy for fear of fetal damage	
Listeriosis	Infants infected either through direct invasion or from birth contamination Generalized disease, skin rash, meningitis, pneumonia, etc. Fetal involvement with scat-tered foci of necrosis (granu-lomatosis infantiseptica) Delayed infection of the new-born infant, usually listerial meningitis	4% of pregnant women har-bor *Listeria monocytogenes* in the cervix or vagina	Mortality and morbidity high, especially from CNS complications; persistent fetal circulation
Malaria	Direct transmission of *P. falci-parum* occurs rarely Diminished growth with placental involvement	Placental involvement 10 times more frequent than fetal involvement	
Mumps	Abortion, premature birth, or stillbirth uncommon ? Cause of endocardial fibro-elastosis		
Poliomyelitis	Abortion Rare congenital or acquired po-liomyelitis Growth retardation in chronic, severe, maternal, paralytic poliomyelitis	Widespread use of immuni-zation procedures has all but eliminated this dis-ease as a pregnancy prob-lem Use of Sabin live virus vac-cine during pregnancy is contraindicated May safely administer Salk vaccine	Fetal and neonatal loss: 33%

Table 18-7 (continued)

Infection	Effect(s) on Fetus and Neonate	Associated Factors	Prognosis of Infant
Rubella	Abortion Congenital malformations of heart, eye, ear, brain; dermatoglyphic abnormalities Systemic involvement with or without malformation, anemia, thrombocytopenia with purpura, jaundice, hepatosplenomegaly, bone changes, myocarditis, encephalitis, pneumonia, etc.	Maternal infection usually mild, occasionally arthritis and/or encephalitis Strict isolation for neonates with congenital rubella as long as virus is present in pharynx or urine for extended period of time	Residua and sequelae for the neonate depend on time during pregnancy when mother acquires the disease, virulence of the virus, and extent of the infectious process Incidence of malformation in the infant is 35% in the first month, 25% in second month, and 16% in third month of gestation. After 4th month, abnormalities are uncommon
Rubeola	Interruption of pregnancy Congenital or neonatal measles, with or without bronchopneumonia (typical dermal lesions are in same stage as those in mother)	Measles vaccine should be given to all nonimmune women prior to but not during gestation	Maternal rubeola at any time during pregnancy is responsible for increased perinatal death rate Great majority of infants are normal
Smallpox and vaccinia	Increased fetal wastage in all stages of pregnancy Congenital malformations not more frequent, but congenital infections with skin lesions reported	Primary vaccination and revaccination against smallpox must be deferred until after delivery because vaccinia often causes fatal widespread fetal visceral and cutaneous lesions	
Syphilis	Major cause of mid-trimester abortion, fetal death in utero, or premature labor and delivery Early congenital syphilis (septicemia, skin lesions, anemia, jaundice, periostitis) Late congenital syphilis	If maternal infection occurs less than 1–2 years prior to gestation, fetus may be affected	40–50% of infants affected in untreated mothers 40% of above show clinical signs at birth
Toxoplasmosis	High incidence of abortion Premature delivery Generalized disease—hepatosplenomegaly, jaundice, chorioretinitis, microphthalmia, convulsions Later manifestations—hydrocephalus or microcephaly, mental retardation, cerebral calcifications		Poor
Tuberculosis	Small infants born to mothers with active disease Congenital tuberculosis (rare) Acquired infection readily contracted	Severe maternal disease and malnutrition Essential to segregate mother with pulmonary tuberculosis from her infant to avoid neonatal infection	Great majority of infants unaffected
Ureaplasma urealyticum (T mycoplasma)	Chronic reproductive failure Low birth weight	Mycoplasma isolated from genital and lower urinary tracts of women and men	Abortion in early pregnancy
Varicella (chicken pox)	Premature delivery Congenital varicella	Low maternal immunity; most mothers have had the disease and developed immunity in childhood; therefore, congenital varicella is rare	Mortality high

Source: M. Klaus, and A. Fanaroff. *Care of the High-risk Neonate*. Philadelphia: Saunders, 1979.

larly weekly for 3 weeks. Aqueous procaine penicillin G, 600,000 units intramuscularly each day for 14 days, is also recommended. For women allergic to penicillin, oral erythromycin, 500 milligrams four times a day for 30 days, is the recommendation.

Following treatment the maternal serologic test may remain positive for 8 months, and the newborn may have a positive test for up to 3 months.

Gonorrhea   ASSESSMENT AND INTERVENTION
Cervical cultures have become a routine part of prenatal care and have been useful in detecting dormant gonorrheal infections. A chronic infection is generally found localized in the urethra, in Skene's and Bartholin's glands, and in the cervix. It usually remains dormant until delivery, when it spreads and may produce endometritis, salpingitis, oophoritis, and/or pelvic peritonitis.

When acute gonorrhea is found during pregnancy, acute inflammation is found in the urethra, vulvar glands, and vaginal and vulvar epithelium. The woman has a greenish-yellow vaginal secretion and her vulva may be red, ulcerated, and covered with a grayish exudate or condylomas. Her cervix is usually swollen and eroded and may secrete a foul secretion in which the gonococci are found. Bed rest is highly recommended and intercourse is halted.

The CDC recommends that the woman receive aqueous procaine penicillin G, 4.8 million units intramuscularly, half in each buttock, following 1 gram of probenecid (Benemid) ingested just before the injections. For women allergic to penicillin or probenecid, spectinomycin, erythromycin, or cefazolin are recommended as follows:

1. Erythromycin, 1.5 grams orally followed by 0.5 grams four times a day for a total of 9.5 grams. This regimen is safe for mother and fetus, but it is not highly effective.
2. Cefazolin, 2 grams intramuscularly with probenecid, 1 gram orally.
3. Spectinomycin, 2 grams intramuscularly.

For the latter two regimes fetal safety has not been established.

The CDC recommends that the term infant of a mother with gonorrhea receive aqueous penicillin G, 50,000 units. For the preterm small infant, 20,000 units is recommended. If the infant's eyes are contaminated with the gonococci during delivery, he develops the eye infection ophthalmia neonatorum.

Urinary Tract   ASSESSMENT AND INTERVENTION
Infections   Because of the physiologic changes in pregnancy, urinary tract infections are common in pregnant women. In the second trimester, the renal pelves, calices, and ureters become dilated. The ureters also exhibit a decrease in peristalsis, and later in pregnancy the heavy uterus places pressure on them at the pelvic brim. All of these factors result in greatly increased collecting space within the urinary tract and urinary stasis, creating optimal conditions for infection. Kass [20] reports that between 5 and 10 percent of all pregnant women have significant bacteriuria, with *Escherichia coli* being the most commonly found organism. Eradication of bacteriuria with antimicrobial agents has been shown to be

effective in preventing ascending urinary tract infections. Many of these women are asymptomatic but approximately one-fourth of them will develop symptomatic urinary tract infections during pregnancy, most commonly acute pyelonephritis. With acute pyelonephritis the woman may have had previous hematuria or bladder irritation. She will usually have chills, a temperature around 38.4°C (103°F), frequent urination, and pain in the abdomen or flank area. Increased fluids (to 3,000 milliliters daily) and short-acting sulfonamides, nitrofurantoin (Macrodantin), or ampicillin are generally prescribed. However, these drugs, such as sulfisoxazole (Gantrisin), may have undesirable fetal effects. In the newborn sulfa drugs compete with unconjugated bilirubin for albumin-binding sites and may increase the level of unbound free bilirubin. Nitrofurantoin can lead to hemolytic anemia in women whose erythrocytes are markedly deficient in G6PD [30].

Tuberculosis   ASSESSMENT AND INTERVENTION
Tuberculosis is difficult to diagnose during pregnancy since diagnostic methods may take months and since the lung becomes compressed as the uterus raises the diaphragm. This compression may conceal a lung cavity. If tuberculosis is found, the usual treatment of isoniazid, ethambutol, or rifampin and possibly streptomycin is begun. With the exception of streptomycin, these drugs do not seem to have an adverse effect on the fetus. Auditory and vestibular abnormalities have been identified after streptomycin therapy, and attempts are made to avoid this drug. The woman is usually hospitalized and encouraged to rest, and her diet is improved so that she gets increased protein, vitamins, and calories. Labor and delivery are carried out normally; however, the infant is isolated from his mother after birth to avoid his becoming infected. It is uncertain whether or not pregnancy aggravates the disease.

PSEUDOCYESIS   Pseudocyesis, or false pregnancy, is usually seen in young women with an intense desire to be pregnant or in women who are nearing menopause. They have many of the symptoms of pregnancy: irregular or absent menses, morning sickness, and increase in abdominal size, the latter occurring as the result of a rapid accumulation of abdominal fat, gas in the intestinal tract, or abdominal fluid. Sometimes their breasts will enlarge and show pigment changes. All of these symptoms may be due to endocrine disorders of the ovary, anterior pituitary, or hypothalamus or to the use of phenothiazines. Contractions of the intestines or abdominal muscles may be misinterpreted as fetal movements. However, when a woman with pseudocyesis is examined, her uterus is found to be small. The most difficult part of her care is convincing her that she is not pregnant, a delusion that may be so strong that it persists for years [30].

DRUG ADDICTION   There has been an apparent increase in the number of infants born to addicted mothers in recent years in the United States. The incidence has risen from 1 out of 200 deliveries to 1 out of 50 in some large urban hospitals [11]. Heroin still appears to be the most common addicting agent, but polydrug use involving amphetamines, tranquilizers, barbiturates, cocaine, methadone, and hallucinogens is now a serious problem, which may actually be adding to the number of pregnancies in addicts. Heroin in high concentrations may suppress ovulation through its action on the pituitary, but some authorities think that amphetamines and marijuana may counteract this heroin effect. In addition, unreliable "cuts" of heroin in bags may not be sufficiently potent to suppress ovulation.

A large number of pregnant addicts are in their teenage years and thus fall into a high-risk group. In addition, because of their life-style as addicts, they often have venereal disease, hepatitis, skin infections, malnutrition, or thrombophlebitis. When a multidisciplinary approach is used to provide care for pregnant addicts, the number of prenatal visits rises above the average for all addicts, which is approximately one per pregnancy [11]. The pregnant addict also faces obstetric problems common to the addict—preeclampsia, abruptio placentae, premature rupture of membranes, postpartum hemorrhage, and an increased incidence of breech birth.

Assessment   The problems faced by the pregnant addict are multiple. She usually lacks self-confidence and self-esteem and appears very anxious and depressed. She may have difficulty with interpersonal relationships, and members of the health team caring for her need to demonstrate patience and understanding when trying to help her. Unless she can establish a trusting relationship with someone on the team at the beginning of her prenatal care, she will not accept and return for care.

In addition to their reluctance to accept prenatal care, addicts commonly arrive at the hospital late in active labor, usually having taken a recent "fix." Sometimes a woman's behavior and physical signs will lead you to suspect that she is an addict; these include her arrival late in labor with a history of little or no prenatal care, the presence of needle marks on the forearm or attempts to hide them with tattoos or scars, burned fingers or holes in her clothing as a result of smoking when she was "high," cellulitis, thrombophlebitis, skin abscesses, signs of jaundice, pinpoint pupils, or an excessive desire for medication. If labor lasts a long time, these women require higher doses of analgesics than usual.

In the postpartum period, if the mother does not receive drugs, she may soon become nervous and unable to sleep. Her eyes may burn, her nose may run, and she may have "gooseflesh" and perspire. She may complain of severe aching in her back, legs, and abdomen, and her muscles may begin to twitch. Her blood pressure, temperature, and respiratory rate increase. If she does not receive drugs, she may sign herself out of the hospital.

Intervention   Many addicted mothers are concerned about their newborns; their anxiety can be lessened while they remain in the hospital by keeping them continually informed about the baby's progress. They also usually need much support in learning adequate mothering practices. Encourage the addicted mother to care for her baby or to assist in his care as much as possible. It is also important to encourage the father of the baby and other family members and friends to visit if they can lend support to the mother.

Explore the addicted mother's feelings concerning her infant and her plans for his care. Here, the multidisciplinary team is invaluable in helping the mother to make realistic plans for discharge and postnatal care of both herself and her infant. The option of temporarily placing the infant in foster care or in an institution until she can assume responsibility for him should be presented to her.

NURSING IN HIGH-RISK PREGNANCY   The focus of nursing care to couples experiencing a high-risk pregnancy is many-faceted. It includes helping the couple promote and maintain the physical health of the woman during pregnancy and delivery; doing everything possible to ensure the delivery of a healthy child; keeping the experience of childbearing as close to normal and as close to the couples idealized pregnancy experience as possible; and making the experience one of personal growth for the couple that strengthens or at least maintains the family unit. Nursing plays the pivotal role in making high-risk childbearing a successful experience for the couple. It is also a time that will challenge you to use all of your nursing skills.

Assessment   You may begin your assessment by determining why the woman or couple is at risk during this pregnancy. What are the implications for the physical care of the woman and for the outcome of the woman and infant? Is this the first time the couple has encountered this risk factor or have they been through another pregnancy with the same problem? Have they known anyone else who has had a similar problem? If so, what effect has it had on their interpretation of their own situation? What is their idealized pregnancy experience? How do they see their current situation differing from the ideal?

You will want to assess the physical changes of pregnancy that the woman is experiencing. Are they within normal ranges? How has the risk factor affected the woman's physical status? What is the woman's and the couple's understanding of these changes?

How have the physical changes of pregnancy and the risk factors affected the couple's life-style? Have they had an effect on normal family functioning, on the couple's sexual needs, their social activities, their employment, their financial situation? What do the couple identify as major problems in their situation [37]?

Interventions   Your interventions will be based upon the findings of your assessment, your own style and knowledge as a practitioner, and your own assertiveness. Having determined the risk factor and the couple's knowledge of and experience with that factor, you can provide the couple with additional information, correct misinformation, and reinforce the normal aspects of the pregnancy. Focus on what can be maintained of their idealized pregnancy experience and help them to feel that they still have control of much of that experience. Are they planning to attend childbirth education classes? Are there pregnancy support groups for the high-risk couple? If the woman is unable to attend, can the father attend several classes and share the information with her? Are they planning a tour of the birthing area? Can you arrange one?

Following your assessment of the physical changes the mother has undergone, explain the changes to the couple and teach them ways of relieving common discomforts during this period. If the woman must rest often, position changes, the use of pillows, and sacral rubs that the father can perform are helpful. Explore ways of ensuring that the father has sufficient rest and support. You may need to review diets with both of them to reinforce the information within the family group. Have them listen to the fetal heart tones. You will also want to teach them the physical changes they can expect the woman to encounter in the months ahead and how they can prepare for them and cope with them.

You may want to have a frank discussion with them on how high-risk pregnancies can put stress on family functioning and ways to cope with those stresses. You may have to help them mobilize a support system of friends and family or community resources; you will want to provide counseling on sexual needs; and you may need to reassure or reinforce to them that no one is to blame for the high-risk pregnancy since guilt is often a common feeling. You may need to help them look realistically at the probable outcome of the pregnancy, since fear of death of the mother or infant is also a common feeling. You may also need to help them identify ways to provide time alone for themselves and for each other, or time with friends if this is something they enjoy. Emphasize the positive things they have done and accomplished thus far: how they have supported one another, how well they have been able to carry out the plan of care, how well the fetus appears to be, how well they have been able to maintain their family functioning. The focus of your interventions here is on strengthening their sense of control over their situation, strengthening their self-esteem, and strengthening the family as a unit. Reassurance and praise, as well as support, will often go far in providing them with additional strength.

Case Study   Cheryl Todd

As Cheryl's primary nurse, develop a plan of care for the Todds including your interventions focused on helping them through this high-risk pregnancy, labor and delivery, and postpartal period. Each of you will develop your own approach and style in providing care to high-risk couples. Applying the nursing process to the outline following the case study will serve as a guide in organizing your approach to the couple during the pregnancy.

Cheryl is a 25-year-old woman who has been married for 3 years. One-and-one-half years ago she spontaneously aborted a 2½-month fetus. She is now pregnant again near the end of her first trimester.

Cheryl is a class C diabetic who was diagnosed at age 18. She is a nurse and is currently teaching in an associate degree nursing program. The semester will be over in 3 weeks. Her husband Philip, 28, is a vice-president in a local consulting firm. His position within the company requires him to travel a great deal. Most of his trips are overnight, but once a month he is required to spend a week away from home. Cheryl's sister is also a nurse who teaches in the same nursing program. She is married with two school-age children and lives 15 minutes away from Cheryl. Another teenage sister lives at home with Cheryl's parents who live 100 miles away. Both parents are in good health. Philip's parents live in Europe. Philip's father is a diabetic.

Cheryl is an independent young woman who has not maintained control of her diabetes. Her lunches commonly consist of a Coke and a candy bar. Following the spontaneous abortion of her first pregnancy, she tried hard to control her blood sugar in anticipation of becoming pregnant again.

During this pregnancy Cheryl has thus far had three periods of hypoglycemia in which she became unconscious. The first occurred during the early morning when she began screaming incoherently. Philip telephoned Cheryl's sister and they drove Cheryl to the hospital where she received glucose intravenously. As she became conscious she began crying and worrying whether the baby would die.

The second episode occurred as she was shopping in a local shopping center. She began screaming incoherently at the checkout counter in a 5-and-10-cent store.

The police were called and took her to a local hospital where she again received glucose intravenously.

The third episode occurred in her office at the college where she teaches. Her sister administered glucagon. When Cheryl became conscious, she was frightened and embarrassed.

Cheryl is currently being cared for both by an obstetrician and by a medical doctor who is treating her diabetes. She is taking 20 units of NPH and 10 units of regular insulin in the morning and an evening dose of half of the same. Her insulin dose has been changed several times in attempts to avoid the hypoglycemic episodes. The fetus appears to be growing appropriately. As the primary nurse working with this family develop your plan of care.

Assessment Form			
Assessment	Plan	Intervention	Evaluation

I. Health History
  A. Age
  B. Family history
    1. Significant health problems
    2. Chronic diseases
  C. Woman's past medical and gynecologic history
    1. Past medical problems
      (a) Infections
      (b) Chronic diseases
    2. Past gynecologic history
      (a) Menstrual history (menarche, length, character, regularity of periods)
      (b) Pap test results
  D. Woman's past obstetric history
    1. Abortions
    2. Deliveries (date, gestation, problems, length of labor, type of delivery, presentation, condition of infant)
    3. Postpartum experience (perception, complications)
  E. Woman's present obstetric history
    1. Gravida, para
    2. EDC
    3. Signs and symptoms present
    4. Unusual signs
    5. Exposure to infections
    6. Current medications, past and current immunizations
  F. Diet history
    1. Weight gain			

Assessment Form			
Assessment	Plan	Intervention	Evaluation

  2. Nutritional pattern
  3. Eating habits
  4. Alcohol consumption
  5. Caffeine consumption
  6. Smoking habits
G. Activities
  1. Rest and sleep (amount, pattern)
  2. Exercise (type, appropriateness)
  3. Sexual (needs met, adjustments needed)
  4. Employment (outside home, possible hazards, plans to continue)
  5. Travel plans
H. Psychosocial
  1. Emotional changes
  2. Reactions to pregnancy (woman's, father's, family's, adjustment required in life-style, planned, motivation for pregnancy, preparations for infant)
  3. Family support system (marital status, who lives with her, significant others, type of support available—financial, emotional —from whom, predominant family style)
  4. Ethnic practices (specific to childbearing, complications common to ethnic group)
  5. Learning style (How does she learn best [method]? Can she read, understand, remember? Does she ask questions? Does she apply knowledge?)

Assessment Form			
Assessment	Plan	Intervention	Evaluation
II. Laboratory Results			
A. Pregnancy test			
B. Hb, Hct			
C. Urine (protein, glucose, acetone)			
D. STS, gonococcal culture			
E. Fetal assessment			
III. Physical Examination			
A. General survey			
B. Vital signs, height, weight			
C. Head			
D. Face (expression, color and condition of facial skin, symmetry of facial structures)			
E. Eye (visual acuity, lids, conjunctivae, sclerae, pupils, optic disc)			
F. Ear (external—size and location; auditory canal, tympanic membrane)			
G. Nose (deviation, discharge, congestion)			
H. Mouth (teeth, gums, mucosal surfaces, tongue)			
I. Throat (tonsils, oropharynx)			
J. Neck (muscles, cervical vertebrae, trachea, thyroid, carotid arteries, jugular veins, cervical lymph nodes)			
K. Skin (color, vascularity, edema, injuries, lesions)			
L. Hair (distribution, quantity, quality)			
M. Nails (shape, texture, curvature, adherence to nail beds)			
N. Respiratory system (shape and symmetry of thorax, respiratory rate, abnormal breath sounds)			
O. Heart and blood volume changes (heart sounds, rate,			

| *Assessment Form* | | | |
Assessment	Plan	Intervention	Evaluation

peripheral pulses, varicosities—legs, vulva, anus)

P. Breasts (symmetry, bulges, retraction, fixation, masses, nipples, color, size, tenderness, discharge)

Q. Abdomen and digestive tract (diastasis, striae, pigmentation, scars, masses, uterine height, lie, presentation and position of fetus, fetal heart rate, nausea, vomiting, heartburn, constipation)

R. Musculoskeletal (posture, deformities, swelling, involuntary movements, pain)

S. External genitalia and pelvis (color, distribution of hairs, signs of infection, position and condition of uterus, ovaries, cervix, vagina, measurements of pelvic inlet, midpelvis, outlet)

T. Anus and rectosigmoid area (adequacy of sphincter, polyps)

U. Urinary system (pain on urination, frequency)

V. Medical treatment plan

IV. Specific Learning Needs to Cope with Physical Changes

V. Needs Identified by Woman, Husband or Baby's Father, Significant Others

VI. Plans and Expectations of Childbirth Experience

   A. Idealized experience

   B. Childbirth education classes

   C. Labor support

   D. Anesthesia

   E. Method of infant feeding

REFERENCES

1. Bates, G. W. Management of gestational diabetes. *Postgraduate Medicine* 55:55, 1974.
2. Beischer, N. The effects of maternal anemia upon the fetus. *Journal of Reproductive Medicine* 6:21, 1971.
3. Boue, A., and Boue, J. Chromosomal Anomalies Associated with Fetal Malformation. In J. Scremgeour (Ed.), *Towards the Prevention of Fetal Malformation*. Edinburgh: Edinburgh University Press, 1978.
4. Cacheris, H. Nutrition for the pregnant diabetic patient. *Arizona Medicine* 36:188, 1979.
5. Cassar, J., Kohner, E., Hamilton, A., Gordon, H., and Joplin, G. Diabetic retinopathy and pregnancy. *Diabetologia* 15:105, 1978.
6. Chesley, L. Severe rheumatic cardiac disease and pregnancy. The ultimate prognosis. *American Journal of Obstetrics and Gynecology* 136:552, 1980.
7. Churchill, J. A., Berendes, H. W., and Nemore, J. Neuropsychological deficits in children of diabetic mothers. *American Journal of Obstetrics and Gynecology* 105:257, 1969.
8. Coustan, D. Managing gestational diabetes. *Contemporary Obstetrics and Gynecology* 8:119, 1976.
9. Daughter's cancers linked to mother's use of estrogen. *Journal of the American Medical Association* 220:653, 1972.
10. Davidson, O. Hemoglobin F in newborn infants of diabetic mothers. *Acta Endocrinologica* 18(Suppl.):73, 1974.
11. Driscoll, J. Metabolic and Endocrine Disturbances. In R. Behrman (Ed.), *Neonatology*. St. Louis: Mosby, 1973.
12. Gabbe, S., Lowenson, R., Wu, P., and Guerra, G. Current patterns of neonatal morbidity and mortality in infants of diabetic mothers. *Diabetic Care* 1:335, 1978.
13. Gallup, D., and Lucas, W. Heparin treatment of consumption coagulopathy associated with intrauterine fetal death. *Obstetrics and Gynecology* 35:690, 1970.
13a. Gant, N., and Worley, R. *Hypertension in Pregnancy: Concepts and Management*. New York: Appleton-Century-Crofts, 1980.
14. Golditch, I., and Boyce, N. E. Management of abruptio placentae. *Journal of the American Medical Association* 212:288, 1970.
15. Greenhill, J. P., and Friedman, E. A. *Biological Principles and Modern Practice of Obstetrics*. Philadelphia: Saunders, 1974.
16. Huber, C. P., Melin, J. R., and Vellios, F. Changes in chorionic tissue of aborted pregnancy. *American Journal of Obstetrics and Gynecology* 73:569, 1957.
17. Hyde, E., Joyce, D., Gurewich, V., Flute, P., and Barrera, S. Intravascular coagulation during pregnancy and the puerperium. *Journal of Obstetrics and Gynecology of the British Commonwealth* 80:1059, 1973.
18. Kajii, T., and Ohama, K. Androgenic origin of hydatidiform mole. *Nature* 268:633, 1977.
19. Karbhari, D. The supine hypertensive test as a predictor of incipient pre-eclampsia. *American Journal of Obstetrics and Gynecology* 127:620, 1977.
20. Kass, E. H. Symposium on the newer aspects of antibiotics: Chemotherapeutic and antibiotic drugs in the management of infections of the urinary tract. *American Journal of Medicine* 18:764, 1955.
20a. Kasser, N. Roll over test. *Obstetrics and Gynecology* 54:411, 1980.
21. Khojandi, M., Tsai, A., and Tyson, J. Gestational diabetes: The dilemma of delivery. *Obstetrics and Gynecology* 43:1, 1974.
22. Kilker, R., and Wilkerson, B. Nursing care in placenta previa and abruptio placentae. *Nursing Clinics of North America* 8:479, 1973.
22a. Leonard, L. Twin pregnancy: Maternal-fetal nutrition. *Journal of Obstetric, Gynecologic and Neonatal Nursing* 11:139, 1982.
23. Lewis, J. Treatment of metastatic gestational trophoblastic neoplasms. *American Journal of Obstetrics and Gynecology* 136:163, 1980.
24. Marshall, G., and Newman, R. Roll over test. *American Journal of Obstetrics and Gynecology* 127:623, 1977.
25. Martin, P. High frequency of hydatidiform mole in native Alaskans. *International Journal of Gynaecology and Obstetrics* 15:395, 1978.
26. Molar pregnancy. *OB World* 3:1, 1974.
27. Morrison, J., Propst, M., and Blake, P. Sickle hemoglobin and the gravid patient: A management controversy. *Clinics in Perinatology* 7:273, 1980.
28. Oakes, G., Chez, R., and Morelli, I. Diet in pregnancy: Meddling with the normal or preventing toxemia. *American Journal of Nursing* 75:1135, 1975.

29. Panayotou, P., Kaskarelis, D., Miettinen, O., Trichopoulos, D., and Kalandidi, A. Induced abortion and ectopic pregnancy. *American Journal of Obstetrics and Gynecology* 114:507, 1972.

30. Pritchard, J., and MacDonald, P. *Williams Obstetrics* (16th ed.). New York: Appleton-Century-Crofts, 1980.

31. Quilligan, E., and Kretchmer, N. *Fetal and Maternal Medicine.* New York: Wiley, 1980.

32. Reid, D., Ryan, K., and Benirschke, K. *Principles and Management of Human Reproduction.* Philadelphia: Saunders, 1972.

33. Smith, C., Gregori, C., and Breen, J. Ultrasonography in threatened abortion. *Obstetrics and Gynecology* 51:173, 1978.

34. Spontaneous abortion's cause studied with fetal tissues. *Journal of the American Medical Association* 197:41, 1966.

35. Tamborlane, W., and Sherwin, R. Man made. *Diabetes Forecast* January/February: 18, 1981.

36. Tapia, H., Johnson, C., and Strong, C. Renin-angiotensin system in normal and in hypertensive disease of pregnancy. *Lancet* 2:847, 1972.

36a.Van Dongen, B. Postural blood pressure differences in pregnancy. *American Journal of Obstetrics and Gynecology* 138:1, 1980.

37. Weil, S. The unspoken needs of families during high risk pregnancies. *American Journal of Nursing* 81:2047, 1981.

38. Weir, R., Fraser, R., Lever, A., Morton, J., Brown, J., Kraszewski, A., McIlwaine, G., Robertson, J., and Tree, M. Plasma renin, renin substrate, angiotensin II, and aldosterone in hypertensive disease of pregnancy. *Lancet* 1:291, 1973.

39. Whittlemore, K., Wright, M., Leonard, M., and Johnson, M. Results of pregnancy in women with congenital heart defects. *Pediatric Research* 14:452, 1980.

40. Williams, S. R. *Essentials of Nutrition and Diet Therapy.* St. Louis: Mosby, 1974.

41. Willis, S. Hypertension in pregnancy: Pathophysiology. *American Journal of Nursing* 82:792, 1982.

FURTHER READING   Alberman, E., et al. Frequency of chromosomal abnormalities in miscarriages and perinatal deaths. *Journal of Medical Genetics* 14:313, 1977.

Allen, E., and Mantz, M. Are normal patients at risk during pregnancy? *Journal of Obstetric, Gynecologic and Neonatal Nursing* 10:348, 1981.

Anderson, C. Enhancing reciprocity between mother and neonate. *Nursing Research* 30:89, 1981.

Avant, K. Anxiety as a potential factor affecting maternal attachment. *Journal of Obstetric, Gynecologic and Neonatal Nursing* 10:416, 1981.

Bampton, B., Jones, J., and Mancini, J. Initial mothering patterns of low-income black primiparas. *Journal of Obstetric, Gynecologic and Neonatal Nursing* 10:174, 1981.

Bank, A., Mears, J. G., and Ramirez, F. Disorders of human hemoglobin. *Science* 207:486, 1980.

Beske, E., and Garvis, M. Research-important factors in breastfeeding success. *American Journal of Maternal-Child Nursing* 7:174, 1982.

Bettoli, E. Herpes: Facts and fallacies. *American Journal of Nursing* 82:924, 1982.

Blake, J. Drugs in pregnancy. *Patient Care* 14:40, 1980.

Boudreaux, M. Maternal attachment of high risk mothers with well newborns: A pilot study. *Journal of Obstetric, Gynecologic and Neonatal Nursing* 10:366, 1981.

Brazy, J. E., Crenshaw, M. C., and Brumley, G. W. Amniotic fluid cortisol in normal and diabetic pregnant women and its relation to respiratory disease in the neonate. *American Journal of Obstetrics and Gynecology* 132:567, 1978.

Brown, Z. A. Diabetes in pregnancy. *FCH Perinatal Health Promotion,* p. 43, 1978.

Bull, M. Change in concerns of first-time mothers after one week at home. *Journal of Obstetric, Gynecologic and Neonatal Nursing* 10:391, 1981.

Butnarescu, G. F., Tillotson, D. M., and Villarreal, P. P. *Perinatal Nursing,* Vol. 2. New York: Wiley, 1980.

Cadwell, K. Improving nipple graspability for success at breastfeeding. *Journal of Obstetric, Gynecologic and Neonatal Nursing* 10:277, 1981.

Carr, K., and Walton, V. Early postpartum discharge. *Journal of Obstetric, Gynecologic and Neonatal Nursing* 11:29, 1982.

Carter, C. Recent advances in genetic counseling. *Nursing Times* 75:1795, 1979.

Cetrulo, C. L., Freeman, R. K., and Kruppel, R. A. Minimizing the risks of twin delivery. *Contemporary OB/GYN* 9:47, 1977.

Connaughton, J. F., Reeser, D., Schut, J., and Finnegan, L. P. Perinatal addiction: Outcome and management. *American Journal of Obstetrics and Gynecology* 129:679, 1977.

Cooper, D. W. Genetic control of severe pre-eclampsia. *Journal of Medical Genetics* 16:409, 1979.

Cranston, J. A Down's baby-nursing care study. *Nursing Times* 75:1792, 1979.

Crosby, W. Automotive trauma and the pregnant patient. *Contemporary Obstetrics and Gynecology* 8:115, 1976.

Dewees, C. Hematologic disorders in pregnancy. *Nursing Clinics of North America* 17:57, 1982.

Diggs, L. W. Sickle cell centers of tomorrow. *Southern Medical Journal* 8:73, 1980.

Dore, S., and Davies, B. Cartharsis for high risk antenatal inpatients. *American Journal of Maternal-Child Nursing* 4:96, 1979.

Duran-Garcia, S., Nieto, J. G., and Cabello, A. M. Effect of gestational diabetes on insulin receptors in human placenta. *Diabetologia* 16:87, 1979.

Eppink, H. Facts and concepts for genetic counseling. *Journal of Obstetric, Gynecologic and Neonatal Nursing* 6:14, 1977.

Foley, K. Caring for the parents of newborn twins. *American Journal of Obstetric, Gynecologic and Neonatal Nursing* 4:221, 1979.

Fuchs, F. Genetic amniocentesis. *Scientific American* 242:47, 1980.

Gabbe, S. G. Application of scientific rationale to the management of the pregnant diabetic. *Seminars in Perinatology* 2:361, 1978.

Gay, J. A conceptual framework of bonding. *Journal of Obstetric, Gynecologic and Neonatal Nursing* 10:440, 1981.

Giefer, M., and Nelson, C. A new method to help new fathers develop parenting skills. *Journal of Obstetric, Gynecologic and Neonatal Nursing* 10:455, 1981.

Golbus, M. Prenatal diagnosis of chromosomal abnormalities and neural tube defects. *Clinics in Perinatology* 9:245, 1979.

Golden, N. L., Sokol, R. J., and Rubin, I. L. Angel dust: Possible effects on the fetus. *Pediatrics* 65:18, 1980.

Gordon, R. S. Transfusions improve outcomes of pregnancies complicated by sickle cell disease. *Journal of the American Medical Association* 231:244, 1980.

Gottlieb, L. Maternal attachment in primiparas. *Journal of Obstetric, Gynecologic and Neonatal Nursing* 7:39, 1978.

Green, M. Outcomes of pregnancy for addicts receiving comprehensive care. *American Journal of Drug Alcohol Abuse* 6(4):413, 1979.

Gromada, K. Maternal-infants attachment: The first step toward individualizing twins. *American Journal of Maternal-Child Nursing* 6:129, 1981.

Hogan, K., and Tcheng, D. The role of the nurse during amniocentesis. *Journal of Obstetric, Gynecologic and Neonatal Nursing* 7:24, 1978.

Horan, M. Genetic counseling, helping the family. *Journal of Obstetric, Gynecologic and Neonatal Nursing* 6:25, 1977.

Horn, B. Cultural concepts and postpartal care. *Nursing and Health Care* 2:516, 1981.

Jarrett, G. Research—Childbearing patterns of young mothers: Expectations, knowledge and practices. *American Journal of Maternal-Child Nursing* 7:119, 1982.

Jones, C. Father to infant attachment: Effects of early contact and characteristics of the infant. *Research in Nursing and Health* 4:193, 1981.

Jones, I. Genetics and inherited disease. *Nursing Times* 74:392, 1978.

Jones, M. Years of life lost through Down's syndrome. *Journal of Medical Genetics* 16:379, 1979.

Jouganatos, D. M., and Gabbe, S. G. Diabetes in pregnancy: Metabolic changes and current management. *Journal of the American Dietetic Association* 73:168, 1978.

Kantor, G. Addicted mother, addicted baby—a challenge to health care providers. *American Journal of Maternal-Child Nursing* 3:281, 1978.

Kelley, M. Maternal position and blood pressure during pregnancy and delivery. *American Journal of Nursing* 82:809, 1982.

Kelley, M., and Mongiello, R. Hypertension in pregnancy: Labor, delivery and postpartum. *American Journal of Nursing* 82:813, 1982.

Kunst-Wilson, W., and Cronenwett, L. Nursing care for the emerging family: Promoting paternal behavior. *Research in Nursing and Health* 4:201, 1981.

Lee, G. Relationship of self-concept during late pregnancy to neonatal perception and parenting profile. *Journal of Obstetric, Gynecologic and Neonatal Nursing* 11:186, 1982.

Leonard, L. Breastfeeding twins: Maternal-infant nutrition. *Journal of Obstetric, Gynecologic and Neonatal Nursing* 11:148, 1982.

Levine, A., and Imai, P. Intrauterine treatment of fetal hydronephrosis. *Association of Operating Room Nurses Journal* 35:655, 1982.

Lieber, M. T. "Nonstress" antepartal monitoring. *Maternal-Child Nursing Journal* 5:335, 1980.

Lotas, M., and Willging, J. Mothers, babies, perception. *Image* 11:45, 1979.

Malter, S. Genetic counseling: A responsibility of health care professionals. *Nursing Forum* 16(1):27, 1977.

Matthews, D. Your fate in your genes. *Nursing Mirror* 12:30, 1978.

McKenzie, C., Canaday, M., and Carroll, E. Comprehensive care during the postpartum period. *Nursing Clinics of North America* 17:23, 1982.

Mercer, R. Ceisis: A baby is born with a defect. *Nursing* 77:45, 1977.

Mercer, R. The nurse and maternal tasks of early postpartum. *American Journal of Maternal-Child Nursing* 6:341, 1981.

Mercer, R. A theoretical framework for studying factors that impact on the maternal role. *Nursing Research* 30:73, 1981.

Merkatz, R. B., Budd, K., and Merkatz, I. R. Psychologic and social implications of scientific care for pregnant diabetic women. *Seminars in Perinatology* 2:373, 1978.

Miskin, N. Ultrasonography in the prenatal diagnosis of spina bifida. *Perinatology/Neonatology* 4:30, 1980.

Moore, D., Bingham, P., and Keesling, O. Nursing care of the pregnant woman with diabetes mellitus. *Journal of Obstetric, Gynecologic and Neonatal Nursing* 10:188, 1981.

Moss, J. Concerns of multiparas on the third postpartum day. *Journal of Obstetric, Gynecologic and Neonatal Nursing* 10:421, 1981.

Naeye, R. L., and Friedman, E. A. Causes of perinatal death associated with gestational hypertension and proteinuria. *American Journal of Obstetrics and Gynecology* 133:8, 1979.

Norr, K., Block, C., Charles, A., and Meyering, S. The second time around: Parity and birth experience. *Journal of Obstetric, Gynecologic and Neonatal Nursing* 9:30, 1980.

Nyman, J. Thrombophlebitis in pregnancy. *American Journal of Nursing* 80:90, 1980.

Patterson, P. Fetal therapy. *Association of Operating Room Nursing Journal* 35:663, 1982.

Paukert, S. Maternal-infant attachment in a traditional hospital setting. *Journal of Obstetric, Gynecologic and Neonatal Nursing* 11:23, 1982.

Penticuff, J. Psychologic implications of high-risk pregnancy. *Nursing Clinics of North America* 17:69, 1982.

Petrowski, D. Effectiveness of prenatal and postnatal instruction in postpartum care. *Journal of Obstetric, Gynecologic and Neonatal Nursing* 10:386, 1981.

Polani, K. Sixteen years experience of counseling, diagnosis and prenatal detection in one genetic centre: Progress, results and problems. *Journal of Medical Genetics* 16:166, 1979.

Rancilio, N. When a pregnant woman is diabetic: Postpartal care. *American Journal of Nursing* 79:453, 1979.

Reiser, S. A tool to facilitate mother-infant attachment. *Journal of Obstetric, Gynecologic and Neonatal Nursing* 10:294, 1981.

Roberts, C. Ethical issues in the treatment of neonates with severe anomalies. *Nursing Forum* 18(4):353, 1979.

Rosenbaum, M. Difficulties in taking care of business: Women addicts as mothers. *American Journal of Drug Alcohol Abuse* 6(4):431, 1979.

Schuler, K. When a pregnant woman is diabetic: Antepartal care. *American Journal of Nursing* 79:448, 1979.

Schuler, K., Wimberly, D., Rancilio, N., and Vogel, M. When a pregnant woman is diabetic: A case study. *American Journal of Nursing* 79:456, 1979.

Schultz, W. Using ultrasonography in the perinatal detection of congenital malformations. *Perinatology/Neonatology* 3:44, 1979.

Schwarz, R. Considerations of antibiotic therapy during pregnancy. *Obstetrics and Gynecology* 58:95s, 1981.

Scott, R. B. Reflections on the current status of the National Sickle Cell Disease Program in the U.S. *Journal of the National Medical Association* 20:71, 1979.

Senie, R. Possible related risks to breastfeeding. *Journal of Obstetric, Gynecologic and Neonatal Nursing* 11:34, 1982.

Sherwen, L. Fantasies during the third trimester of pregnancy. *American Journal of Maternal-Child Nursing* 6:398, 1981.

Sicuranza, B. J., Tisdall, L. H., Sarreck, R., and DeStefano, R. Thalassemia minor. *New York State Journal of Medicine* 9:1691, 1978.

Simpson, J. L. Genetics of diabetes mellitus and anomalies in offspring of diabetic mothers. *Seminars in Perinatology* 2:383, 1978.

Soler, N. G., Soler, S. M., and Malins, J. M. Neonatal morbidity among infants of diabetic mothers. *Diabetes Care* 1:340, 1978.

Sonstegard, L. Pregnancy-induced hypertension: Prenatal nursing concerns. *American Journal of Maternal-Child Nursing* 4:90, 1982.

Spellacy, W. N. Family planning and the diabetic mother. *Seminars in Perinatology* 2:395, 1978.

Symonds, E. M., and Pipkin, F. B. Pregnancy hypertension, parity, and the renin-angiotensin system. *American Journal of Obstetrics and Gynecology* 132:473, 1978.

Szekely, P., and Snaith, L. Cardiac disorders. *Clinics in Obstetrics and Gynecology* 4:265, 1977.

Taubenheim, A. Paternal-infant bonding in the first time father. *Journal of Obstetric, Gynecologic and Neonatal Nursing* 10:261, 1981.

Thompson, C. E. Legal aspects of genetic screening. *Journal of Obstetric, Gynecologic and Neonatal Nursing* 6:34, 1977.

Tibbetts, E., and Cadwell, K. Selecting the right breast pump. *American Journal of Maternal-Child Nursing* 5:262, 1980.

Tichy, A., and Chong, D. Placental function and its role in toxemia. *American Journal of Maternal-Child Nursing* 4:84, 1979.

Tison, C. A. Possible acceleration of neurological maturation following high risk pregnancy. *American Journal of Obstetrics and Gynecology* 138:303, 1980.

Ueland, K., and Metcalfe, J. Heart disease in pregnancy. *Clinics in Perinatology* 1:349, 1974.

Vestal, K. A proposal: Primary nursing for the mother-baby dyad. *Nursing Clinics of North America* 17:3, 1982.

Warshaw, J. B. Insulin influences on fetal growth. *Mead-Johnson Symposium on Perinatal Developmental Medicine* 13:40, 1978.

Weingold, A. B., Yonekura, M. L., and O'Kieffe, J. Fetus, placenta, and newborn: Nonstress testing. *American Journal of Obstetrics and Gynecology* 138:195, 1980.

Welt, S. I., and Crenshaw, M. C., Jr. Concurrent hypertension and pregnancy. *Clinical Obstetrics and Gynecology* 21:619, 1978.

Wetzel, S. Are we ignoring the needs of the woman with a spontaneous abortion? *American Journal of Maternal-Child Nursing* 7:258, 1982.

Wheeler, L., Duxbury, M., Raff, B., and Carroll, P. Fetal assessment. White Plains, N.Y.: National Foundation March of Dimes, 1979.

Wheeler, L., and Jones, M. Pregnancy-induced hypertension. *Journal of Obstetric, Gynecologic and Neonatal Nursing* 10:212, 1981.

Willis, S., and Sharp, E. Hypertension in pregnancy: Prenatal detection and management. *American Journal of Nursing* 82:798, 1982.

Chapter 19 Complications of Labor

PREMATURE LABOR
Assessment

Premature or preterm labor is labor that occurs prior to 38 weeks' gestation. The causes are numerous. They include spontaneous rupture of membranes; cervical incompetency; uterine abnormalities such as two distinct horns or a septum in the central uterine cavity; an overdistended uterus such as occurs in twinning and polyhydramnios; bleeding such as abruptio placentae or placenta previa; maternal infection such as urinary tract infections; chronic maternal diseases such as hypertension and diabetes; and fetal death. In many instances the cause of preterm labor is unknown. A history of preterm deliveries may be associated with increased risk for premature labor.

The decision facing the clinician and the woman is whether an early delivery of the fetus is more advantageous to his survival than remaining in utero. When the mother's labor is active and has progressed beyond 4 centimeters' dilatation or if there is severe bleeding, gross fetal anomaly, or conditions that place the mother in jeopardy, such as severe hypertensive disease or ruptured membranes with the risk of uterine infection, preterm labor is not stopped [10].

In other instances attempts are made to halt labor to provide more time for fetal maturation. This also provides additional time for the woman and family to ready themselves for the birth of the infant. The mother is placed on bed rest and may receive a number of pharmacologic agents used to arrest labor (Table 19-1). While attempts are being made to halt labor, the amniotic fluid may be tested to assess fetal maturity. The woman may also receive a glucocorticoid intramuscularly (betamethasone or dexamethasone) to accelerate fetal lung maturation if delivery is projected to be postponed at least 24 hours. In this situation the incidence of respiratory distress may be reduced by 50 percent [19]. Long-term effects of steroid treatment on the fetus require further investigation.

The benefits of agents used to arrest premature labor remain controversial. According to the analysis of Hemminki and Starfield [8], who evaluated the evidence provided in 16 published controlled clinical trials in which pharmacologic agents were used, only two of the therapeutic trials were more effective than a placebo in postponing delivery. In only one therapeutic trial were the outcomes of the infants more favorable than the controls. In the opinion of Pritchard and MacDonald [14], improvement in perinatal morbidity and mortality is more likely to be achieved by concentrating on (1) the identification of pregnancies in which preterm labor is likely to develop, (2) early hospitalization, (3) optimal delivery, and (4) appropriate intensive neonatal care.

Interventions

When attempts to arrest labor fail and delivery of a preterm infant is imminent, vaginal delivery is the preferred method. Often forceps are used to protect the fragile vessels in the head of the preterm infant, and an episiotomy is performed to reduce pressure on the fetal head. Cesarean birth may be performed if the infant is in a transverse lie or a breech presentation. Resuscitation equipment should be available to assist the infant's respiratory effort if necessary, and the staff and other equipment required to care for both mother and infant should be readied. Keep the mother and father informed of each phase of the plan of care and help them to retain as much control over their situation as possible.

Table 19-1.
Pharmacologic Agents
Used for Preterm Labor

Agent	Dose and Method of Administration	Maternal Side Effects	Fetal Effects
Ethanol	10% solution of ethanol in 5% aqueous dextrose is infused at the rate of 7.5 ml/hr for each kg of body weight. After infusing this loading dose for 2 hr, the rate of infusion is reduced from 7.5 ml to 1.5 ml/hr, which is then maintained for up to 12 hr	Nausea, vomiting, overt intoxication, hypoglycemia, lactic acidemia	Intoxication, metabolic derangements, respiratory distress if labor cannot be arrested
Magnesium sulfate	4 g as a loading dose intravenously, followed by a continuous infusion of 2 g/hr in a 10% or 20% solution (not very effective)	Hypermagnesemia: flushing, sweating, extreme thirst, hypotension, sedation, confusion, depressed reflexes, muscle weakness	Hypermagnesemia
Beta-mimetic drugs: Isoxsuprine	Initial intravenous infusion followed by oral or intramuscular doses; oral 10 to 20 mg 3 or 4 times daily; intramuscular 5 to 10 mg 2 or 3 times a day	Increase in heart rate, drop in diastolic blood pressure	Increase in heart rate, drop in diastolic blood pressure
Ritodrine	Intravenously administered by calibrated infusion pump; initial dose 50 to 100 μg/min, increased by 50 μg/min every 10 min until contractions stop, unacceptable side effects develop, or the maximum dose of 350 μg/min is reached	Increase in heart rate, decrease in blood pressure, widening pulse pressure, tremor, palpations, nervousness, restlessness, ketoacidosis in diabetics	Increase in heart rate Increase in blood pressure
	Oral therapy is started 30 min before the infusion is stopped with a dosage of 10 mg; 10 mg every 2 hr or 20 mg every 2 hr for first 24 hr (max. dose, 120 mg/day)		

Sources: G. Aumann, and G. Blake. Ritodrine hydrochloride in the control of premature labor. *Journal of Obstetric, Gynecologic and Neonatal Nursing* 11:75, 1982; T. Barden et al. Ritodrine hydrochloride. *Obstetrics and Gynecology* 56:1, 1980; I. Merkatz, et al. Ritodrine hydrochloride. *Obstetrics and Gynecology* 56:7, 1980; and J. Pritchard and P. MacDonald. *Williams Obstetrics* (16th ed.). New York: Appleton-Century-Crofts, 1980.

INDUCTION OF LABOR   Induction, the deliberate initiation of uterine contractions prior to their spontaneous onset, is performed at or near term for a variety of reasons. Induction is used when the woman's life or well-being is in danger or if the fetus may be compromised by remaining in the uterus any longer. Labor is often induced when the woman has hypertensive disease, diabetes, premature rupture of the membranes, or a renal disorder or when the fetus is postmature, has erythroblastosis, or is being compromised by placental insufficiency. Labor is often also electively induced for the convenience of the physician and the woman, particularly when the woman lives far away or has a history of rapid labors.

The advantages of induction in this latter situation are that the mother is well rested, has time to organize her family for her absence, and is psychologically ready for labor. In addition, it can be assured that her bowel, bladder, and stomach are empty, and the risk of excessively rapid labor and possible delivery en route to the hospital is avoided. This method ensures that the physician is present and that labor and delivery take place when adequate personnel are available.

Assessment   For labor to be induced successfully, the woman must be near term with a mature fetus. Her cervix must be soft with a moderate amount of effacement and dilatation (a ripe cervix). The fetal head should be fixed in the pelvic inlet, and there must be no cephalopelvic disproportion. Women with cephalopelvic disproportion, previous uterine surgery including cesarean delivery malpresentation, placenta previa, abruptio placentae, herpesvirus type 2, or uterine overdistention should not have induced labor. Complications of induction are those associated in major part with uterine overstimulation. They include tetanic contractions, uterine rupture, abruptio placentae, cervical lacerations, postpartum hemorrhage, fetal distress, birth injuries, and delivery of a premature infant if the infant's maturity has been miscalculated.

Interventions   One of the most commonly used methods of inducing labor is by artificial rupture of the membranes, or *amniotomy*. Approximately 80 percent the time a woman whose cervix is ripe and the fetal head is in the pelvis will go into active labor within 24 hours after amniotomy. The woman's perineum and vulva are washed with antiseptic solution. Using sterile gloves, the physician inserts two fingers into the woman's vagina and into the cervix, separates the membranes from the lower uterine segment, and ruptures the membranes with an amnihook, toothed forceps, or stylet. Take the fetal heart sounds immediately prior to rupture and immediately afterward to determine what effect the procedure has had on fetal oxygenation. If the cord has washed down with the amniotic fluid or has become compressed between the bony pelvis and the presenting part, a fetal bradycardia can be detected promptly and appropriate intervention begun. The color and amount of amniotic fluid expelled should also be noted and recorded.

If the woman's cervix is effaced and partially dilated and the fetal head is deep in the pelvis, labor usually will begin. The procedure is most successful if performed within 2 weeks of the woman's expected date of confinement. If labor must be induced before this time for medical reasons, amniotomy is preceded by stripping of the membranes and is followed by oxytocin induction. If the woman does not go into labor after the procedure, she may become infected by an ascending amnionitis. This woman, like those whose membranes rupture prematurely during the latter weeks of pregnancy, may be placed on antibiotic therapy and delivered within a few days if the fetus is mature. The incidence of infection increases significantly if the membranes have been ruptured for over 24 hours.

Stripping the membranes from the lower uterine segment without rupturing them is another method used to induce labor. When the membranes are separated as described previously, labor may be initiated by the release of oxytocin in response to the cervical manipulation that occurs. The loosened membranes also act as a wedge in dilating the cervix. This method does not always work; also, it may increase the incidence of infection and result in accidental rupture of the membranes. The method is also not effective if the presenting part of the fetus is high in the woman's pelvis. This procedure may be more painful than amniotomy for some women.

Another widely used method of inducing labor is the *administration of oxytocin*. The purpose of induction by oxytocin is to elicit normal uterine activity—that is, three contractions in 10 minutes, averaging 50 millimeters of mercury in intensity. For administration, a solution of 10 I.U. of oxytocin is added to 1 liter of usually a 5% dextrose in water or a balanced salt solution. When 10 I.U. (10,000 milliunits) are added to 1 liter (1,000 ml) of intravenous solution, each milliliter of this solution will provide 10 milliunits of oxytocin [2]. The solution is administered intravenously usually by means of a constant infusion pump. A two-bottle system is used: One bottle of fluid without oxytocin is used so that if the oxytocin solution must be discontinued suddenly the alternate fluid can be used to keep the woman's vein open. As the medication is begun, it is administered at 2 milliunits per minute, and the dose is increased slowly every 15 to 20 minutes until the dose is 20 milliunits per minute. It is rarely necessary to exceed this rate, and if satisfactory uterine contractions have not been established with 30 to 40 milliunits per minute, it is unlikely that a greater dose will induce them [14].

The mean half life of oxytocin in plasma is approximately 3 minutes. For any one rate of infusion, the plasma level reaches a plateau after about 20 minutes, as the rate of infusion and rate of destruction by oxytocinase achieve equilibrium. Oxytocin also possesses a potent antidiuretic action. At infusion rates of 20 milliunits per minute or more, free water clearance by the kidney decreases significantly, and infusion of appreciative amounts of intravenous fluids, especially dextrose in water, poses the possibility of serious water intoxication that can lead to convulsions, coma, and death [1, 9].

When the infusion begins, record the rate of infusion, the woman's blood pressure and pulse, and fetal heart rate every 15 minutes, and observe her closely for the beginning of uterine contractions. When contractions begin, evaluate and record them every 15 minutes for interval, duration, and intensity. Ideally fetal heart rate is monitored continuously. If the fetal heart rate is taken at 15-minute intervals, check it immediately following contractions in order to evaluate the fetus's response to the stress of the contraction. Oxytocin is a powerful drug and can cause rupture of the uterus or hypoxia for the fetus from markedly hypertonic uterine contractions.

If the fetal heart rate indicates distress or if contractions last 70 seconds or more, reduce or discontinue the intravenous solution immediately. If tetanic contractions result (hypersensitivity), they will usually occur within the first five contractions. Should this occur, take the fetal heart tones and immediately administer oxygen to the woman. While blood pressure elevation rarely occurs with the use of synthetic oxytocin, monitor the woman's blood pressure nevertheless for any changes, in view of the possibility of water intoxication.

Induction of labor with intramuscular, intranasal, or sublingual administration of oxytocin is not commonly used because of problems in controlling the rate of absorption via these routes. Because of these problems the use of transbuccal oxytocin to induce labor has been disapproved by the Food and Drug Administration.

Many clinicians have objected to the frequency of elective induction of labor and its possible effects on the fetus. The main hazard associated with artificial induction of labor is premature delivery. While one study [12] of almost 3,000 elective inductions found only 0.7 percent of the perinatal deaths to be related to the induction, Schwarz and colleagues [17] reported an increased incidence of early deceleration of the fetal heart rate and increased intensity of uterine contractions in women with induced labor. They questioned the effect this may have on the child's future growth and development.

Recently prostaglandin E_2 vaginal suppositories have been used to ripen unfavorable cervixes of women in whom labor was to be induced. In one study a suppository containing 3 milligrams of prostaglandin E_2 was administered the evening before induction. If the woman's cervix remained unfavorable, a second dose was administered the next morning. Labor often followed the administration of the first or second suppository. If labor did not begin and the cervix was ripened, amniotomy was performed or oxytocin was administered intravenously, usually successfully [18].

DYSTOCIA

The term *dystocia* refers to a labor that is difficult because of mechanical or functional factors, or both. Mechanical causes of dystocia include maternal elements, such as a contracted pelvis (passage). Fetal (passenger) causes of mechanical dystocia include failure to rotate from an occiput transverse or posterior position, malpresentation, malformation such as hydrocephalus, and excessive size.

Functional Dystocia

ASSESSMENT

Functional dystocia (or dysfunctional labor) results from contractions that deviate from normal. These contractions may be extremely forceful, with a rapid and traumatic labor and precipitate delivery. More commonly, the contractions are ineffectual. In the majority of cases there is no apparent cause, although contributing conditions include uterine anomalies, overdistention such as is found in multiple pregnancy or hydramnios, delayed labor or postmaturity, cervical scar tissue from previous surgery, or chronic disease. Cervical resistance may be an important contributing factor, although this is usually restricted to first labors. Once the cervix has been dilated, it is no longer that resistant.

The contractions of functional dystocia may differ in quality and synchronization of activity. They may be localized to one portion of the uterus rather than involving the entire organ. They may be stronger in the lower uterine segment than in the upper uterine segment or may move upward over the uterus rather than downward. On the other hand, they may be properly synchronized and have a normal pattern but may exert so little pressure on the cervix that it does not dilate.

Desultory or prolonged labor may be evident within 6 to 8 hours of the onset of labor, particularly if the woman's progress is plotted on a graph that features a normal labor curve for comparison (Fig. 19-1). Once labor begins, its progress should be definite and sustained until the baby is successfully delivered within the period of time defined for normal labor—20 hours. If it goes beyond that time, there is a resulting increase in fetal and maternal morbidity and mortality. In order to avoid these misfortunes, supportive measures and uterine stimulation are often used if the pattern of labor becomes abnormal.

Figure 19-1. Abnormal labor can be detected early when plotted against a normal labor curve. This graph shows a prolonged latent phase.

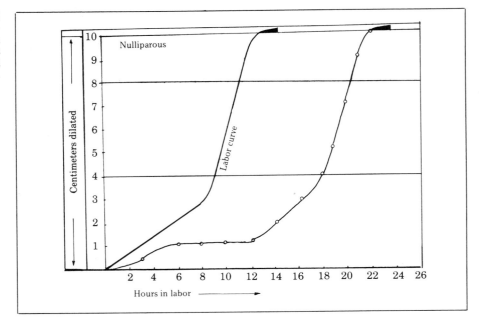

INTERVENTIONS

For functional dystocia labor is stimulated by the common methods used for artificial induction. Amniotomy is chosen with the knowledge that delivery should occur within 24 hours if increased fetal and maternal morbidity is to be avoided. Oxytocin also is frequently used to prevent and treat functional dystocia by producing uterine contractions that are strong enough to dilate the cervix and by demonstrating over a short time whether or not the uterus will contract effectively to complete at least the first stage of labor. Usually progress is evident in 3 to 4 hours; if none occurs, the oxytocin stimulation process is abandoned, since an increase in fetal morbidity is likely to follow. With the use of oxytocin tetanic contractions may occur, with the resulting hazards of uterine rupture or fetal asphyxia. Monitor the fetal heart rate and the woman's uterine contractions as you would if she were being induced.

Decisions regarding delivery for a woman with functional dystocia depend on the degree of cervical dilatation and the station of the fetal presenting part. If the woman's cervix is more than half dilated, if the presenting part is near her pelvic floor, and if her outlet is ample, vaginal delivery may be possible. Otherwise, a cesarean delivery is less traumatic and far safer.

LATENT PHASE

Assessment. Functional causes of labor abnormalities may be divided into three types according to the phase of labor affected—latent, active, or deceleration. The latent phase of dilatation is prolonged if it lasts more than 20 hours in a nullipara and more than 14 hours in a multipara. Almost half of the time prolonged labor during this phase is due to excessive or untimely sedation or anesthesia. About 20 percent of the time a thick, uneffaced, undilated, and unyielding cervix is the cause. In another 10 percent of cases false labor is diagnosed in retrospect, and in an additional 10 percent of women the cervix just dilates very slowly [7]. In many instances the cause is unknown.

The uterine contractions that occur when the latent phase is prolonged are often hypertonic and uncoordinated, with an improper gradient and transmission over the uterus. The woman becomes exhausted, emotionally discouraged, and anxious, since these contractions can be very painful and result in little progress of labor.

Interventions. The usual treatment involves giving the woman a significant period of rest and suspending labor temporarily by the use of a narcotic such as morphine. When the effects of the narcotic wear off and contractions resume, they are almost always likely to be of normal quality; in addition, the woman is usually well rested, emotionally rejuvenated, and better able to cope with the labor ahead of her. In the rare instances in which the contractions do not resume normally, intravenous administration of oxytocin is sometimes helpful. In some instances where the woman's uterus fails continuously to respond with coordinated contractions, a cesarean delivery may be performed.

ACTIVE PHASE

Assessment. When labor is prolonged in the active phase, there are abnormally slow rates of cervical dilation and descent of the fetus. The cervix dilates at a rate of less than 1.2 centimeters per hour in nulliparas and less than 1.5 centimeters per hour in multiparas. Such small degrees of dilation are impossible to determine at each individual examination, of course, but over a period of time they may be determined in retrospect, and plotting the mother's progress of labor on a graph will facilitate keeping track of these changes. Labor is also considered to be prolonged in the active phase if descent of the fetus occurs at a rate of less than 1 centimeter per hour in nulliparas and less than 2 centimeters per hour in multiparas.

The underlying pathogenesis for prolonged labor in the active phase is essentially unknown. Associated factors include minor fetal malposition, excessive sedation, or conduction anesthesia given at a high level or administered too early. Cephalopelvic disproportion is a contributory factor in about one-fourth of the situations.

The contractions associated with this type of dysfunctional labor are likely to be hypotonic, exerting less than the pressure of 15 millimeters of mercury necessary for progress to occur. The woman becomes exhausted, and there is a substantial risk of ascending infection, since it is likely that the membranes ruptured previously.

Interventions. Maintenance of the woman's fluid and electrolyte balance is a special consideration. Following a careful evaluation of the fetopelvic relationship, oxytocin is usually administered. Most of these women can then deliver vaginally. If there is fetopelvic disproportion or if progress in labor does not result from the oxytocin administration, a cesarean is performed to decrease fetal and maternal risks.

DECELERATION PHASE (TRANSITION)

Assessment. Labor can also be prolonged in the deceleration phase of the first stage of labor, or cervical dilation and/or descent of the fetus may come to a standstill at this time. The deceleration phase is prolonged if it lasts over 3 hours in nulliparas and over 1 hour in multiparas. Dilation is said to be arrested when expected progress ceases for at least 2 hours. Arrested descent exists when descent is interrupted for at least 1 hour; it usually occurs in the second stage. When arrest develops, a cesarean delivery becomes a likely possibility, although about 60 percent of women can deliver vaginally if given the opportunity [7]. The most ominous cause of arrested dilation or descent is cephalopelvic disproportion, occurring in about 40 percent of cases and necessitating a cesarean birth. Other causes of arrested dilation or descent include minor malpositions, excessive sedation, or conduction anesthesia. Before any therapy for functional dystocia is instituted, x-ray pelvimetry should be done to rule out cephalopelvic disproportion. If the cause of the difficulty is excessive sedation or anesthesia, normal labor is likely to ensue when the effects wear off. If the woman needs to be given oxytocin stimulation, she will probably respond with additional progress in dilation and descent in less than 3 hours. The earlier the diagnosis and the more careful the treatment, the less likely the woman and fetus are to suffer serious consequences.

Intervention.   When caring for women with functional dystocia, be particularly aware of their general physical and emotional status, paying careful attention to the intensity of contractions, signs of fetal distress, and signs of maternal distress, such as a rising temperature with prolonged rupture of membranes, exhaustion, or dehydration. Since patterns of dysfunctional labor are very discouraging to parents and usually increase their levels of anxiety and tension, include careful explanations of the treatment and words of reassurance and encouragement. It is important to promote the woman's relaxation and make her as comfortable as possible so she can conserve her strength. You may want to give her a sponge bath, change her position, rub her back, and keep her clean and dry. She may also find some diversionary activity helpful. Since a full bladder or rectum can block the woman's labor progress or may be traumatized during the labor and delivery process, provide for adequate elimination.

Probably one of the most important elements in helping parents to cope with the crisis situation of abnormal labor is your calm, knowledgeable, and supportive presence. You will also need to inform postpartum and nursery personnel about the particular stresses that the couple has already encountered.

DYSFUNCTION OF ABDOMINAL MUSCLES.   In order for the second stage of labor to progress normally, some voluntary pushing by the woman, using her abdominal muscles, is usually required. Sometimes the second stage is prolonged if, for some reason, the mother is unable to push effectively. Possible causes of this inability are relaxed abdominal musculature (in the multipara), an anesthesia-blocked perineal reflex, weakness from exhaustion, or the woman's refusal to push if her discomfort is severe. Relieve her discomfort as much as possible, support and coach her to push properly. Forceps are commonly used to shorten the second stage of labor if the mother is exhausted.

Mechanical Dystocia   ASSESSMENT AND INTERVENTION

Maternal Pelvic Contraction.   In 75 percent of nulliparas with a vertex presentation, engagement has occurred by the thirty-eighth week of gestation; in 95 percent, by the onset of labor. If the vertex is engaged at the onset of labor, a vaginal delivery can be anticipated in 99 percent of pregnant women. A contracted pelvis may be the cause of nonengagement of the vertex at the onset of labor. The definition of a contracted pelvis is somewhat arbitrary, since the type of pelvis in the individual woman is an important consideration. Enlargement in one pelvic diameter may compensate for narrowing in another and may actually permit vaginal delivery. Other factors that affect pelvic adequacy are the size of the fetus, the hardness and moldability of the fetal head, and the fetal presentation, position, and attitude. It is possible for all three planes of the pelvis to be contracted, either singly or in combination.

INLET.   Contraction of the pelvic inlet is suspected when the anterior-posterior diameter (diagonal conjugate) is less than 11 centimeters (average, 12.5 centimeters). The contracted conjugate vera is generally considered to be below 10 centimeters (average, 11 centimeters), although a nullipara with a conjugate vera of 9.0 to 9.5 centimeters is usually permitted a trial labor, especially if the fetus is not large.

If there are consistently strong labor contractions but no descent of the fetal head through the pelvis, the head will develop large caput succedaneum; in addition, there may be placental insufficiency, fetal cerebral injury and hemorrhage, or a ruptured uterus. Hopefully the contracted pelvis is usually suspected and diagnosed, and a cesarean delivery is done before the mother or infant suffers such consequences.

MIDPELVIS.   The average bispinous diameter of the midpelvis is 10.5 centimeters. A measurement of less than 9.5 centimeters between the ischial spines usually results in a contracted pelvis. This measurement is one that can be accurately obtained only by x-ray pelvimetry.

OUTLET.   The pelvic outlet has an average bituberous diameter of 10.5 centimeters; it is usually contracted when the diameter is less than 8.5 centimeters. Ordinarily the coccyx can be forced back 2.5 centimeters or more during delivery, adding to the available outlet space. When the sacrococcygeal joint is healthy, no problems result. If it is ankylotic, the bone may be fractured or the joint may break open. Chronic arthritis may develop as a result.

The mother who has a fractured coccyx may be unable to sit comfortably. She may complain of pain running up her back and down her thighs and of difficulty in walking. The fracture usually heals by itself within 6 months. The application of heat or the injection of procaine around the joint and nerve supply will probably relieve the associated discomfort. Rarely will the mother need to have the bone excised.

Although the pelvic planes are described separately, the midpelvis and outlet are usually considered together in evaluating pelvic adequacy. Their contraction may actually be more dangerous than a contracted inlet, since it may not be discovered until late in labor or when an attempt is made to deliver the baby vaginally. This problem is commonly associated with android pelves. Contractures are less often seen with the anthropoid type, and the low incidence of platypelloid (flat) pelves makes pelvic contraction associated with this type relatively rare. In general, the most common problem seen clinically is that of pelvic inlet contraction.

A pelvic contraction is diagnosed when labor is not progressing normally, when the presenting part of the fetus is high and undescending, or when a dysfunctional labor pattern develops. X-ray pelvimetry is used to confirm the diagnosis. This procedure involves a small amount of radiation but not enough to discourage its use for this purpose, for placentography, or to determine fetal position; however, if possible, it should not be repeated.

Abnormal fetal presentations are four times as frequent with contracted pelves as with normal ones. Prolapse of the fetal arm, foot, and cord are therefore relatively common, and at the beginning of labor the fetal head is likely to be high and not engaged. Since a contracted pelvis often causes a large caput succedaneum to form, it may be incorrectly surmised that the head is actually engaged when in reality it is still high. Caput often obscures the landmarks of the head and makes accurate diagnosis of its position difficult. Because the head may not fill the lower uterine segment normally, the membranes over the cervical os may be exposed to the full force of the uterine contractions. As a result, they may rupture prematurely, predisposing the fetus to prolapsed cord and the mother to uterine infection. Sometimes the cervix is compressed between the bony surface of the fetal head and the maternal pelvis and becomes edematous.

If the pelvic contraction is a serious one, the fetal prognosis is actually better since the abnormality is likely to be recognized early and a cesarean delivery can be performed before the fetus is distressed. If the contraction is very slight, usually the woman will deliver spontaneously, provided the fetus is of moderate size, fetal presentation and position are normal, and uterine contractions are strong.

In countries such as Africa where facilities to perform a cesarean operation may not be readily available when pelvic contraction exists, the cartilage between the woman's symphysis is cut. This allows greater expansion of the bony pelvis. Ambulation is often difficult postpartum until healing occurs.

Any problem that causes a delay in the progress of labor increases the parents' anxiety level; therefore, careful explanations of the procedures involved in the diagnosis and of the alternative methods of treatment to ensure maternal and fetal safety are reassuring.

Trial Labor.   As already mentioned, when the adequacy of a woman's pelvis is borderline or functional dystocia is diagnosed, she may undergo a trial labor. Trial labor usually is a period of 6 to 12 hours during which the obstetrician concludes that the woman can be safely delivered vaginally or that she will have to be delivered by cesarean.

It is rare that cephalopelvic disproportion is absolute, given the fact that the pelvis does expand somewhat during the process of labor. In addition, if the woman is permitted to have a trial labor, the obstetrician can be more certain that the labor has progressed as long as possible and that a cesarean operation is not done unnecessarily.

A trial labor is probably most anxiety-producing in the primigravida who fears surgery, is disappointed regarding the outcome of her pregnancy, and wishes to avoid a primary cesarean delivery in light of future childbearing. Your constant presence and support are helpful. In order to ensure maximum pelvic space, it is important that the woman's bladder and bowel remain as empty as possible.

Soft Tissue Dystocia   While a narrow bony pelvis can be a serious cause of dystocia, another possible cause is an anomaly of the maternal soft parts. Sometimes the woman's cervix is very rigid. This may be caused by chronic cervicitis, deep cauterizations, or previous surgical procedures. Digital dilation or softening with intravenous oxytocin stimulation may be the clinician's choice of treatment. Sometimes a cesarean delivery is necessary.

Tumors, congenital deformities, edema, scars, or hematomas may contribute to vulvar or vaginal stenosis. Usually the obstruction clears spontaneously as the tissues soften during pregnancy and labor. An episiotomy often solves the problem. Rarely, a cesarean becomes necessary.

Fetal Causes of Mechanical Dystocia

PERSISTENT OCCIPUT POSTERIOR

Assessment. A common cause of arrested labor is the failure of the fetal occiput to rotate anteriorly, so that it remains posterior or transverse. Generally, this occurs in pelves other than the gynecoid type. If the occiput is posterior, the fetal head meets resistance at the sacrococcygeal platform and the ischial spines and becomes deflexed. Complete descent is prevented, so that the head is arrested between the spines and the perineum. If the head is deflexed, the cervix may fail to dilate completely and may become edematous from being pressed between the presenting part and the symphysis pubis. The progress of labor will slow as a result, especially in the deceleration phase of the first stage and in the second stage. As a rule, if delivery does not occur within an hour, the vertex will only extend further and the cervix will become more edematous.

Generally, the persistent occiput rotates spontaneously once it reaches the slinglike musculature of the pelvic floor. If this does not happen, there is less risk of maternal soft tissue damage if the vertex can be rotated and delivered in an anterior position. In addition, the amount of force necessary for delivery is three times less if the occiput is anterior. Rotation of the fetal head can be accomplished either manually or by forceps. Manual rotation is often possible and results in fewer vaginal lacerations. If manual rotation is not possible, rotation by forceps is necessary. (Rotation of the fetal head by forceps and application of another set of forceps for delivery is referred to as the *Scanzoni maneuver.*)

If the head presents posteriorly, spontaneous delivery requires more uterine and abdominal effort than if the head presents anteriorly. The sinciput passes well below the inferior aspect of the symphysis pubis, and the vertex is delivered face up by flexion. In the posterior position, the larger occipitofrontal diameter (11.5 centimeters or more) of the vertex appears at the outlet rather than the suboccipitobregmatic diameter, a difference of 2.5 to 3 centimeters, causing the woman's perineum to become greatly distended. The underlying endopelvic fascia often separates despite an extensive mediolateral episiotomy unless the outlet is exceptionally large. Thus, rather severe perineal lacerations commonly occur unless the fetus is small or the woman is a multipara. Since a large caput succedaneum generally forms, there may be fetal head damage as well.

Intervention. The woman who is carrying a fetus in the posterior position often has severe pain in her back with contractions, as the fetal head presses against her sacrum. Back rubs and position changes are sometimes helpful. Some clinicians feel turning the woman from side to side will assist rotation of the fetal head; however, there is no supporting documentation. Side lying will increase blood flow to the uterus and fetus while a modified knee-chest position will decrease pressure on the woman's sacral nerves. In this presentation, fetal heart tones are heard best deep in the mother's flank. Her labor contractions commonly follow a pattern of alternating large and small contractions.

Occiput posterior fetal positions do not per se increase maternal morbidity or infant mortality; however, they are commonly associated with prolonged labor, arrested descent, or operative deliveries and thus can be contributing factors.

PERSISTENT OCCIPUT TRANSVERSE

Assessment and Intervention. Transverse arrest occurs when the occiput, which is originally in a transverse position, fails to rotate. This is usually no problem if the woman's pelvis is gynecoid, since rotation to the anterior position is easily accomplished and forceps extraction of the head is not difficult. If her pelvis is android, or possibly if her midpelvis and outlet are contracted, a cesarean delivery is usually done to avoid traumatizing the fetus or the woman's soft tissues. Severe vaginal lacerations may follow the use of forceps in the case of persistent occiput transverse.

Nursing interventions with both persistent occipital posterior and transverse arrest positions include support and comfort measures for the woman and monitoring uterine contractions, vital signs, and fetal heart rate patterns. Helping the mother and her partner cope with the stress of this situation is likewise very important.

SINCIPUT PRESENTATION

If the amount of head deflexion is only slight, the fetus's sinciput will present (Fig. 19-2). In this presentation the woman's labor and her treatment are like that

Figure 19-2. Sinciput presentation with slight head flexion, forcing a larger fetal head diameter to present.

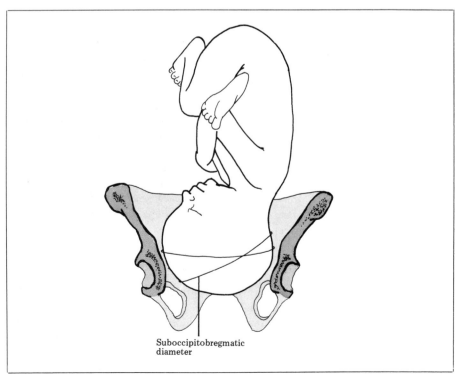

Suboccipitobregmatic
diameter

for the occiput posterior presentation. The occiput still remains the point of reference. Usually, when the fetal head reaches the pelvic floor, contractions improve, the head flexes, and the child is born without further difficulty.

BROW AND FACE PRESENTATIONS

Assessment and Intervention.   Generally, brow and face presentations have the same etiology and are diagnosed by the same methods. Pelvic contracture, fetal abnormalities, or a very large maternal pelvis are contributing factors. These presentations are two to three times as frequent in multiparas as in nulliparas, probably due to the multipara's decreased abdominal and pelvic muscle tone. A fetus with excessive muscle tone in the extensor muscles of the back and neck can also be a cause of brow and face presentations.

Deflexion to the greatest degree results in a face presentation, and anencephaly accounts for 5 percent of these cases. The chin, or mentum, is the point of reference. Early diagnosis of the extended vertex depends on abdominal palpation, and a brow or face presentation is suspected when the most prominent portion of the vertex is on the same side as the fetal back or opposite the fetal small parts. X-ray or vaginal examination, or both, confirms the diagnosis.

If the woman's pelvis is normal and the membranes are intact, her labor progress is observed carefully, with no specific intervention, since spontaneous conversion of a brow presentation to a face presentation or flexion to a more desirable vertex presentation may occur. The obstetrician may attempt to flex the fetal head manually, with the woman under anesthesia, but extension frequently recurs. With more manipulation, cord prolapse becomes more of a possibility. Usually the delivery of the infant is accomplished with the aid of forceps and a deep episiotomy to minimize maternal and fetal injuries. In about 30 percent of cases, either the membranes rupture early or progress is unsatisfactory, and a cesarean birth becomes a necessity.

Needless to say, in brow and face presentations the baby's head becomes molded and a large caput succedaneum develops. Fetal morbidity and mortality are high due to hypoxia, cranial compression with tentorial or falx tears, compression of the neck against the mother's pubis, and fractures of the trachea and larynx. Maternal mortality is also increased because of a longer labor, a greater danger of infection, and the increased frequency of a contracted pelvis and need for operative procedures.

After birth the baby's face is often disfigured and bruised, especially if the labor has been prolonged and the mother's membranes have been ruptured. There may be edema over his cheek and eye. His eyes may bulge, may have a mucoserous discharge, and may be swollen. The baby often lies on his side with his head extended and his back straight. Parents should be reassured that their infant's features will regain a normal appearance within 2 weeks.

BREECH PRESENTATION

Assessment.   Since vertex presentations of the fetal head constitute 95 percent of all deliveries, any other presentation—breech, face, brow, shoulder—is considered a deviation from normal. In about 3 to 4 percent of all deliveries, the breech will be the presenting part, with the fetal head in the woman's fundus and the buttocks in her lower uterine segment. The point of reference is the sacrum. The most common breech positions are left sacroanterior (LSA) and right sacroposterior (RSP).

The fetus does not necessarily assume the final presentation and position in the uterus until the last weeks of pregnancy, when it must accommodate itself to available space. Therefore, breech presentations are more common in premature labor than in full-term labor, since the law of accommodation is not operative yet. They are also more common in hydramnios or multiple pregnancy, in which excessive distention of the uterine cavity or the presence of another fetus can interfere with the development of normal uterine polarity. Anencephalic or hydrocephalic fetuses commonly present in the breech position, often with accompanying hydramnios. Breech presentations are also linked with placenta previa, which occupies space in the lower uterine segment, although transverse lie is probably more common in association with this disorder.

There are three varieties of breech presentations. In the *frank breech*, the fetus's thighs are flexed on the abdomen and the legs are extended in such a way that the feet are at the level of the thorax or shoulders. The buttocks are in the woman's lower uterine segment. The frank breech provides a better dilating wedge than the complete breech.

The *complete* or *full breech* has almost the same attitude as a vertex presentation but with reversed polarity. The fetus's thighs are flexed on the abdomen and the lower legs are on the thighs. The feet appear in the woman's birth canal at the same level as the buttocks. This presentation is considered more satisfactory for immediate delivery, since one of the feet may be brought down readily for traction, if necessary.

If the infant is in a *footling breech* presentation, one leg is extended and the foot is in the woman's birth canal before the buttocks. If both legs are extended, it is a double footling breech.

Breech presentations are diagnosed by abdominal palpation and vaginal examination in the later weeks of pregnancy, and the diagnosis is verified by x-ray studies. With Leopold's maneuvers, you will feel the round fetal head in the woman's fundus and the back on either side; the irregular breech is usually well above the pelvic brim, but occasionally it is fixed in the inlet. You will find fetal heart tones at or above the woman's umbilicus.

If the membranes are ruptured, the fetal landmarks are more distinguishable on vaginal examination. The gluteal cleft and anus are palpable, with the two ischial tuberosities on either side. Sometimes the gluteal cleft is mistaken for the mouth, and a face presentation is wrongly diagnosed. Exact differentiation of genitalia by palpation may be obscured by compression and edema (although the examiner is often tempted to predict the sex of the infant). After birth, genitalia may be ecchymotic. If one of the fetus's legs has been in the woman's birth canal, it may be swollen and ecchymotic. All of these sequelae disappear within a week.

Usually the breech does not enter the pelvis until labor begins. Descent may be slow since the breech is not as firm a dilating wedge as the head, but the overall time of labor is not appreciably longer than in a vertex presentation [6]. After the largest diameter of the breech (bitrochanteric—9 centimeters) clears the pelvic outlet, the fetus is easily borne to the umbilicus. Usually the legs slip out of the birth canal spontaneously and the fetal sacrum then normally rotates 45 degrees or more anteriorly, thus favoring anterior rotation of the occiput of the aftercoming head. The shoulders are usually delivered with the widest diameter (bisacromial—12 centimeters) passing through the anterior-posterior dimension of the pelvic outlet by lateral flexion. This diameter can be shortened a bit by compression and by the range of mobility of the shoulder girdle. The anterior shoulder appears beneath the pubic arch, and the posterior shoulder then passes over the perineum.

If the infant's arms remain flexed on his chest, they are beside the thorax as it emerges. It is possible for one or both of the arms to become extended above the shoulders, especially if the woman's pelvis is contracted. This situation demands the assistance of the obstetrician; otherwise, the fetus is subjected to increasing hypoxia from compression of the umbilical cord after the umbilicus has passed through the woman's pelvic outlet.

Normal engagement of the aftercoming head takes place with the occiput in the anterior position. As descent occurs, the fetus's cervical spine, the region of maximum flexibility, is brought into the curve of the lower birth canal. The suboccipital region of the head is the fulcrum around which the chin, mouth, face, vertex, and finally the occiput pass over the woman's perineum. Usually a deep episiotomy is performed to avoid delay in delivering the fetal head and shoulders and to prevent severe maternal perineal lacerations. Sometimes Piper forceps are used to facilitate the head's delivery (Fig. 19-3).

In general, maternal morbidity is higher in breech presentations than in vertex. The associated perinatal loss is between 12 and 15 percent. The breech does not fill the lower uterine segment as completely as the vertex; therefore, there is greater opportunity for the umbilical cord to prolapse when the membranes rupture. Premature rupture of the membranes is frequent in breech presentation, and amniotic fluid may be stained with meconium. The latter is a rather insignificant fact of breech presentation, however, since meconium may be

Figure 19-3. Fetal head delivered with Piper forceps in breech delivery.

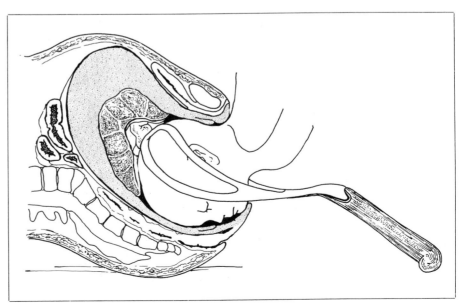

pressed out naturally by the increased intrauterine pressure on the breech during a contraction.

During the usual delivery process in a breech presentation, the umbilical cord is subjected to greater degrees of pressure, leading to fetal hypoxia. The fetal prognosis is also more hazardous in breech presentations because the largest part of the infant, the fetal head, is delivered last, and cephalopelvic disproportion may become apparent only after delivery of the breech and shoulders, leaving the head remaining in the birth canal. Attempts to extract the head are usually traumatizing to the fetus. Also, after the delivery of the hips and shoulders the uterus decreases in size, and this may facilitate placental release while the head is still in the birth canal.

Intervention. For all of the previously mentioned reasons, monitor the fetal heart tones constantly during labor and delivery. Fetal complications include anoxia, intracranial damage from rupture of the tentorium with or without associated hemorrhage, and traumatic injury of the spinal cord. Fractures of the infant's clavicle or extremities may occur. A cesarean delivery may be the delivery of choice if the breech infant is large or if the woman's pelvis is small.

It is common for a breech presentation to convert to a vertex presentation spontaneously. If this does not happen, sometimes the obstetrician will attempt an external cephalic version [15]. In order for this to be done, there should be an accurate diagnosis of presentation and position, a nonirritable uterus, an unengaged breech, and enough amniotic fluid to allow the fetus to be turned. Before the version is attempted, the fetal heart rate and rhythm are carefully noted. The obstetrician grasps the fetal caudal pole and cephalic pole through the woman's abdominal wall and turns them slowly and intermittently. The fetal heart tones are checked frequently throughout the procedure, since the change in fetal position may place tension on the umbilical cord or compress it between the fetus and the uterine wall. If the heart tones decrease or become irregular, the fetus is reconverted to a breech presentation.

The best time for attempting an external cephalic version is between 34 and 35 weeks' gestation. At that time the fetus can be turned with a minimum amount of force, and there is less chance that it will spontaneously reconvert to a breech presentation, since the woman's abdominal wall is comparatively relaxed. If the version is done later in pregnancy, there is greater likelihood of trauma to the umbilical cord and placenta and a chance that premature labor might be initiated. However, if rupture of the membranes accidently occurs, the fetus is more likely to be mature enough to survive. Conversion at 34 to 35 weeks' gestation is more likely to be successful in the multigravida who has relaxed abdominal walls and a large amount of amniotic fluid [16].

Since expectant parents may be aware of the complications involved in breech presentations or may be alerted to the fact that something is unusual based on the extra-careful monitoring of the woman's condition, their anxiety level will be high. Frequent explanations and reassurance regarding the status of the fetus and the woman are important psychologic elements of nursing actions in this situation.

TRANSVERSE LIE

Assessment and Intervention. If the fetus is in a transverse lie, the acromial process of the shoulder is commonly the presenting part (Fig. 19-4). The etiology

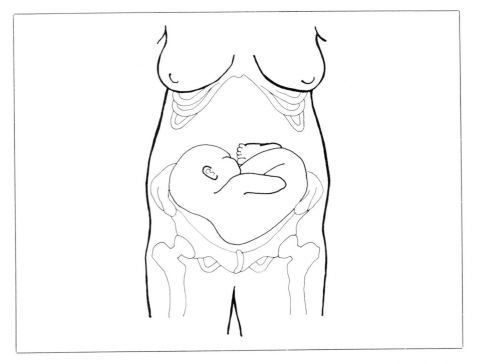

Figure 19-4. Transverse lie with shoulder presenting.

of this presentation is any condition that prevents engagement of the fetal head in the mother's pelvis or that permits the fetus to be very mobile. Placenta previa is a contributing factor in about 27 percent of the cases, and other factors are the same as those contributing to the face and brow presentations.

With the fetus in a transverse lie, the uterus is a transverse ovoid. Nothing is felt over the inlet and nothing is in the inlet. The head may be felt on one side of the uterus, the breech on the other. X-ray or ultrasound studies verify the diagnosis and often reveal the prolapse of a fetal arm or elbow. External version is often attempted to convert either one of the fetal poles to the inlet, but the fetus often reverts to the transverse position and a cesarean delivery must be performed.

The prognosis for the mother and fetus is good if the transverse lie is diagnosed early. Unfortunately, it is too frequently discovered late in labor, and the prognosis for both is then considerably worse. The woman is at risk of prolonged labor and uterine rupture. The fetus is at risk for asphyxia, prolapsed cord, and trauma. The prognosis is improved if a cesarean delivery is done, and the classic incision is the one of choice.

COMPOUND PRESENTATION

On rare occasions one of the fetal extremities prolapses alongside the presenting part so that both enter the pelvic cavity at the same time, resulting in a compound presentation. Associated factors that contribute to compound presentation include twinning, prematurity, and an unengaged or persistently high presenting part, with ruptured membranes.

If a hand presents with the vertex, it will usually slip back as the cervix dilates and the fetal head descends. If the head is engaged with the arm down, nothing particular is done, since there is obviously enough room for both. The labor is longer, however, and the mechanisms of descent and rotation may be abnormal.

OVERSIZE INFANT
Assessment and Intervention

Fetal morbidity and mortality are increased significantly in vaginal deliveries when the fetus weighs more than 4,500 grams (10 pounds). During pregnancy the woman's abdomen is usually overdistended, and once her labor begins, it progresses very slowly. The fetal head, which may be more ossified than usual, is less moldable and does not readily engage.

If the fetus's shoulders are very large, the dystocia is apparent immediately after the head is delivered. The woman must bear down strongly, and the excessive abdominal, uterine, and suprasymphyseal pressure applied to deliver the shoulders may cause the rupture of her lower uterine segment. In addition, excessive traction on the infant's neck may result in permanent damage to his brachial plexus, Erb's palsy, the dislocation of his cervical vertebrae, spinal cord damage, or even death. His humerus or clavicle may be fractured (sometimes intentionally) in order to reduce the size of his shoulder girdle.

HYDROCEPHALUS

The skull of the hydrocephalic fetus may hold several liters of cerebrospinal fluid. This condition is commonly diagnosed when the fetal head overrides the pelvis, and it is confirmed by x-ray or ultrasound studies. The large head provides a mechanical obstruction to labor, and as the overdistended lower uterine segment thins, the uterus may rupture. A cesarean delivery is usually done since the large head often makes vaginal delivery impossible. Postpartum hemorrhage from uterine atony or lacerations frequently occurs.

PATHOLOGIC
RETRACTION RING
(BANDL'S RING)

If a prolonged labor is neglected, a palpable ring may develop at the point where the upper and lower uterine segments meet, and the woman's uterus may develop an hourglass shape and is in danger of imminent rupture. As a rule, a cesarean delivery is less hazardous than a vaginal delivery in such cases, and anesthesia is used to provide maximum uterine relaxation.

The woman whose labor reaches this point is understandably exhausted and extremely apprehensive. Her lack of progress contributes to her loss of morale. The fact that she is predisposed to develop a uterine infection from prolonged rupture of membranes, or an electrolyte imbalance from dehydration, should be considered when her care is being planned. Since fetal morbidity and mortality are increased with this condition, it is fortunate that it occurs infrequently in current practice.

UTERINE RUPTURE
Assessment and Intervention

Uterine rupture results in massive hemorrhage. It rarely occurs during pregnancy but may happen during labor, when it may be spontaneous or traumatic, in an intact uterus or in one previously incised. Uterine rupture occurs eight or nine times as often in multiparas as in nulliparas.

In the past 20 years the overall incidence of uterine rupture has remained relatively constant, while its causes have changed. There has been a decrease in those caused by obstetric trauma, since procedures such as x-ray pelvimetry have indicated a sound basis for not allowing an unproductive labor to continue. In practice today, many hazardous maneuvers, such as manual dilation of the cervix and internal podalic version, have been largely eliminated. As a result, the number of cesarean deliveries being performed has increased, so that a previous cesarean scar is becoming a more frequent cause of uterine rupture.

The most frequent cause of spontaneous rupture of an intact uterus is labor that is obstructed by any of the conditions discussed previously. Another cause of uterine rupture is the use of oxytocin, which may stimulate violent uterine contractions, causing rupture at a point where the uterine wall happens to be weak. Traumatic rupture of the uterus may be caused by internal podalic version, application of forceps and extraction of the fetus before the cervical os is completely dilated, or excessive fundal pressure to deliver a large baby.

Spontaneous uterine rupture is likely to begin in the lower uterine segment and extend into the body. The onset is usually sudden and without warning, although in prolonged or obstructed labor the woman experiences increasing tenderness over her lower uterus. Her contractions may be tetanic, and she may reflexively support her uterus with her hand during each contraction. Her mouth may be dry and she may have the desire to void frequently. Her respirations and pulse will be rapid. When the uterus ruptures, she will have a sudden, stabbing abdominal pain, with the sensation of something giving way. She may or may not have vaginal bleeding, but she will begin to appear to be in shock due to intraperitoneal hemorrhage. Contractions and pain cease when the uterus ruptures; the fetal heart tones disappear, and the fetus may become palpable in the abdominal cavity if the rupture is complete. If the rupture is incomplete, the uterine muscle is torn but the peritoneum remains intact and a hematoma develops.

Uterine rupture can be prevented by careful evaluation of the woman's pelvis before labor and by avoiding a prolonged labor once it begins. Once the uterus has ruptured, it may be repaired or an immediate abdominal hysterectomy may be necessary, depending on the extent of the tear. If the uterus is repaired, the woman is advised to have elective cesarean births with future pregnancies.

Fetal prognosis is very poor unless delivery can be accomplished immediately. Maternal prognosis is grave, especially if the rupture is traumatic. Although associated maternal mortality used to be close to 25 percent, it is now about 5 to 10 percent. This improvement is due to improved obstetric practice, antibiotics, blood transfusions, and earlier recognition and treatment.

PRECIPITATE LABOR
Assessment

A precipitate labor is one that lasts less than 3 hours from the time of the first contraction to delivery of the baby. It is also defined as one in which cervical dilatation in the active phase is greater than 5 centimeters per hour in nulliparas or greater than 10 centimeters per hour in multiparas. Obviously, it is abnormally fast and tumultuous. When the maternal soft tissues offer little resistance and the uterus contracts strongly and frequently, both fetal and maternal trauma may result. Since the uterus relaxes for only a short time between contractions, the intervillous blood flow may be impaired enough to cause fetal hypoxia. Rapid passage of the fetal head through the birth canal may result in intracranial hemorrhage. Because a precipitate labor may be unexpected and thus the delivery may be unattended, the baby may not receive necessary resuscitation. The woman may have cervical and vaginal lacerations as well as rupture of her lower uterine segment. In most instances, however, the trauma is restricted to her perineum, labia minora, urethra, and clitoris. As a result of excessively strong contractions, she may develop an amniotic fluid embolism.

Intervention   Women with a history of precipitate labor are often induced electively so that their labor may be somewhat controlled. Amniotomy is commonly done to initiate contractions, which are then carefully monitored along with the fetal heart rate. Because these contractions can be very stressful and because the woman's condition may change very rapidly, do not leave her alone. Sometimes anesthesia (e.g., pudendal block) is administered to decrease the strength of contractions or to abolish the woman's perineal reflex, thus preventing her from pushing with her abdominal muscles at delivery. No attempt should be made to hold back the fetal head.

Because the passage through the birth canal is so rapid and stressful, evaluate the baby very carefully for any injury immediately after birth, and inform other staff of the stresses the infant has undergone. Observe the mother carefully for signs of hemorrhage from undetected or unrepaired lacerations.

INJURIES TO THE BIRTH CANAL
Assessment and Intervention

Vulvar lacerations occur commonly in nulliparas and in many multiparas. They appear most frequently around the vulvar orifice, in the vagina, and around the urethra but are seldom deep enough to cause serious problems.

Some lacerations of the perineal body occur in most first deliveries, but these are less important than deeper tears of the pelvic floor (levator ani and its fascia). If they are unrepaired or improperly repaired, the woman's pelvic supports will not be as strong, leading to the development of a rectocele or cystocele, which will require surgical repair at a later date. When these deeper structures are torn, the skin often remains intact, thus giving the clinician a false sense of security.

The cervix undergoes some injury during almost every labor. This can result from too rapid or forceful dilation or from very large fetal diameters. Many times cervical lacerations are not discovered until after delivery, when an unusual amount of bright red blood is noticed. Repair of the lacerations prevents further blood loss.

AMNIOTIC FLUID EMBOLISM
Assessment

Amniotic fluid embolism is a major cause of the few maternal deaths that occur during labor. Predisposing factors include tetanic uterine contractions and multiparity, especially if the fetus is very large. Sudden dyspnea, chest pain, tachycardia, hypotension, and cyanosis are the initial signs and symptoms, and the woman may die within 30 minutes after the symptoms appear. If she survives the initial shock, she may still die from postpartum hemorrhage.

It is believed that the particulate matter in amniotic fluid causes embolization of the pulmonary arterioles and capillaries. In addition, since amniotic fluid has thromboplastic qualities, death may result from extensive disseminated intravascular clotting (DIC) and subsequent postpartum hemorrhage.

The generally accepted route by which amniotic fluid enters the woman's circulation is through rupture of membranes in the upper uterine segment, with escape of the fluid through the vessels of the placental site. This process can be accentuated if uterine contractions are especially forceful and if conditions exist in which the myometrial vessels are exposed, such as marginal placental separation, uterine rupture, or hysterotomy.

Intervention   The amniotic fluid may also enter the maternal circulation through the endocervical veins, which are normally torn in labor as the cervix dilates. Probably the most significant contributing factor is a very forceful and rapid labor; the improper administration of oxytocic medications may be responsible for this. Vigorous and immediate treatment will help some mothers to survive by relieving their respiratory distress, preventing the development of or correcting a coagulation problem, and maintaining their normal blood volume. This will require oxygen administration and fresh whole blood and fibrinogen for treatment of DIC, and plasma and intravenous fluids to combat decreased blood volume. The fetus is in great danger and should be delivered as soon as possible.

INVERSION OF THE UTERUS
Assessment and Intervention

Inversion of the uterus is a very rare complication of the third stage of labor. In this condition the corpus virtually turns inside out. It usually occurs after the distended uterus empties very suddenly and some forceful pressure or traction is placed on the uncontracted fundus, such as from improper placental expression or traction on the umbilical cord. Maternal symptoms of shock and profuse hemorrhage are readily apparent. Generally, manual replacement of the uterus to its normal position with the woman under deep anesthesia is successful if the inversion is recognized at the time it occurs. Following its replacement, an intravenous drip of oxytocin helps to keep the uterus well contracted and in position. Blood volume is replaced, intake and output and vital signs are monitored, and an indwelling urinary catheter is inserted.

CORD PRESENTATION
Assessment

In approximately 1 of every 200 deliveries, the umbilical cord prolapses in front of or alongside the presenting part (funic presentation). The presentation may be occult (at or near the mother's pelvis but not reachable on vaginal examination) or prolapsed (in the vagina or even outside the vulva following membrane rupture).

Anything that favors an abnormal adaptation of the presenting part to the lower uterine segment or prevents head engagement will contribute to the incidence of funic presentations. These factors include a contracted pelvis, placenta previa, an unusually long cord, multiple pregnancy, hydramnios, or breech presentation.

The actual course of the woman's labor is not affected by cord presentations. However, for the fetus the situation is life-threatening; about one-sixth do not survive. Compression of the cord between the presenting part and the bony pelvis greatly restricts the flow of oxygen to the fetus. If the cord is exposed to cold room air, there may be a reflex constriction of umbilical blood vessels with the same end result.

Many times cord presentations are diagnosed by an irregular fetal heart rate pattern, with periodic bradycardia of *variable* duration and *variable* association with maternal contractions.

Intervention   If the woman's pelvis is contracted or if an immediate vaginal delivery is impossible, an immediate cesarean delivery is done. While preparations are being made, the woman is given oxygen and is placed in the Trendelenburg, elevated Sims', or knee-chest position. If the cord is outside the vulva and the fetus is alive and viable, the fetal head may be held up out of the woman's pelvis by the clinician's hand in her vagina. Attempts to replace the cord are of questionable value, since handling the cord may cause spasm of the umbilical vessels. In the home, a protruding cord should be covered with clean, wet dressings soaked in a mild salt solution, the woman's hips elevated, and she should be immediately transported to the hospital.

It is easy to understand that cord presentation can be a very frightening experience for the prospective parents. The nurse who remains by the couple's side, calmly and efficiently providing the care necessary for their baby's safety, should encourage them to verbalize their fears and can reassure them that everything is being done to ensure a favorable outcome.

It is interesting to note that formerly, when a woman's membranes ruptured early and the fetal presenting part was high, she was always kept prone in the belief that the upright position would predispose the cord to prolapse. With the woman in the standing position, however, the presenting part actually dips farther below the pelvic inlet than when she is recumbent; theoretically, then, this leaves less room for the cord to prolapse. It would seem that the more rational approach would be to encourage ambulation in such a woman, providing she does not have a shoulder presentation or true cephalopelvic disproportion. Also remember, whenever a woman's membranes rupture, take the fetal heart tones for a full minute and observe the fetal response for signs of cord prolapse or cord compression.

OPERATIVE OBSTETRICS
Forceps Deliveries

ASSESSMENT

Forceps are used in instances in which the life or well-being of the woman or fetus may be compromised, and when the danger may be relieved by more rapid delivery. This occurs in cases of uterine dysfunction in which oxytocin has been ineffective and the fetal head is well down in the pelvis. It may also be indicated in eclampsia, heart disease, acute pulmonary edema, hemorrhage from placental abruption, maternal exhaustion, and intrapartum infection. Excessive analgesics and certain types of anesthesia interfere with the woman's voluntary expulsive efforts, increasing the number of forceps deliveries. Forceps deliveries also are performed for fetal indications, including cord prolapse, abruptio placentae, excess pressure on the fetal head from arrested descent, and fetal distress.

Forceps are designed for extracting or rotating the fetal head. They consist of two pieces: a right blade, which is slipped into the right side of the mother's pelvis, and a left blade, which is slipped into the left side. Each piece consists of a blade, handle, shank, and lock. The blades have two curves: that on the outer edge conforms to the curve of the birth canal (pelvic curve), while the inside of the blade conforms to the curve of the fetal head (cephalic curve). The blade may be solid or have a window; the latter type is referred to as *fenestrated*. The two blades articulate at the lock, which is designed to prevent excessive pressure on the fetal head.

While there are more than 600 types of forceps, there are only two major classifications of classic forceps (Fig. 19-5). The Simpson type has separated shanks and is used to extract fetuses with elongated, molded heads. This type is used commonly with nulliparas who have long labors; the DeLee forceps is an example. The second major type is the Elliot forceps, which has overlapping shanks and is used to deliver infants with unmolded, rounder heads. This type is

Figure 19-5. The classic types of forceps. A. Simpson forceps. B. Elliot forceps. C. Forceps blade, at angle to show fenestration.

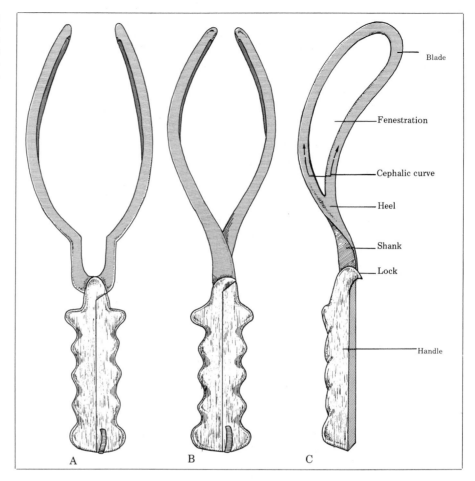

used commonly with multiparas who have briefer labors; the Tucker-McLean forceps is an example. In addition to these major types, there are also special forceps. The Piper forceps is used to deliver the aftercoming head in a breech presentation. Kielland and Barton forceps are used to rotate the head from a transverse or occipital position to an anterior position. Kielland forceps commonly are used to deliver women with anthropoid pelves, while Barton forceps are designed to be used in women with flat pelves with the fetal head in a transverse position.

Conditions for a forceps delivery include that: the fetal head be engaged; the fetus be in a vertex presentation with the chin anterior; the position of the head is known; there is no cephalopelvic disproportion; the cervix is completely dilated and the membranes ruptured; and that the mother's bladder and preferably also her rectum are empty. Anesthesia is required. When these criteria are met, a low or midforceps delivery may be effected.

INTERVENTION

The delivery is classified as low or midforceps according to the level and position of the fetal head when the blades are applied. In a low forceps delivery, the forceps are applied after the fetal head has reached the perineal floor, with the sagittal suture in the anterior-posterior diameter of the outlet. When the head is on the perineal floor, a low forceps delivery, preceded by episiotomy, is a simple, safe procedure, requiring only gentle traction. It is usually performed when the mother has insufficient expulsive forces or abnormally great perineal resistance.

In midforceps deliveries, the forceps are used to grasp the fetal head after engagement has taken place but before the head reaches the perineal floor. Any forceps delivery requiring rotation, regardless of the station, is considered a midforceps delivery. Since the fetal head is higher in the pelvis before rotation takes place, greater traction is required.

Some compression of the fetal head is inevitable. The widest dimension between the two blades of the forceps when they are articulated is 7.5 centimeters, while the biparietal diameter of the average term infant's head is 9.5 centimeters. Compression can be harmful since circulation may be impaired, causing asphyxia and hemorrhage, in addition to possible direct injury to the cranial bones, tentorium, falx, vessels, and brain. It should be remembered that the diameters of the fetal head are reduced during forceps delivery and during spontaneous delivery by overriding of the cranial bones. Fetuses vary in their ability to withstand compression, full-term infants being able to withstand greater compression than preterm infants. The physician avoids compression by placing a finger between the handles of the forceps.

In high forceps applications, the forceps are applied to the fetal head before engagement has occurred. This procedure had a place when cesarean delivery was dangerous, but it is not used today.

When a forceps delivery has been decided on, the forceps are slipped into the right and left sides of the woman's pelvis. The physician then slides two fingers along the forceps blades to examine the application and to ensure that no cervical tissue has been grasped. Explain to the mother that she will feel pressure but should not feel pain. Keep her informed at each step in the procedure, and help her to breathe and relax as much as possible to avoid pushing. Monitor the fetal heart rate. When the blades are on correctly, the handles are held in the physician's hand, and gentle, intermittent, horizontal traction is exerted with each contraction until the perineum begins to bulge. As soon as the vulva is distended by the occiput, the handles are gradually elevated, eventually pointing upward as the parietal bones emerge.

Occasionally, the Scanzoni maneuver is used for posterior presentation. The fetal head is rotated anteriorly with forceps. Then, since the position of the forceps is not one in which the fetal head could be extracted, the forceps are removed and another pair is applied for extraction.

The perinatal mortality associated with forceps delivery depends on the condition of the fetus and on the station of the head during delivery. There usually is no mortality when the head is at or very near the perineum. Use of forceps at higher stations of the head is attended by perinatal loss or damage in direct proportion to the height of the skull. Examine the newborn carefully after delivery since he may sustain injuries to the face, eyes, and skull. Evaluate the mother's condition carefully following delivery since she may sustain injuries from a difficult forceps delivery, including cervical laceration and injury to the bladder, rectum, or vagina. She may also experience hemorrhage or infection as a result of the trauma. There are usually few complications following low forceps delivery.

Vacuum Extraction   With the use of a vacuum extractor, suction applied to the fetal head creates an artificial caput within the suction cup and allows adequate traction for delivery of the infant's head (Fig. 19-6). This method is used mainly in dysfunctional labor, fetal distress, maternal cardiopulmonary disease, hypertensive disorders of pregnancy, abruptio placentae, and fetal malpositions. It has the advantage over forceps of avoiding the use of an instrument that would occupy space between the fetal head and maternal pelvis; vacuum extraction carries less potential risk of damage to the infant.

This method is not used extensively in most of the United States, perhaps because of reports of fetal damage, including lacerations of the scalp, cephalhematomas, intracranial hemorrhage, and infant mortality. The mother may suffer lacerations and should be observed postpartally for hemorrhage. In Europe the vacuum extractor is more widely used and is felt to be superior to forceps on the basis of comparisons of perinatal mortality and morbidity of infants and mothers.

Cesarean Birth   Legend holds that Julius Caesar was born by cesarean delivery. In his time, however, and as late as the seventeenth century, the operation is believed to have been invariably fatal to the mother, even though Caesar's mother lived for many years after his birth. As described in ancient mythology, birth in this extraordinary manner was believed to confer supernatural powers and elevate those so born above the ordinary level of humanity to the heroic level.

The extraordinary maternal mortality (85 percent in 1865) continued until Max Sanger, in 1882, introduced the technique of suturing the uterine wall. This reduced the death rate due to hemorrhage, but generalized peritonitis remained a major cause of maternal death. Today, for cesarean deliveries performed by competent practitioners the maternal mortality is 0.2 percent or less [14].

Figure 19-6. Delivery using the vacuum extractor.

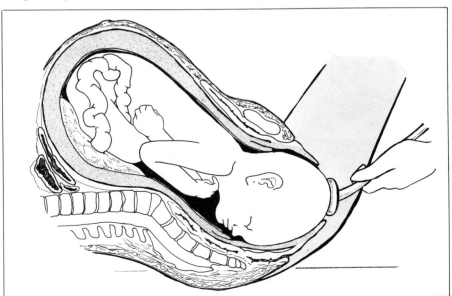

During the 1970s, the cesarean birth rate in the United States increased about threefold, from 5.5 percent in 1970 to 15.2 percent in 1978, and appears to be continuing to increase [2]. In response to the increase in cesarean births, the National Institutes of Health held a conference to address issues that have arisen concerning cesarean childbirth.

They cited many factors to account for the increase in cesarean birth rates. In the 1960s, the decline in the overall birth rate was accompanied by an increasing emphasis on the health of the fetus. With couples choosing to have fewer children, greater attention was given to favorable pregnancy outcome. There were societal demands for prevention of death of the fetus and neonate and for improvement in the quality of life for the newborn survivors. The nation's infant mortality rate was used as a yardstick of the quality of health care, and great emphasis was placed on improving infant survival. Advances in medical care—such as improved anesthetic techniques, blood products and blood transfusions, and better medical control of maternal illnesses such as diabetes, hypertension, and heart disease—made maternal death from cesarean childbirth a rare occurrence. The safer the procedure became, the easier it became to decide to perform the operation. Thus, cesarean delivery was one approach applied to try to improve fetal outcome [2].

But have the increased number of cesarean deliveries improved fetal outcomes? The NIH panel concluded that there is insufficient data to draw this conclusion; in particular, there is no morbidity data available and no data on fetal brain damage difference. They did offer several recommendations, however. In reviewing the cesarean rates for dystocia, the task force reported that there seems to be no survival advantage for babies delivered by cesarean rather than vaginally because of difficult labor, but that morbidity data are not available. It recommended that physicians consider measures such as sedating the woman, stimulating her uterine contractions with oxytocin, or having her walk about to facilitate labor.

In reviewing the cesarean rates for breech deliveries, the task force concluded that full-term fetuses in breech presentation can be delivered vaginally when the fetuses weigh less than 8 pounds, the physician is experienced in breech deliveries, the woman has a normal pelvis, and the fetus's head is not bent back. For premature breech babies, it is not clear whether vaginal or cesarean deliveries are safer.

The task force also recommended delivering women vaginally following a primary low-segment cesarean operation if staff and facilities are adequate. This approach would decrease the number of secondary cesarean operations.

In evaluating cesarean deliveries for reasons of fetal distress, the task force felt that it had insufficient data on fetal mortality and morbidity to recommend decreasing the number of cesareans performed for this reason.

The group also noted that with the increasing popularity of prepared childbirth classes, nonmedicated childbirth, the presence of husbands in delivery rooms, home births, and hospital birthing centers, many couples look forward to idealized vaginal deliveries and feel cheated and disappointed by cesarean deliveries. The task force recommended that childbirth classes discuss the possibility of cesareans and that hospitals consider allowing fathers in operating rooms to observe cesarean deliveries. The group also recommended that hospitals reconsider the practice of routinely separating healthy babies delivered by cesarean from their parents so that the babies reportedly can be observed in special nurseries.

ASSESSMENT

Cesarean birth, the delivery of a fetus through an incision in the abdominal and uterine wall, is a major surgical procedure. It has been performed historically when a woman cannot deliver vaginally without seriously jeopardizing her life or health or that of the fetus. Cesarean birth is also performed if a woman has had a previous cesarean delivery or other extensive uterine or vaginal surgery. It is also necessary in cases of cephalopelvic disproportion, fetal distress, malpresentation, obstructive tumors, and certain chronic disorders, such as diabetes or hypertension.

While previous cesarean birth has been the most common indication for cesarean operations, not all women who have had a previous cesarean have deliveries this way. The baby may be delivered vaginally if the reason for the original cesarean operation no longer exists (e.g., an abruptio placentae), if the previous cesarean operation was in the lower uterine segment, and if the woman is monitored very carefully during labor, with standby facilities for an emergency operation if it becomes necessary. Cesarean birth is avoided if the fetus is dead or if the woman has a full stomach or an upper respiratory infection, is in ketoacidosis or cardiac decompensation, or has recently convulsed.

In the United States, the diagnoses having the largest effect on the increase in the cesarean birth rate between 1970 and 1978 are dystocia, repeat cesarean, breech presentation, and fetal distress (Table 19-2).

There are four types of cesarean operations: classic cesarean, low-segment cesarean, extraperitoneal cesarean, and cesarean hysterectomy (Fig. 19-7). The low-segment cesarean operation is the one most commonly performed. The incision is made either transversely or vertically in the lower uterine segment; since this is a fibrous rather than a muscular area, there is less chance of hemorrhage, subsequent rupture infection, or postpartum adhesion formation. The surgery takes longer than the classic cesarean, but the skin scar is often hidden by the hair on the mons.

Speed is the main advantage of the classic approach, in which a vertical incision is made into the upper portion of the uterus. Since this is a muscular part of the uterus, there is a greater chance of hemorrhage, rupture, hematoma, adhesion formation, poor healing, and febrile morbidity. This method may be

Table 19-2. Diagnoses Resulting in Cesarean Birth

Indications	Percent of Cesareans Performed for This Indication (1978)	Percent of Contribution to Rise in Cesarean Rate
Dystocia	31	30
Repeat cesarean	31	25–30
Breech presentation	12	10–15
Fetal distress	5	10–15

Source: National Institutes of Health Consensus Development Conference Summary (0341-132/3553), Vol. 3, No. 6. U.S. Government Printing Office, 1981.

Figure 19-7. A. Low-segment cesarean section with transverse uterine incision into lower uterine segment. B. Classic cesarean section with vertical uterine incision into upper, more muscular portion of the uterus. C. Extraperitoneal cesarean section with vertical uterine incision. Surgeon's fingers separate peritoneum and bladder from uterus.

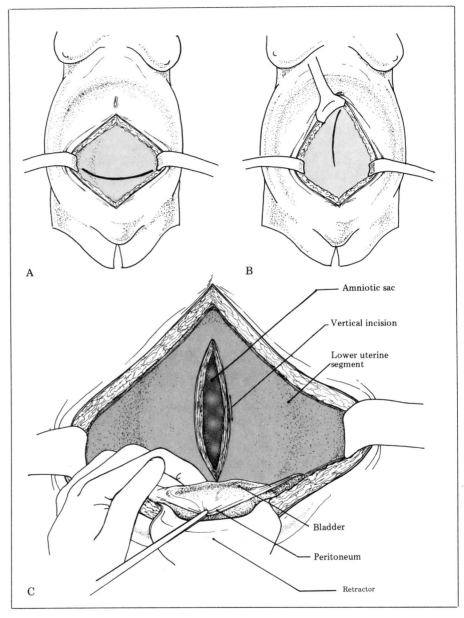

used in emergencies in which rapidity is important or in instances in which the lower uterine segment has tumors, adhesions, or a low-lying placenta.

The incision for the extraperitoneal cesarean section is in the lower uterine segment, after the peritoneum has been dissected away from the uterine wall. The peritoneum is not incised. This method has been used in the past to prevent infection in the uterus from being introduced into the peritoneal cavity. It is a difficult procedure which often results in bladder or ureteral injury and is not commonly used today.

Cesarean hysterectomy may be performed as a method of sterilization after a woman has had several cesarean operations. It also may be performed if the woman's uterus fails to contract, as with a Couvelaire uterus, or in placenta previa, when bleeding is uncontrolled. After delivery of the baby and the placenta, the woman's uterus is removed.

INTERVENTION

Preparing a woman for a cesarean operation involves a number of measures. Both she and her partner will need assessment, information, and reassurance regarding the surgery itself. They need to be clear on the reasons for the surgery, what can be expected to happen, whether the father or support person is permitted to be with the mother during surgery, and what the mother can expect following surgery.

If the cesarean birth is planned, there will be ample time to prepare the couple and to teach the mother how to splint her abdominal muscles, cough and deep breathe, and the activities that she will need to do following surgery. There will also be time to have the couple share their feelings regarding a cesarean birth and what it means to them. Often this method of birth engenders feelings on the part of the woman of having been cheated of participation in a vaginal delivery or of having failed in her reproductive function. According to one study the woman may also be concerned about her body image and the accompanying scar following the surgery and her ability to fulfill her mothering role [3]. The father may have guilt feelings because he impregnated the woman and sees himself as the cause of her pain or discomfort. The authors' clinical observations suggest that women having their first cesarean delivery seem to focus their fears and concerns on the fetus's well-being whereas women having a second cesarean delivery express more fear and concern about themselves and a fear of dying. These observations require formal data collection for confirmation.

Just as couples have fantasies of the ideal child, they also tend to have preconceived ideas regarding their role and actions during the labor and delivery of their child. You need to understand their expectations, and when there is a disparity between those expectations and the reality of their upcoming experience, you need to help them work toward resolution of possible disappointments. As client advocate, once you know the couple's desires and expectations regarding the birth experience, you can help them achieve some of their original goals when the unexpected occurs. These may include the father being with the mother during surgery, the father and mother holding and becoming acquainted with their newborn almost immediately after its birth and stabilization, or the parents being together during the mother's immediate recovery period. If the cesarean birth is an emergency, you will need to help the couple work through many of their feelings after the birth. Even in this instance many of their original desires and goals may still be achieved.

The nursing research of Cranley et al. [4], Fawcett [5], and Marut and Mercer [11] indicates that couples experiencing cesarean birth report negative responses to childbirth. Marut and Mercer note that in addition the cesarean mothers displayed greater hesitancy in naming their infants and tended to view their deliveries as abnormal and having a social stigma. Cranley, Hedahl, and Pegg report that women having emergency cesareans have more negative perceptions of the birth than women whose surgery is planned. When the surgical method of delivery is anticipated, however, and when women perceive themselves as having some control over the course of events, their perceptions of giving birth more closely approximate those of women who deliver vaginally. Fawcett reports similar findings.

The use of regional anesthesia and having the husband present at delivery also improves perceptions of the cesarean experience, as does informing the couple of the flow of events surrounding the cesarean delivery. Even when a cesarean birth is necessary, many of the couple's original desires and goals may still be achieved.

Physical preparation of the mother for surgery is also required. Prepare the mother's skin surface by shaving her abdomen from under her breasts to her midthighs. Make sure that blood has been drawn for type and cross match and for hemoglobin and hematocrit if these are not available. Her hemoglobin should be at least 10 and her hematocrit 30, and the results of her urinalysis should indicate no signs of infection. Her vital signs should be within normal limits. Be sure her operative permit has been signed. Preoperative medication usually includes atropine, but do not give a narcotic, since it would cause depression in the infant. As in all pelvic surgery, insert a Foley catheter prior to surgery to keep the woman's bladder deflated. When the surgery is imminent, notify the woman's pediatrician so that he or she may be present to resuscitate the baby if it becomes necessary. Also notify the nursery staff so that they are prepared for the infant's arrival.

Following the surgery and the delivery of the infant, the woman will be given oxytocin to keep her uterus contracted. Monitor her vital signs until they are stable, and monitor the rate and flow of her intravenous fluids. Observe her urine output for volume and for any bleeding that might indicate bladder trauma during surgery. Her urinary output should be 30 milliliters per hour at the minimum. Observe her abdominal incision for signs of bleeding. Gently palpate the height of her fundus and determine if it is well contracted. Observe the character and amount of lochia to determine if it is excessive. Encourage the mother to get out of bed the day following surgery; this improves her circulation, the aeration of her lungs, and her muscle tone as well as lochial drainage. Take her to see her infant and to hold and feed him as soon as possible.

The incidence of respiratory distress is higher in infants born by cesarean delivery than in those delivered vaginally. This may be because of the need to deliver the infant prior to term, or because the thorax is not compressed during delivery and therefore the respiratory tract is not drained of fluids prior to birth. It has been noted that delivery by cesarean eliminates the stress of labor to the infant; thus, his cortisol levels are not raised as are those of infants born vaginally, and the lower cortisol levels may allow the infant's lungs to be less ready to aerate at birth [13, 2].

Case Study   Sarah Morton

As Sarah's primary nurse, develop a plan of care for the Mortons, including your interventions aimed at helping them through this emergency and through the transitional postpartum period. Each of you will develop your own approach and style in providing care to laboring couples. Applying the nursing process to the outline following the case study will serve as a guide in organizing your approach to the couple during labor and delivery.

Sarah (age 27) and Greg (age 29) Morton moved to the area a little more than a year ago from the Midwest with their 4-year-old son, Mark. Mark was born at home aided by a nurse midwife. The Mortons chose a home delivery in part for financial reasons and in part because they wanted the family togetherness that it provided. They were very pleased with the experience and with their healthy son.

The Mortons moved to their current urban setting because Greg completed his Ph.D. in geophysics and found a good position in the local public university. Sarah, who completed her Ph.D. in English literature, found a position in one of the small private colleges in the area. Mark is attending a nursery school. All of the Mortons' extended family live on the West Coast.

When Sarah became pregnant again, the Mortons looked for a midwife who would deliver their child in their home. They were unsuccessful. Shortly after their initial search, Greg met an obstetrician in the university faculty club who convinced him that the university hospital could provide all the Mortons were looking for. The hospital had a birthing room where Greg could be with Sarah during the labor and delivery. The obstetrician would deliver Sarah and discharge her in 48 hours if that was their wish.

Sarah had her doubts after visiting the obstetrician but went along with the plan mainly because she felt Greg respected the doctor and his position of power within the university. Sarah's pregnancy was uneventful and both she and Greg attended the hospital's childbirth education classes.

Sarah's labor began one evening after her membranes ruptured. She and Greg went to the hospital. She was admitted but the birthing room was occupied. The physician assured her that she could have almost everything the birthing room offered "except the wallpaper and drapes." He would deliver her in the labor room.

Sarah was in actual labor for 12 hours and had dilated to only 5 centimeters. Her temperature was now 100°F. She refused intravenous fluids. The physician told the Mortons he would like to use fetal monitoring to evaluate the fetal response to Sarah's contractions in light of her progress and her elevated temperature. Sarah and Greg reluctantly agreed, with the understanding that it would be for an hour and no longer. Although tired, Sarah was coping well with her labor and effectively using her breathing techniques.

Twenty minutes after the internal fetal monitor had been in use, the fetal heart rate indicated severe and persistent late decelerations. The leaking amniotic fluid was meconium-stained despite the vertex presentation. After 15 minutes the fetal heart rate baseline was falling, and the physician told the Mortons an emergency cesarean delivery was indicated to deliver a healthy live infant. They were incredulous and now very frightened. They consented after a brief discussion, and the emergency delivery is now about to be performed. Greg will not be allowed to be with Sarah because it is an emergency situation.

Assessment Form			
Assessment	Plan	Intervention	Evaluation

  I. Significant Factors from Pregnancy
      A. Specific problems during current pregnancy
          1. Planned or unplanned
          2. Bleeding
          3. Hypertension
          4. Severe nausea or vomiting
          5. Weight gain
          6. Anemia
          7. Infections
      B. Problems during previous pregnancies
      C. Previous or existing health problems
      D. Childbirth education preparation
          1. Type
          2. Length
          3. Educator
 II. Admission
      A. Gravida, para
      B. EDC
      C. Membranes ruptured, color, amount, odor
      D. Bloody show
      E. Vital signs
          1. Temperature
          2. Pulse
          3. Respirations
      F. Fetal heart rate
      G. Contraction pattern
          1. Duration
          2. Frequency
          3. Intensity
          4. When did contractions begin
          5. Amount of discomfort
      H. Cervical dilation and effacement
      I. Blood type and Rh
      J. Allergies
III. Labor Progress
      A. Physical changes

Assessment Form			
Assessment	Plan	Intervention	Evaluation
1. Vital signs—temperature, blood pressure, pulse, respirations			

1. Vital signs—temperature, blood pressure, pulse, respirations
2. Contraction pattern
   (a) Duration
   (b) Frequency
   (c) Intensity
3. Cervical dilation and effacement
   (a) Normal progress according to normal labor curve (graph)
4. Rupture of membranes, color, amount, odor
5. Fetal heart rate
   (a) Baseline rate
   (b) Variability
   (c) Response to uterine contractions
6. Fetus
   (a) Lie
   (b) Presentation
   (c) Position and rotation
   (d) Station and descent

B. Comfort measures
1. Mother
   (a) Positioning
   (b) Mouth care
   (c) Back rub and sacral counterpressure
   (d) Effleurage
   (e) Pain relief
      (1) Breathing techniques
      (2) Analgesia
      (3) Anesthesia
   (f) Safety precautions
   (g) Hydration
   (h) Urinary elimination
   (i) Perineal hygiene
   (j) Restful environment, soft lights
   (k) Sponge bath (face, neck, upper chest)

Assessment Form			
Assessment	Plan	Intervention	Evaluation

    2. Father or support person

      (a) Rest

      (b) Nutrition

      (c) Relief from support role

C. Woman's expectations regarding:

    1. Labor

    2. Delivery

    3. Type of delivery

    4. Type of anesthesia

    5. Fetal monitoring

    6. Position for delivery

    7. Episiotomy

    8. Support person during labor, delivery

    9. Interaction and time with infant following delivery

  10. Breast or bottle feeding

D. Father's or support person's expectations regarding above

E. Couple's need for information regarding:

    1. Labor

    2. Delivery

    3. Institutional routines and alternatives

    4. Unforeseen emergency measures

F. Behavioral

    1. Coping of mother

    2. Coping of father or support person

    3. Communication pattern, verbal, nonverbal

    4. Dependent functioning

    5. Need for control

    6. Measures to enhance self-esteem of mother and father:

      (a) Information to make informed choices

      (b) Reassurance

      (c) Praise

      (d) Help to achieve expectations and goals

Assessment Form			
Assessment	Plan	Intervention	Evaluation

G. Needs identified by:
  1. Mother
  2. Father
IV. Delivery
  A. Preparation for:
    1. Physical
    2. Informational
  B. Vital signs
  C. Contractions
  D. Fetal heart rate
  E. Mother's ability to push
  F. Parents' ability to:
    1. View delivery process
    2. See and hold newborn
V. Recovery Period
  A. Vital signs
  B. Uterus
    1. Position
      (a) Height in relation to um-
          bilicus
      (b) Midline
      (c) Firmly contracted
  C. Lochia
    1. Amount
    2. Character
  D. Perineum
    1. Episiotomy
    2. Swelling
    3. Ecchymosis
  E. Comfort measures
    1. Adequate warmth
    2. Hydration
    3. Voiding
    4. Relief of:
      (a) Pain
      (b) Nausea or vomiting
    5. Restful environment
  F. Opportunity and privacy to in-
    teract with:
    1. Newborn
    2. Each other
  G. Opportunity to have questions
    answered			

REFERENCES

1. Aladjem, S. *Obstetrical Practice*. St. Louis: Mosby, 1980.
2. *Cesarean Childbirth*. National Institutes of Health Consensus Development Conference Summary. (0341-132/3553), Vol. 3, No. 6, U.S. Government Printing Office, 1981.
3. Clark, A., and Affonso, D. *Childbearing: A Nursing Perspective* (2nd ed.). Philadelphia: Davis, 1979.
4. Cranley, M., Hedahl, K., and Pegg, S. Women's Perceptions of Giving Birth: A Comparison of Vaginal and Cesarean Deliveries. Presented at the Biennial Convention of Sigma Theta Tau, Minneapolis, Minnesota, November 4, 1981.
5. Fawcett, J. Needs of cesarean birth parents. *Journal of Obstetric, Gynecologic and Neonatal Nursing* 10:372, 1981.
6. Friedman, E. A., and Kroll, B. Computer analysis of labor progression v. effect of fetal presentation and position. *Journal of Reproductive Medicine* 8:117, 1972.
7. Greenhill, J. P., and Friedman, E. A. *Biological Principles and Modern Practice of Obstetrics*. Philadelphia: Saunders, 1974.
8. Hemminki, E., and Starfield, B. Prevention and treatment of premature labor by drugs: Review of controlled clinical trials. *British Journal of Obstetrics and Gynecology* 85:411, 1978.
9. Johnson, G. *Oxytocics for the Induction of Labor*. White Plains, N.Y.: The March of Dimes Birth Defects Foundation, 1981.
10. Lauersen, N., and Wilson, K. How to treat premature labor. *The Female Patient* 4:91, 1977.
11. Marut, J., and Mercer, R. Comparison of primiparas' perceptions of vaginal and cesarean birth. *Nursing Research* 28:260, 1979.
12. Niswander, K. R., and Patterson, R. J. Hazards of elective induction of labor. *Obstetrics and Gynecology* 22:228, 1963.
13. Pokoly, T. B. The role of cortisol in human parturition. *American Journal of Obstetrics and Gynecology* 117:549, 1973.
14. Pritchard, J., and MacDonald, P. *Williams Obstetrics* (16th ed.). New York: Appleton-Century-Crofts, 1980.
15. Ranney, B. The gentle art of external cephalic version. *American Journal of Obstetrics and Gynecology* 116:239, 1973.
16. Reid, D., Ryan, K., and Benirschke, K. *Principles and Management of Human Reproduction*. Philadelphia: Saunders, 1972.
17. Schwarz, R., Beliyan, J., Cifuentes, J., Cuadro, J., Marques, M., and Caldeyro-Barcia, R. Fetal and maternal monitoring in spontaneous labors and in elective inductions. *American Journal of Obstetrics and Gynecology* 120:356, 1974.
18. Shepherd, J., Pearce, J., and Sims, C. Induction of labor using prostaglandin E_2 pessaries. *British Medical Journal* 2:108, 1979.
19. Thornfeldt, R., et al. The effect of glucocorticoids on the maturation of premature lung membranes. *American Journal of Obstetrics and Gynecology* 131:143, 1978.

FURTHER READING

Affonso, D., and Stichler, J. Cesarean birth: Women's reactions. *American Journal of Nursing* 80:468, 1980.
Applegate, J., Haverkamp, A., Orleans, M., and Taylor, C. Electronic fetal monitoring: Implications for obstetrical nursing. *Nursing Research* 28:369, 1979.
Babson, S. G., Pernoll, M. L., and Benda, G. I. *Diagnosis and Management of the Fetus and Neonate at Risk: A Guide for Team Care* (4th ed.). St. Louis: Mosby, 1979.
Barden, T., Peter, J., and Merkatz, I. Ritodrine hydrochloride: A betamimetic agent for use in preterm labor. *Obstetrics and Gynecology* 56:1, 1980.
Berkowitz, R. L., et al. The relationship between premature rupture of the membranes and the respiratory distress syndrome. *American Journal of Obstetrics and Gynecology* 131:503, 1978.
Boyd, S., and Mahon, P. The family-centered cesarean delivery. *American Journal of Maternal-Child Nursing* 5:176, 1980.
Brazy, J. E., and Pupkin, M. J. Effects of maternal isoxsuprine administration on preterm infants. *Journal of Pediatrics* 94:444, 1979.
Britton, G. Early mother-infant contact and infant temperature stabilization. *Journal of Obstetric, Gynecologic and Neonatal Nursing* 9:84, 1980.
Caire, J. Are current rates of cesarean justified? *Southern Medical Journal* 71:571, 1978.
Carmack, B., and Corwin, T. Nursing care of the schizophrenic maternity patient during labor. *American Journal of Maternal-Child Nursing* 5:107, 1980.

Cogan, R., and Edmunds, E. P. The unkindest cut. *Contemporary Obstetrics Gynecology* 9:55, 1977.

Cohen, W. Influence of the duration of second stage labor on perinatal outcome and puerperal morbidity. *Obstetrics and Gynecology* 49:266, 1977.

Csapo, A. I., and Herczeg, J. Arrest of premature labor by isoxsuprine. *American Journal of Obstetrics and Gynecology* 129:482, 1977.

Danforth, D. *Obstetrics and Gynecology.* Hagerstown, Md.: Harper & Row, 1977.

Epstein, M. F., et al. Neonatal hypoglycemia after beta-sympathomimetic tocolytic therapy. *Journal of Pediatrics* 94:449, 1979.

Friedman, E., et al. Dysfunctional labor. XII: Long term effects on infant. *American Journal of Obstetrics and Gynecology* 127:779, 1977.

Friedman, E., and Sachtleben, M. R. Station of the fetal presenting part. VI: Arrest of descent in nulliparas. *Obstetrics and Gynecology* 47:129, 1976.

Gardner, S. The mother as incubator—After delivery. *Journal of Obstetric, Gynecologic and Neonatal Nursing* 8:174, 1979.

Hart, G. Maternal attitudes in prepared and unprepared cesarean deliveries. *Journal of Obstetric, Gynecologic and Neonatal Nursing* 9:243, 1980.

Heath, D. Freedom of choice for cesarean parents—Vaginal birth after cesarean. *International Childbirth Education Association News* 20:3, 1981.

Hedahl, K. Cesarean birth: A real family affair. *American Journal of Nursing* 80:471, 1980.

Hill, S., and Shronk, L. The effect of early parent-infant contact on newborn body temperature. *Journal of Obstetric, Gynecologic and Neonatal Nursing* 8:287, 1979.

Hobel, C. Problem-oriented risk assessment during labor. *Contemporary Obstetrics and Gynecology* 8:120, 1976.

Hodnett, E. Patient control during labor: Effects of two types of fetal monitors. *Journal of Obstetric, Gynecologic and Neonatal Nursing* 11:94, 1982.

Hott, J. Best laid plans: Pre- and postpartum comparison of self and spouse in primiparous Lamaze couples who share delivery and those who do not. *Nursing Research* 29:20, 1980.

Johnson, J. Teaching self-hypnosis in pregnancy, labor and delivery. *American Journal of Maternal-Child Nursing* 5:98, 1980.

Kauppila, A., et al. Effects of ritodrine and isoxsuprine with or without dexamethasone during late pregnancy. *Obstetrics and Gynecology* 51:288, 1978.

Kennel, J. H., and Trause, M. A. Helping parents cope with perinatal death. *Contemporary Obstetrics and Gynecology* 12:53, 1978.

Kochenour, N. The management of breech presentations. *PCC News* 3:32, 1977.

Miller, J. M., et al. Premature labor and premature rupture of the membranes. *American Journal of Obstetrics and Gynecology* 132:1, 1978.

Nicolls, E., Corke, B., and Ostheimer, G. Epidural anesthesia for the woman in labor. *American Journal of Nursing* 81:1826, 1981.

Niebyl, J. R., et al. The pharmacologic inhibition of premature labor. *Obstetrical and Gynecological Survey* 33:507, 1978.

Ryden, G. Effect of salbutamol and terbutaline in the management of premature labor. *Acta Obstetricia et Gynecologica Scandinavica* 56:293, 1977.

Saylor, D. E. Understanding presurgical anxiety. *Association of Operating Room Nurses* 22:624, 1975.

Shannon-Babitz, M. Addressing the needs of fathers during labor and delivery. *American Journal of Maternal-Child Nursing* 4:378, 1979.

Shnider, S. Choice of anesthesia for labor and delivery. *Obstetrics and Gynecology* 58:24s, 1981.

Spellacy, W. N., et al. The acute effects of ritodrine infusion on maternal metabolism: Measurements of levels of glucose, insulin, glucagon, triglycerides, cholesterol, placental lactogen and chorionic gonadotrophin. *American Journal of Obstetrics and Gynecology* 131(6):637, 1978.

Stichler, J., and Affonso, D. Cesarean birth. *American Journal of Nursing* 80:466, 1980.

Stubblefield, P. G. Pulmonary edema occurring after therapy with dexamethasone and terbutaline for premature labor: A case report. *American Journal of Obstetrics and Gynecology* 132:341, 1978.

Vadurro, J., and Butts, P. Reducing anxiety and pain of childbirth through hypnosis. *American Journal of Nursing* 82:620, 1982.

Wagner, P. Continuous fetal tissue pH monitoring. *Journal of Obstetric, Gynecologic and Neonatal Nursing* 10:164, 1981.

Wallace, R. L., et al. Inhibition of premature labor by terbutaline. *Obstetrics and Gynecology* 51:387, 1978.

Young, B. K., et al. Intravenous dexamethasone for prevention of neonatal respiratory distress: A prospective controlled study. *American Journal of Obstetrics and Gynecology* 138:203, 1980.

Young, D. Policy reversal for vaginal delivery after cesarean. *International Childbirth Education Association News* 21:1, 1982.

Chapter 20 Complications During the Postpartum Period

PUERPERAL
INFECTION A puerperal infection is an infection of the genital tract that appears in the postpartum period, although the invasion of organisms may have occurred during labor. It remains a serious problem today despite the use of antibiotics and is one cause of maternal death. Clinicians and researchers attribute the problem to the evolution of resistant organisms, the sensitivity that some women have developed to antibiotic drugs, and a periodic relaxation of aseptic technique and preventive care by health care workers who have come to rely too heavily on antibiotics to combat the organisms; historically this cavalier attitude has been one of the major contributing factors in puerperal infection.

Prior to the mid-nineteenth century, it was commonplace for medical students and physicians returning from cadaver dissection to attend women in labor without so much as washing their hands. No precautions were taken when examining more than one woman in labor, even when some were already infected. The reasons postulated for the high maternal mortality in those days (often between 10 and 20 percent) were numerous, ranging from retained lochia to an act of Divine Providence. It was not until the work of Holmes, Semmelweis, and Pasteur demonstrated the etiology of puerperal or childbed fever to the satisfaction of the medical community that changes were effected in caring for women in labor.

Oliver Wendell Holmes, in 1843, read a paper before the Boston Society for Medical Improvement entitled "The Contagiousness of Puerperal Fever." In it he demonstrated that at least the epidemic forms of the infection could be traced to inadequate precautions taken by the nurse or physician attending women in labor or women who had just given birth. His work was not well received, nor was that of Ignaz Semmelweis 4 years later. Semmelweis noted a striking contrast in maternal mortality between women delivered in their homes and those delivered in the Vienna Lying-In Hospital, where he was an assistant. As a result of his own careful investigations, he concluded that childbed fever was essentially a wound infection caused by septic material introduced during vaginal examination. He then required physicians, medical students, and midwives to wash their hands with chlorine water prior to examining women in labor. The mortality dropped dramatically from 10 to 1 percent—yet he, like Holmes, was ridiculed by some of the most prominent men of his time. Many physicians thought it an intellectual insult for them to be expected to believe that the problem could be caused by something invisible to the naked eye. It was not until Pasteur later demonstrated in women with puerperal fever what are now known as *Streptococcus* organisms that Holmes's and Semmelweis's work slowly became accepted and their recommendations adopted.

Modes of Infection Today, infection is still introduced into the uterus through vaginal examinations, and as the number of examinations during labor increases so does the incidence of infection. Organisms already present in the vagina may be carried to the uterus. In hospitals, the examiners' hands or instruments may become contaminated as a result of droplet infection dispersed by them or other staff members. Personnel working with the mother may be carriers of streptococci and may spread the organism by coughing, sneezing, or just talking. Since the nasopharynx is one of the most common sources of extraneous bacteria brought to the birth canal, all personnel in the delivery room wear masks that cover the nose and mouth. Anyone with an upper respiratory infection should not be present.

Infection may also result from instruments that are insufficiently sterilized or contaminated prior to use. Bedpans should be cleansed and sterilized after each use. Heat lamps and other pieces of equipment that are taken from one woman to another should first be thoroughly cleansed. Infection may also be caused by bacteria-laden dust carried from one part of a hospital to another via air currents in ventilating ducts. Thus, infectious material from one part of the institution can easily flow and settle on sterilized tables, towels, instruments, and bedclothes.

The woman may also carry infectious organisms on her fingers from various parts of her body to her genitals. Following delivery the birth canal represents a wound for many days. It is vitally important that the woman observe adequate hygiene measures accompanying perineal care, such as cleansing from her vulva to her anus and not back over the area. It is important that perineal pads be sterile and changed frequently, at least every 4 hours. It is also wise to separate any woman with a puerperal infection from other women who have just given birth.

Infection is more likely to occur in women with severe anemia, malnutrition, debilitating or chronic illness, or infection elsewhere in the body. Prolonged labor with exhaustion and dehydration, particularly when accompanied by prolonged rupture of the membranes, traumatic delivery, the use of instruments and intrauterine manipulation, retention of placental fragments, blood clots in the uterus, lacerations, or hemorrhage, are associated with the development of puerperal sepsis.

Analysis of the predisposing factors makes clear the extent to which puerperal sepsis can be prevented by good health care during pregnancy, by sufficient rest and fluids during labor, by minimizing obstetric trauma, by prevention of hemorrhage, and by careful examination of the uterovaginal tract after delivery, as well as by proper aseptic technique.

Puerperal morbidity is generally diagnosed according to the definition advanced by the Joint Committee on Maternal Welfare in the United States. They define morbidity as a temperature of 38.0°C (100.4°F) or higher occurring on any two of the first 10 days post partum, excluding the first 24 hours. The woman's temperature, according to the Committee, should be taken by mouth at least four times a day. Researchers [4] have questioned the validity of morbidity statistics prepared from these criteria. They note that the majority of women who develop fevers are immediately given antibiotics, causing their temperatures to drop before they can be included in the statistics.

Causative Organisms   In the great majority of cases of puerperal infection, the causative organisms are those that normally inhabit the bowel and lower genital tract. These are potentially pathogenic anaerobic and aerobic organisms, including *Bacteroides*, *Peptostreptococcus*, and *Clostridium* [3].

Historically, anaerobic *Streptococcus* has been identified as the most common organism causing puerperal morbidity [2]. More recently, researchers [4] have reported the gram-negative aerobic rod *Escherichia coli* to be the most common organism. They also found *Peptostreptococcus*, alpha-hemolytic streptococci, *Bacteroides*, enterococci, and coagulase-negative *Staphylococcus* as causative organisms and noted the increasing importance of gram-negative organisms in hospital-acquired infections. Occasionally *Clostridium*, beta-hemolytic streptococci, *Klebsiella, Pseudomonas*, and *Neisseria* are also involved in postpartum sepsis. Mixed flora are common. The causative organisms appear to depend upon the population studied.

Following traumatic delivery, lacerations and contusions are commonly found in the external genitalia. The vulva may become edematous, and if the wounds become infected, they are covered with a grayish or greenish exudate and may ulcerate. Infected wounds in the vagina cause the mucous membrane to become swollen and red and, in many instances, to begin sloughing. If the discharge produced is unable to drain properly, the woman may experience high fever, chills, urinary retention, dysuria, and pelvic pain.

Cervical lacerations may also become infected; deep lacerations may be the origin of extensive infections such as lymphatic infection, bacteremia, and parametritis. Episiotomy wounds may become infected, with the suture line becoming red and swollen and later containing areas that will slough and ooze serum and pus. The woman may have difficulty voiding as well as local pain, discomfort, and an elevated temperature. The infection is usually treated by removing the sutures and promoting drainage of the exudate. Sitz baths several times a day relieve much of the discomfort.

Sites and Types of Infections

ASSESSMENT

Endometritis. Almost all postpartum infections involve the endometrium. The organisms invade the area particularly at the placental site, which takes a longer time to heal than the surrounding endometrium. Blood and lymphatic vessels in the infected area become engorged, and in some instances the necrotic mucosa sloughs. If the lochial discharge is obstructed by the debris or by clots, the woman usually experiences a severe chill and fever until free drainage is established.

In addition to noting an increased pulse and temperature, symptoms that usually appear on the third to fifth day post partum, carefully check the woman's uterus and lochial discharge. If she has endometritis, her uterus is usually larger than would be expected for that postdelivery day and it is usually soft and tender. The lochia may be more profuse, bloody, and have a foul odor, depending on the type of infecting organism. The mother's abdomen may also appear distended.

Occasionally the infection spreads from the endometrium to the myometrium, parametrium, fallopian tubes, peritoneum, and blood. Rarely the infection spreads to involve abscess formation in the tubes or ovaries. Mild salpingitis may occur unnoticed and account for secondary infertility.

Pelvic Cellulitis (Parametritis). Infection of the pelvic connective tissue may result from an infected wound in the cervix, vagina, perineum, or lower uterine segment, or as an extension of pelvic thrombophlebitis. The symptoms, which usually occur about the fourth postdelivery day, include chills, high fever, tachycardia, severe local pain in one or both sides of the abdomen, and tenderness on vaginal examination. Initially the fever is high, but as the infection progresses it may become intermittent. On examination, the mother's uterus appears to be unusually large for that postdelivery day and is sensitive to the touch. As the infection becomes more severe, her uterus becomes fixed. Her pelvic area is warm and soft, with one extremely sensitive spot; the abscess is usually located under this area. If suppuration is present, pointing usually occurs, with the skin over the area becoming red, edematous, and tender. Pointing may also occur in the posterior cul-de-sac, or the abscess can be felt bulging into one of the fornices. When the symptoms of suppuration become apparent, incision and drainage is performed. Most often, however, the infected mass heals by absorption in several weeks.

Thrombophlebitis. Puerperal infection spreads most commonly along the veins, resulting in thrombophlebitis. The veins most commonly infected are those of the uterine wall and broad ligament. The resulting condition is called *pelvic thrombophlebitis*, while infection of the leg veins is known as *femoral thrombophlebitis*. The vein most commonly involved in pelvic thrombophlebitis is the ovarian. If the left ovarian vein is extensively involved, renal complications may occur because of its junction with the renal vein.

As the inflammatory process in the veins spreads, the thrombus may increase in size in an attempt to wall off the infecting organisms. Occasionally small emboli break loose and lodge in other parts of the body, such as the kidneys, heart valves, and lungs. In the lungs these emboli cause pneumonia, pleurisy, abscesses, infarctions, or, in severe cases, death.

Danger of thrombosis in the puerperium is high when both blood fibrinogen content and platelet count increase and when those platelets present become more sticky [1]. Risk factors include inactivity (bed rest following cesarean delivery), estrogen preparations to suppress lactation, maternal age over 30, family tendency, obesity, and previous thromboembolic disease.

The onset of symptoms of pelvic thrombophlebitis usually occurs during the second week after delivery. The mother generally has repeated severe chills and fever, with her temperature rising to 40.6°C (105°F). Between the episodes she may look and feel well. Specimens of blood for cultures should be taken during the chill to isolate the causative organism.

The signs and symptoms of femoral thrombophlebitis are generally the same as those found during the nonpregnant state. They include pain, tenderness, and turgidity of the calf, redness, increased skin temperature, positive Homan's sign, and edema of the calf or thigh. If there is reflex arterial spasm, the affected leg may be cool and pale with decreased peripheral pulses.

Pulmonary Embolism. The greatest danger of a pulmonary embolism in the postpartum period comes from a venous thrombosis. Even though it occurs only once in about 3,000 to 7,000 deliveries, it is still a very serious postpartum complication because it is life-threatening. Be on the alert for significant symptoms: chest pain (even if it is transient) accompanied by shortness of breath, air hunger, tachypnea, or just apprehension. Lung scans are useful diagnostic tools. If the embolus is large, a pulmonary artery embolectomy could be lifesaving. Oxygen, sedatives, and preparation of the woman for emergency surgery may be necessary.

A pulmonary embolism may also be caused by amniotic fluid in the maternal circulation. After the membranes have ruptured, and particularly just after delivery, amniotic fluid may enter venous sinuses in the uterine wall and travel to the pulmonary vessels. Since the fluid contains vernix and other solid material, it may form small emboli in the lungs and contribute to maternal shock and sudden death. It is also instrumental in producing fibrinogenopenia as a result of intravascular clotting. Amniotic fluid embolism tends to occur in rapid labors in which there are powerful contractions and may be seen in conjunction with the use of oxytocin.

Bacteremia.   As a result of infected thrombi breaking loose, usually from the uterine veins, or because of lymphatic spread of bacteria from an endometritis, the mother can become extremely ill. She usually has a severe chill, fever, and rapid respirations. Her skin is pale, her lips and fingers may become cyanotic, and she may soon develop symptoms of peritonitis. Her lochial discharge may increase and have a foul odor. When blood cultures are grown, *Streptococcus* is the organism found most frequently. With treatment the condition rarely lasts more than 10 days.

Peritonitis.   The signs and symptoms of puerperal peritonitis resemble those of surgical peritonitis except that abdominal rigidity is slight or absent. The mother has chills, high fever, rapid pulse, vomiting, and severe abdominal pain. Paralytic ileus leads to abdominal distention, although severe diarrhea may follow. The mother is treated immediately with antimicrobial agents, gastrointestinal suction, fluid and electrolyte replacement, analgesics, and sedation. Oral feedings are generally resumed when bowel sounds return.

INTERVENTIONS

In general, puerperal infection is treated by isolating the infected woman to prevent spread of the infection. Supportive medical therapy is given, including appropriate fluid and electrolyte replacement, blood to combat anemia, and antibiotics to which the organism is sensitive. If the mother is unresponsive to specific antibiotic therapy, septic thrombophlebitis or abscess formation is suspected. When the abscess is found, drainage is usually instituted. If the mother has thrombophlebitis, anticoagulant therapy is begun.

Nursing interventions include continued evaluation of the woman's temperature, pulse, respiration, and laboratory studies that monitor the course of her infection. Carefully monitor the site of infection for signs and symptoms such as pain, rigidity, edema, redness, and elevated skin temperature in order to evaluate progress of the infection. Monitor the amount, color, and odor of lochia or other wound drainage. The mother's diet should emphasize increased calories to meet the needs of an elevated temperature and metabolic rate as well as increased protein and vitamins, particularly vitamin C, to promote healing of infected tissues. The mother will also need additional fluids to meet the needs of her increased metabolism and analgesics to relieve pain. Pay particular attention to the mother's hygiene and comfort needs. A fresh clean mouth, dry, clean linens and perineal pad, skin care over bony prominences, and a soothing back rub do much to help the mother over this difficult period.

Minimize the number of visitors to prevent excessive maternal fatigue. While many institutions continue to separate mother and infant, breast-feeding may continue if the infection is localized. If breast-feeding is temporarily discontinued, instruct the mother to express her milk on a regular basis, either manually or with a breast pump.

Pay particular attention to measures that support the family unit. This can be accomplished by helping the mother make telephone calls to children at home, helping and encouraging her to hold her newborn if her infection is localized, and assisting the couple find solutions to problems raised by the extended hospitalization of the mother.

POSTPARTUM
HEMORRHAGE

Postpartum hemorrhage is the loss of more than 500 milliliters of blood, either measured or estimated. It occurs in about 10 percent of all deliveries and is a major cause of maternal mortality. Whether the blood flows freely or seeps slowly, the blood loss may be great. In fact, it is more often fatal when it occurs slowly, since it tends to be neglected.

Factors predisposing a woman to immediate postpartum hemorrhage are high parity, previous obstetric trauma, third-stage complications of labor, and coagulation disorders. The three most common causes are lacerations of the birth canal, uterine atony, and retention of placental fragments.

Lacerations of the birth canal commonly follow operative deliveries, especially when forceps have been improperly applied. The vaults or lateral fornices of the vagina and the vaginal wall behind the pubic arch and lateral to the urethra are frequently involved. Perineal and cervical lacerations also occur. Lacerations of the birth canal are suspected when the woman's uterine tone is good but she still has bright red bleeding. The lacerations must be located and repaired to stop the blood loss.

Uterine atony (uterine hypotonia) occurs when the myometrium fails to constrict the endometrial blood vessels. It is often precipitated by failure of the placenta to separate normally and be completely expelled. Other contributing factors include deep inhalation anesthesia, prolonged labor, marked distention of the uterus, the presence of fibroid tumors, and hypotension.

*Assessment and
Nursing Intervention*

Normally the woman's uterus is firm, well contracted, and found in the midline at or below her umbilicus immediately following delivery. If her uterus is boggy and does not remain well contracted, and she is losing an abnormal amount of blood, massage her fundus frequently and palpate it deeply to express blood and clots. Examine the discharge for pieces of tissue. Since massage and palpation of the woman's uterus can be a painful, disturbing procedure that can increase her anxiety, make the necessary observations of uterine size and position and blood loss as quickly and as efficiently as possible. The couple's concern can be somewhat allayed by appropriate explanations of what is being done and why. Take vital signs every 5 or 10 minutes, but remember that marked fluctuations in blood pressure and pulse will not occur until the woman has lost a large amount of blood. Charting should include a pad count and saturation description. Intravenous fluids may be started containing an oxytocic drug, or she may be given a dose of oxytocin, usually ergonovine, intramuscularly.

In the treatment of hemorrhage, recognition of the cause and restoration of the blood volume to normal are very important. Adequate inspection of the placenta for completeness upon delivery can often prevent hemorrhagic problems due to retention of placental fragments by indicating the need for a curettage. The value of uterine packing in the control of blood loss is a controversial issue; presently, packing is not often used.

Postpartum hemorrhage can also occur after the first 24 hours, even as late as the fifth month post partum. Secondary bleeding may result on or about the tenth postpartum day from lacerations of the birth canal, coinciding with absorption of sutures used to control a primary hemorrhage.

If placental tissue has been retained, the hemorrhage usually occurs about the tenth day post partum, when the decidua of the placental site undergoes maximum slough, or even weeks or months later. A curettage is usually curative.

In the case of placental subinvolution, due perhaps to a low-grade endometritis, some of the thrombosed portions of the decidual blood vessels slough away, leaving the ends of the spiral arteries open. Profuse bleeding may occur suddenly around the sixth to tenth week post partum. As in the case of retained placental tissue, a curettage is usually curative.

Anxiety may be high for the couple, since the situation presents as an emergency and arrangements may have to be made for care of the infant and other family members if the mother's hospitalization is extended. Their anxiety may be decreased by supporting them through the emergency period followed by support while they identify their problems and then helping them work out solutions acceptable to them.

POSTPARTUM HEMATOMAS
Assessment and Nursing Intervention

Hematomas may develop during the postpartum period in the loose connective tissue beneath the skin that covers the external genitalia (without apparent laceration of the skin), beneath the vaginal mucosa, or in the broad ligaments. They occur once in about every 500 to 1,000 deliveries; it may be several hours before they are noticed.

Vulvar hematomas, particularly those that develop rapidly, may cause excruciating pain, which is often the first symptom to appear. The pain is accompanied by the sudden development of a fluctuant and sensitive tumor of varying size, covered by discolored skin. Vaginal hematomas usually present with symptoms of pressure and inability to void. To assess the woman for a vaginal hematoma, ask her to assume a side-lying position, raise her upper buttock, and ask her to bear down. A large purple mass may be seen at the introitus. Hematomas have a varied etiology, including the trauma of a spontaneous labor or forceps application, failure to suture far enough beyond the upper angle of the episiotomy or laceration, or even rough uterine massage.

The prognosis for most women who develop hematomas is favorable. Small hematomas are treated expectantly, as they are absorbed spontaneously. If the pain is severe or the hematoma continues to grow, incision and drainage with ligation of the bleeding points is necessary. Sometimes vaginal packing for 24 hours is useful. Since blood loss is almost always more than the clinical estimate, observe the mother carefully for signs of needed blood replacement.

SUBINVOLUTION
Assessment and Nursing Intervention

Subinvolution is the slowing or stopping of the normal autolytic process of involution. Anything that interferes with myometrial contraction may be a contributing factor, including retention of placental fragments, endometritis, myomas, fibroid tumors, and pelvic infection.

Symptoms of subinvolution are prolonged lochial discharge (after a month or more), followed by prolonged leukorrhea or irregular uterine bleeding and sometimes by profuse hemorrhage. The woman's uterus is larger or softer than would be expected for the given time post partum, and she may have subjective complaints of backache or a sensation of weight in her pelvis.

Treatment with ergonovine maleate (Ergotrate) or methylergonovine maleate (Methergine), 0.2 milligram every 3 to 4 hours over 2 to 4 days, may cause improvement by increasing contractions and thus improving drainage. If there are retained secundines, curettage is indicated and is usually curative. Instruct the woman to save any tissue passed for her midwife or physician to inspect.

UTERINE
DISPLACEMENTS
*Assessment and
Nursing Intervention*

As soon as the uterus involutes to the point of entry into the pelvic cavity, retroversion may occur, particularly if some degree of subinvolution is present. In the early postpartum period, uterine retrodisplacement may cause lochia to be retained (lochiometra).

Symptoms of retrodisplacement may include backache, sometimes with increased or persistent lochia. Relief in many patients is obtained with bimanual or instrument anteflexion of the uterus, followed by the introduction of a pessary during the third to sixth week post partum. In some cases, knee-chest exercises are also helpful.

RELAXATION OF THE
VAGINAL OUTLET
AND PROLAPSE OF
THE UTERUS
*Assessment and
Nursing Intervention*

Frequently, improperly repaired lacerations of the perineum may be followed by relaxation of the vaginal outlet. Changes in the pelvic supports during pregnancy and delivery predispose the woman to the development of a cystocele or rectocele, urinary stress incontinence, and a prolapsed uterus. Operative procedures for the correction of these conditions are not done until at least 3 to 6 months post partum and are usually postponed until the end of the childbearing period unless urinary stress incontinence becomes a serious problem. Perineal tightening is a good prophylactic exercise that can help to maintain the tone of the pelvic supports.

DISORDERS OF THE
URINARY TRACT
*Assessment and
Nursing Intervention*

Several situations that may occur during or following delivery, such as trauma to the bladder, residual urine, and the need for catheterization, predispose the new mother to the development of urinary tract infections. The administration of large volumes of intravenous fluids during labor may contribute to rapid overdistention of the bladder. Additionally, the use of general anesthesia and especially conduction anesthesia acts to delay normal bladder function. Symptoms that suggest cystitis include suprapubic or perineal discomfort, dysuria, urinary frequency, and an elevated temperature of around 37.8° to 38.3°C (100°–101°F). If the mother has flank pain and higher fever accompanied by chills, pyelitis may be the cause. Following urine culture and sensitivity studies, treatment includes increasing fluid intake, complete emptying of the bladder, appropriate antibiotics, urinary tract antispasmotics and analgesic drugs, and, if her condition warrants it, bed rest.

OBSTETRIC
PARALYSIS
*Assessment and
Nursing Intervention*

When the fetal head begins to descend into the pelvis or forceps pressure is applied, the mother may complain of intense neuralgia or cramping in one or both legs. In some instances the pain persists after delivery and may be accompanied by muscle paralysis. In this case the fibers of the popliteal nerve may have been injured where they pass over the brim of the pelvis, causing dysfunction of the ankle flexor and toe extensor muscles. (Fortunately, this rarely occurs in the modern practice of obstetrics.) The prognosis for the woman with localized paralysis is good; it is poor if the paralysis is generalized. Generalized paralysis might also be suggestive of a cerebral vascular accident.

A more common but preventable problem is that of footdrop, which may occur when a woman is improperly positioned in stirrups or leg holders. In addition, a neuritic-type pain may also be caused by a separated symphysis pubis or looseness of the sacroiliac joints. In this instance, locomotion may be difficult as well as painful.

DISORDERS OF THE BREASTS
Assessment and Nursing Intervention

MASTITIS

Mastitis, inflammation of the breast tissue, is sometimes seen during lactation in the postpartum period. Symptoms seldom appear before the end of the first postpartum week and generally not until the third or fourth week. They may include varying degrees of engorgement, chills, increased temperature (usually not above 39.4°C, or 103°F), and increased pulse. The mother's breasts are hard, reddened, and painful.

Mastitis may at first be confined to the areola, with the formation of a subareolar abscess in the underlying milk glands, around the nipple, or in one of the tubercles of Montgomery (Fig. 20-1). It may also involve the lactiferous tubules (parenchymatous or glandular mastitis), which is probably the most common form. Further extension of the process involves the connective tissue and

Figure 20-1. Mastitis.

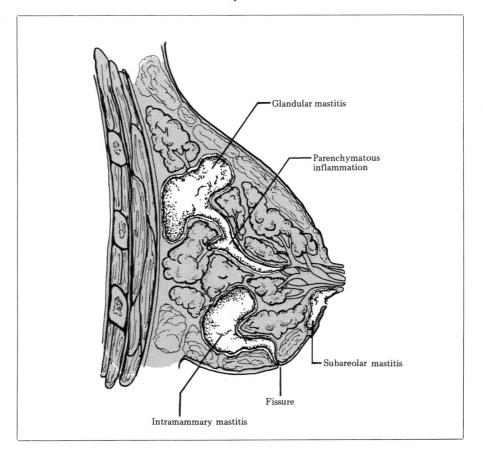

Glandular mastitis

Parenchymatous inflammation

Subareolar mastitis

Fissure

Intramammary mastitis

the fat around the lobes and lobules (intramammary or phlegmonous mastitis). Cellulitis may be superficial or deep.

The causative organism is most often *Staphylococcus aureus* and the source is almost always the infant's nose and throat. The organism travels through the nipple at the site of a fissure or abrasion (which may be very small), although some believe that the organism may still enter the lactiferous ducts even though the skin is intact. In the hospital the infant typically becomes a carrier while he is in the nursery, where he comes in contact with personnel who are carriers themselves. Needless to say, the hands of such personnel are a major source of contamination for both the infant and the mother.

Prevention of mastitis may depend on the exclusion of all personnel who are known or suspected *Staphylococcus* carriers from the care of mothers and babies. You are in an excellent position to prevent the development of mastitis by making sure that mothers are aware of the need for cleanliness, i.e., that mothers wash their *own* hands before handling their breasts. In addition, they should know how to prevent injured or fissured nipples—proper cleansing, proper sucking by the infant, and the mode of his removal from the breast. Perform a close daily inspection of every infant and isolate those with developing infections of the umbilical cord or skin.

If mastitis is promptly treated within 48 hours (following a culture of the milk), the infection is usually aborted. If the fever persists for more than 48 hours, suppuration usually appears. Physical comfort measures include proper support—a tight breast-binder or bra—and applications of cold or heat to allay the inflammation. Heat is preferred if suppuration is present.

Whether or not actual breast-feeding should be discontinued in the presence of mastitis is a matter of controversy. Advocates of its discontinuation propose that with less stimulation the infection will disappear more quickly and that reinfection may recur if breast-feeding is continued. Breast-feeding may be painful and the milk may be contaminated. An infant who harbors the infectious organisms may cause reinfection of the mother or develop a frank infection himself, and so should be closely observed.

Alternatively, if the mother does not stop breast-feeding, she avoids the distention of the breast tissue and milk stasis that occurs when nursing is suddenly discontinued. Additionally, while bacteria may be present in the breast milk, the antibiotic the mother is taking also passes into the milk. If the decision is made to continue lactation, breast-feeding may be temporarily stopped on the affected side and the breast emptied by manual expression or by an atraumatic breast pump. The expressed milk is usually discarded during the time the mother has a fever. Breast-feeding is resumed within 24 hours after the mother's temperature returns to normal, which is commonly within 1 to 3 days unless her recovery is unusually slow.

If a frank abscess forms, its incision and drainage, in addition to antibiotic therapy, are necessary for a rapid cure. Healing may require weeks or even months. When this is the case, if the mother chooses to resume breast-feeding, close supervision is essential.

Nipple Abnormalities   On rare occasions the nipples are so inverted that the lactiferous ducts open directly into a depression in the center of the areola. This makes breast-feeding extremely difficult, if not impossible. More commonly, the nipple may be very flat, making it difficult for the infant to grasp and retain. Treatment success is greatest when it is initiated during the antenatal period. Use of Woolwich Shields or Netsy Swedish Milk Cups may draw the inverted nipple out by applying gentle pressure around the areolar border.

Sore nipples are a common complication of the early weeks of nursing, especially if erosions, blisters, cracks, fissures, or ulcerations develop. The pain that results from breast-feeding with any of these disorders may have an inhibiting effect on secretory function. Primiparas seem to have more problems with sore nipples, especially if they are fair-skinned or older, or if their nipples are deformed. Once again, prenatal preparation of the nipple is one of the greatest preventive interventions.

If nipples are cracked or fissured, infection may easily develop, not only in the mother but also in the baby. If the nipples are bleeding and the baby swallows some blood, he may develop a false melena as a result.

Management of sore or cracked nipples begins with a careful assessment of the mother and baby. Improper positioning of the infant at the breast as well as traumatic removal from the breast contribute to the development of nipple problems. Mothers are instructed with two principles in mind: prevention of milk stasis and avoidance of moisture build-up against the nipple. In general, harsh soaps or astringent agents should be avoided, and the nipple should be kept dry by exposure to air after each nursing for at least 20 minutes. Varying nursing positions should be encouraged to avoid excessive trauma at one point on the areola. Additionally, infants should be permitted to nurse on demand; this prevents an aggressively hungry baby from sucking too vigorously. Also, with more frequent feedings the number of minutes at each breast can be decreased. Application of a water-soluble cream such as hydrous lanolin may be applied after each nursing and air drying. This cream is readily absorbed into the skin, maintains nipple suppleness, and need not be removed. Nipple shields may be used as a last resort; specific instructions to the mother in their proper use is essential.

SECRETION ABNORMALITIES

Agalactia, a rare phenomenon, is complete lack of mammary secretion. It may be due to many factors—febrile disorders, ill health, malformation, occlusion or disease of the milk ducts, atrophy or destruction of tissue from mastitis, or insufficient stimulation of the breasts. The infant of a mother with agalactia loses weight and may appear to be in distress.

Polygalactia is an excessive amount of milk secretion. *Galactorrhea* is a constant leakage of milk bearing no relationship to breast-feeding and persisting after weaning. It, too, occurs rarely and may be associated with a pituitary or hypothalamic dysfunction associated with low estrogen levels and decreased follicle-stimulating hormone. It may also be related to a blockade of the hypothalamic prolactin-inhibiting center by an unknown agent. In some women persistent abnormal or erogenous stimulation of the breasts may be a contributing factor. Galactorrhea may be unilateral or bilateral, slight or profuse. Treatment includes compression of the breasts with a binder and administration of clomiphene, levodopa, or ergot alkaloids on a chronic schedule.

GALACTOCELE

A galactocele is a collection of milk in one or more lobes of the breasts and its symptoms are related to increased pressure. If the galactocele is small, it can be effectively treated by massage; if large, a tight binder is usually effective.

SUPERNUMERARY BREASTS

One in every few hundred persons has one or more accessory breasts, a condition called *polymastia*. Such breasts, which may have distinct nipples, are sometimes mistaken for pigmented moles. They are commonly situated in pairs (usually two to four) on either side of the midline of the thoracic or abdominal wall, usually below the main breasts. Sometimes they are found in the axillae. Usually they are of no significance during pregnancy, although they may enlarge, secrete milk, and cause discomfort. These changes usually regress after delivery [3].

EMOTIONAL COMPLICATIONS

The stresses of pregnancy and delivery and the accompanying new responsibilities are precipitating factors in the development of postpartum psychosis in about 1 out of every 1,000 new mothers. Although postpartum psychosis is not in itself a distinct clinical entity, its symptoms usually can be identified within 6 months after delivery, most commonly in the first postpartum month. About half of the patients with postpartum psychosis demonstrate schizophrenic characteristics, while another 40 percent are manic-depressive in behavior. Primiparas and multiparas appear to be affected equally, and about one-third of them have probably had a mental illness prior to pregnancy.

In the majority of cases the onset of the psychosis is rather sudden, with a variety of affective symptoms—clouding of consciousness, withdrawal, depression, hostility, suspicion, unreasonable fear, and feelings of inadequacy. The woman may also have hallucinations or delusions regarding the child, her delivery, her mothering role, or her relationship with the baby's father.

Because the early symptoms are very similar to those of the common postpartum "blues," do not be too quick to treat their appearance in a superficial manner, since in some cases they may develop into more serious psychiatric difficulties. The fact that some postpartum psychoses may be prevented by antepartal therapy highlights the importance of your assessment of the woman's ability to cope with stresses while she is pregnant. Nurses in community settings as well as hospital settings are in a good position to offer support to family members during the crisis period. The adjustments that the family must make if the mother becomes psychotic are tremendous.

About 20 percent of women with postpartum psychosis recover within a month. In 40 percent recovery takes longer than 6 months, and about 15 percent remain chronically ill. For about half of the women it will remain an isolated event in their lives; the incidence of recurrence in subsequent pregnancies is about 1 in 7 women.

CONCERNS OF PARENTS
Assessment and Nursing Intervention

When postpartum complications arise, the family faces stress from a number of sources. The mother has recently experienced the stress of delivery and now faces an increased physical and emotional burden. The father, who is generally shouldering more responsibility in the home during the mother's hospitalization, faces the possibility of doing so over a longer period in addition to his concern about her condition. There is an added financial burden and the possibility that the newborn may be discharged before the mother. The mother in this situation may not be able to interact with the newborn or to establish a relationship with him. Other young children the couple may have will wonder why "mommy" is not coming home and may be particularly upset if "daddy" spends much time away from the home to be with his wife.

You can be invaluable in this situation. Start by acknowledging to the parents that this is often a difficult time for couples. Mention that many couples find that, in addition to worry created by the mother's condition, the home responsibilities can be very demanding and other children at home often become concerned. This approach opens the door for the parents to share their feelings and possible anxiety. Assess the couple's response to the woman's state of health, the father's ability to cope with the home situation, and the response of other children at home. If the father needs additional help, discuss with the couple the possibility of friends or relatives helping out or explain the services available from agencies in the community. This is particularly important if the newborn is to be discharged before the mother. Such planning should be done well in advance of the discharge so the family is spared the added stress of last-minute crisis arrangements.

While the newborn is in the hospital, support his incorporation into the family unit. The mother should see him as much as possible. Whenever feasible, she should be taken to the nursery not only to see him but, as soon as permitted, to hold and feed him. If she is confined to her room, give her daily reports on his progress, including personal characteristics that make him unique. When the father visits, encourage him to hold and feed his child and tell him of the baby's progress.

When there are other young children in the home, the mother can maintain contact with them by phone. Small gifts such as a pack of gum or a lollipop from "mommy" help a great deal. The children can be encouraged to draw pictures or write her a note that "daddy" can deliver. When she is able, take the mother to an area of the hospital where she can visit with the children. In short, support the family in any activity that helps them to maintain their unity.

Case Study   Julie Thomas

As Julie Thomas's primary nurse, develop a plan of care for her, including your interventions aimed at helping her through her current difficulty and in making the transitional postpartum period at home successful. Each of you will develop your own approach and style in providing care to newly delivered women. Applying the nursing process to the outline following the case study will serve as a guide in organizing your approach to this group of clients for as long as they are in the hospital and in your subsequent follow-up care.

Julie Thomas, gravida 2, para 2, delivered a 7-pound baby girl 4 days ago. Her pregnancy was uneventful until 3 days prior to her EDC when her membranes ruptured. She remained at home for 2 days without notifying her physician since she believed she had voided and was simply "dribbling urine" afterward. On the third day following the rupture of her membranes she went into labor, notified her physician, and went to the hospital. Julie labored for 16 hours and was delivered of her infant via low forceps. The newborn's Apgar scores were 8 at 1 minute and 9 at 5 minutes after delivery. The infant's next 4 days were uneventful, and she is now bottle-feeding and functioning well. The baby is scheduled to be discharged tomorrow morning.

For the past day and a half Julie has been having periodic chills with a temperature of 101°F to 103°F, and her pulse rate is increased. Her lochia has been dark red, profuse, and foul-smelling for the past 24 hours. Her uterus is soft and one fingerbreadth below her umbilicus. A cervical and a urine culture have been taken, and she is receiving a broad-spectrum antibiotic. Julie complains of being very fatigued, has lost her appetite, and is extremely irritable when interacting with the staff. When her husband, Jason, visited her several hours ago, she accused him of neglecting her, argued with him, and then burst into tears.

The Thomases live in an apartment building in the center of a large city. Julie, 27, teaches English in a community college but has 4 months of maternity leave before she is scheduled to return to class. She plans to continue teaching. Her husband, Jason, 30, is a lawyer who has just opened his own practice. Their only other child, Jason, Jr., is 3 years old. Jason, Sr., has been caring for their son during Julie's hospitalization. Julie's parents are dead; those of Jason, Sr. live approximately 2 miles from the Thomases' apartment. While Julie and her father-in-law have a close relationship, the relationship between Julie and her mother-in-law is strained. They frequently argue over how Jason, Jr., should be reared. Jason, Sr., supports his wife during these arguments.

Assessment Form

Assessment	Plan	Intervention	Evaluation
I. Physical Changes			
A. Breasts			
1. Contour			
2. Areolae			
3. Nipples			
4. Colostrum or milk			
5. Brassiere			
B. Cardiovascular			
1. Hb, Hct			
2. Varicosities			
C. Abdomen			
1. Diastasis			
2. Distended			
D. Skin			
1. Perspiration			
2. Pigmentation			
E. GI system			
1. Appetite			
2. Food and fluid intake			
3. Bowel movements			
F. Genital tract			
1. Uterus			
(a) Firm			
(b) Location			
2. Lochia			
(a) Character			
(b) Amount			
(c) Clots			
(d) Odor			
3. Cervix			
4. Perineum			
(a) Episiotomy			
(b) Hematomas			
(c) Discomfort			
G. Urinary system			
1. Voiding			
(a) Character			
(b) Frequency			
(c) Pain			
H. Medical treatment plan			
1. Drug therapy			
(a) Antibiotics			

Assessment Form			
Assessment	Plan	Intervention	Evaluation

       (b) Analgesics
       (c) Drugs, dose, possible
          side effects
     2. Monitoring of vital signs
       (a) Laboratory studies
          (WBC, cultures)
       (b) Intake and output
     3. Isolation
       (a) Of mother
       (b) Of infant from mother
  I. Comfort measures
    1. General hygiene
    2. Positioning
    3. Measures to promote rest
      and sleep
  J. Specific learning needs to cope
    with physical changes
II. Behavioral Changes
  A. Taking-in
    1. Dependency needs
  B. Taking-hold
    1. Reaching out to others
    2. Increased independence
  C. Mood swings
    1. Elation
    2. Blues
    3. Tearfulness
    4. Severe depression
III. Needs Identified by
  A. Mother
  B. Father
IV. Needs Identified for Successful
  Incorporation of Newborn
  into Family and the Return of Normal
  Family Functioning
  A. Rest and assistance for
    1. Mother
    2. Father
  B. Special time
    1. For mother alone
    2. For father alone

Assessment Form			
Assessment	Plan	Intervention	Evaluation
3. For couple			
C. Reestablishment of sexual relations and contraceptive method chosen			
D. Interaction with newborn			
1. Comfort and expertise in feeding, bathing, dressing, cord care, circumcision care			
2. Comfort and character of interaction with newborn—holding, cuddling, talking to, ability to soothe			
E. Sibling interaction with newborn			
1. Sibling rivalry			
F. Resumption of employment of father and mother			
G. Reestablishment of social relationships			
V. Specific Discharge Information			
A. Nurse and physician who can be contacted regarding further questions or concerns			
B. Date of return visit for check-up			
C. Information reinforcing activity level at home			
1. Regarding child care			
2. Regarding breast self-examination			
3. Regarding untoward signs and symptoms to be reported			
D. Community resources available			
1. Parent groups			
2. Nursing mothers groups			
3. Visiting nurse service			

REFERENCES
1. Cooper, K. Thrombosis and embolism in obstetrics. *Nursing Mirror* 142:65, 1976.
2. Gibbs, R. S., O'Dell, T. N., MacGregor, R., Schwarz, R. H., and Morton, H. Puerperal endometritis: A prospective microbiologic study. *American Journal of Obstetrics and Gynecology* 121:919, 1975.
3. Pritchard, J., and MacDonald, P. *Williams Obstetrics* (16th ed.). New York: Appleton-Century-Crofts, 1980.
4. Sweet, R. L., and Ledger, W. J. Puerperal infectious morbidity. *American Journal of Obstetrics and Gynecology* 117:1093, 1973.

FURTHER READING
Aladjem, S. *Obstetric Practice*. St. Louis: Mosby, 1980.
Bash, D., and Gold, W. *The Nurse and the Childbearing Family*. New York: Wiley, 1981.
Butnarescu, G., Tillotson, D., and Villarreal, P. *Perinatal Nursing*. Vol. 2 (Reproductive Risk). New York: Wiley, 1980.
Carmack, B., and Corwin, T. Nursing care of the schizophrenic maternity patient during labor. *American Journal of Maternal-Child Nursing* 5:107, 1980.
Focusing on today's issues in perinatal care. Postpartum depression (with a commentary by Niles Newton). *I.C.E.A. Review* 4:2, 1980.
Jensen, M., Benson, R., and Bobak, I. *Maternity Care* (2nd ed.). St. Louis: Mosby, 1981.
Marraro, R. V., and Harris, R. E. Incidence and spontaneous resolution of postpartum bacteria. *American Journal of Obstetrics and Gynecology* 128:722, 1977.
Olds, S., London, M., Ladewig, P., and Davidson, S. *Obstetric Nursing*. Menlo Park, Calif.: Addison-Wesley, 1980.
Paydar, M., and Ostooarzaden, M. Late postpartum hemorrhage. *International Journal of Gynaecology and Obstetrics* 12:141, 1974.
Quilligan, E., and Kretchmer, N. *Fetal and Maternal Medicine*. New York: Wiley, 1980.
Richardson, W. W. Breast abscess. *Nursing Times* 61:557, 1977.
Uddenberg, N., and Englesson, I. Prognosis of postpartum mental disturbance: A prospective study of primiparous women and their 4-year-old children. *Acta Psychiatrica Scandinavica* 58:201, 1978.

Chapter 21 Complications of the Newborn

PRETERM AND LOW
BIRTH WEIGHT
INFANTS

In the past, classifications for newborns were based mainly on the infant's weight at the time of birth (Table 21-1). Recognizing that all newborns weighing 2,500 grams or less at birth are not born prematurely, the World Health Organization recommended a new classification. As a result *low birth weight* is the designation applied to infants of less than 2,500 grams birth weight, regardless of the cause of their light weight and the length of their gestation.

Babies are also classified according to gestational age. Babies who grew at a normal rate in utero, whether they are born at term (beginning of 38th to end of 41st week), preterm (born before beginning of 38th week), or postterm (born at the onset of 42nd week or later), are referred to as *appropriate for gestational age (AGA)*. If they grew at a retarded rate, they are labeled *small for gestational age (SGA)*, while if the rate of their intrauterine growth was accelerated (above the 90th percentile on intrauterine growth charts), they are *large for gestational age (LGA)*. Finally, if the infant was growth retarded and preterm, he is referred to as *a small for gestational age, premature*. When infants of low birth weight (less than 2,500 grams) are properly classified, about one-third are SGA (growth retarded) and two-thirds are AGA (preterm).

Assessment of Gestational Age

Because the problems of preterm and low birth weight babies may be different, it is important to assess their gestational age and to project the difference in their care and treatment. For instance, an infant weighing over 2,500 grams (5.5 pounds) may be assumed to be full term when he is actually LGA and preterm (e.g., the infant of a diabetic mother). Several tools that you can easily use have been developed to assess gestational age (Fig. 21-1, 21-2; Table 21-2); they are based on the appearance of external characteristics that develop in orderly fashion during gestation and the use of a neurologic evaluation. This latter examination is done when the infant is in a resting state. The scores from each part of the evaluation are combined, and the result is plotted on a rating scale, yielding an approximate gestational age (Fig. 21-3).

THE PRETERM
INFANT

The characteristics of the truly preterm infant are most noticeable in babies with the shortest gestational age. Factors associated with prematurity are, of course, involved with the onset of premature labor, which may have many causes, including placental malfunction and maternal or fetal disease such as chronic hypertensive disease, preeclampsia, placenta previa, abruptio placentae, cervical incompetence, multiple gestation, or blood group incompatibility. Other factors include low socioeconomic status, short maternal stature, absence of prenatal care, malnutrition, and a history of previous premature delivery. In the United States, approximately 8 percent of all live births are before term, and prematurity still ranks as the leading cause of infant death.

The preterm baby usually weighs from 1,000 to 2,500 grams (2.2–5.5 pounds), with a vertex-heel length of under 48 centimeters (19 inches) and a head circumference of 25 to 31 centimeters (10–12 inches). The baby's head appears large in proportion to the rest of his body. His chest circumference is relatively small—less than 30 centimeters (12 inches), generally 3 centimeters (1½ inches)

Table 21-1.
Classifications for
Newborns

Classification	Weight	Gestational Age
Abortus	Under 500 g	20 weeks or under
Immature	500–999 g	21–26/27 weeks
Preterm	1,000–2,500 g	27–36 weeks
Full-term	Over 2,500 g	37–42 weeks
Postterm	—	Over 42 weeks

smaller than his head. The lower his gestational age, the weaker his activity and the less frequent his cry. His loss of weight (10–15 percent) in the first week of extrauterine life is greater than that of the term infant (7–10 percent). As a rule weight is regained more slowly, sometimes not until the third week.

Respiratory System In general, respirations in the preterm infant are irregular, rapid, and sometimes shallow, with periods of apnea and cyanosis. Periodic breathing (short pauses in respiration) is a common pattern and is differentiated from true apnea. Apnea involves either a given time period without any respirations (15–30 seconds) or a time without respiration after which functional changes in the infant, such as cyanosis, hypotonia, or acidosis, are noted.

The heart rate drops 10 to 15 seconds after respirations cease and is usually below 100 beats per minute within 30 seconds. No theory completely explains the occurrence of apneic spells, although it is known that changes in the excitatory state of the immature respiratory center can alter breathing remarkably. Therefore, either restraining the extremities of the small, preterm infant and thus changing the sensory input from bones and joints, or increasing the isolette temperature and thus altering skin temperature receptors, will sometimes induce or increase the number of his apneic episodes [11].

The more immature the infant, the more likely he is to have apneic spells, sometimes not beginning until 5 to 7 days of age. Since even short periods of apnea may produce brain damage in very small infants, it is essential that their respirations be carefully monitored. Apnea in these infants can also be a sign of infection, hypoglycemia, or cold stress.

RESPIRATORY DISTRESS SYNDROME

Assessment. An infant's lung development depends on the length of gestation. The very young premature baby may have small alveoli and few blood vessels, since there is a great increase in the lung capillary network between 26 and 36 weeks. He often has difficulty in initiating normal respiration, which may result in lung collapse (primary atelectasis). This problem is related to sparsity of pulmonary elastic tissue and general anatomic immaturity of alveoli; weak respiratory muscles and a soft yielding thoracic cage, leading to reduced intratho-

Figure 21-1. Assessing gestational age in the newborn; external criteria. (From L. M. S. Dubowitz, V. Dubowitz, and C. Goldberg. Clinical assessment of gestational age in the newborn infant. *Journal of Pediatrics* 77:1, 1970.)

External Sign	Score*				
	0	1	2	3	4
Edema	Obvious edema hands and feet; pitting over tibia	No obvious edema hands and feet; pitting over tibia	No edema		
Skin texture	Very thin, gelatinous	Thin and smooth	Smooth; medium thickness. Rash or superficial peeling	Slight thickening. Superficial cracking and peeling especially hands and feet	Thick and parchment-like; superficial or deep cracking
Skin color (infant not crying)	Dark red	Uniformly pink	Pale pink: variable over body	Pale. Only pink over ears, lips, palms, or soles	
Skin opacity (trunk)	Numerous veins and venules clearly seen, especially over abdomen	Veins and tributaries seen	A few large vessels clearly seen over abdomen	A few large vessels seen indistinctly over abdomen	No blood vessels seen
Lanugo (over back)	No lanugo	Abundant; long and thick over whole back	Hair thinning especially over lower back	Small amount of lanugo and bald areas	At least half of back devoid of lanugo
Plantar creases	No skin creases	Faint red marks over anterior half of sole	Definite red marks over more than anterior half; indentations over less than anterior third	Indentations over more than anterior third	Definite *deep* indentations over more than anterior third
Nipple formation	Nipple barely visible; no areola	Nipple well defined; areola smooth and flat diam. <0.75 cm	Areola stippled, edge not raised diam. <0.75 cm	Areola stippled, edge raised diam. >0.75 cm	
Breast size	No breast tissue palpable	Breast tissue on one or both sides <0.5 cm diam.	Breast tissue both sides; one or both 0.5–1.0 cm	Breast tissue both sides; one or both >1 cm	
Ear form	Pinna flat and shapeless, little or no incurving of edge	Incurving of part of edge of pinna	Partial incurving whole of upper pinna	Well-defined incurving whole of upper pinna	
Ear firmness	Pinna soft, easily folded, no recoil	Pinna soft, easily folded, slow recoil	Cartilage to edge of pinna, but soft in places, ready recoil	Pinna firm, cartilage to edge; instant recoil	
Genitalia Male	Neither testis in scrotum	At least one testis high in scrotum	At least one testis right down		
Females (with hips half abducted)	Labia majora widely separated, labia minora protruding	Labia majora almost cover labia minora	Labia majora completely cover labia minora		

* If score differs on two sides, take the mean.

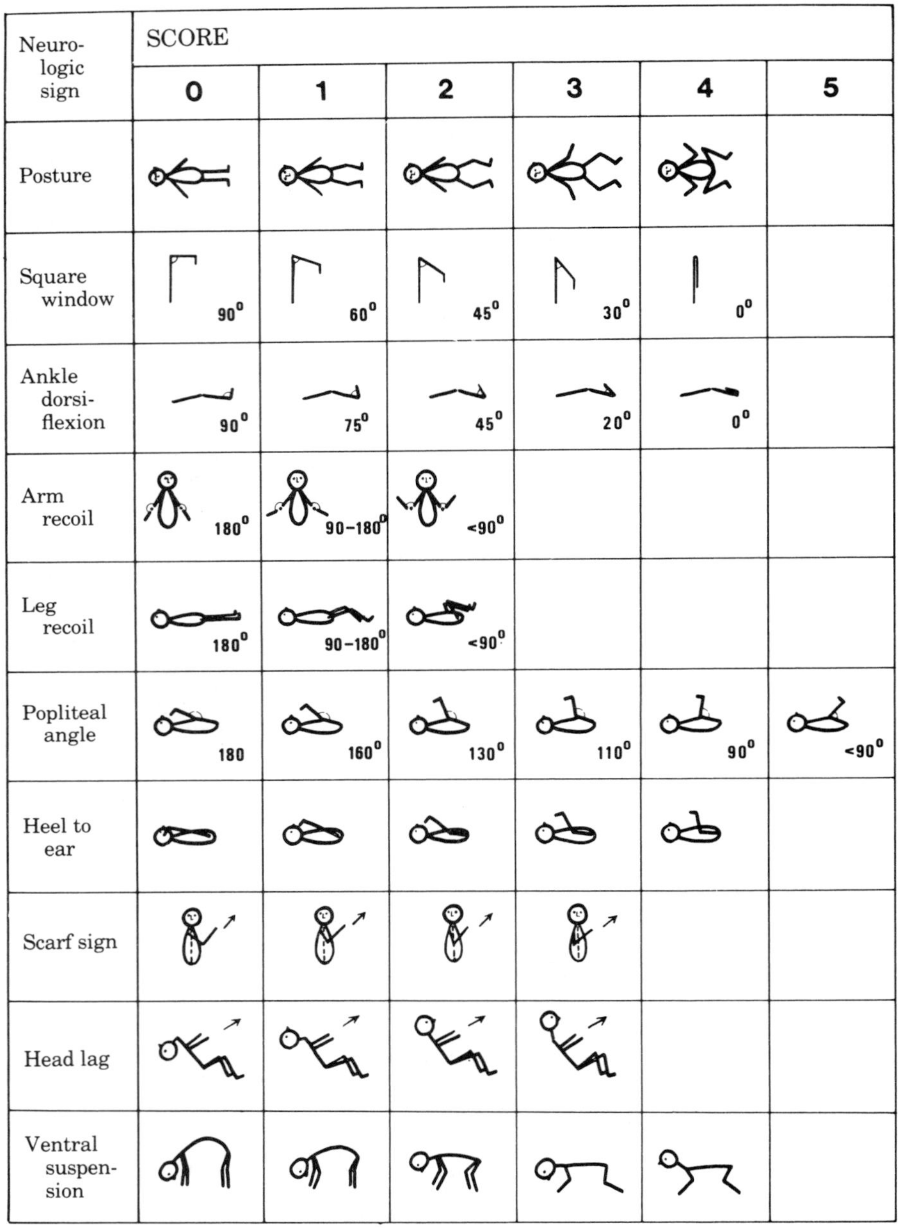

Figure 21-2. Assessing gestational age in the newborn: Neurologic signs. (See Table 21-2 for explanation of scores.) (From L. M. S. Dubowitz, V. Dubowitz, and C. Goldberg. Clinical Assessment of gestational age in the newborn infant. *Journal of Pediatrics* 77:1, 1970.)

Neurologic sign	SCORE					
	0	1	2	3	4	5
Posture						
Square window	90°	60°	45°	30°	0°	
Ankle dorsiflexion	90°	75°	45°	20°	0°	
Arm recoil	180°	90–180°	<90°			
Leg recoil	180°	90–180°	<90°			
Popliteal angle	180	160°	130°	110°	90°	<90°
Heel to ear						
Scarf sign						
Head lag						
Ventral suspension						

racic pressure; and a poorly developed respiratory center that requires strong afferent stimuli for response.

In addition to having difficulty in initiating respiration, approximately 10 to 20 percent of all preterm babies develop respiratory distress syndrome (RDS), also known as hyaline membrane disease [12]. Its symptoms are evident at birth or shortly thereafter, and the disease course usually lasts 3 to 5 days. The infant develops tachypnea, with his respiratory rate usually over 60 breaths per minute.

Posture   Observed with infant quiet and in supine position. Score 0: arms and legs extended; 1: beginning of flexion of hips and knees, arms extended; 2: stronger flexion of legs, arms extended; 3: arms slightly flexed, legs flexed and abducted; 4: full flexion of arms and legs.

Square Window   The hand is flexed on the forearm between the thumb and the index finger of the examiner. Enough pressure is applied to get as full a flexion as possible, and the angle between the hypothenar eminence and the ventral aspect of the forearm is measured and graded according to Fig. 21-2. (Care is taken not to rotate the infant's wrist while doing this maneuver.)

Ankle Dorsiflexion   The foot is dorsiflexed onto the anterior aspect of the leg, with the examiner's thumb on the sole of the foot and other fingers behind the leg. Enough pressure is applied to get as full flexion as possible, and the angle between the dorsum of the foot and the anterior aspect of the leg is measured.

Arm Recoil   With the infant in the supine position, the forearms are first flexed for 5 seconds, then fully extended by pulling on the hands, and then released. The sign is fully positive if the arms return briskly to full flexion (score 2). If the arms return to incomplete flexion or the response is sluggish, it is scored as 1. If they remain extended or are only followed by random movements, the score is 0.

Leg Recoil   With the infant supine, the hips and knees are fully flexed for 5 seconds, then extended by traction on the feet, and released. A maximal response is one of full flexion of the hips and knees (score 2). A partial flexion scores 1, and minimal or no movement scores 0.

Popliteal Angle   With the infant supine and his pelvis flat on the examining couch, the thigh is held in the knee-chest position by the examiner's left index finger and thumb supporting the knee. The leg is then extended by gentle pressure from the examiner's right index finger behind the ankle and the popliteal angle is measured.

Heel To Ear Maneuver   With the baby supine, draw the baby's foot as near to the head as it will go without forcing it. Observe the distance between the foot and the head as well as the degree of extension at the knee. Grade according to Fig. 21-2. Note that the knee is left free and may draw down alongside the abdomen.

Scarf Sign   With the baby supine, take the infant's hand and try to put it around the neck and as far posteriorly as possible around the opposite shoulder. Assist this maneuver by lifting the elbow across the body. See how far the elbow will go across and grade according to illustrations. Score 0: elbow reaches opposite axillary line; 1: elbow between midline and opposite axillary line; 2: elbow reaches midline; 3: elbow will not reach midline.

Head Lag   With the baby lying supine, grasp the hands (or the arms if a very small infant) and pull him slowly towards the sitting position. Observe the position of the head in relation to the trunk and grade accordingly. In a small infant the head may initially be supported by one hand. Score 0: complete lag; 1: partial head control; 2: able to maintain head in line with body; 3: brings head anterior to body.

Ventral Suspension   The infant is suspended in the prone position, with the examiner's hand under the infant's chest (one hand in a small infant; two in a large infant). Observe the degree of extension of the back and the amount of flexion of the arms and legs. Also note the relation of the head to the trunk. Grade according to Fig. 21-2.

With each inspiration his chest wall retracts, his nares flare, and he may have accompanying respiratory grunting. Soon he may become cyanotic in room air and experience periods of apnea. His general skin color may appear pale due to vasoconstriction. Upon auscultation of his chest, air entry appears diminished. Edema may develop in his extremities because of altered vascular permeability but usually subsides by the fifth day.

If the disorder is severe, he may have bradycardia and difficulty in maintaining his temperature. In severe cases the infant is extremely hypoactive and flaccid. He develops severe retractions in the first 6 hours and shows no improvement of air exchange after 24 hours. In addition, he remains cyanotic while receiving oxygen. Often he assumes a froglike position with his head turned to one side and

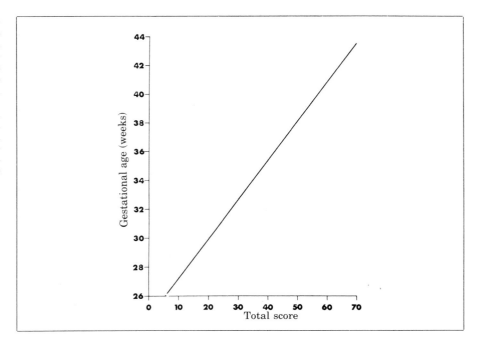

Figure 21-3. Scores obtained from assessment of external criteria and neurologic signs are totaled. The total score is plotted on the graph to obtain the gestational age. (From L. M. S. Dubowitz, V. Dubowitz, and C. Goldberg. Clinical assessment of gestational age in the newborn infant. *Journal of Pediatrics* 77:1, 1970.)

his mouth open. After 72 hours, death is unlikely unless the infant encounters further complications, such as pneumonia, pulmonary hemorrhage, or intracranial hemorrhage. In most cases of RDS, retractions begin to improve in approximately 72 hours, and tachypnea a day or two thereafter.

The etiology of RDS involves deficient or absent pulmonary surfactant, a lipoprotein produced by cells in the alveolar wall. As the fetus matures, phospholipids necessary for lung expansion and gas exchange at birth are present in the alveoli of the lung. Prior to lung maturity, two important lipoproteins, lecithin and sphingomyelin, are in equal concentrations. Lecithin is produced in two major pathways, the choline and methylation pathways. Until the thirty-fifth week of gestation, methylation is the primary pathway, while after 36 weeks of gestation lecithin is produced through the choline pathway. The choline pathway yields a more stable and effective form of lecithin, while lecithin produced by the methylation reaction is easily inhibited by hypothermia, hypoxia, and acidosis, and possibly by cesarean delivery. After 34 to 35 weeks of gestation the concentration of lecithin usually increases in amniotic fluid, while that of sphingomyelin remains the same. When the ratio of lecithin to sphingomyelin in amniotic fluid is 2 : 1, the choline pathway of lecithin synthesis is functional, the fetal lung is considered mature, and the chances that the infant will develop respiratory distress syndrome are low [4, 22]. Two other phospholipids found in smaller quantities in amniotic fluid, phosphatidyl glycerol (PG) and phosphatidyl inositol (PI), are important in stabilizing lecithin in the surfactant layer that lines the alveoli. When they are present, the infant very rarely develops respiratory distress [13].

Surfactant acts at the air-liquid interface of the alveoli, decreasing surface tension and thus preventing the alveoli from collapsing during expiration. This allows the infant to establish a functional residual capacity. In normal infants, therefore, approximately 25 percent of the alveolar volume remains expanded after expiration; this is not the case with the infant with RDS. An infant with inadequate surfactant and little or no residual capacity requires higher pressures to reinflate his alveoli during the next inspiration.

The resistance within the pulmonary circuit causes reduced blood flow to the alveolar capillaries, and the lungs are therefore ischemic as well as collapsed. As this atelectasis continues, it enhances hypoxia, hypercapnia, and acidosis, which cause an additional increase in pulmonary vasoconstriction and ischemia and decreases the alveolar cells' ability to produce surfactant. As these events continue, the lung collapse becomes more extensive, requiring more pressure to inflate the infant's lungs and more energy on the infant's part to breathe [12].

Pulmonary vasoconstriction effects further changes in the heart. Normally after birth the pulmonary vessels dilate, and there is a decrease in the vascular resistance in the lungs. The increased blood flow through the lungs leads to an increased flow and pressure in the left atrium. The pressure in the left atrium, which is higher than that in the right, closes the foramen ovale, eliminating a right-to-left shunt. Pulmonary vasoconstriction reverses this effect and opens the shunt.

In addition, as the infant's arterial PO_2 normally increases, the ductus arteriosis gradually begins to close, thus causing more blood flow to the lung. Hypoxia, which constricts the pulmonary vasculature, also reverses closing of the ductus. It is also believed that hypoxia damages the capillary endothelium, and, when accompanied by high negative intrathoracic pressure, helps to promote transudation of fluid into the alveoli. Fibrin forms a matrix that traps the necrotic alveolar duct epithelium, red blood cells, serum proteins, and so forth. These coalesce to form hyaline membranes that line the alveolar ducts and terminal bronchioles. Unfortunately, the young premature infant lacks the fibrinolysins necessary for dissolution of the membrane. This leads to airway obstruction and further compounds the problem. Hypoxia also induces a metabolic acidosis as lactic acid increases, which results in impaired metabolic response to cold stress and ultimately a low systemic blood pressure from diminished cardiac output [12].

Intervention. The treatment and care of infants with RDS is complex and requires constant observation on your part. The infant will receive oxygen, but it may be administered in a number of ways. If it flows into an isolette (Fig. 21-4), the percentage of oxygen in the infant's environment will be increased. It may be administered via a hood or dome placed over his head, or, in the very ill infant who has been intubated, it may flow through his endotracheal tube. However it is administered, it must be given cautiously, since excessive levels may lead to eye or lung damage. The infant's retina may scar, resulting in blindness (retrolental fibroplasia). The lung tissues may fibrose under excessive oxygen administration, impairing oxygen diffusion from the alveolar lumen to the capillaries.

If the infant can breathe spontaneously and atelectasis is no problem, oxygen may be delivered via a head hood. If the infant has atelectasis but is able to breathe spontaneously, a system such as continuous positive airway pressure (CPAP) may be used to maintain some degree of positive pressure throughout the respiratory cycle. Continuous positive airway pressure is also referred to as

Figure 21-4. Twin preterm infants receiving oxygen via respirators. (Courtesy of Pennsylvania Hospital, Philadelphia, Pa.)

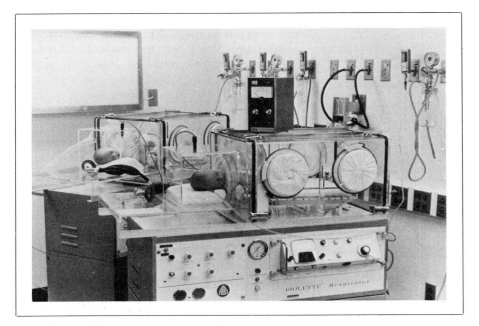

continuous distending pressure (CDP) and is a form of positive end-expiratory pressure. It maintains alveolar stability.

Positive end-expiratory pressure can also be achieved by maintaining continuous negative pressure (CNP) to the chest by enveloping the chest or upper abdomen in a dome. The sustained negative pressure expands the chest, and the continuous pull on the alveoli prevents their collapse at end expiration.

If the infant is frequently apneic and does not respond to CPAP or CNP, a mechanically assisted ventilator may be used. Two types of positive pressure respirators are used. One type controls the volume of gas by limiting inspiratory pressure created in the respiratory tract during delivery. The other type limits the volume of gas delivered and can be pressure-restricted as well. Negative pressure respirators are used less often. This type encloses the body from the neck down and moves gas in and out of the lungs by intermittently creating negative pressure around the body. Oxygen is delivered in the head chamber.

In the infant, PaO_2 over 100 millimeters of mercury is currently considered hyperoxemic; under 50 millimeters of mercury it is hypoxemic. Arterial blood levels are determined at least every 4 hours for sick babies, at shorter intervals for the very sick, and every 6 hours for babies not acutely ill. Blood for blood gas determinations is usually drawn from an umbilical artery catheter or from the radial, brachial, or temporal arteries by needle puncture. Another method used to measure oxygen tension is the transcutaneous oxygen sensor, an electrode secured to the skin. This device can produce PO_2 values from the warmed skin (tc PO_2) that are generally well correlated with arterial PO_2. Continuous readouts of oxygen tensions on the infant's skin can be done.

Oxygen administered to infants should be moist and warm no matter what method is used to deliver it. When oxygen to the infant can be decreased, it is usually well tolerated if decreased 5 to 10 percentage points every 4 hours, but some infants may require a slower weaning.

Cyanosis is not used as a method of determining oxygen levels in sick infants since it is an unreliable indicator of hypoxia in the infant. As Korones notes, several factors influence the recognition of cyanosis including color and thickness of skin, number of capillaries, hemoglobin level, serum bilirubin, and the type and intensity of light present [12].

RETROLENTAL FIBROPLASIA AND BRONCHOPULMONARY DYSPLASIA

Assessment. In the early 1950s it was discovered that the oxygen used to treat RDS in the premature baby was also the source of another of his major complications, retrolental fibroplasia, which develops as a result of inordinately high levels of oxygen in the retinal capillaries. The effect of oxygen on the retinal vessels depends on the duration of their exposure to oxygen, the stage of their development, and the oxygen concentration in the infant's arterial blood.

The first stage of reaction involves constriction of retinal vessels. It is felt that the vasoconstrictor effects of short periods of high oxygen are reversible. If vasoconstriction lasts longer than several hours, the process may not be reversible, although the point at which this occurs is not known. Severe vasoconstriction is not seen when the retina is fully vascularized. The younger the infant, the less vascularization is present. Retinal damage is greatest when the infant's gestational age is less than 36 weeks or when he weighs less than 2,000 grams (4.4 pounds).

The second stage begins within 1 or 2 months after oxygen treatment is terminated. At this time there is a proliferation of new blood vessels from the retinal capillaries. They sprout through the retina into the vitreous body. These vessels are often permeable, and hemorrhage and edema sometimes occur. Organization of these hemorrhages can produce pressure on the retina and may result in its detachment. Detachment of the retina is followed by absorption of the vitreous body, pulling together of the retina, and formation of a membrane behind the lens, which ultimately leads to blindness. The process reaches this point in approximately 25 percent of infants with retinal vasospasm during early oxygen therapy. It is important, therefore, to have an ophthalmologist examine these babies periodically and to decrease the oxygen as much as possible if vasospasm is noted [8, 9]. Also monitor the PaO_2 levels closely, particularly as the infant's condition improves and PaO_2 levels increase rapidly. Recent research indicates vitamin E given to premature infants provides some protection against retinopathy [20].

High oxygen concentrations can also injure the infant's lungs. While eye injury is due to high PaO_2, bronchopulmonary dysplasia (BPD) is a result of a high FiO_2 and perhaps other factors as well. It is a progressive chronic lung disease which is virtually always associated with long periods of mechanical ventilation with high concentrations of oxygen administered through an endotracheal tube.

Lung changes include thickening and necrosis of alveolar walls, basement membranes, and broncheolar epithelial lining layers. Atelectasis and fibrosis also occur, impairing diffusion of oxygen from alveolar lumens to capillaries.

BPD may become apparent when increased oxygen and ventilatory pressure requirements are needed at a time when recovery from RDS should occur. Retractions and diminished breath sounds persist, and crepitant rales become audible. As the disease progresses, oxygen and ventilatory pressures increase, emphysema progresses, CO_2 retention increases, respiratory acidosis results, and right heart failure may occur. About 30 percent of infants with BPD die by 7 to 8 months of age, while young children who have had less severe lung changes survive but may experience recurrent episodes of pulmonary infections and wheezing [12].

Intervention.   Because arterial levels of oxygen over 100 millimeters of mercury lead to eye and lung impairment, the American Academy of Pediatrics recommends that infants' PO_2 levels be kept between 60 and 80 millimeters of mercury when infants are receiving oxygen for more than brief periods. As mentioned previously, in monitoring the infant's oxygen levels, keep in mind that as his ventilation improves, his PO_2 level will rise. He therefore needs very close observation. His position is important, since it can maintain or obstruct his airway. The head of his bed may be elevated 10 degrees, and his shoulders may be raised. If necessary, his head may be kept in slight hyperextension. In addition to proper positioning, suction should be used as necessary to maintain an open airway.

Infants with RDS usually develop some degree of acidosis. In the early stages respiratory acidosis predominates, but as the infant works harder to breathe, lactic acid levels increase and metabolic acidosis appears. If the acidosis is not corrected, it may lead to pulmonary vasoconstriction, irregular heartbeat, depression of myocardial function, dilatation of cerebral vessels that can lead to cerebral hemorrhage, further impairment of surfactant activity, and detachment of bilirubin from albumin, causing kernicterus at low serum bilirubin concentrations. Levels of blood gases and pH are usually used to determine the amount of sodium bicarbonate that will be given to the acidotic infant. The accepted normal pH values of arterial blood in newborns 24 hours old is 7.35 to 7.44. The range compatible with life is 6.8 to 7.8. Clinically important deviations occur between 7.00 and 7.25 [12].

Keeping the infant warm is essential, since cold stress increases the need for oxygen. In an infant who is already having difficulty maintaining an adequate oxygen level, cold stress can be disastrous. Cold increases the metabolic rate and the production of lactic acid, thereby aggravating hypoxia and acidosis, increasing pulmonary vasoconstriction, and possibly impairing production and activity of surfactant.

Circulatory System   The preterm infant's heart is relatively large at birth compared to his overall body size, and murmurs are not uncommon. Because of immature cardiac conductile tissue, his heartbeat may be arrhythmic; therefore, his pulse rate is most accurately obtained by listening to the apical rate for 1 full minute. His blood pressure is lower than the term infant's (45–60/30–45 millimeters of mercury), and his peripheral circulation is poor.

The proportion of fetal hemoglobin to adult hemoglobin is higher than in the mature baby, and the fetal hemoglobin tends to disappear more slowly. Since fetal hemoglobin releases oxygen to peripheral tissues less readily than the adult type, and since the preterm infant's capillaries may be fewer in number, oxygen perfusion of some of his tissues is marginal, at best. The walls of his blood vessels are known to be very fragile, especially those of the intracranial vessels. This, plus a decrease in several clotting factors (particularly prothrombin), predisposes him not only to bruising but also to hemorrhage, especially in the ventricles of the brain. The precipitate births, breech presentations, and hypoxia associated with premature delivery raise the risks of intracranial bleeding.

The fall in the preterm infant's red blood cell level and hemoglobin concentration is greater and the final rise of these two values is slower than in the full-term infant. This results in a more prolonged physiologic anemia in the preterm baby, whose hemoglobin level may drop as low as 6 to 7 grams per 100 milliliters in 4 to 8 weeks. This is particularly due to a reduced rate of hematopoiesis and the shortened life span of his red blood cells, poor iron stores, and a greater growth rate after birth with a corresponding greater increase in blood volume. The rapid destruction of his immature red cells, together with the immaturity of his liver, predisposes him to a more prolonged course of hyperbilirubinemia and jaundice than that which the full-term infant is likely to experience.

Nervous System

The development of the nervous system depends on the baby's length of gestation. The young preterm baby lies quietly, and external stimulation elicits weak, uncoordinated, purposeless movements and perhaps a feeble cry. He may first lie in the fetal position but gradually uncurls to lie on his back with his head rolled to one side, hips flexed and abducted, and knees and ankles flexed (frog position) (Fig. 21-5). His centers for vital functions (respiration and temperature) as well as vital reflexes (cough, swallow, and suck) may be poorly developed. The Moro, tonic neck, Chvostek, and Babinski reflexes are usually present, but tendon reflexes are variable.

Gastrointestinal System

ASSESSMENT

Digestion is rudimentary in an infant of 26 to 28 weeks' gestation but becomes more effective as his age increases. Even though fat-splitting enzymes are present at birth, the infant fails to absorb 20 to 40 percent of the saturated fat from his milk feedings. Except for a possible decrease in bile salts, no chemical cause for the poor absorption is obvious. However, unsaturated fats of vegetable origin are better absorbed than animal fats. Both preterm and full-term infants are born with low levels of lipoproteins, which transport fat. These apparently are synthesized in the liver within the first 2 or 3 weeks after feeding is begun. The

Figure 21-5. Usual position of the preterm infant.

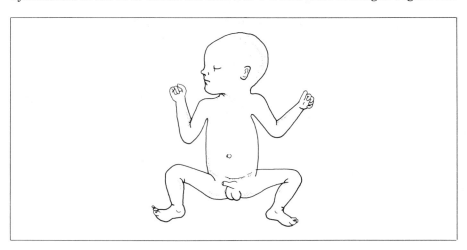

preterm infant may also have difficulty metabolizing lactose because lactase is a late-appearing enzyme.

The larger preterm infant (33–34 weeks) has good sucking and swallowing reflexes. Even so, regurgitation may be common, since he is likely to have a limited stomach capacity, a poorly developed cardiac sphincter, and a relatively strong pyloric sphincter. The musculature of his bowel wall is weak and easily distended, so constipation and abdominal distention may be special problems. Normal gastric peristalsis can be seen through his thin abdominal wall.

His liver is relatively large, but its function is poorly developed. Because his liver enzymes are decreased, he is unable to conjugate and excrete bilirubin satisfactorily (tendency to jaundice). Other liver-related problems involve his small glycogen stores (tendency to hypoglycemia), lower serum protein (tendency to edema), decreased blood clotting factors (hemorrhagic disease), and inability to conjugate and detoxify certain drugs. In addition, he has received less than the usual antibody complement from his mother, and his own poor formation of antibody protein predisposes him to infection. He synthesizes IgG poorly and his rate of IgM synthesis is slower than that of the full-term infant.

Premature infants are also prone to developing necrotizing enterocolitis (NEC). Its etiology remains unknown but it is believed to be caused by ischemic injury to the intestine from mesenteric vasoconstriction. This may result from fetal or infant stresses such as hypoxia, hypovolemia, and hypothermia. Enteric bacteria gain access to the bowel wall and spread. Air is produced in the bowel wall (pneumatosis intestinalis), and pneumobilia (pylephlebitis with air in the portal venous system from gas forming gram-negative organisms) can be identified. Subsequently the infant's intestine perforates, and air and intestinal contents leak into the peritoneal cavity [10].

The early symptoms of NEC include abdominal distention, loose seedy stools often positive for occult blood, and bile-stained vomiting or gastric contents. Signs of sepsis such as apnea, bradycardia, and hypothermia may occur at the same time.

INTERVENTION

The infant's bowel is rested by means of nasogastric decompression. Intravenous antibiotic therapy and fluid and electrolyte therapy are begun. The baby is kept warm. Bowel rest is usually required for at least 3 weeks. If the infant's bowel has perforated, surgery is required to resect the perforated and gangrenous section. He is also given broad-spectrum antibiotics effective against gram-negative organisms.

The research of several nurses has important implications for the prevention of necrotizing enterocolitis in prematures. In 1976 two nurses, Measel and Anderson, noted that restless premature infants developing intestinal distention would become relaxed and could be tube-fed successfully if allowed to suck on a pacifier during and following each feeding. Their study of 59 premature infants randomly assigned to treatment and control groups showed that treated infants were ready for bottle-feeding 3.4 days earlier and therefore required 27 fewer tube feedings, gained 2.6 grams more per day, and were discharged an average of 4 days sooner than the control group [15].

Their research has been replicated and extended twice. In one study Dr.

Anderson collaborated with a group of developmental psychologists, and their findings were essentially the same regarding weight gain and infant readiness for bottle-feeding. Additionally, the 30 treated infants went home 8 days sooner than the controls at an actual cost saving of over one hundred thousand dollars [9]. The second extension of their work was conducted by a pediatrician, Dr. Judy Bernbaum, and her associates [2]. Their findings regarding infant weight gain, earlier bottle-feeding, and earlier discharge were similar to the earlier studies. In addition, they found the infants' intestinal transit time was 12 hours for the treated infants and 32 hours for the controls. This work has important implications for necrotizing enterocolitis which occurs so often in prematures.

Genitourinary System   The preterm infant's urine is scanty and infrequent for a few days after birth because of his limited intake. Since tubules continue to be formed during the entire 40 weeks of normal gestation, the baby's ability to excrete sodium and chlorides is compromised, making him more susceptible to electrolyte imbalance, edema, and a more marked and prolonged acidosis. These factors may also affect the excretion of medication he may receive. The preterm baby has more extracellular fluid than the term infant and less renal capacity for concentrating urine, a fact that is of clinical importance when the baby is suffering from diarrhea, vomiting, or other conditions involving loss of water.

Preterm infants have a special tendency to develop inguinal hernias. In girls, the labia minora are not usually covered by the labia majora. In boys, the testes may be in the abdomen, inguinal canal, or scrotum, depending on the infant's gestational age.

Eyes, Ears, Nose,   The premature infant's eyes appear prominent and widely spaced. By 24 weeks'
Mouth   gestation, retinal vessels have grown close to the optic nerve. From 24 to 30 weeks no further growth occurs, and the fundus is immature. Growth then resumes, so that by 34 weeks the fundus is usually mature [6]. The eyes are most likely to develop retrolental fibroplasia before 34 weeks.

The preterm infant's nose is small and short. His small ears lack cartilage and can be folded with little resistance. His tongue appears large in his mouth and the fat pads in his cheeks are absent. In general, his head looks large and out of proportion to his relatively short neck and extremities and elongated trunk.

Skin, Hair, Nails   The preterm infant's skin is often red and wrinkled, since he usually has little subcutaneous fat. In the smallest babies the nipples are flat, pigmented areas. It is only after 36 weeks' gestation that they rise above the surrounding skin. Engorgement of the breast is rare. The skin on the soles of the feet is likely to be uncreased.

Lanugo is plentiful until 28 weeks; then it decreases in amount. The back, face, and extensor surfaces of the limbs are the most likely to remain covered. The hair on the head is usually soft, short, and scanty. Eyebrows are often absent. The nails are softer than those of the full-term infant but reach to his fingertips as early as 28 weeks' gestation.

Caring for the Preterm   In general, care of the infant is based on providing him with warmth, meticulous
Infant   physical care, gentleness, precise and careful feeding, and protection from

infection. It is also based on the satisfaction of his emotional needs, so necessary for the growth and development of all infants.

FEEDING

Assessment and Intervention.   There are considerable differences of opinion among competent pediatricians concerning some aspects of feeding premature infants—choice of food, number of calories per pound of body weight, time at which the feedings are started. One food choice, breast milk, has the advantages of easy digestibility and reduced incidence of abdominal distention and regurgitation, in addition to its effectiveness in preventing enteric infections. However, it may lack sufficient protein for the rapid growth of the small preterm infant [31].

Formulas for the preterm infant contain 2.2 grams of protein per 100 milliliters and 24 calories per ounce. The infants are usually fed 120 to 130 calories per kilogram, which means they receive 3.3 to 3.6 grams of protein per kilogram. The carbohydrate content of formulas for prematures consists of lactose and glucose polymers, and the fat content consists of 40 to 50 percent medium chain triglycerides [1]. The SGA infant has a higher metabolic rate and may require more calories; he may also require a vitamin supplement because of his rapid growth as will the preterm infant because of his poor vitamin stores, although the minimum daily requirement of the rapidly growing preterm infant is not known.

In addition to his poor tolerance of fat, the preterm infant often has mechanical difficulties. If he is very small, he may have weak buccal, tongue, and palate muscles. Incomplete nervous system development may result in weak suck and swallow reflexes, so he may have to be gavage-fed. His small stomach capacity sometimes requires that he be fed as little as 5 cubic centimeters at a time initially to avoid overfeeding. Nurses often use early feedings to judge the individual infant's volume tolerance and make adjustments in his feeding schedule accordingly. Continuous gastric (nasogastric or oralgastric) feedings may be used in infants less than 1,000 grams rather than a bolus feeding.

Because the preterm infant tires very quickly, his sucking becomes less efficient, especially if the feeding is prolonged beyond 15 minutes. Sometimes his sucking reflex can be stimulated if the nipple is moved about; this must be done very gently to avoid injuring the mucous membrane in his mouth. If the nipple is pressed down on his tongue or gentle upward pressure is applied under his chin, he often begins sucking with renewed vigor (Fig. 21-6).

Despite the fact that feeding time is usually the only time a preterm baby is removed from his isolette and can be cuddled in the traditional sense, nurses should remember the importance of other modes of sensory stimulation, such as the sound of a voice and touch, which are just as effective inside the isolette (Fig. 21-7). While the temptation to hold the preterm infant close is hard to resist, you will find that the more "comfortable" the baby is, the sooner he will go to sleep and not complete his feeding. Holding him in a semi-erect position away from the body will facilitate both feeding and burping and allow for more direct observation of how he is handling the formula. Burp the baby in this position with one hand supporting his head and chest, while the other hand gently pats or rubs his back (Fig. 21-8). If the baby is burped in the over-the-shoulder manner, he cannot be observed as well. In addition, he is pressed against the bony shoulder, which may be somewhat traumatic, and he is placed dangerously close to the nurse's nasopharynx, a potential source of contamination.

Figure 21-6. Preterm infant bottle-feeding. The nurse stimulates the infant's senses by talking to him, rubbing him, and fondling him even if he must remain in the isolette. (Courtesy of Thomas Jefferson University, Philadelphia, Pa.)

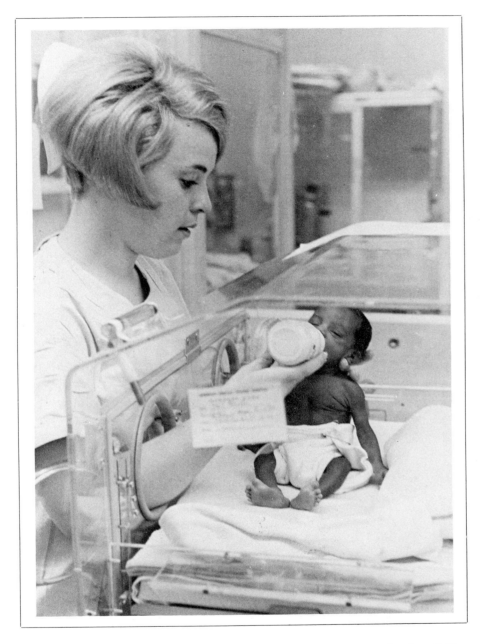

Small infants who cannot suck or swallow or who become cyanotic when fed by bottle are usually fed by gavage (Fig. 21-9). A polyethylene French catheter (No. 5 or 8) is used for the feeding and may be indwelling (changed every 2 to 3 days) or may be inserted at each feeding and then removed. If the infant is very small, an indwelling nasojejunum or gastric tube can be used to provide continuous feedings.

Prepackaged sterile gavage tubes are usually premarked for insertion point, but to be on the safe side they should be remeasured and marked prior to insertion

Figure 21-7. A day in an isolette can be boring. A soft voice and gentle touch help so much.

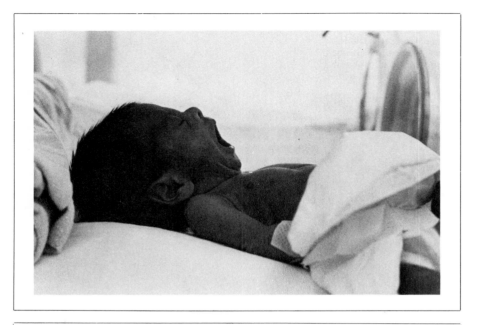

Figure 21-8. Position for burping the infant.

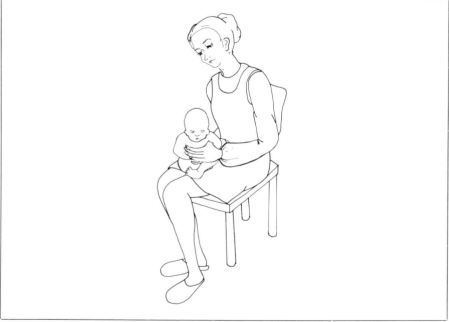

in order to estimate distance into the stomach. If the tube is to be passed through the nose, the distance from the nares to the earlobe and from the earlobe to the xiphoid process is marked off. If it is to be passed through the mouth, the distance from the bridge of the nose to the xiphoid process is measured. This method is often preferred, since the narrow nasal passage may be easily injured or infected.

Prior to insertion of the gavage tube or gavage feeding, the infant is positioned

Figure 21-9. Preterm infant with indwelling nasal gavage tube. (Courtesy of Thomas Jefferson University, Philadelphia, Pa.)

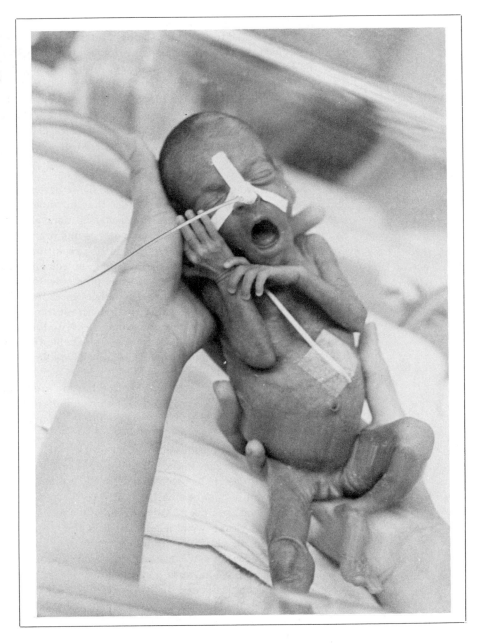

on his back, with his shoulders elevated by placing a rolled diaper under them and his neck hyperextended. As the catheter is passed, he is observed for dyspnea and cyanosis (tube in trachea). To determine that this has not occurred, the open end of the gavage tube is placed in a medicine glass containing sterile water. If the tube is in the trachea, air bubbles will appear as the infant exhales.

Another way to test if the tube is in the stomach involves injecting 2 cubic centimeters of air through the tubing. The flow of air can be heard as a rushing sound when a stethoscope is placed over the infant's stomach.

Before the feeding is begun, a syringe is attached to the feeding tube and is gently aspirated to estimate residual contents of the stomach. If there is residual, it is refed to the baby and the new feeding, reduced by this amount, is poured into the barrel of the syringe and allowed to flow slowly into the infant's stomach. With a No. 5 feeding tube, it may be impossible to get the formula flowing freely. If so, it may be pushed at a rate of 3 milliliters per minute using a syringe with a large barrel to minimize the pressure generated. When the catheter is to be removed, it is pinched off, withdrawn, and discarded. The infant is turned on his right side when the feeding is completed or on his abdomen with his head elevated.

LOW BIRTH WEIGHT BABIES (SGA)

Low birth weight babies, who are small for gestational age, require as much special care as preterm babies. Since they have been subject to stress in utero, they are prone to develop a number of conditions neonatally. Most commonly, a baby who is SGA has suffered from severe and prolonged intrauterine malnutrition. This may be caused by any condition resulting in poor placental growth or function (e.g., poor maternal nutrition, preeclampsia, smoking, high-altitude residence, drug addiction, or multiple pregnancy). Chromosomal abnormalities and congenital malformations as well as intrauterine infections may also be contributing factors to intrauterine growth retardation (IUGR).

Intrauterine growth retardation may be of two types. If the stress occurs in the initial stage of growth (as with chromosomal abnormality and congenital malformation), mitosis is impaired, fewer new cells are formed, and the body organs are small and of subnormal weight. Individual cells have a normal amount of cytoplasm. If there is fetal malnutrition later in pregnancy (due to preeclampsia, smoking, or placental insufficiency, for example), the total number of cells will be normal but decreased in size because of lower amounts of cytoplasm. Most cases of IUGR fall into this category. If malnutrition occurs during the period of very rapid brain growth (the last few months of pregnancy), it may be associated with a permanent decrease in the total number of cells. In general, the brain, skeleton, heart, and lungs are least affected by IUGR, while the adrenals, liver, spleen, and thymus are likely to be smaller in size.

Infants who are SGA usually appear thin and wasted, with little subcutaneous tissue. Their skin is wrinkled, loose, often dry, frequently scaling, and commonly meconium-stained. Their umbilical cords may be withered, appearing dull, yellow, and dry. In extreme cases, the trunk (buttocks particularly) and extremities may not have as much musculature as would be expected. Usually the body length is not affected and the head size may be normal, although the hair on the head will be sparse, coarse, and longer than that of the preterm infant. The skull sutures may be wider than normal because of impaired bone growth. Infants who are SGA are often alert and active, and seem hungry.

These babies are particularly subject to neonatal asphyxia, especially if they have been exposed to chronic intrauterine hypoxia. In utero or at birth they commonly aspirate amniotic fluid, which often contains meconium. With amniotic fluid aspiration, the fluid portion is absorbed by the pulmonary circulation, but the solid particles become lodged in the alveoli and small tubes leading to them. The debris causes mechanical obstruction and hypoxia; the meconium, if present, is irritating and may cause an inflammation of the bronchial mucosa. Meconium aspiration may be complicated by pneumothorax due to partially blocked, overexpanded areas of the lungs. Pneumonia and pulmonary hemorrhage occur frequently.

The infant who has aspirated meconium may be depressed and require resuscitation. Gasping respirations are sometimes observed; the chest may appear enlarged; respirations are rapid; and rales may or may not be heard. The lungs can remove meconium rapidly, and improvement is often marked after 48 hours [11].

Babies who are SGA may also have polycythemia, with a hematocrit of over 60 percent. The cause of this is unknown, although it may be related to hypoxia in utero. No specific congenital abnormalities are associated with SGA neonates. Both preterm and SGA babies are prone to suffer from hypoglycemia and heat loss.

Hypoglycemia   ASSESSMENT

The SGA infant's hypoglycemia is a result of his limited or depleted glycogen stores, and gluconeogenesis in his undergrown liver may be inadequate to support his relatively well-grown brain. The preterm infant is prone to hypoglycemia because of increased energy consumption caused by hypothermia, anoxia, acidosis, or respiratory distress, any of which may exhaust his limited glycogen stores.

In utero, glucose is transferred across the placenta and is the main source of fetal energy. Hepatic gluconeogenesis probably does not occur in utero even though the necessary enzymes are present in the liver at birth. Fat catabolism in utero is not a significant energy source, and plasma-free fatty acids exist at low levels.

The placenta begins to accumulate glycogen as early as the eighth week of gestation. As term approaches, glycogen is increasingly stored in the fetal liver and heart and not in the placenta. Such stores are essential to the infant's survival during labor and immediately after birth, but with intrauterine malnutrition or anoxia, they may either fail to accumulate or be utilized before birth [30].

At birth the placental glucose supply is abruptly cut off. At the same time, energy demands increase, and the newborn's responses are directed toward maintaining blood glucose levels. His system's first reaction is rapid glycogenolysis. Almost all the hepatic glycogen is used in the first 2 or 3 hours after birth. Gluconeogenesis, which begins in the first few hours, becomes increasingly important as a source of glucose for his brain. As the glucose is used, plasma-free fatty acids begin to increase.

Newborn blood glucose levels at birth are approximately 70 to 80 milligrams per 100 milliliters. A rapid decline occurs for the first 2 hours; then the blood level rises to 50 to 60 milligrams per 100 milliliters at 4 to 6 hours. However, if the infant's temperature is low, his glucose level is likely to be 40 to 50 milligrams per 100 milliliters. At 4 to 6 hours after birth a low birth weight infant will have a glucose level of approximately 40 milligrams per 100 milliliters.

INTERVENTION

Hypoglycemic infants have whole blood glucose levels below 30 milligrams per 100 milliliters if they are full-term and below 20 milligrams per 100 milliliters if they are of low birth weight [12]. To be diagnostic these values must appear in two sequential samples taken at least 1 hour apart during the first 3 days of life; after this, 40 milligrams per 100 milliliters is the diagnostic level. Clinical symptoms usually appear at these levels and are associated with jitteriness, cyanosis, convulsions, apnea, apathy, high-pitched or weak cry, limpness, refusal to feed, or temperature instability. If hypoglycemia is untreated, it may result in central nervous system damage of varying degrees. Treatment consists of careful observation, blood glucose determinations, and, if oral feeding is not sufficient, intravenous infusions of glucose. If the infant shows signs of hypoglycemia, a 25% glucose solution is given in a dose of 2 to 4 milliliters per kilogram of body weight followed by a solution that delivers glucose at 7 to 8 milligrams per kilogram per minute. A 15% dextrose solution at 80 milliliters per kilogram per 24 hours will deliver glucose at a rate of 8 milligrams per kilogram per minute as will a 10% dextrose solution at 120 milliliters per kilogram per 24 hours [12]. Hypoglycemic infants are fed as soon as possible after birth.

Heat Loss   ASSESSMENT
Both SGA and preterm infants lack the insulating effect of subcutaneous fat, and as a result they are prone to lose heat rapidly. The preterm baby is particularly susceptible due to the poor development of his heat-regulating center, sluggish circulation, poor reflex control of skin capillaries, feeble respirations with poor oxygen consumption, muscular inactivity, and poor food intake. Additionally, the premature's large body surface area compared to his mass, his nonflexed position, and his lack of brown fat all contribute to rapid heat loss.

INTERVENTION
Temperature maintenance is even more difficult in a cool environment for the small preterm infant whose caloric intake is already limited by a small stomach capacity. Since fewer calories are required for maintenance of body temperature if the baby is kept in a warmer environment, he is placed in an isolette where the environmental temperature can be regulated to keep his body temperature in the range of 97.6° to 98.8° rectal or 97° to 98° skin temperatures.

While isolettes are expensive equipment, they supply correct heat, humidity, and concentration of oxygen to suit individual babies. They also save nursing time and allow easier observation of the baby from a distance. On the other hand, they allow the naked infant to lose heat by radiation, and their humidity reservoirs are probably one of the greatest sources of bacterial growth in the nursery. For this reason, the water is changed frequently or the reservoir is kept empty. Isolettes are kept scrupulously clean, and the infant is moved to a new one every few days if water is being used. Careful monitoring by an observant nurse is just as essential for infants in isolettes as for those in open cribs, and the same precautions for their safety and freedom from infection must be taken.

Currently temperature-control isolettes are being used frequently. These can provide a more sensitive temperature regulation, since their heating element is activated by a probe placed on the infant's anterior abdominal wall. Skin temperature is considered to be a more reliable index than rectal temperature, because the latter only increases or decreases when the infant's own thermostatic mechanism is failing. Unfortunately, an infant can become overheated in an isolette if the servo-control temperature probe slips off his skin. Therefore, it is important that the infant's body temperature be adequately monitored.

Hypocalcemia   ASSESSMENT AND INTERVENTION

Hypocalcemia is often an additional problem of preterm infants as well as of those babies subjected to an abnormal intrauterine environment (e.g., maternal diabetes or hyperparathyroidism) or suffering from a postnatal infection. In fetal life the plasma levels of glucose and calcium are regulated by placental exchange. Perhaps as a result, the baby's regulatory mechanisms for both these substances are somewhat immature. He shows rapid changes in his plasma glucose, as already noted, and in his plasma calcium during the first days after birth, with a delay of 1 or 2 weeks before the levels characteristic of maturity are reached.

In utero, the fetus accumulates most of his calcium during the last trimester, so that 75 percent of the calcium in a full-term infant is acquired after the twenty-eighth week of gestation. Fetal calcium concentration is higher than the maternal concentration, and fetal calcification proceeds normally despite poor maternal nutrition and even placental insufficiency and fetal malnutrition. Therefore, SGA babies normally have adequate calcium stores at birth. The true preterm infant, however, has missed most of his intrauterine calcium accumulation and is born relatively calcium-deficient. In addition, the baby's immature kidney cannot reabsorb sufficient calcium from the tubules and responds poorly to parathyroid hormone, thereby causing retention of phosphate. As a result, the calcium level decreases and the phosphorus level increases during the first days after birth [30].

Certain factors besides the degree of prematurity and calcium deficiency in the bones tend to predispose the newborn to hypocalcemia. If the infant has been stressed due to obstetric trauma or asphyxia, the endogenous corticosteroid his body releases will tend to decrease his serum calcium. If his acidosis is treated with bicarbonate, the ionized fraction of serum calcium will be decreased as a result. If his diet is low in calcium and high in phosphorus, the risk of hypocalcemia is increased. Cows' milk has a particularly high phosphorus level and a low calcium-to-phosphorus ratio, and the low dose of vitamin D in some commercial formulas encourages calcium transport into the bone and could potentiate a resulting hypocalcemia. If the infant has received an exchange transfusion with citrated blood, the ionized calcium level is likely to be decreased, whether or not calcium gluconate is given to him.

Symptoms of hypocalcemia are nonspecific in the newborn. Twitching, jitteriness, and convulsions are most frequent, followed by cyanosis and vomiting. Chvostek's and Trousseau's signs, which are present in older children with hypocalcemia, occur in only 20 percent of hypocalcemic neonates. Chvostek's sign in particular is not very reliable, since it is present in many normal newborns.

Hypocalcemia, defined as calcium levels below 7 to 7.5 milligrams per 100 milliliters, peaks on the first day after birth and again at around 5 or 6 days. After 7 to 10 days, most infants achieve a calcemia level of 9 milligrams per 100 milliliters. The incidence of hypocalcemia is said to be highest in late winter and early spring, presumably due to the increased maternal parathyroid activity to compensate for lack of sunlight and decreased vitamin D.

Treatment consists of a slow intravenous injection of calcium gluconate. Unless the hypocalcemia results in convulsions, which are an immediate threat to life, there is usually no structural damage to the central nervous system associated with it.

Sequelae of Low Birth Weight

Preterm infants are likely to have lower average heights and weights than full-term babies of the same age during the first 1 or 2 years of life unless allowances are made for the length of gestation. A number of infants will take longer than that to reach average growth and development norms, and a few will never reach them, perhaps due to genetic causes or socioeconomic factors. Preterm infants are notoriously late within this time period in reaching developmental milestones—smiling, sitting without support, standing, walking, talking, and bladder control. Again, this developmental lag is largely eliminated if age is calculated from the estimated date of confinement. SGA babies are more likely to be mentally retarded than preterm infants because of the intrauterine anoxia to which they were subjected.

Other sequelae of premature birth include reduced intellectual ability, neurologic deficits (spastic diplegia), vision and hearing difficulties, and a greater risk of infectious disease in the first year of life. The majority of premature infants are remarkably well adjusted and normal in behavior, although a short attention span, lack of confidence, and emotional instability were noted in some studies. Some of these findings may be the result of damage to the central nervous system, but others may result from an overprotective or rejecting attitude of the parents toward the child or may be due to the innate personality characteristics of the individual. Infant stimulation programs have been effective in decreasing developmental delays associated with prematurity.

POSTMATURITY

An infant is postmature if he is born during or after the forty-second week of gestation. By this definition, approximately 12 percent of all pregnancies are prolonged. The postmature infant may be appropriately sized but quite often he is SGA because of a decrease in placental function. In this case he may actually have a wasted appearance. Vernix is virtually absent from his loose skin, which becomes dry, cracked, and parchment-like soon after birth. His subcutaneous fat is likely to be decreased so that his body appears thin and long. Frequently his long nails, skin, and cord are meconium-stained. Usually he has a profuse amount of long scalp hair. He often appears alert and wide-eyed, indicating chronic intrauterine hypoxia. As a result of this, perinatal mortality is higher for postmature infants than for full-term infants [12].

Approximately 75 to 85 percent of the deaths among postmature babies occur during the stress of labor [12]. Often the infant's oxygen supply was marginal for days before delivery. When postmaturity is suspected, nonstress tests, maternal urinary estriol determinations, and oxytocin challenge tests are often used as an index of fetal well-being and placental function so that measures may be taken to deliver the baby before the stress becomes too great.

HEMOLYTIC DISORDERS

Hemolytic disease in the newborn is a result of fetal erythrocyte antigens' gaining access to the maternal circulation. The mother's body responds by producing antibodies, which may then cross the placenta, attach themselves to fetal cells bearing the antigen, and cause these cells to be removed from the fetal circulation; they are subsequently destroyed. Stevenson [25] noted that at least 50 genetically determined erythrocyte agglutinogens exist, and that maternal-fetal incompatibility for one or more of these antigens probably occurs in all pregnancies. Fortunately, not all agglutinogens are sufficiently antigenic to result in clinically significant isoimmunization. The Rh and ABO antigens evoke a strong response and therefore are the most important.

Rh Incompatibility   ASSESSMENT

What is commonly referred to as the Rh (Rhesus) antigen is found on the erythrocytes of 85 percent of all Caucasians, approximately 95 percent of all black people, and virtually all Orientals. Rh is really not one antigen but a group of six antigens designated C, D, E, c, d, e. Because of the strong antigenicity of D, individuals are classified as Rh-negative or Rh-positive according to whether or not they possess this particular antigen.

In order for hemolytic disease to become a problem for the fetus or infant, the fetus must possess the antigen (Rh+) on his erythrocytes while his mother does not (Rh−). The father of the baby must be either homozygous (DD) or heterozygous (Dd) for the gene in order for the infant to inherit the antigen. The fetal antigen in turn must reach the maternal circulation and produce an antibody response. Fetal transfusion of 0.5 milliliters or more will produce primary maternal sensitization; after this, smaller amounts will evoke an antibody response. In addition to occurring with a pregnancy, sensitization may also follow an abortion, a ruptured ectopic pregnancy, or an improperly matched blood transfusion.

In order for the fetus to be affected, the maternal antibody must cross the placenta. In Rh immunization, the IgG fraction of these antibodies is readily transferred to the fetus, attaching to his Rh-positive erythrocytes. The red blood cells are then removed from his circulation—primarily by the spleen—and destroyed. With the destruction of many of his erythrocytes, the fetus becomes anemic. In utero most of the bilirubin produced by the fetus is transported across the placenta in an unconjugated form and conjugated and excreted by the mother's liver and intestine so the infant is rarely jaundiced at birth. If the fetus is severely affected (hydrops fetalis), his hematopoietic tissue cannot compensate for the anemia. He may be stillborn, or, if born alive, suffer from severe anemia, generalized edema, and cardiac failure.

After birth the excessive bilirubin resulting from the erythrocyte breakdown leaves him with hyperbilirubinemia. If the anemia is severe, the fetus or infant may have cardiac failure and generalized edema. In an effort to compensate for the anemia, hematopoietic tissue in the fetus's liver and spleen becomes active, partially explaining why these organs become enlarged.

In most instances, however, the infant or fetus is not so severely compromised, but after birth he must cope with hyperbilirubinemia. With rapid hemoglobin breakdown, the rate of bilirubin production exceeds the capacity of the infant's liver to conjugate it. Normally, the bilirubin is transported via albumin to the liver, where hepatic cells conjugate it with glucuronic acid, changing it to a water-soluble form. Some of the conjugated form (direct bilirubin) again attaches to albumin for transport through the circulation and excretion by the kidneys. Much more conjugated bilirubin is transported to the gastrointestinal tract where it is metabolized to urobilinogen and excreted in the urine and stool. With very rapid breakdown of the erythrocytes, excessive amounts of unconjugated bilirubin (indirect bilirubin) accumulate in the blood, rapidly attaching to the albumin for transport. Once the albumin-binding sites are saturated, the excess unconjugated bilirubin remains free. This fraction is fat-soluble and diffuses across vascular membranes into tissues, especially those of the brain. Bilirubin deposits in the brain (kernicterus) produce irreversible damage. Since in this instance a large amount of bilirubin is present, there is a high indirect bilirubin (unconjugated) but some of the bilirubin is conjugated and this exceeds the body's ability to excrete it from the gut and perhaps the liver as well after conjugation. Therefore, the infant's direct bilirubin (conjugated) may be elevated as well.

Usually on the first prenatal visit a woman's blood type and Rh factor are determined. If she is Rh-negative, a serum screening test for antibodies is done. Even if no antibodies are detected, the screening may be repeated at monthly intervals throughout the pregnancy.

Since the intensity of the disease is likely to be greater with rising serum titers, generally the higher the titer, the more dangerous the outcome for the infant. Chances for the infant's survival have been reported to be excellent if the mother's titer is 1 : 64 or less; however, when it rises above this, chances of his survival decrease [22]. The use of antibody titers to accurately predict fetal outcome is limited. Antibodies may not rise significantly in some severe cases, and occasionally a mother's titer may rise even though she carries an Rh-negative fetus. While some physicians still feel that serum antibody titers are of value in predicting fetal prognosis, many now feel that they serve only to indicate whether or not the mother is sensitized. Since the bilirubin levels rise in the amniotic fluid of an affected fetus, amniocentesis is now used more frequently to determine fetal prognosis.

Since the mother must have prior sensitization with antibody formation in order for the fetus to be affected, first pregnancies are usually not associated with problems. If an Rh-negative primigravida has previously become sensitized, perhaps by incompatible blood transfusion, an amniocentesis will be performed at approximately 28 weeks' gestation. For women who have shown moderate to severe sensitization previously, the procedure is performed earlier.

Amniotic fluid is analyzed for the breakdown products produced during erythrocyte destruction, mainly bilirubin. The amount of blood pigments in the amniotic fluid closely parallels the severity of the hemolytic process. When analyzed using a spectrophotometer, a spectral absorption curve is obtained by plotting optical density against the wavelength of visible light spectrum. The breakdown products of hemoglobin absorb monochromatic light at a wavelength range of 400 to 500 millimicrons, with the cumulative peak seen at 450 millimicrons. Using this technique, researchers have developed a number of graphs that are used to predict the severity of the hemolytic disease. The graph proposed by Liley (Fig. 21-10) contains three zones: Zone A indicates mild or no hemolytic disease; zone B, moderate disease; and zone C, severe disease. A moderately affected fetus (zone B) has a good chance of survival if labor is induced at 35 to 37 weeks of gestation, or if delivery by cesarean birth is performed at 36 to 37 weeks if induction of labor fails. A severely affected fetus (zone C) may require delivery as early as 33 weeks if death is to be avoided [21]. Those fetuses severely affected prior to a time of viability may be transfused in utero to prevent fetal death.

Figure 21-10. Spectrophotometric analysis of amniotic fluid of an erythroblastotic fetus taken at 31.5 and 32.5 weeks' gestation. Analysis indicates progression from moderate to severe disease. The infant will be delivered if mature; if not, he may receive an intrauterine transfusion. (From S. G. Babson and R. Benson. *Management of High-Risk Pregnancy and Intensive Care of the Neonate.* St. Louis: Mosby, 1971.)

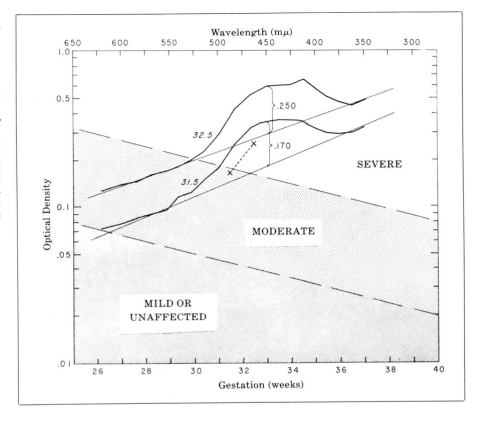

INTERVENTION

In utero transfusion is indicated when the fetus is severely affected (Liley's zone C) and will die prior to 32 to 34 weeks of pregnancy if not transfused. A minimum of 5 hours prior to transfusion, 10 to 15 milliliters of a radiopaque contrast medium is injected into the amniotic fluid. The fetus swallows the medium, thus providing an outline of his intestines on x-ray 5 to 24 hours later. Using local anesthesia, the physician passes an open lumen needle through the mother's abdominal and uterine walls into the fetal abdominal cavity. After further x-rays or ultrasound scanning to confirm the position of the needle, polyethylene tubing is threaded through the needle into the fetal abdomen and the needle is removed. With a three-way stopcock attached to the catheter, 50 to 150 milliliters of packed red cells are injected into the fetus over a 2-hour period. The packed red cells are from freshly drawn O-negative blood that is compatible with the mother's blood. The amount injected depends on the estimated fetal weight. Since the fetus is now being maintained on transfused blood, transfusions may be repeated every 7 to 10 days until a total of about 350 milliliters is given or until the fetus is believed to have a good chance of survival if delivered.

The erythrocytes are absorbed from the fetal peritoneal cavity, elevating the fetal hemoglobin and preventing cardiac failure and generalized edema. The fetus who is already hydroptic, as evidenced by thickening of the scalp on ultrasound, does not benefit from the procedure, and it is felt that it should be reserved for fetuses that are not so severely affected. The incidence of maternal complications from the procedure is 2 to 3 percent from hemorrhage, infection, and further sensitization because of damaged placenta. Fetal loss is 10 to 15 percent due to cardiac failure (overload), infection, serum jaundice, and needle trauma.

At birth, a sample of cord blood from infants of Rh-negative mothers is routinely sent to the laboratory. Samples of anticoagulated blood are used for hemoglobin and hematocrit measurements, reticulocyte count, white blood cell count, and blood smears. Clotted blood samples are used for blood typing, Coombs' test, and measurements of serum bilirubin. The umbilical cord is clamped as early as possible during delivery to avoid the infant's receiving extra antibodies and erythrocytes from the placenta. Should he receive them, these extra erythrocytes place an added strain on his liver's conjugating system when they are broken down. The umbilical cord is usually left about 10 centimeters (4 inches) long to facilitate introduction of umbilical catheters in case exchange transfusions become necessary in the next few days.

The infant is carefully observed for signs of pallor, jaundice, and an enlarged liver and spleen. The jaundice, which commonly appears during the first 24 hours, may be evident in the sclera, umbilical cord, skin, and mucous membrane. With increasing jaundice, the infant may appear lethargic and feed poorly, and his activity and muscle tone may decrease. As the bilirubin levels climb, signs of central nervous system irritability develop; the infant has a high-pitched cry, muscle spasticity, retraction of the head, and later, convulsions.

In order to avoid central nervous system involvement, serum bilirubin levels are carefully monitored. Generally infants do not exhibit signs of kernicterus if bilirubin levels remain below 18 to 20 milligrams per 100 milliliters of blood. However, the preterm infant whose liver is especially immature may develop symptoms at levels as low as 9 milligrams per 100 milliliters of blood [3].

The amount of free bilirubin may be increased if hypoxia, acidosis, hypothermia, or hypoglycemia occurs. In acidosis the binding of albumin is impaired. In hypothermia and hypoglycemia, the level of nonesterified fatty acids increases, and the acids then compete with bilirubin for the albumin-binding sites. Low albumin levels increase the danger of kernicterus. Sulfonamides and salicylates compete with bilirubin for protein-binding sites, and caffeine sodium benzoate uncouples bilirubin from albumin.

Infants who are born with a positive Coombs' test, a cord hemoglobin of 14 grams per 100 milliliters of blood or less, and a cord unconjugated bilirubin level of 4.5 milligrams per 100 milliliters of blood or more need exchange transfusion. Infants whose bilirubin levels indicate a rise of more than 0.5 milligrams per 100 milliliters of blood per hour during the first 48 hours of life or whose bilirubin levels are projected to exceed 20 milligrams per 100 milliliters need treatment [21]. O-negative compatible blood, 500 milliliters, is used for exchange transfusion. It is preferable to have freshly drawn blood, since 110 milliliters of acid citrate dextrose added to a pint of blood to preserve it lowers the albumin and erythrocyte volume. It also contributes to the production of postexchange hypoglycemia by stimulating insulin secretion.

While receiving an exchange transfusion, the infant is placed in an incubator or on a working surface with a radiant overhead heater so that his temperature is carefully maintained. A piece of plastic tubing is placed in his umbilical vein. The other end of the tubing contains an adaptor (Tuohy) and two stopcocks. One stopcock is connected to a bag of blood and the other to a bottle or bag for collecting the waste blood. Five to 20 milliliters of blood is injected into the infant at a time, depending on his size and condition, and the same amount is withdrawn and discarded after each injection. His apical rate is monitored continuously, and his respirations and skin color are meticulously observed. His blood sugar is monitored with a Dextrostix since the procedure may aggravate hypoglycemia. A pacifier can be used during the procedure to keep the infant from crying. After transfusion of each 100 milliliters of blood, 0.5 to 1 milliliter of 10% calcium gluconate solution may be given intravenously to prevent hypocalcemia. The amount of blood given to the infant is twice the volume of his blood (170 ml of blood/kg) [12] (Fig. 21-11).

While the exchange transfusion corrects the anemia, decreases the bilirubin level, and removes Rh antibodies, the procedure is not without complications. Mortality has been reported to be as high as 5 percent, but a significant portion of these deaths were of already moribund, hydropic, and kernicteric infants. Complications from the procedure include air or thrombotic emboli; sepsis, hypothermia, bradycardia, or cardiac arrest from low pH of donor blood; heart failure from hypervolemia or hypovolemia; and hypocalcemia from citrate binding.

An alternate way to reduce increased bilirubin levels is by the use of phototherapy (Fig. 21-12). This procedure eliminates the need to perform exchange transfusions on some infants and reduces the number of transfusions

Figure 21-11. Infant receiving an exchange transfusion.

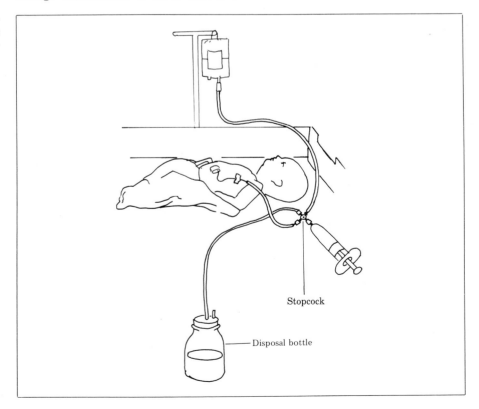

Stopcock

Disposal bottle

Figure 21-12. Infant receiving phototherapy. The infant's eyes are well protected from the light rays, which may cause retinal damage. (Courtesy of Thomas Jefferson University, Philadelphia, Pa.)

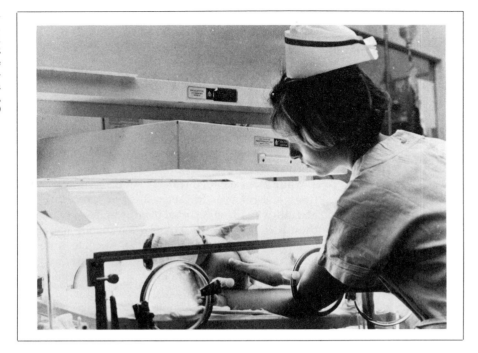

Figure 21-12. Infant receiving phototherapy. The infant's eyes are well protected from the light rays, which may cause retinal damage. (Courtesy of Thomas Jefferson University, Philadelphia, Pa.)

needed for others [14]. Light therapy can reduce serum levels of unconjugated bilirubin by as much as 25 to 50 percent. Bilirubin is thought to produce photoisomers, which are excreted in urine and also passed through the liver into the gut without conjugation [5].

The effectiveness of phototherapy is in the blue light segment of the light spectrum. The intensity of blue light can be demonstrated by measuring energy in the 400 to 500 nanometer range. The units of energy are expressed as microwatts per square centimeter per nanometer ($\mu W/cm^2/nm$). A minimum of 4 microwatts per square centimeter per nanometer is considered necessary for effective phototherapy. The FDA recommends the use of a protective plastic barrier between phototherapy lights and babies, since ultraviolet light can cause skin erythema. A bronze baby syndrome has been reported in infants with liver damage and high direct bilirubin. These infants developed gray-brown skin, serum, and urine; discoloration regressed 3 weeks after phototherapy was discontinued [12].

To prevent retinal damage, the infant's eyes should be protected from the light rays by cotton and gauze pads, with a head bandage to keep them in place. It is essential that the bandage cover the eyes but keep the eyeballs and soft cranium of preterm infants free of pressure. It is also essential that the infant's bilirubin and hemoglobin levels be carefully monitored, for the changes in skin color may mask increasing levels of bilirubin and anemia. Loose stools, rashes, and changes in activity are common side effects of light therapy. The infant also experiences water loss because of an increased metabolic rate, loose stools, and water loss via the skin while under phototherapy. Overheating may also occur as a result of heat production from the light. Since little is known about the long-term effects of light therapy, it should not be used prophylactically or indiscriminately.

In women who have not yet become sensitized, Rh sensitivity can be prevented by the use of $Rh_o(D)$ immune globulin (RhoGAM), which confers passive immunity to the woman by neutralizing the Rh-positive antigen. (As a blood product, RhoGAM may be refused by certain groups of people.) When given within 48 hours after delivery, it neutralizes and later destroys the Rh-positive antigen of the fetal erythrocytes that have entered the mother's circulation during delivery; her own immune system is therefore not activated. The globulin will remain for several months, and during that period she will have positive antibody titers, which gradually decrease in potency. The immunization must be repeated after each delivery or abortion of an Rh-positive fetus. RhoGAM is not effective for and should not be given to a woman who is already sensitized. Therefore, mothers must have a negative Coombs' test prior to its administration. Crossmatching is also done to ensure compatibility of the anti-D preparation and the mother's own erythrocytes.

While hemolytic disease most commonly occurs in response to the Rh D antigen, it can also occur in response to c(hr), C (rh), E (rh), and e(hr), or in response to the ABO blood-group antigens.

ABO Incompatibility   ASSESSMENT AND INTERVENTION

While ABO incompatibility occurs more often than Rh incompatibility during pregnancies, its clinical problems are far less severe. Antibodies formed against A and B antigens are of two immunoglobulin fractions. A naturally occurring type (IgM) is formed in response to a variety of antigenic stimuli (e.g., food proteins); this type does not cross the placental barrier. The second type, an immune one (IgG), does cross the barrier. Mothers with type-O blood usually produce anti-A and anti-B antibodies of the IgG type that pass through the placenta to the fetus, causing hemolysis of the fetal erythrocytes if fetal blood type is A, B, or AB.

Mothers with type A or B blood produce anti-B or anti-A antibodies of the IgM variety. It is believed that certain amounts of immune types (IgG) of anti-A or anti-B antibody may exist at all times in the circulation of type-O mothers and therefore may cross the placenta during a woman's first pregnancy. This explains why firstborn children represent 40 to 50 percent of the cases of ABO disease. The next born is usually affected less than the first. The reasons for this are unknown. Most cases of ABO incompatibility occur with a woman whose blood type is O, while her fetus's blood type is A or B.

The infant with ABO incompatibility may become jaundiced within the first 24 hours after birth, but his anemia is usually not as severe as that seen with Rh incompatibility. There is usually no pallor or cardiovascular stress in the infant. After birth, antibody may be detected by the Coombs' test. Treatment is the same as that for the infant with hyperbilirubinemia due to Rh; however, exchange transfusion is rarely necessary.

NEONATAL   Asymptomatic maternal infection usually precedes fetal infection, which occurs
INFECTIONS   antepartally or intrapartally. The infection may be transmitted through infected amniotic fluid, from the maternal bloodstream across the placenta, or from direct contact with infected maternal tissue in the birth canal. After birth the infant may become infected by the people or objects used to save his life. Infections that are mild or asymptomatic in children or adults may be devastating to the neonate. Physical signs of infection in the neonate are unique in their subtlety

and lack of specificity. Although antibiotics are the mainstay of therapy for infections in the newborn, supportive therapy is also essential to meet normal infant needs. It includes the maintenance of body temperature, the administration of oxygen as indicated, and the administration of fluids to maintain normal fluid, electrolyte, and acid-base balance, as well as the interaction necessary for the foundation of a basic trust relationship.

Bacterial Infections　　ASSESSMENT AND INTERVENTIONS

Bacterial agents are responsible for three major clinical disorders—pneumonia, septicemia, and meningitis. Before the emergence of group B streptococci in the early 1970s as the most frequent etiologic agents, gram-negative rods caused 75 to 85 percent of bacterial infections. *Escherichia coli* was the predominant organism. *Pseudomonas aeruginosa* (often found growing on nursery equipment) was the next most common causative organism. The remaining infections were caused most often by staphylococci.

Bacterial infections may be acquired in utero, during the infant's descent through the birth canal, or after birth in the delivery room or nursery. Most are of the ascending type, resulting in amniotic fluid infection following passage of bacteria from the perineum, vagina, or both through a ruptured amniotic membrane. Sometimes, however, the organisms pass through an intact membrane. From the amniotic fluid they gain entry to the fetus, primarily through the oral cavity, and move to the lungs, gastrointestinal tract, and middle ear, although their presence in the amniotic fluid does not necessarily mean that the fetus will become infected. Since early rupture of membranes predisposes the fetus to exposure to intrauterine infection, it is better if delivery can be accomplished within 24 hours of the rupture. If an infection is suspected in the newborn, the best sites for specimen collections for culture are the throat, axillae, inguinal folds, or external auditory canals, preferably 1 to 2 hours after birth [12]. A frozen section of the umbilical cord will show infiltration by polymorphonuclear leukocytes. The gastric contents of the neonate may also be examined for neutrophils and bacteria. A microscopic examination of amniotic membrane will show the presence of infiltrate.

In general, if the infection is manifested during the first 48 hours, it is likely to have been congenitally acquired (most likely caused by coliforms and group B streptococci) and is best treated with gentamicin and ampicillin. Onset at a later age is usually related to hospital-acquired organisms (*Staphylococcus* and *Pseudomonas*). The treatment in this case is often a combination of gentamicin, carbenicillin, and nafcillin, for late infections [12].

Pneumonia. Pneumonia is the most common of the serious neonatal infections and has been given as a cause of death in 10 to 20 percent of autopsies. The peak incidence is during the second and third days after birth. Congenital pneumonia is commonly associated with obstetric abnormalities such as premature rupture of membranes, uncomplicated premature delivery, prolonged labor, and maternal infection. The bacteria most frequently involved are *E. coli* and other enteric organisms, staphylococci, and group B streptococci. Symptoms, which are evident at birth or within 48 hours after birth, include rapid, shallow respirations, slight retractions, apnea, pallor or cyanosis, and flaccidity. Crepitant rales are sometimes detectable. Body temperature is likely to be elevated in a full-term infant, whereas a preterm baby may have a subnormal temperature.

If the infection is acquired postnatally, *Pseudomonas* is the most common cause along with penicillin-resistant staphylococci and enteric organisms. Clinical signs appearing 48 hours after birth or later include tachypnea and poor feeding or aspiration during feeding. Recovery is more common from this type of pneumonia than from the congenitally acquired variety [12].

Septicemia. Septicemia is a generalized infection that is characterized by growth of bacteria in the infant's bloodstream. Presently, coliform organisms and group B streptococci are the most frequent causes. Early symptoms are vague and nonspecific—loss of appetite, inactivity, loss of weight, vomiting, diarrhea, abdominal distention, abnormal respirations, jaundice, or skin lesions. Meningitis occurs in about one-third of these infants. Septicemia is usually diagnosed from a blood culture, although centrifuged spinal fluid or urine is sometimes used. When the identity of the causative organism is unknown, kanamycin (Kantrex), or gentamicin (Garamycin), and ampicillin may be given immediately. The use of antibiotics has reduced mortality from septicemia from 90 percent to a range of 13 to 45 percent [12].

Meningitis. Almost half of the cases of meningitis in children occur during the first year of life, with the highest incidence occurring in the neonatal period, most frequently in preterm and male infants. Causative organisms are the same as those for septicemia, and the systemic symptoms are similar. Fullness of the anterior fontanelle is the most specific sign, while neck stiffness (Kernig's sign) is rare in the neonate. Opisthotonos may be seen in about 25 percent of infected infants, and coma and convulsions in about 50 percent.

Diagnosis of meningitis is confirmed by abnormalities in the spinal fluid. Treatment is the same as for septicemia. Fatality rates from meningitis range from 35 to 60 percent—and 30 to 35 percent of survivors have some form of central nervous system handicap [12].

Diarrhea. Diarrhea is another important bacterial infection most frequently caused by *E. coli,* although *Salmonella, Shigella,* and *Staphylococcus* are sometimes involved. *E. coli* and *Salmonella* infections produce a stool that is green and slimy, while *Shigella* infections produce watery stools that lack odor and contain blood-tinged mucus. Early symptoms of the infection are loss of appetite, weight loss, and listlessness—all of which may precede diarrhea by 1 or 2 days. *Shigella* infections tend to start explosively. As diarrhea continues, the infant becomes dehydrated and acidotic (metabolic acidosis), and the process is more rapid if vomiting is also present. Milder forms of infectious diarrhea are not unusual.

Diarrheal stools should be cultured as soon as they appear. Neomycin or polymyxin is commonly administered orally before the results of the culture are returned. Diarrhea can become epidemic in a nursery, since the organisms are easily transferred from baby to baby, particularly from unwashed hands of personnel and from gowns; therefore, scrupulous aseptic technique is absolutely essential. In addition, any abnormal stools in infants should be reported, so that isolation precautions may be taken if necessary.

Because these babies may not be given to their mothers to be fed, it is important for you to keep the parents informed about their baby's status. Since the changes in the appearance of an infant who has diarrhea can be quite startling and anxiety-provoking, the parents will need extra support in coping with this additional stress.

Omphalitis. Omphalitis, infection of the umbilical stump, causes the umbilical area to become edematous and red, with a purulent exudate (in mild forms there usually is no exudate). Cultures of the blood and umbilicus should be done. Since omphalitis may herald septicemia, treatment for this infection should be initiated immediately.

Syphilis. Untreated syphilis during pregnancy is a major cause of abortion, fetal death in utero, and premature labor and delivery. Since penicillin crosses the placenta, treatment of the mother almost always successfully treats the fetus also. As a screening device, a serologic test for syphilis (STS) is commonly included in the examination a mother receives at her first prenatal visit. Penicillin is also the treatment of choice for the neonate who shows signs of rhinitis, skin eruptions of the copper-colored macular variety, and x-ray evidence of osteochondritis or periostitis.

Rhinitis (snuffles), caused by a swelling of the nasal mucous membrane, is one of the most frequent signs of congenital syphilis. It tends to make breathing and sucking difficult and is accompanied by a profuse nasal discharge that is extremely irritating to the skin it contacts. Skin lesions may appear on all or part of the infant's body. The palms of his hands and soles of his feet are commonly affected, becoming erythematous, swollen, and peeling. Fissures may appear in all directions about the mouth, anus, and vulva. Infection of the central nervous system occurs in approximately one-third of all syphilitic infants, and a large proportion of such babies have splenomegaly.

Symptoms in early infancy correspond to secondary stages of syphilis in the adult. If he is untreated, the child will show other manifestations of disease later, such as condylomas, peg-shaped and notched (Hutchinson's) incisor teeth, nerve deafness, pupillary abnormalities, tabes, paralysis, and dementia.

Diagnosis of syphilis in the newborn is made on detection of spirochetes in the nasal discharge, open skin ulcers, and a positive *Treponema pallidum* inhibition test (TPI). The TPI test offers more conclusive evidence of true infection than the STS, which may react positively to maternal antibodies that have been transmitted across the placenta to the infant. Usually these antibodies disappear within 3 or 4 months.

Since the nasal discharge and exudate from skin lesions is potentially contagious, it is wise to observe good isolation technique, including the use of gloves when working with infected infants. Although the need for additional therapy beyond the initial treatment is remote, generally it is agreed that children should be followed for 1 or 2 years after treatment.

Skin Infection—Impetigo. Impetigo contagiosa is a bacterial skin infection caused by streptococci or staphylococci that invade the superficial layers of the skin. It tends to spread from one spot to another and is easily transmitted to other persons by direct or indirect contact, so isolation precautions are essential. The skin vesicles, which are most likely to develop in body folds, creases, and moist surfaces, contain purulent material and rupture easily, with the exudate forming a crust that eventually drops off. Because of continued auto-inoculation, the lesions may persist for several weeks. When the infection occurs in the newborn (pemphigus neonatorum), large blisters form over the skin.

Antibiotic ointments are usually quite effective in the treatment of impetigo; they are applied at least twice daily to areas that cannot be protected by a dressing. Before application of the ointment, crusts of the lesions are removed by washing them gently with warm saline solution.

Viral Infections   ASSESSMENT AND INTERVENTION

Viral infections in the newborn occur less frequently than bacterial ones. Generally they are transmitted from the mother, but they may be acquired after birth. Many of the infants who survive these infections are left with varying degrees of damage to the central nervous system. The most important intrauterine viral infections are caused by rubella, cytomegalovirus, and herpesvirus.

Congenital Rubella Syndrome.   Rubella causes a chronic infection of the fetus and neonate that begins in the first trimester of pregnancy and may persist for months after birth. Some infants may harbor the virus for as long as 3 months or more, and if pregnant women who are not immunized are exposed to them, they run the risk of becoming infected themselves.

It is estimated that about 10 to 20 percent of pregnant women are susceptible to rubella. A history of having or not having had the infection is often unreliable, since the clinical signs mimic other viral infections and in many cases infected older children and adults are asymptomatic. Serology is the best diagnostic method, and among the various serologic procedures, the test for hemagglutination inhibition (HI) is the most sensitive one. The presence of HI antibody in serum indicates immunity to rubella. A minimum fourfold rise in titer is necessary to diagnose the infection. Since the HI test is not easy to perform, it should be done by properly trained personnel. It would be disastrous to erroneously tell a susceptible pregnant woman that she is immune, or vice versa.

Because the teratogenic effect of rubella occurs almost exclusively during the first trimester of pregnancy, the exposed pregnant woman should find out as soon as possible whether or not she is immune to the infection. A sample of her serum should be collected immediately for rubella HI titer, and if results are strongly positive, no further test is necessary. If the antibody titer is low or if the original test is sero-negative, a second sample is tested 3 weeks later. A fourfold rise or more in HI titer or its initial appearance signifies recent infection and the possibility of damage to the fetus.

In general, maternal infection in the first month of pregnancy causes infection and congenital malformations in 33 to 50 percent of exposed fetuses; in the second month, 25 percent; and in the third month, 9 percent. If the mother becomes infected in her fourth month, only about 4 percent of the fetuses are affected, primarily by permanent hearing impairment. The chief clinical signs of congenital infection are hypoplastic intrauterine growth retardation, congenital heart disease, and cataracts. The most common cardiac malformations are patent ductus arteriosus and narrowing of the peripheral pulmonary arteries. In a few instances there may be severe myocardial degeneration. Cataracts, which may be unilateral or bilateral, are usually present at birth but sometimes do not appear for a few days or weeks. Microphthalmia and glaucoma are other eye abnormalities that may develop.

Thrombocytopenia and petechiae occur in 40 to 80 percent of infected infants. Hepatosplenomegaly is common, and hyperbilirubinemia due to hemolysis is frequent. Sometimes rubella hepatitis develops, and pneumonia is not uncommon. Neurologic abnormalities, which are present in a few neonates, most often appear later in infancy.

The diagnosis of congenital rubella is indicated by the combination of cataracts and congenital heart disease in the neonate. Although elevated IgM levels are not always detectable at birth, serologic diagnosis is possible by demonstrating the rubella antibody in the serum immunoglobulin M (IgM) [12].

The best method of treatment is prevention, by having all women of childbearing age vaccinated against the infection. If a woman is diagnosed as having rubella during early pregnancy, therapeutic abortion is an alternative for some parents. Since infected babies can communicate the virus to others, the immune status of female nursery personnel of childbearing age should be determined at the time of their employment. If they are susceptible to rubella, they should be vaccinated.

Cytomegalovirus Infection.   Congenital infection caused by the cytomegalovirus may be transmitted from asymptomatic mothers across the placenta or by the ascending cervical route. The results of a congenital infection range from extensive tissue damage that is incompatible with life, particularly if the infection has occurred early in pregnancy, to survival with serious brain damage or survival with a total absence of sequelae.

An infant who has this infection is often SGA and hypoplastic. The principal tissues and organs affected are the blood, brain, and liver. Hemolysis leads to anemia and hyperbilirubinemia, and thrombocytopenia with petechiae and ecchymoses occurs frequently. Hepatosplenomegaly is common. Encephalitis with signs ranging from lethargy to hyperactivity and convulsions may result. Microcephaly may be present at birth, and 10 to 20 percent of symptomatic infants will have chorioretinitis.

Diagnosis involves recovery of the virus from the urine, elevated IgM levels, and identification of cytomegalovirus antibodies within the serum IgM fraction. Of the antiviral drugs used in treatment of this infection, none as yet have been proved particularly effective [12].

Herpesvirus Infection.   About 95 percent of neonatal infections with the herpesvirus are due to type 2, which causes most infections involving the cervix, vagina, and external genitalia. (Type 1 causes lip lesions in older children and adults and skin lesions above the waist.) The infant is infected either when the organism ascends into the uterus or by direct contact during his passage through the birth canal, in a manner similar to infection by gonorrhea. Infection by the transplacental route is rare. If the pregnant woman is known to have active lesions of herpesvirus type 2, the fetus is usually delivered by cesarean to avoid infection.

Neonatal herpesvirus infection presents a wide array of clinical signs. One variety of the infection is usually fatal to almost all affected infants; it involves the adrenals, liver, brain, blood, and lung. Symptoms, which are present at birth or by 3 or 4 weeks of age, include fever, hepatosplenomegaly, hepatitis with jaundice, a bleeding tendency, and neurologic abnormalities. Vesicular skin lesions indicative of the disease are seen in about one-third of the infected infants. They appear occasionally in clusters and are thinly spread over the entire body.

Other, more localized varieties of neonatal herpesvirus infection are less severe, resulting in death in about 25 percent of the infants. The central nervous system, eyes, and skin are most commonly affected, either singly or together. Over one-half of the infants who survive have residual neurologic or visual damage. Clinical signs include convulsions, abnormal muscle tone, opisthotonos, bulging fontanelle, and lethargy or coma. Eye signs include conjunctivitis, chorioretinitis, and a cloudy cornea (keratitis). Sometimes skin lesions are the only manifestation of the infection.

When there are no skin lesions, diagnosis is often difficult, since the symptoms are otherwise nonspecific and very similar to those of septicemia. The most reliable diagnostic procedures are cultures of the virus from the baby's skin lesions and throat and identification of herpes antibodies in the serum IgM fraction. Research is being performed to determine the effectiveness of antiviral drugs as therapy for neonatal herpesvirus.

Protozoan Infection   Toxoplasmosis, the most common protozoan infection, is transmitted to the fetus transplacentally, particularly during the second and third trimesters. The mother, who may be asymptomatic, usually contracts the organism from eating raw or poorly cooked meat or by contact with infected animals. Signs, which appear at birth or soon after, include neurologic abnormalities such as convulsions, coma, hypotonia, microcephaly, or hydrocephalus. The infected infant may also have intracranial calcifications, chorioretinitis, microphthalmia, hepatosplenomegaly, jaundice, petechiae, ecchymoses (thrombocytopenia), and pallor (anemia). The fatality rate is about 12 percent; neurologic disorders in survivors are common. Toxoplasmosis is diagnosed by demonstration of specific antibodies in serum IgM [12]. More information is needed on the potential value of therapy for pregnant women and newborns who are diagnosed as having toxoplasmosis.

DRUG ADDICTION   While the addicted mother faces multiple problems, approximately 50 percent of
Assessment   the live-born infants of mothers who use "hard" drugs experience symptoms of neonatal addiction. Maternal use of 6 to 12 milligrams of heroin daily will usually result in withdrawal symptoms in the newborn. In addition, many newborns, half in some populations, have birth weights of less than 2,500 grams (5.5 pounds). A significant portion of these babies (40 percent in some populations) are full-term infants who are SGA. The perinatal mortality in these groups ranges from 15 to 20 percent [1,21], with the infants succumbing to respiratory difficulties, intracranial hemorrhage, inadequate hydration, electrolyte imbalance, and congenital anomalies. Recent studies show a mortality of 3 to 4.5 percent in rigorously treated infants.

The higher the daily dose of narcotic, the longer the mother has had her habit, and the closer to delivery she had her last "fix," the greater the chances are that her infant will have withdrawal symptoms. Most infants (60 percent) show withdrawal symptoms within 24 hours, practically all within 4 days. Rarely, an infant will show symptoms 7 to 10 days after birth. Excitement of the autonomic nervous system and gastrointestinal and respiratory distress are the most common signs of withdrawal in the newborn (Table 21-3). Two complications that addicted infants appear to be spared are RDS and jaundice. Heroin and phenobarbital are believed to increase bilirubin glucuronyl transferase activity, thus decreasing the incidence of jaundice. Heroin, thought to be an important enzyme inducer, also is reported to speed maturation of pulmonary function [28]. If the health care team is not aware of the mother's addiction, neonatal diagnosis may present a problem, since many of these signs are the same as those found with sepsis, hypocalcemia, hypoglycemia, and cerebral hemorrhage (Figure 21-13).

Table 21-3. Common Signs and Care of Addicted Infants

Infant Behavior	Intervention
Hypertonicity	Observe body prominences for skin breakdown Use sheepskin Change position frequently Check temperature because of increased activity; if it is elevated, decrease environmental temperature
Tachypnea	Watch for signs of progressive respiratory distress Hyperextend head to assure patent airway Maintain in semi-Fowler's position Maintain warmth
Sneezing and nasal stuffiness	Observe for respiratory distress Suction as necessary Feed slowly, allowing for periods of rest as necessary
Poor feeding	Observe sucking quality Feed small amounts frequently
Inability to sleep	Observe character of sleeping pattern Reduce environmental stimuli Swaddle Feed frequently
Fist sucking	Observe for character, occurrence, or precipitating Keep skin area clean Apply mittens
Regurgitation, vomiting, or diarrhea	Observe for character, occurrence or precipitating factor (medication, handling) Observe for fluid and electrolyte balance Maintain side-lying position to prevent aspiration Give good skin care Maintain fluid balance
Tremors or convulsions	Observe character, location, frequency, and any predisposing factor Decrease environmental stimuli Maintain airway Prevent self-trauma Frequent skin care and position changes
High-pitched cry	Note character, duration, or other reasons for cry Decrease environmental stimuli Feed frequently Swaddle tightly in blankets Hold close to nurse's body

Source: L. P. Finnegan and B. A. Macnew. Care of the addicted infant. *American Journal of Nursing* 74:685, 1974. Copyright April, 1974, The American Journal of Nursing Company. Reproduced by permission.

Intervention   Once symptoms appear, treatment with chlorpromazine, phenobarbital, methadone, or paregoric is begun (Table 21-4). In addition to drug therapy, the infant is given supportive treatment. Because of his increased activity, his caloric requirements are increased. Small frequent feedings of a concentrated formula may be given, since larger feedings may not be retained. In the very ill infant, parenteral feeding may be necessary to prevent aspiration and dehydration. With adequate therapy and swaddling the infant will decrease crying and activity, begin sleeping between feedings, maintain a normal temperature, and begin to gain weight.

In attempting to combat the problems of addicted mothers, health care professionals have organized methadone maintenance programs for them. Moth-

Figure 21-13. Common withdrawal signs of an addicted newborn. A. Normal newborn head lag. B. Hypertonicity of newborn addict. C. Standing position of normal newborn. D. Newborn addict supports his own weight with little help. E. Startle reflex in normal newborn. F. Tremors of addicted newborn.

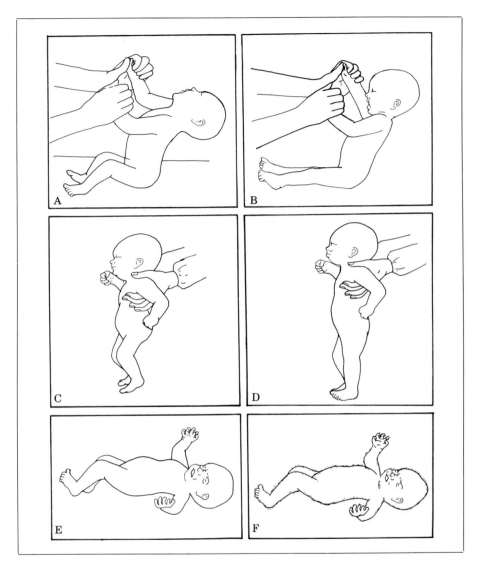

Table 21-4. Drugs Used in Neonatal Addiction

Drug	Dosage and Administration
Chlorpromazine	1–2 mg/kg/day, IM, for 2–4 days; may then be given orally for about 7 days in lesser doses; currently used less frequently
Phenobarbital	8–10 mg/kg/day, IM, for 2–3 days; may then be given orally for about 7 days in lesser doses
Paregoric (for gastrointestinal symptoms)	3–5 drops every 3 hours until infant appears drowsy or encounters respiratory depression; dosage is tapered slowly over 7 days

Source: S. Pierog, and A. Ferrara. *Approach to the Medical Care of the Sick Newborn*. St. Louis: Mosby, 1971.

ers who participate in these programs generally receive better prenatal care, and as a rule their newborns fare better than those of the street addict. The infants' hospital stays are shorter, and the mothers have shown improved attention to child care. Symptoms in these babies may not appear until the end of the first day and on rare occasions may not appear until the first or second week of life.

There have also been attempts at drug withdrawal during pregnancy or attempts to extend the intervals between doses in late pregnancy. When this was attempted, mothers reported violent fetal kicking, which was interpreted by the medical team to be a sign of fetal withdrawal. There appeared to be no damage to the fetus, but some authorities now advocate no withdrawal attempts after the seventh month of pregnancy [25]. Others prefer women to be detoxified during pregnancy to improve infant birth weight and to avoid neonatal withdrawal symptoms [24].

Infants addicted to barbiturates usually are full-term and are of adequate weight. They have a later onset of withdrawal signs (6½ hours to 7 days), and the signs last longer than those of the heroin-addicted infant. Infants whose mothers were on barbiturates for medical reasons tend to have symptoms that last for briefer periods than babies whose mothers were addicted.

FETAL ALCOHOL
SYNDROME

Chronic maternal alcoholism during pregnancy can result in fetal wastage. It can also result in the birth of a fetus who is growth retarded or has microcephaly, short palpebral fissures and microphthalmia, epicanthal folds, micrognothia, malformed and immobile joints, dislocated hips, cardiac malformations, and malformations of the brain. Approximately 50 percent of these infants are at least mildly retarded and 20 percent of the affected infants die [12].

After birth and for up to 3 days, the newborn of an alcoholic mother may exhibit withdrawal symptoms of agitation, hyperactivity, tremors, and seizures. Withdrawal may be followed by 24 to 48 hours of lethargy.

DISORDERS OF
METABOLISM
*Infant of the Diabetic
Mother*

ASSESSMENT

Infants of diabetic mothers are routinely subjected to stresses not normally encountered by other newborns. There is an increased incidence of intrauterine deaths and premature deliveries. In addition to facing the problems encountered by the preterm infant, these infants are frequently large for gestational age and appear plethoric and cushingoid. They are also subject to hypoglycemia, hypocalcemia, electrolyte imbalance, respiratory distress syndrome, polycythemia, hyperbilirubinemia, and possibly a greater incidence of congenital anomalies. The overall survival rate of these infants is 80 to 90 percent. Korones notes that diabetic women in classifications A and B tend to have large-for-dates babies whereas mothers in classes C through R tend to have small-for-dates babies [12].

The LGA infant of the mother with uncontrolled diabetes was formerly thought to be edematous; these babies are now believed to be macrosomic, with an increased number of total body cells. The reasons for this are not totally clear, but it may be due to increased insulin levels in the fetus, resulting in an increase in protein synthesis. Hyperadrenocorticism may play a part. It has also been suggested that the fetus's hyperinsulinism and hyperglycemia in utero lead to excessive growth and deposition of fat. Another theory is that the infant's large size is due to pituitary growth hormone.

These infants in utero have hypertrophy and hyperplasia of the beta cells in the islets of Langerhans and are in a state of hyperinsulinism, perhaps due to the mother's hyperglycemia. At birth, their hyperinsulinism causes their blood sugar levels to drop rapidly, especially during the first 2 to 4 hours after birth. Hypocalcemia frequently accompanies the hypoglycemia; the reasons for this are not fully understood, but it is believed to be caused by depressed fetal parathyroid function that persists temporarily in the neonate.

The frequent incidence of respiratory distress in these infants may be due to asphyxia in utero because of placental insufficiency or to the fact that many are preterm infants often delivered by cesarean operation. Reportedly the enzyme systems of these infants mature more slowly than those of infants of nondiabetic mothers, and this may be a contributory factor. Additionally Smith et al. [25] have noted that insulin abolishes the stimulatory effect of cortisol on the synthesis of lecithin, which may explain the increased incidence of RDS observed in some infants of diabetic mothers. Approximately 50 percent of infants of diabetic mothers develop tachypnea soon after birth, unassociated with RDS.

It has been reported by many authorities that infants of diabetic mothers have a higher incidence of congenital anomalies. These infants often have congenital heart defects such as coarctation of the aorta, ventricular septal defect, transposition of the great vessels, and enlarged hearts. They also have caudal regression and defects of the pelvis and lower limbs, ureteral duplication, and renal agenesis [17].

INTERVENTION

In caring for the infant of a diabetic mother observe the baby carefully, especially for signs of hypoglycemia, hypocalcemia, RDS, and hyperbilirubinemia. Keep the infant warm in an isolette. Tests for blood glucose level begin with a cord blood at birth followed by levels at 1, 2, 4, and 6 hours after birth. Early feedings of 5 to 15 percent glucose should be started, often within an hour of birth, and should be given every 2 hours approximately three times; formula is then given if tolerated. If hypoglycemia is present (serum glucose level below 30 milligrams per 100 milliliters), a parenteral glucose infusion of 10 to 15% dextrose in water should be started, usually in the umbilical vein. Distressed infants and infants of diabetic mothers classes B through F should be given 10% dextrose intravenously immediately after birth at a rate of 65 to 70 milliliters per kilogram of body weight [23].

Phenylketonuria   ASSESSMENT

Phenylketonuria (PKU) is inherited as an autosomal recessive disorder. An infant receives an abnormal gene from each of his heterozygous parents. It occurs in approximately one in 10,000 to 20,000 births and is more common in Caucasians from northern Europe and the United States.

The basic defect in PKU is deficient amounts of the liver enzyme phenylalanine hydroxylase, which converts phenylalanine to tyrosine. In carriers, enough enzyme is present to prevent high concentrations of phenylalanine and its metabolites, which are formed from alternate pathways, from accumulating in the blood, urine, sweat, cerebral spinal fluid, and tissues. The infant who is homozygous for the gene is defenseless. When normal levels of phenylalanine (1–

4 milligrams per milliliter) are exceeded as the newborn feeds during the first few weeks of life, a metabolite of phenylalanine, phenylpyruvic acid, can be detected in the urine. The urine can be tested with Phenistix (paper impregnated with ferric salt) or a few drops of 5% ferric chloride placed on a wet diaper. The diaper will turn green in the presence of phenylpyruvic acid. These tests, however, are not felt to be reliable until the infant is 4 to 6 weeks of age. With earlier hospital discharge, an affected infant may not be identified because phenylalanine levels have not increased sufficiently to be detected in the urine. Earlier diagnosis can be made if increased levels of phenylalanine are found in the infant's blood. The blood test (Guthrie test) is performed using blood from a heel prick. Many states now require routine blood screening for PKU just prior to the newborn's discharge from the hospital.

Infants with the defect may become severely mentally retarded. The exact cause of this is unknown, but it has been attributed to a neurotoxic agent that has an inhibitory effect on development before myelinization in the central nervous system is complete. It has also been postulated that brain damage may already have begun by the time the phenylpyruvic acid is detected in the urine. The children may also have seizures, become hyperactive, and exhibit erratic and unpredictable behavior. Untreated infants also fail to thrive and suffer from skin rashes, vomiting, and irritability. The decreasd tyrosine leads to decreased melanin production and reduced pigment in skin, hair, and eyes, explaining in part why the majority of these infants have fair skin, blonde hair, and blue eyes.

INTERVENTION

Treatment is aimed at eliminating from the infant's diet foods that are high in phenylalanine. Therapy with exogenous enzyme has been of no value. The diet is begun in infancy, maintained during the period of rapid myelinization, and continued during childhood.

Since virtually all vegetable and animal protein contains phenylalanine, the infant is placed on a special protein formula (Lofenalac) that contains essential amino acids but is low in phenylalanine. During pregnancy, mothers with PKU should also be placed on diets with decreased levels of phenylalanine, since phenylalanine will cross the placenta and may cause mental retardation in infants who are themselves only carriers of the gene.

Galactosemia   ASSESSMENT AND INTERVENTION

Galactosemia is transmitted as an autosomal recessive trait and is not common, occurring in approximately 1 in 35,000 births.

Lactose (milk sugar) is normally broken down in the digestive tract into galactose, which is absorbed and converted to glucose in the liver. When the enzyme galactose 1-phosphate uridyl transferase is absent, galactose accumulates in blood and tissues. Affected infants appear normal at birth but within a few days begin to vomit, have diarrhea, lose weight, become jaundiced and drowsy, and have an enlarged liver.

Diagnosis is made on the finding of increased levels of galactose in the blood or urine and/or low levels or absence of galactose 1-phosphate uridyl transferase in red blood cells. Carriers of the disease have decreased levels of the enzyme in their erythrocytes.

Treatment is aimed at eliminating all milk and galactose-containing foods from the diet. Nutramigen and soybean preparations such as Sobee or Mull-Soy are substituted. Untreated infants who survive develop irreversible cataracts and mental retardation.

CHROMOSOMAL ABNORMALITIES
Trisomy 21 Syndrome

Trisomy 21 syndrome is also known as trisomy G syndrome, mongolism, or Down's syndrome. In approximately 95 percent of all affected infants, the syndrome is due to meiotic nondisjunction of one of the G-group chromosomes, usually in the maternal gamete. The infant thus inherits an extra chromosome in this group and a total cell complement of 47 chromosomes.

The incidence of this type of nondisjunction increases with advancing maternal age. The frequency in young mothers is approximately 1 in 1,000 to 2,000 births; at 35 years of age, 1 in 300 births; and at 45 years of age, 1 in 50 births. Many authorities believe that the ova of women over 30 have a greater chance of mechanical error when they proceed through both meiotic divisions than the ova of younger women.

A smaller number of cases of Down's syndrome are due to translocation, in which chromosome 21 attaches to another chromosome, often chromosome 22 or one of the D group. Advanced maternal age is not a factor in these cases, and in fact the parents are usually younger, one of them possibly being a carrier of the disorder. The parent in this case appears normal and has 45 chromosomes. The chance of this couple's producing another affected child is significant. Theoretically, each pregnancy carries a 33 percent chance of recurrence.

An even smaller percentage of children with Down's syndrome may result from mosaicism, in which the child has a mixture of two cell types, one with 46 chromosomes and the other with 47.

Down's syndrome is usually diagnosed at birth. The infant has hypotonic muscles, hypermobility of the joints, short broad hands with stubby fingers, a transverse palmar crease (simian line), a small round head with low-set ears, a flattened occiput, and a small mouth with a protruding tongue (Fig. 21-14). As the child grows, he is usually of short stature, has some degree of mental retardation, and is susceptible to many respiratory diseases. Infants with Down's syndrome often have associated cardiac, renal, and gastrointestinal defects. While male children with the disorder are believed to be sterile, female children may reproduce and have a 50 percent chance of having an infant similarly affected.

Trisomy 18 Syndrome

Trisomy 18 syndrome (E syndrome) occurs in approximately 1 in 3,500 births and is far more frequent in females than in males [18]. It is easily recognizable at birth due to the infant's facial features, which include low-set ears, a prominent occiput, wide-spaced eyes, and micrognathia. The infant also has rocker-bottom feet and a characteristic overlapping of his index finger over the third finger. Usually these infants fail to thrive and rarely survive beyond a few months.

BIRTH INJURY
Assessment and Intervention

The most common and serious form of birth injury is *intracranial injury*. Prolonged labor, difficult delivery requiring use of forceps, precipitate delivery, and breech extraction are likely to result in a sudden change in the shape of the skull rather than the gradual molding process that takes place throughout a normal labor. Intracranial hemorrhage results.

Figure 21-14. Neonate with Down's syndrome. A. Note upward slant of the eyes and epicanthal folds. B. Characteristic grimace. C. Relative broadening of the face. D. Fat pad at the back of the neck and helical distortion of the ear. (From E. L. Potter and J. M. Craig. *Pathology of the Fetus and Infant* [3rd ed.]. Copyright © 1975 by Year Book Medical Publishers, Inc., Chicago. Used by permission.)

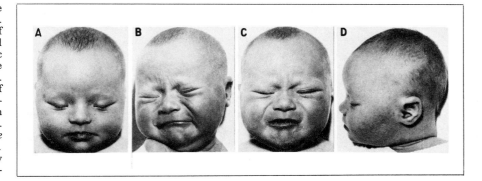

The edema or hemorrhage accompanying intracranial injury leads to a compromise in the blood supply to various portions of the brain, which may suffer temporary or permanent damage. Large hemorrhages occur most commonly in the falx cerebri, which separates the two halves of the cerebrum, or in the tentorium cerebelli, which divides the cerebellum from the cerebrum. In the preterm infant, the vessels of the choroid plexus may be injured, resulting in a hemorrhage into the ventricular system of the brain.

The infant with intraventricular injury may be asymptomatic or his symptoms may be extreme, depending upon the severity of damage. With severe damage, the infant may die within a few hours. The infant may be hypotonic and difficult to arouse, with little spontaneous movement, a depressed or absent Moro reflex, and poor sucking and/or swallowing reflexes. With significant injury his intracranial pressure is high, his respirations may be slow, grunting, irregular, and periodic. Bradycardia exists, his fontanelle bulges, and he may be cyanotic. There may be twitching, or even generalized convulsions. He may have a subnormal body temperature and his cry, although weak, is likely to be sharp and shrill. Blood is usually present in cerebral spinal fluid. Opisthotonic posture, coma, and fixed dilated pupils are frequent. Metabolic acidosis is severe and persistent. Infants who are less affected most frequently exhibit lethargy and hypotonia; they may also show unexplained jaundice, metabolic acidosis, and hyper- or hypoglycemia. A CT scan is used to grade the severity of the lesion (Table 21-5). The prognosis varies with the severity of the injury. Mortality is high when large or vital areas of the brain are affected. Infants who survive are likely to have significant neurologic handicaps [29].

General supportive measures are used in treatment to remedy the hypoxemia, acidosis, and hypotension. Infants are handled gently and sparingly. Sometimes a spinal tap or subdural tap in the area of the fontanelle may be done to relieve

Table 21-5. Grades of Severity of Intraventricular Hemorrhage

Grade I	Isolated subependymal hemorrhage
Grade II	Intraventricular hemorrhage without ventricular dilatation
Grade III	Intraventricular hemorrhage with ventricular dilatation
Grade IV	Intraventricular hemorrhage with ventricular dilatation and hemorrhage into the parenchyma of the brain

Source: G. Fenichel. *Neonatal Neurology*. New York: Churchill Livingstone, 1980.

some intracranial pressure. The best treatment is prevention through careful obstetric management of the mother.

Three other common birth injuries, previously discussed in Chapter 16, are *caput succedaneum, cephalhematoma,* and *facial nerve paralysis.* A fourth is *brachial palsy.* When the nerve fibers running from the neck through the shoulder and toward the arm are injured during obstetric maneuvers, a partial paralysis of the arm results. Most often this involves the muscles of the upper arm and not those of the hand and fingers. The infant holds his arm at his side with his elbow extended and the hand rotated inward (Fig. 21-15). If the nerve fibers have not broken, recovery is usually rapid and complete within a few weeks. If the nerve fibers are broken, recovery depends on their regeneration, which may take from 2 to 3 months or may never occur. During this time the muscles of the shoulder are exercised gently to prevent contractures from forming.

Sometimes *fractures* occur during birth, most often of the clavicle when the shoulder is extracted. No special management is required since they usually heal rapidly without producing much pain or disability. Breaks of an extremity (humerus, femur) are rare and are usually apparent from their abnormal appearance. They heal well when immobilized in the correct position by splints or slings. Since parents may be fearful of hurting the baby by handling him, instruct them in his care and encourage them to hold, fondle, and talk to him.

CONGENITAL
MALFORMATIONS

Malformations of the fetus range from very small defects, such as supernumerary digits, to those that are incompatible with life. The incidence of congenital malformations may be affected by maternal race (more common in Caucasians than in blacks except for supernumerary digits), age (more frequent in infants of mothers over 35—mongolism, central nervous system malformations), parity (anencephalus and spina bifida are more common with first births and those after the sixth), and fetal sex (the majority of anencephalics are female).

Figure 21-15. Brachial palsy.

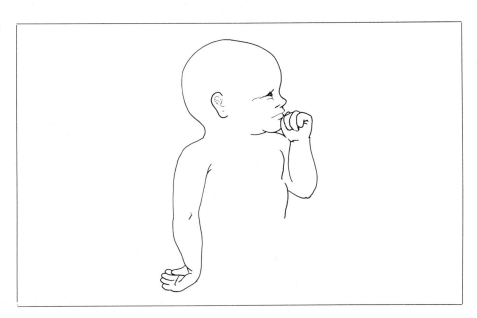

In general, if a woman has given birth to a malformed child, there is an increased likelihood of subsequent malformed infants. Since congenital malformations are often multiple, the presence of one deformity may mean that another is present as well. Current theory indicates that both genetic and environmental factors play a part in the etiology of most congenital anomalies.

Central Nervous System

ASSESSMENT AND INTERVENTION

The nervous system of the newborn is immature anatomically, chemically, and physiologically. In the preterm infant there is little myelination, and polysynaptic connections are just beginning to form. Neurologic function is largely at the brain stem and spinal cord level. The primitive reflexes represent primitive released neuronal function, largely uninhibited by higher cerebral control. Deep tendon reflexes are normally symmetrical; patellar, biceps, and triceps are the most easily elicited.

The three most common congenital anomalies of the central nervous system involve either abnormal size of the head or defects in closure of the bony spine. They are anencephalus, hydrocephalus, and spina bifida.

Anencephalus, the most common cause of gross hydramnios, is a malformation characterized by complete or partial absence of the pituitary gland, brain, and overlying skull. The condition is incompatible with life. The infant's face is very prominent as a result of the absence of the skull, his eyes often protrude markedly from their sockets, and his tongue hangs from his mouth. About 70 percent of anencephalics are female. It is believed that both genetic and environmental factors play a part in the etiology of this defect. Diagnosis, which is suggested by the inability to palpate a fetal head abdominally, is confirmed by x-ray or ultrasound. Increased amounts of alpha-fetoproteins, formed in the fetal liver, are found in the amniotic fluid of fetuses with anencephaly, probably because of leakage of their cerebrospinal fluid.

Hydrocephalus involves an excessive accumulation of cerebrospinal fluid in the ventricles of the brain with resulting enlargement of the cranium. It accounts for about 12 percent of all malformations found at birth, and about 33 percent of the time it is associated with spina bifida, although other defects are also common. It is often the result of meningitis, head trauma, intraventricular hemorrhage, or subdural hematoma in the newborn.

The volume of the fluid involved is usually 500 to 1,500 milliliters, and since the fetus's head in utero is often too large to enter the pelvis, breech presentations are common. Cephalopelvic disproportion is the rule, and dystocia is the result, with uterine rupture a definite risk. Hydrocephalus is suspected if, on abdominal and vaginal examination, the floating fetal head feels unusually broad or if during labor the head remains high despite a normal pelvis and good contractions. Diagnosis of hydrocephalus may be confirmed by x-ray or ultrasonic cephalometry.

Often the disorder is not manifested until several weeks after birth, when the infant's head rapidly begins to increase in size—sometimes 2.5 centimeters (1 inch) or more a month—and signs of increased intracranial pressure appear in the infant. For most babies surgical intervention provides the only hope of relief.

In instances of *spina bifida,* the posterior portion of the bony canal containing the spinal cord is completely or partially absent because of failure of the vertebral laminae to develop or to fuse. This defect is relatively common, particularly in the lumbar or sacral region.

Sometimes the meninges protrude through the defect to form an external cystic tumor (meningocele) that contains cerebrospinal fluid and is present at birth. Occasionally the cord as well as the meninges protrudes (myelomeningocele). The prognosis is generally not good, since hydrocephalus often occurs following surgical repair. In addition, there may be residual rectal or bladder paralysis, with spasticity and deformity of the infant's legs.

Circulatory System—
Congenital Heart
Disease

ASSESSMENT AND INTERVENTION

The most common causes of death in pediatric referral hospitals, excluding problems specifically related to prematurity, are congenital heart defects, despite the fact that there has been rapid advancement in their diagnosis and management. Most of these deaths occur in the neonatal period, particularly during the first 2 weeks after birth.

About 70 percent of newborns with fatal heart defects will have one of the following five structural defects because of errors of embryogenesis in the first 2 months of gestation: hypoplastic left ventricle syndrome (hypoplasia of left ventricle, aortic atresia, or mitral atresia); complicated coarctation of the aorta; transposition of the great arteries; hypoplastic right ventricle syndrome (with pulmonary arterial atresia or stenosis); or severe tetralogy of Fallot. Statistically, the low-risk cardiac newborn is likely to have a simple left-to-right shunt lesion— commonly a ventricular septal defect. Atrial septal defect and patent ductus arteriosus may also occur.

Signs and symptoms of various defects vary with the type and severity. In general, the cardinal signs are cyanosis, respiratory distress, systemic venous congestion (hepatosplenomegaly), and diminished cardiac output. A heart murmur is not usually a presenting sign. Tachypnea is a sign of cardiorespiratory difficulty, and when little respiratory effort is associated with it, congenital heart disease is suggested as the cause. Marked respiratory effort, especially with grunting, suggests lung disease, but there may be much overlap in these two areas. Other observations may include reluctance to feed, easy exhaustion, or changes in color (pallor, grayishness, or cyanosis).

The diagnosis may be made from history, physical findings, x-ray, and electrocardiogram results. Sometimes cardiac catheterization or angiography supplies confirmation. When these infants remain in the newborn nursery while diagnosis is being completed, the staff will take special precautions to prevent infection and unnecessary stresses. Signs such as cyanosis and respiratory distress may be treated symptomatically by the use of oxygen administration and positioning. Frequent small feedings will avoid the possibility of gastric distention and increased pressure on the diaphragm and heart. In the presence of heart failure, digitalis is often prescribed.

Musculoskeletal
System

ASSESSMENT AND INTERVENTION

Clubfoot (talipes equinovarus) is relatively common, occurring in about 1 in 1,000 births. It involves extension and inversion of the foot so that the tarsal bones are displaced and the foot cannot be passively restored to normal position. This defect may occur alone or in association with spinal or central nervous system anomalies (particularly spina bifida) or oligohydramnios. There is some evidence that there may be an underlying genetic defect in the formation of connective tissue. Plaster boots applied to the feet in the correcting position are used to remedy the defect.

Talipes calcaneovalgus and *metatarsus varus* are milder deformities that may be treated by passive manipulation of the foot in the opposite direction and maintenance of the correct position for a minute at a time. This is done frequently during the day, and parents may be taught to do the exercise at home.

Congenital dislocated hip, as discussed in Chapter 16, is a fairly common malformation that is six times more frequent in girls than in boys. X-rays reveal lateral displacement of the upper end of the femur and poor development of the acetabulum on that side. A dislocated hip is treated by maintaining abduction of the hips during the early months of life, usually by application of a cast. Frequently, the application of a triple layer of diapers will maintain the recommended abduction.

In addition to the skeletal fractures already discussed, injury to the sternocleidomastoid muscle may occur during delivery, particularly if the fetus's presentation is breech. The damaged muscle is less elastic and does not elongate at a normal rate during growth, with the result that the child's head is gradually turned to one side, producing *torticollis* or *wry neck*. Surgery can be used to correct the muscle contraction. If the initial injury was slight, healing is usually spontaneous.

Gastrointestinal Disorders

ASSESSMENT AND INTERVENTION

Cleft Lip and Cleft Palate. Cleft lip occurs in approximately 1 in 800 births and results when the embryo's lateral and medial nasal processes fail to fuse between the fifth and eighth week of intrauterine life. The incomplete cleft may be little more than a notch in the lip, or it may extend up into the nostril. The incidence is higher in males and in families with a history of the defect. The deformity may also occur in infants whose mothers had rubella in the first trimester of pregnancy.

Should the palatal processes fail to fuse (usually 1 month later than the nasal processes), the infant is born with a cleft palate. More than 40 percent of the time these two defects occur in conjunction with one another.

Corrective treatment for these disorders is surgery. The cleft lip is usually repaired as soon as the infant can tolerate surgery. The cleft palate is usually not closed until 1½ to 2½ years of age.

Prior to closure of a moderate to severely affected cleft lip, feeding is a problem since the infant cannot create a vacuum in his mouth which enables him to suck. Many infants with cleft lip and palate can adapt to breast-feeding. They learn to place their tongue over the cleft to create a suction or squeeze the nipple with the tongue against the remaining hard palate. Nursing is most successful when the breast is full and firm. Styler and Freeh suggest having the mother massage her breast from the shoulder and armpit to the lower breast to help the milk flow more freely [27].

When breast-feeding is not possible, a soft nipple with a large hole, a specialized nipple such as a Brecht feeder, a Beniflex Disposal Nurser made especially for infants with clefts, or a rubber-tipped medicine dropper may be used to feed him. Styler and Freeh report that parents of infants with clefts find that holding the infant in an upright to semiupright position works best for them. They also suggest feeding the infant slowly, directing the flow of milk to the side of the infant's mouth, giving smaller, more frequent feedings, burping the infant often, and giving him good oral hygiene.

Esophageal Atresia.   Esophageal atresia is a serious anomaly and most commonly involves the upper (proximal) end of the esophagus, which ends in a blind pouch. In approximately 85 percent of the affected infants, the lower end of the esophagus is connected to the trachea by a fistulous tract. The infant may also have associated cardiac defects and anal atresia.

As the infant swallows fluid and mucus, the pouch fills and soon overflows. The infant froths and drools and may aspirate the material into his trachea, resulting in pneumonia. Pneumonia also commonly results when gastric contents gain entrance to the lungs via the fistula. The infant must be positioned with his head up and suctioned frequently to keep his nasopharynx clear of secretions; otherwise, he becomes cyanotic and experiences respiratory distress. He should be kept in an isolette with humidity to keep the secretions liquified. He should also be kept warm and precautions should be taken to keep him free from infection. A gastrostomy may be performed to provide for his nutrition.

The condition is usually diagnosed by x-ray after a catheter is passed through the infant's nose into his trachea. The x-ray shows the catheter coiled on itself in the blind pouch. Treatment consists of surgical anastomosis of the esophageal segments. If there is too large a gap between the segments, the upper segment may be brought to the skin surface, a gastrostomy performed, and later a colon transplant used to join the segments.

Pyloric Stenosis.   Pyloric stenosis is not actually a congenital malformation but is a common functional anomaly present at or soon after birth. The musculature of the pyloric sphincter hypertrophies, thus hindering the passage of stomach contents into the duodenum. It occurs in approximately 1 in 350 births, and about 80 percent of the affected infants are male. It is far more common in Caucasians than in blacks or Orientals and is more common in firstborn children.

Although the anomaly may be present at birth, symptoms usually begin at 2 to 3 weeks of age when the infant begins vomiting. The vomiting, which occurs during or shortly after feeding, becomes progressively more marked and projectile in character. If the infant is untreated, the probability of death is high. Surgical relief of the obstruction consists of longitudinal splitting of the pyloric muscle (Ramstedt's operation).

Imperforate Anus.   During the eighth week of embryonic life the membrane separating the rectum from the anus is normally absorbed. When this does not occur, imperforate anus results (see Chapter 6). The infant is unable to pass stool and abdominal distention occurs. If the anal opening is blocked by a thin membrane, perforation of it may be all the treatment that is necessary. When there is a distance between the anal dimple and the end of the colon, surgical repair includes either a temporary colostomy or joining of the colon to the anal dimple by an abdominal perineal operation. Whatever procedure is used, following surgery the infant is positioned on his side and turned frequently to prevent tension on the suture line. Skin care is very important postoperatively to prevent skin breakdown and subsequent infection. An aluminum paste or zinc oxide ointment may be applied to the skin for this purpose.

Genitourinary Disorders

ASSESSMENT AND INTERVENTION

Undescended Testicles. Usually testicles descend into the scrotum in the eighth month of fetal life. If only one has descended, the scrotal sac appears uneven; if both have failed to descend, the sac appears small. Newborns with undescended testicles may be preterm infants.

Descent may be spontaneous during the first few weeks of life or up to the age of puberty. Correction is necessary prior to puberty, since the undescended testis is at a higher temperature in the abdomen and the sperm-forming cells may degenerate because of this. Surgical intervention (orchiopexy) may be performed during infancy or the school years. It is usually avoided during the preschool years because of the child's fear of bodily intrusion.

Hydrocele. A hydrocele is an accumulation of fluid around the testis or along the spermatic cord. It appears as a swollen, oval, translucent sac. The fluid is gradually absorbed.

Phimosis. In phimosis the foreskin of the male infant has a very narrow orifice. It does not obstruct the flow of urine but may cause some straining during urination. It also prevents proper cleaning of the penis, since retraction of the foreskin is impossible. Treatment consists of circumcision or stretching the foreskin with a hemostat.

PARENTAL REACTIONS TO PROBLEM NEWBORNS

The image of the expected baby represents self and loved ones to the prospective parents. In most instances there will be some discrepancy between the parents' fantasized ideal child and the actual child; coming to an acceptance of that discrepancy is one of the developmental tasks of parenthood. When the discrepancy is great, as in the birth of a defective or prematurely born child or when the parents' wishes are too unrealistic, a problem may develop in the establishment of a healthy parent-child relationship. The parents' reactions, of course, are shaped by the type and degree of defect and their own past experiences with parents and siblings, as well as by the acceptance and emotional support that the two partners give each other and that is given by other important people in their environment.

As Elsas notes, the infant who requires intensive care immediately following birth and his parents face many hazards that may result in emotional, psychological, and developmental deviations [7]. The birth of an ill or premature infant constitutes a crisis event for the family, one for which they may not have been prepared. How they will be able to handle the crisis depends in part on the state of organization or disorganization of the family, the resources at their disposal, and the previous experiences of the family with crises.

During a crisis the family is more susceptible to influence. Nurses working in neonatal units can assess the family's strengths and weaknesses according to the factors previously mentioned and plan appropriate interventions to aid the family's move toward healthy crisis resolution. In addition, nurses can be alert to characteristics frequently associated with child abuse. These include: less mature infants (average 31.5 weeks), low birth weight (average 1,477 grams), congenital defects (especially if more than one), an infant who has surgery for a defect, infants whose nursery stay exceeds 40 days, and infants who are visited infrequently by their parents.

Elsas also notes that the infant is not passive and that his reciprocal interactions with his parents influence their behaviors toward him. According to the work of Medoff-Cooper and Schrader and others, very low birth weight infants demonstrate difficult temperaments [16]. They are difficult to soothe, less adaptable, have negative moods, and tend to withdraw. The low soothability and negative mood in the infants studied by Medoff-Cooper and Schrader were associated with less maternal responsiveness and involvement. Include in your nursing interventions with these parents a discussion of the uniqueness of their infant and an assessment of his characteristics, focusing on his assets. Help the parents understand differences in temperaments so they avoid focusing on their own possible inadequacies in parenting and move toward meeting their infant's needs and maximizing his potential.

If the expected ideal child is defective, parents' goals, fantasies, and idealizations have to be modified in relation to reality. This adaptation takes the form of grief work—a readjusting to the real situation and a redefinition of relationships to compensate for the unexpected. Grief over the loss leads to mourning, with the sadness, withdrawal, resentment, and self-blame inherent in the mourning process. If you are aware of these developments, you will have an increased understanding of the impact of disappointment, the feeling of helplessness, and the sense of failure that these parents are experiencing, and you will be able to help them to eventually begin to build on the strengths in the situation.

In a culture that emphasizes success, a defective child presents an extremely stressful situation. If a parent views the child as an extension of self, he may consider the defective child as proof of a defect within himself. Therefore, the parent may be a person whose ego is threatened and can be expected to build up strong defenses against the pain that comes with recognition of a child's anomaly. Parents may develop excessive concern about the child, which suggests that they perceive him as a defective child—not merely a child with a defect. This can prolong dependent ties instead of helping the child in the process of gradual separation, which is so necessary for the development of his emotional autonomy.

Some parents may feel that with enough love the child will be "whole," and in lavishing love and attention on him they may fail to relate adequately to other members of the family. At the other extreme, some parents and family members show an intolerance of the child and an almost irresistible urge to deny their relationship to him. Just as the infant's imperfection has an effect upon his total family, the ways in which they react to him and accept him affect his total personality development.

Parents often react initially by feeling shock, hurt, disappointment, and a helpless resentment at the revelation that they have a child who is not perfect. Since the baby is regarded as part of themselves, their efforts toward rehabilitation are motivated not only by reality but also by a desire for restitution for the child and themselves. As soon as most parents are able to master the expression of acute grief, they tend to regard as unacceptable any negative feelings they have toward the baby. This frequently leads to a denial of difficulties and a hiding of anxieties.

Denial of the defect is often reflected in the parents' "shopping around" for a more acceptable diagnosis, hostility toward professional workers, overprotection of the child, or projection of difficulties onto other people or circumstances. The depression sometimes associated with recognition of the handicap may result in denial of the fact that the defective child has the same needs as any other child and that with help he can often develop a degree of independence and social acceptability as well as a sense of achievement. The parents' acceptance of a referral for special help is often accompanied by a feeling of inadequacy, since, if one denies a problem, he need not seek or accept help related to it.

Lack of opportunity to discuss the diagnosis can create a situation in which parents feel overwhelmed and unable to gauge the reality of their child's retarded development. Denial then serves to forestall anxiety and depression.

A repetitive aspect of the mourning process in the parents' reactions—the need to grieve about the loss—indicates the need for repeated opportunities to review the situation. Your availability to them and encouragement of a trusting environment can make this task easier and more completely accomplished. Guilt feelings commonly enter into the mourning process. Parents ask, "Where did I fail? Was it someone else's fault? Why me?" Expressions of guilt take many forms—anger, aggression, hostility—and demonstrate how important the child's appearance and wholeness really are. Parents search for the cause of the malformation, and since explanations do not always relieve anxieties, they often resort to fantasies. Mothers recall significant fears that they had during pregnancy and may blame the defect on procedures that were performed before or during pregnancy or delivery or on the obstetrician and health team. In addition, parents may have fears about subsequent pregnancies or about their ability to give adequate care to this baby or may feel the need to prove that they are "good" parents.

The father of a defective child sometimes changes his work habits, working day and night, following the birth. It is suggested that this may illustrate his desire to prove himself as an adequate man, partner, and father. Another practical interpretation involves the financial burden and need for money that a child with special problems might represent. The extra time spent at work is also time spent away from the home situation, which is a constant reminder of the child's defect.

In the hospital the mother sometimes shows a vagueness or detachment when she is at the point of verbalizing her loss but is not realistically able to feel it. She wants someone to care about her, share her grief, and guide her in the acceptance of her loss, and so she often turns to the nurse.

We grieve over the parents' loss but do not always realize this. We often attempt to deny our feelings and respond by acting in a formalized way, reinforcing the loneliness the parents are experiencing. As long as we are unable to accept our own grief in a realistic context, we will have little alternative but to inhibit the expression of grief in the parents. The hospital is the place for crying for many parents—for getting it out of their systems. They need one of us who will stand by, letting them cry, and letting them feel that it is good for them to cry. The initial mourning period is not the time to accentuate the positive nor to tell parents that they have other perfect children or time to have more. This baby is the important one at that moment, not the ones they have already or could have in the future.

Review pertinent hospital regulations and routines. In situations in which parents are not permitted to see their defective baby immediately because the staff wants to spare them the pain, consideration should be given to whether or not the parents are really being done a service. Are we in reality sparing ourselves the difficulties inherent in giving the parents support at this time? Is it a good idea to isolate the mother from other mothers with healthy newborns, whether it is by room placement itself or by confinement to her own room when babies are out of the nursery? We often assume that she prefers to be alone, but sometimes we neglect to ask her is this is so, an apparent direct violation of respect for her individuality.

Gauge the parents' mourning reaction in order to know how and when to help them take an active role in planning the child's care. If the parents' mourning reaction is not understood and if the care of the child is carried out without their active participation or they are kept separated from him, their mourning may resolve into a persistently depressed, self-reproachful state. But if their own needs for support are met, they will be able to look realistically at the needs of the child. Demonstrate that you value the infant by giving him complete and expert care. Sometimes this is all that is needed to open the channels of communication for the parents to express their disappointment and grief and to begin to recognize the strengths and normal aspects of the child. Accurate listening and observation should alert you to the parents' needs. If the parents begin to feel that they are doing the best possible for the infant with the resources they have, their thinking usually changes from despair and guilt to more positive feelings. As they participate in the care of the child, help them to accept what cannot be changed, find satisfaction in improvement, and prepare to appreciate what the child offers.

In an atmosphere of trust and confidence, parents should be able to express their critical questions to members of the health care team who can describe what is known or not known regarding the child's defect. It is important that we do not give parents unrealistic hope for the future and that we tell the parents *together* about the prognosis, especially if it is poor, since neither one is in any better condition to accept the news. Communication between parents and nursery personnel and between nursery personnel and staff on the postpartum unit is essential if the parents are to receive the support they need.

If the baby is stillborn or dies in the neonatal period, parents react similarly. Initial responses commonly involve disbelief and shock, anger, inadequacy, and guilt, especially if the pregnancy was not wanted. The last phases of the mourning process—resolution and idealization—take the longest (6 months to a year), as thoughts of the loss become replaced with other interests and relationships. At the time of the baby's death it is recommended that the couple be told together so that they may give each other mutual support. Sometimes, even if they have communicated well before the birth of the baby, they have such strong feelings after the infant's death that they are unable to share them. Since this can only hinder the resolution of grieving, they should be encouraged to talk together about their loss. Parents will have a better chance of successful grieving if they have seen the child, especially if he was abnormal. If they do not, they tend to mourn on the basis of fantasy, and the fantasized abnormality may be far worse than the actual defect.

In the hospital setting, it is most often nurses upon whom parents rely for acceptance, support, and encouragement. If we are aware of our own feelings of grief and helplessness in the situation, we will be better able to work more effectively with the parents.

Premature Birth   Parent's reactions to premature birth have been reported to revolve around four psychologic tasks that they must accomplish. The first is anticipatory grief, or preparing for the infant's death. Their anxieties are increased at this time, not only concerning whether the baby will live, but, if he does, whether he will be deformed or mentally retarded. The second task is realization and acceptance of the mother's failure to carry the infant to term. This phase is often accompanied by guilt feelings that one or both parents might have done something to cause the premature labor.

The third task is the resumption of the process of relating to the infant. The support required here is very similar to that needed by parents of children with defects. We can establish a supportive relationship by talking with the parents together, by finding out what they believe is going to happen or what they know about the infant's problem. What the baby and his equipment will look like and why it is necessary should be discussed before the parents are taken to the nursery to see him. Whenever possible, encourage the parents to scrub, gown, and enter the nursery and to touch, hold, or feed the baby. Extended visiting hours should be made available for them (Fig. 21-16).

While the parents are there, describe their infant's individual behavioral characteristics, since this helps to emphasize his individuality, that he is somebody "special" from the very beginning. Describe the infant's equipment and what is being done for him, staying by the parents' side to answer their questions. If the baby is under the bili-light, turning it off and removing his eye patches for a

Figure 21-16. Parents of preterm infants need help in developing confidence in their ability to hold and to care for their newborn.

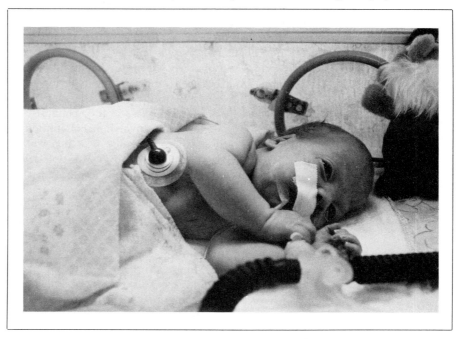

brief period will allow the parents to establish eye contact with him, to get the feeling that the baby is really theirs.

The final task the parents must accomplish is that of learning the special needs of the baby. They need to develop confidence in their ability to care for the infant; feeding will be one of the first experiences in which they can base this feeling. Reassure and guide parents so that their attempts to feed and care for their baby meet with success. Since the parents usually must go home without the baby, it is important that they be encouraged to return to the nursery to visit and feed the baby, or to call whenever they wish for information about his condition.

Involve public health or visiting nurses and hospital home-care coordinators in the planning of care for the family as soon as possible after the birth of the child. Noga suggests home visits by the community nurse prior to the infant's discharge, within 3 days of a high-risk infant's discharge, a second within 2 weeks of his discharge, a visit at 3, 6, and 12 months followed by a visit at 2, 3, and 4 years of age [19]. In this way a relationship is established between the parents and the nurse, who can provide continued guidance once the family is together in the home following the infant's discharge.

Case Study   Baby Amy

As Amy Michaels' primary nurse, develop a plan of care for her and her family including your interventions focused on her immediate care and her incorporation into the family unit. Each of you will develop your own approach and style in providing care to infants and families at risk. Applying the nursing process to the outline following the case study will serve as a guideline in organizing your approach to the infant and family.

Baby Girl (Amy) Michaels was born at 6:32 A.M. on October 19th. She was delivered vaginally with low forceps and epidural anesthesia following a 14-hour labor to a 20-year-old primigravida. Ms. Michaels' EDC was October 25. Her membranes ruptured spontaneously 10 hours prior to delivery. Amy's Apgars were 7 at 1 minute and 9 at 5 minutes. She received routine newborn care in the delivery room and was transferred to the normal nursery.

The baby was admitted to the nursery at 6:55 A.M. Initial nursing assessments found an awake, active, crying but consolable infant: temperature 96.4°F (rectal); heart rate 172 beats per minute; respiratory rate 70 per minute (irregular); weight 5 pounds 12 ounces; head circumference 13 inches; chest circumference 12 inches; head-to-toe length 18½ inches. The baby was noted to be covered with vernix and had lanugo on her back and shoulders and in small amounts on her forehead. She was placed in a heated Kreisselman bed.

At 8 A.M. Amy was sleeping. Her vital signs were temperature 98.4° (ax), heart rate 142, respiratory rate 38; Amy's breath sounds were somewhat wet sounding, especially in the bases. The baby's hands and feet were cyanotic, and suctioning Amy's mouth yielded moderate amounts of clear mucus. Amy did not react strongly to this suctioning; in fact, a superficial neurologic examination showed Amy to be somewhat hypotonic. Amy exhibited a delayed root, weak suck, an easily broken grasp, and a good deal of head lag when an attempt was made to pull her to a sitting position.

At 12 noon Amy was awake and crying. She was suctioned for a moderate amount of white mucus. Her vital signs were temperature 97.6° (rectal), heart rate 146, respiratory rate 48. Amy took one ounce of 5% glucose water, her first feeding, and regurgitated a moderate amount of yellowish mucus. At 2 P.M. Amy was taken to her mother for a feeding of half-strength formula. The nurse stayed with them for part of the feeding. She noted that Amy took one half-ounce of the formula and her mother handled her easily and confidently. She had voided three times and passed a meconium stool by 4 P.M., October 19th. She continued to take 1 to 1½ ounces of formula every 4 hours through her first day.

On October 20th, Amy Michaels weighed 5 pounds 7 ounces. Her vital signs were temperature 98.2° (ax), heart rate 146, respiratory rate 44. Amy was slightly jaundiced so when routine bloodwork (PKU and thyroid screening) was done a newborn bilirubin measurement was also obtained. Amy's bilirubin was reported as 12 milligrams. Phototherapy was ordered and begun.

That evening the nurse noted that Amy was irritable and crying much of the time. The baby took 3 ounces of formula at 6 P.M. but vomited a large amount afterwards. Since she remained irritable she was refed 1 ounce. She took 3 ounces at 10 P.M. without vomiting, but her abdomen was noted to be distended after the feeding. She had three watery stools between 6 P.M. and 10 P.M. The nurse assumed she voided in these diapers as well, although it was difficult to differentiate urine from the water ring of the stools.

The next morning Amy weighed 5 pounds 3 ounces. Her vital signs were temperature 99.8° (ax), heart rate 164, respiratory rate 58. She is noted to be jaundiced but very pink and irritable. She is difficult to console. Her serum bilirubin, drawn at 8 A.M., was 14 milligrams. Although her mother is scheduled for discharge, Amy is to remain hospitalized and phototherapy continued.

Assessment Form			
Assessment	Plan	Intervention	Evaluation

I. Pertinent History
  A. Mother's age, socioeconomic level, ethnic cultural group, education, marital status
  B. Mother's/family's past medical history
  C. Mother's past obstetric history
  D. Mother's present prenatal history
  E. Labor and delivery

II. Physical Findings
  A. Posture, length, weight
  B. Gestational age
  C. Skin
    1. Hair distribution
    2. Turgor
    3. Color
      (a) Cyanosis
      (b) Pallor
      (c) Plethora
      (d) Jaundice
      (e) Pink
      (f) Meconium staining
    4. Vernix
    5. Dryness or peeling
    6. Other
      (a) Edema
      (b) Ecchymoses
      (c) Petechiae
      (d) Erythema toxicum
      (e) Hemangiomas
      (f) Telangiectatic nevi
      (g) Milia
      (h) Harlequin color change
      (i) Mongolian spots
      (j) Café-au-lait spots
      (k) Nails
  D. Head
    1. Biparietal circumference
    2. Symmetry, shape, swelling
      (a) Caput succedaneum

Assessment Form			
Assessment	Plan	Intervention	Evaluation

(b) Cephalohematoma
(c) Molding
(d) Facial movements, asymmetry
3. Fontanelles—anterior, posterior
    (a) Enlarged
    (b) Bulging
    (c) Sunken
    (d) Size
4. Sutures
    (a) Overriding
    (b) Separation
E. Face
    1. Eyes
        (a) Color
        (b) Hemorrhagic areas
        (c) Edema
        (d) Discharge
        (e) Conjunctivitis
        (f) Jaundice
        (g) Pupils
        (h) Size
    2. Nose
        (a) Patency
        (b) Nasal flaring
        (c) Discharge
    3. Ears
        (a) Formation
        (b) Position in relation to eye
        (c) Cartilage
        (d) Hearing
    4. Mouth
        (a) Size
        (b) Palate lip
        (c) Size of tongue in relation to mouth
        (d) Predeciduous teeth
        (e) Epstein's pearls
        (f) Frenulum linguae
        (g) Sucking blisters

Assessment Form			
Assessment	Plan	Intervention	Evaluation

       (h) Infections (thrush)
       (i) Gums
  F. Neck
    1. Mobility
    2. Torticollis
    3. Length
    4. Goiter
  G. Chest
    1. Circumference
    2. Symmetry
    3. Breast
      (a) Engorgement
      (b) Nipples
      (c) Areola
      (d) Accessory nipples
    4. Respiratory system
      (a) Rate
      (b) Rhythm
      (c) Type of respiration
      (d) Grunting
      (e) Retraction
      (f) Lungs
        (1) Rhonchi
        (2) Rales
    5. Cardiovascular
      (a) Rate
      (b) Rhythm
      (c) Murmurs
      (d) Capillary filling time
      (e) Pulses
        (1) Radial
        (2) Brachial
        (3) Femoral
      (f) Blood pressure
  H. Abdomen and back
    1. Appearance
      (a) Shape
      (b) Distention
        (1) Abdominal
        (2) Bladder

Assessment Form			
Assessment	Plan	Intervention	Evaluation

    2. Liver, kidney, spleen
      (a) Size
      (b) Shape
    3. Umbilicus
      (a) Infection
      (b) Hernia
      (c) Cutis navel
      (d) Vein and arteries
      (e) Bleeding
    4. Bowel sounds
    5. Spinal column
      (a) Curvature
      (b) Pilonidal cyst
      (c) Masses
I. Genital-anal
    1. Appearance
      (a) Male
        (1) Testicles
        (2) Scrotum
          a. Rugae
          b. Edema
        (3) Urethral patency
        (4) Hypo- or epispadias
        (5) Foreskin
        (6) Ambiguities
      (b) Female
        (1) Prominence of labia majora/minora
        (2) Vaginal discharge
        (3) Hymenal tag
        (4) Urethral patency
        (5) Ambiguities
    2. Anus
      (a) Patency
      (b) Stool transition
J. Musculoskeletal
    1. Posture, muscle tone
    2. Extremities
      (a) Contour
      (b) Symmetry

Assessment Form			
Assessment	Plan	Intervention	Evaluation

    (c) Fractures (clavicle, scapula, humerus, femur)
    (d) Range of motion
    (e) Paralysis
    (f) Irregular position
    (g) Polydactyly, syndactyly
  3. Hip
    (a) Hip click
    (b) Gluteal folds
K. Neurologic
  1. Muscle tone
  2. Head control
  3. Cranial nerves
  4. Reflexes
    (a) Tonic neck
    (b) Grasp
    (c) Rooting
    (d) Sucking
    (e) Moro
    (f) Stepping
    (g) Babinski
    (h) Baby doll
    (i) Tendon
    (j) Truncal incurvation
    (k) Anal wink
III. Behavioral Assessment
  A. Response to stimulation
  B. State
    1. Quiet deep sleep
    2. Light active sleep
    3. Drowsy awake
    4. Quiet alert
    5. Active alert
    6. Crying
  C. Sleeping pattern
  D. Feeding pattern
    1. Type of feeding
    2. Intake
  E. Voiding pattern
  F. Stool pattern

Assessment Form			
Assessment	Plan	Intervention	Evaluation

    G. Temperature regulation
    H. Relationship with parents
        1. Parental interest
        2. Eye-to-eye contact
        3. Refusal to handle baby
        4. How refer to baby
        5. Support systems at home
        6. Need for referral to clinical or community resources
        7. Date for return visit to pediatrician or pediatric nurse practitioner
IV. Medical Treatment Plan
    A. Medications
    B. IV fluids
    C. Oxygen

REFERENCES

1. Babson, S., Pernoll, M., and Benda, G. *Diagnosis and Management of the Fetus and Neonate at Risk*. St. Louis: Mosby, 1980.
2. Bernbaum, J., Pereira, G., Watkins, J., and Pecklam, G. Enhanced growth and gastrointestinal function in premature infants given nonnutritive sucking (NNS). *Pediatric Research* 15:650, 1981.
3. Brain damage in newborn may be due to kernicterus. *Journal of the American Medical Association* 212:45, 1970.
4. Brown, B. Respiratory distress syndrome surfactant biochemistry and acceleration of fetal lung maturity: A review. *Obstetrical and Gynecological Survey* 30:71, 1975.
5. Cohen, A., and Ostrow, J. New concepts in phototherapy: Photoisomerization of bilirubin IXa and potential toxic effects of light. *Pediatrics* 65:740, 1980.
6. Crosse, V. M. *The PreTerm Baby and Other Babies with Low Birth Weight*. Edinburgh: Churchill Livingstone, 1971.
7. Elsas, T. Family mental health care in the neonatal intensive care unit. *Journal of Obstetric, Gynecologic and Neonatal Nursing* 10:204, 1981.
8. Fenichel, G. *Neonatal Neurology*. New York: Churchill Livingstone, 1980.
9. Field, T., Ignatoff, E., Stringer, S., Brennan, J., Greenberg, R., Widmayer, S., and Anderson, G. Effects of nonnutritive sucking during tube feedings of ICU preterm neonates. *Pediatrics* (in press).
10. Filston, H., and Izant, R. *The Surgical Neonate*. New York: Appleton-Century-Crofts, 1978.
11. Klaus, M., and Fanaroff, A. Respiratory Problems. In M. Klaus and A. Fanaroff (Eds.), *Care of the High Risk Neonate*. Philadelphia: Saunders, 1979.
12. Korones, S. B. *High Risk Newborn Infants*. St. Louis: Mosby, 1981.
13. Kulovich, M., Hallman, M., and Gluck, L. The lung profile. *American Journal of Obstetrics and Gynecology* 135:57, 1979.
14. Lucey, J., Ferreiro, M., and Hewitt, J. Prevention of hyperbilirubinemia of prematurity by prototherapy. *Pediatrics* 41:1047, 1968.
15. Measel, C., and Anderson, G. Nonnutritive sucking during tube feedings: Effect upon clinical course in premature infants. *Journal of Obstetric, Gynecologic and Neonatal Nursing* 8:265, 1979.
16. Medoff-Cooper, B. and Schraeder, B. Developmental trends and behavioral styles in very low birth weight infants. *Nursing Research* 31:68. 1982.
17. Miller, H. The effect of diabetic and prediabetic pregnancies on the fetus and newborn infant. *Landmarks in Perinatology and Neonatology* 14:455, 1981.
18. Moore, K. *The Developing Human* (2nd ed.). Philadelphia: Saunders, 1977.
19. Noga, K. High risk infants: The need for nursing follow-up. *Journal of Obstetric, Gynecologic and Neonatal Nursing* 11:112, 1982.
20. Phelps, D., and Rosenbaum, A. Observations of vitamin E in experimental oxygen-induced retinopathy. *Ophthalmia* 86:1741, 1978.
21. Pierog, S., and Ferrara, A. *Approach to the Medical Care of the Sick Newborn*. St. Louis: Mosby, 1971.
22. Pritchard, J., and MacDonald, P. *Williams Obstetrics* (16th ed.). New York: Appleton-Century-Crofts, 1980.
23. Quilligan, E., and Kretchmer, N. *Fetal and Maternal Medicine*. New York: Wiley, 1980.
24. Salerno, L. Treating the drug-addicted mother and neonate. *Symposia Reporter* 4:17, 1981.
25. Smith, B., Giroud, C., Robert, M., and Avery, M. Insulin antagonism of cortisol action on lecithin synthesis by cultured fetal lung cells. *Journal of Pediatrics* 87:953, 1975.
26. Stevenson, R. *The Fetus and Newly Born Infant*. St. Louis: Mosby, 1971.
27. Styler, G., and Freeh, K. Feeding infants with cleft lip and/or palate. *Journal of Obstetric, Gynecologic and Neonatal Nursing* 10:329, 1981.
28. Sweet, A. Classification of the Low Birth Weight Infant. In M. Klaus and A. Fanaroff (Eds.), *Care of the High Risk Neonate*. Philadelphia: Saunders, 1973.
29. Volpe, J. *Neurology of the Newborn*. Philadelphia: Saunders, 1981.
30. Wald, M. Problems in Chemical Adaptation. In M. Klaus and A. Fanaroff (Eds.), *Care of the High Risk Neonate*. Philadelphia: Saunders, 1973.
31. Williams, S. R. *Essentials of Nutrition and Diet Therapy*. St. Louis: Mosby, 1974.

FURTHER READING

Anderson, C. Enhancing reciprocity between mother and neonate. *Nursing Research* 30:89, 1981.
Avant, K. Anxiety as a potential factor affecting maternal attachment. *Journal of Obstetric, Gynecologic and Neonatal Nursing* 10:416, 1981.

Bernardo, M. Craniosyntosis: The child's care from detection through correction. *American Journal of Maternal-Child Nursing* 4:234, 1979.

Bowen, S., and Miller, B. Paternal attachment behavior. *Nursing Research* 29:307, 1980.

Cordell, A., and Apolito, R. Family support in infant death. *Journal of Obstetric, Gynecologic and Neonatal Nursing* 10:281, 1981.

Dingle, R., Grady, M., Lee, J., and Paul, S. Continuous transcutaneous O_2 monitoring in the neonate. *American Journal of Nursing* 80:829, 1980.

Eager, M. Long-distance nurturing of the family bond. *American Journal of Maternal-Child Nursing* 2:293, 1977.

Eager, M., and Exoo, R. Parents visiting parents for unequaled support. *American Journal of Maternal-Child Nursing* 5:35, 1980.

Fagin, C., and Nusbaum, J. Parental visiting privileges in pediatric units: A survey. *Journal of Nursing Administration* 8:24, 1978.

Gennaro, S. Listerial infection: Nursing care of mother and infant. *American Journal of Maternal-Child Nursing* 5:390, 1980.

Giefer, M., and Nelson, C. A new method to help new fathers develop parenting skills. *Journal of Obstetric, Gynecologic and Neonatal Nursing* 10:455, 1981.

Glassano, M. Infants who are oxygen dependent—sending them home. *American Journal of Maternal-Child Nursing* 5:42, 1980.

Gottlieb, L. Maternal attachment in primiparas. *Journal of Obstetric, Gynecologic and Neonatal Nursing* 7:39, 1978.

Haddock, N. Blood pressure monitoring in neonates. *American Journal of Maternal-Child Nursing* 5:131, 1980.

Haire, M., Davidson, K., and Boehm, F. Perinatal nursing education in Tennessee: A regional approach. *Journal of Obstetric and Gynecologic and Neonatal Nursing* 10:451, 1981.

Hall, L. Effects of teaching on primiparas' perceptions of their newborns. *Nursing Research* 29:317, 1980.

Hall-Johnson, S. *High Risk Parenting: Nursing Assessment and Strategies for the Family at Risk.* Philadelphia: Lippincott, 1979.

Hansen, F. Nursing care in the neonatal intensive care unit. *Journal of Obstetric, Gynecologic and Neonatal Nursing* 11:17, 1982.

Hawkins-Walsh, E. Diminishing anxiety in parents of sick newborns. *American Journal of Maternal-Child Nursing* 5:30, 1980.

Iyer, P. My baby was premature. *Journal of Obstetric, Gynecologic and Neonatal Nursing* 10:304, 1981.

Jacobson, S. Stressful situations for neonatal intensive care nurses. *American Journal of Maternal-Child Nursing* 3:144, 1978.

Jones, C. Father to infant attachment: Effects of early contact and characteristics of the infant. *Research in Nursing and Health* 4:193, 1981.

Klopf, J. Please don't go away. *Nursing Clinics of North America* 9:77, 1974.

Knafl, K., Deatrick, J., and Kodadek, S. How parents manage jobs and a child's hospitalization. *American Journal of Maternal-Child Nursing* 7:125, 1982.

Kowalski, K., and Bowes, W. Parent's response to a stillborn baby. *Contemporary Obstetrics and Gynecology* 8:53, 1976.

Kubler-Ross, E., and Warshaw, M. *To Live Until We Say Goodbye.* Englewood Cliffs, N. J.: Prentice-Hall, 1978.

Kunst-Wilson, W., and Cronenwett, L. Nursing care for the emerging family: Promoting paternal behavior. *Research in Nursing and Health* 4:201, 1981.

Kushner, L. Infant death and the childbirth educator. *American Journal of Maternal-Child Nursing* 4:231, 1979.

Lee, G. Relationship of self-concept during late pregnancy to neonatal perception and parenting profile. *Journal of Obstetric, Gynecologic and Neonatal Nursing* 11:186, 1982.

Levine, A., and Imai, P. Intrauterine treatment of fetal hydronephrosis. *Association of Operating Room Nurses Journal* 35:655, 1982.

McKeever, P. Fathering the chronically ill child. *American Journal of Maternal-Child Nursing* 6:124, 1981.

Marshall, R. E., and Kasman, C. Burnout in the neonatal intensive care unit. *Pediatrics* 65:1161, 1980.

Martin, T., and Burnett, P. Development of a neonatal intensive care orientation program. *Journal of Obstetric, Gynecologic and Neonatal Nursing* 11:175, 1982.

Naegle-McGowan, M. Post-partum disturbance. A review of the literature in terms of stress response. *Journal of Midwifery* 22:27, 1977.

Norbeck, J. Young children's ability to conserve facial identity when facial emotion varies. *Nursing Research* 30:329, 1981.

O'Pray, M. Developmental screening tools: Using them effectively. *American Journal of Maternal-Child Nursing* 5:126, 1980.

Patterson, P. Fetal therapy. *Association of Operating Room Nurses Journal* 35:663, 1982.

Pirong, G., and Smith, M. An in-house program of continuing education for perinatal nurses. *Journal of Obstetric, Gynecologic and Neonatal Nursing* 11:109, 1982.

Poland, R., and Odell, G. Physiologic jaundice: The enterohepatic circulation of bilirubin. *New England Journal of Medicine* 284:1, 1971.

Price, E., and Gyotoku, S. Using the nasojejunal feeding technique in a neonatal intensive care unit. *American Journal of Maternal-Child Nursing* 3:361, 1978.

Quinn, S. The competence of babies. *The Atlantic Monthly* 249:54, 1980.

Rumack, C., Guggenheim, M., Rumack, B., Peterson, R., Johnson, M., and Braithwaite, W. Neonatal intracranial hemorrhage and maternal use of aspirin. *Obstetrics and Gynecology* 58:52s, 1981.

Schodt, C. Grief in adolescent mothers after an infant death. *Image* 14:20, 1982.

Schraeder, B. Attachment and parenting despite lengthy intensive care. *American Journal of Maternal-Child Nursing* 5:37, 1980.

Snyder, C., Eyres, S., and Barnard, K. New findings about mothers' antenatal expectations and their relationship to infant development. *American Journal of Maternal-Child Nursing* 4:354, 1979.

Spenner, D. When the baby is sick and the mother's concerns are ignored. *American Journal of Nursing* 80:2222, 1980.

Stagno, S. Toxoplasmosis. *American Journal of Nursing* 80:720, 1980.

Sullivan, R., Foster, J., and Schreiner, R. Determining a newborn's gestational age. *American Journal of Maternal-Child Nursing* 4:38, 1979.

Trotter, C., Chang, P., and Thompson, T. Perinatal factors and the developmental outcome of preterm infants. *Journal of Obstetric, Gynecologic and Neonatal Nursing* 11:83, 1982.

Vogel, M. When a pregnant woman is diabetic: Care of the newborn. *American Journal of Nursing* 79:458, 1979.

Voyles, J. Bronchopulmonary dysplasia. *American Journal of Nursing* 81:510, 1981.

Wheeler, L., Duxbury, M., Raff B., and Carroll, P. *Fetal Assessment*. White Plains, N.Y.: National Foundation March of Dimes, 1979.

Wong, D. Bereavement: The empty-mother syndrome. *American Journal of Maternal-Child Nursing* 5:384, 1980.

Yaffe, S. Antimicrobial therapy and the neonate. *Obstetrics and Gynecology* 58:85s, 1981.

Yates, S. Stillbirth—What a staff can do. *American Journal of Nursing* 72:1592, 1972.

Ziemer, M., and Carroll, J. Infant gavage reconsidered. *American Journal of Nursing* 78:1543, 1978.

APPENDIXES

Appendix 1 Midwifery Programs Accredited by the American College of Nurse Midwives

Institution	Type of Program
Booth Maternity Center 6051 Overbrook Avenue Philadelphia, Pa. 19131	R, I
College of Medicine and Dentistry of New Jersey School of Allied Health Professions Nurse-Midwifery Program 100 Bergen Street Newark, N.J. 07103	CB
Columbia University Graduate Program in Maternity Nursing and Nurse-Midwifery Department of Nursing, Faculty of Medicine Columbia-Presbyterian Medical Center 622 West 168th Street New York, N.Y. 10032	MB
Cleveland Metropolitan General Hospital Nurse-Midwifery Service c/o Department of Ob-Gyn 3395 Scranton Road Cleveland, Ohio 44109	I
Emory University School of Nursing Atlanta, Ga. 30322	MB
Frontier School of Midwifery and Family Nursing Frontier Nursing Service Hyden, Ky. 41749	CB
Georgetown University School of Nursing Graduate Program, Growing Family-Nurse-Midwifery 3700 Reservoir Road, N.W. Washington, D.C. 20007	MB
Medical University of South Carolina Nurse-Midwifery Program, College of Nursing 171 Ashley Avenue Charleston, S.C. 29425	MB, CB
St. Louis University Department of Nursing Graduate Program in Nurse Midwifery 3525 Caroline Street St. Louis, Mo. 63104	MB

Institution	*Type of Program*
State University of New York Downstate Medical Center College of Health Related Professions Nurse-Midwifery Program, Box 93 450 Clarkson Avenue Brooklyn, N.Y. 11203	CB
United States Air Force (USAF nurses only) Nurse-Midwifery Program Malcolm Grow USAF Medical Center Andrews Air Force Base, Md. 20331	CB
*University of Arizona College of Nursing Nurse-Midwifery Program Tucson, Ariz. 85721	CB
University of California at San Diego Primary Care Nurse Practitioner Program Nurse-Midwifery Component University Hospital, H-813 225 Dickinson Street San Diego, Calif. 92103	CB
University of California at San Francisco San Francisco General Hospital Room 6B30 1001 Potrero Avenue San Francisco, Calif. 94110	CB
*University of Colorado Health Sciences Center School of Nursing Graduate Program Nurse-Midwifery Tract Box C 288 4200 East 9th Street Denver, Colo. 80262	MB
The University of Illinois at the Medical Center College of Nursing Department of Maternal-Child Nursing P.O. Box 6998 Chicago, Ill. 60680	MB
University of Kentucky College of Nursing 760 Rose Street Lexington, Ky. 40536-0232	MB
University of Miami School of Nursing 1540 Corniche Coral Gables, Fla. 33124	MB, R

Institution	*Type of Program*
University of Minnesota 5-140 Unit F 308 Harvard Street Minneapolis, Minn. 55455	MB
University of Mississippi Nurse-Midwifery Education Program 265 Woodland Hills Bldg. Jackson, Miss. 39216	CB
*University of Oregon Health Services Center School of Nursing, Department of Family Nursing Nurse-Midwifery Program 3181 S.W. Sam Jackson Park Road Portland, Oreg. 97201	MB
University of Pennsylvania School of Nursing Nursing Education Building 420 Service Drive S2 Philadelphia, Pa. 19104	MB
*University of Southern California LA County–USC Medical Center Women's Hospital Room 8L1 1240 N. Mission Road Los Angeles, Calif. 90033	CB, I
University of Utah College of Nursing Graduate Major in Maternal and Newborn Nursing and Nurse-Midwifery 25 South Medical Drive Salt Lake City, Utah 84112	MB
Yale University Maternal-Newborn (Nurse-Midwifery) Program 855 Howard Avenue, Box 3333 New Haven, Conn. 06510	MB, CM

CB = certificate basic program. MB = master's basic program. CM = combined RN/master's program. R = refresher program. I = internship. For students who have graduated from programs accredited by Division of Accreditation (ACNM) and who have sat for the ACNM certification examination.

* Preaccreditation status—a program initiating a nurse-midwifery curriculum that demonstrates that its planning is within the guidelines established by the Division to assure development of a quality education program. Programs are evaluated for accreditation status upon completion of the first class of students enrolled.

American College of Nurse-Midwives, 1522 K Street, N.W., Suite 1120, Washington, D.C. 20005

Appendix 2   Resources for Parents

General Information
Newsletter of Parenting
P.O. Box 2505
2300 W. Fifth Avenue
Columbus, Ohio 43216

Family Journal
RD 2, P.O. Box 165
Putney, Vt. 05346

Single Dad's Lifestyle
P.O. Box 4842
Scottsdale, Ariz. 85258

Practical Parenting
18318 Minnetonka Blvd.
Deephaven, Minn. 55391

Games for Children
Building Blocks
Box 31
Dundee, Ill. 60118

Totline
Warren Publishing
1004 Harborview Lane
Everett, Wash. 98203

Parenting Center Newsletter
92nd Street Y
1395 Lexington Avenue
New York, N.Y. 10028

Mothering
P.O. Box 2046
Albuquerque, N.M. 87103

Nurturing News
187 Caselli Avenue
San Francisco, Calif. 94114

Pediatrics for Parents
P.O. Box 1069
Bangor, Me. 04401

Appendix 3 Conversion of Pounds and Ounces to Grams*

Pounds	Ounces 0	1	2	3	4	5	6	7	8	9	10	11	12	13	14	15
	Grams															
0	—	28	57	85	113	142	170	198	227	255	283	312	340	369	397	425
1	454	482	510	539	567	595	624	652	680	709	737	765	794	822	850	879
2	907	936	964	992	1,021	1,049	1,077	1,106	1,134	1,162	1,191	1,219	1,247	1,276	1,304	1,332
3	1,361	1,389	1,417	1,446	1,474	1,503	1,531	1,559	1,588	1,616	1,644	1,673	1,701	1,729	1,758	1,786
4	1,814	1,843	1,871	1,899	1,928	1,956	1,984	2,013	2,041	2,070	2,098	2,126	2,155	2,183	2,211	2,240
5	2,268	2,296	2,325	2,353	2,381	2,410	2,438	2,466	2,495	2,523	2,551	2,580	2,608	2,637	2,665	2,693
6	2,722	2,750	2,778	2,807	2,835	2,863	2,892	2,920	2,948	2,977	3,005	3,033	3,062	3,090	3,118	3,147
7	3,175	3,203	3,232	3,260	3,289	3,317	3,345	3,374	3,402	3,430	3,459	3,487	3,515	3,544	3,572	3,600
8	3,629	3,657	3,685	3,714	3,742	3,770	3,799	3,827	3,856	3,884	3,912	3,941	3,969	3,997	4,026	4,054
9	4,082	4,111	4,139	4,167	4,196	4,224	4,252	4,281	4,309	4,337	4,366	4,394	4,423	4,451	4,479	4,508
10	4,536	4,564	4,593	4,621	4,649	4,678	4,706	4,734	4,763	4,791	4,819	4,848	4,876	4,904	4,933	4,961
11	4,990	5,018	5,046	5,075	5,103	5,131	5,160	5,188	5,216	5,245	5,273	5,301	5,330	5,358	5,386	5,415
12	5,443	5,471	5,500	5,528	5,557	5,585	5,613	5,642	5,670	5,698	5,727	5,755	5,783	5,812	5,840	5,868

* Grams = pounds × 454.

Appendix 4 The Pregnant Patient's Bill of Rights

American parents are becoming increasingly aware that well-intentioned health professionals do not always have scientific data to support common American obstetric practices and that many of these practices are carried out primarily because they are part of medical and hospital tradition. In the last 40 years many artificial practices have been introduced which have changed childbirth from a physiologic event to a very complicated medical procedure in which all kinds of drugs are used and procedures carried out, sometimes unnecessarily, and many of them potentially damaging for the baby and even for the mother. A growing body of research makes it alarmingly clear that every aspect of traditional American hospital care during labor and delivery must now be questioned as to its possible effect on the future well-being of both the obstetric patient and her unborn child.

One in every 35 children born in the United States today will eventually be diagnosed as retarded; in 75 percent of these cases there is no familial or genetic predisposing factor. One in every 10 to 17 children has been found to have some form of brain dysfunction or learning disability requiring special treatment. Such statistics are not confined to the lower socioeconomic group but cut across all segments of American society.

New concerns are being raised by childbearing women because no one knows what degree of oxygen depletion, head compression, or traction by forceps the unborn or newborn infant can tolerate before that child sustains permanent brain damage or dysfunction. The recent findings regarding the cancer-related drug diethylstilbestrol have alerted the public to the fact that neither the approval of a drug by the U.S. Food and Drug Administration nor the fact that a drug is prescribed by a physician serves as a guarantee that a drug or medication is safe for the mother or her unborn child. In fact, the American Academy of Pediatrics' Committee on Drugs has recently stated that there is no drug, whether prescription or over-the-counter remedy, which has been proven safe for the unborn child.

The Pregnant Patient has the right to participate in decisions involving her well-being and that of her unborn child, unless there is a clearcut medical emergency that prevents her participation. In addition to the rights set forth in the American Hospital Association's "Patient's Bill of Rights" (which has also been adopted by the New York City Department of Health), the Pregnant Patient, because she represents two patients rather than one, should be recognized as having the additional rights listed below.

1. *The Pregnant Patient has the right*, prior to the administration of any drug or procedure, to be informed by the health professional caring for her of any potential direct or indirect effects, risks or hazards to herself or her unborn or newborn infant which may result from the use of a drug or procedure prescribed for or administered to her during pregnancy, labor, birth or lactation.

2. *The Pregnant Patient has the right*, prior to the proposed therapy, to be informed, not only of the benefits, risks and hazards of the proposed therapy but also of known alternative therapy, such as available childbirth education classes which could help to prepare the Pregnant Patient physically and mentally to cope with the discomfort or stress of pregnancy and the experience of childbirth, thereby reducing or eliminating her need for drugs and obstetric intervention. She should be offered such informa-

tion early in her pregnancy in order that she may make a reasoned decision.

3. *The Pregnant Patient has the right*, prior to the administration of any drug, to be informed by the health professional who is prescribing or administering the drug to her that any drug which she receives during pregnancy, labor and birth, no matter how or when the drug is taken or administered, may adversely affect her unborn baby, directly or indirectly, and that there is no drug or chemical which has been proven safe for the unborn child.

4. *The Pregnant Patient has the right* if cesarean birth is anticipated, to be informed prior to the administration of any drug, and preferably prior to her hospitalization, that minimizing her and, in turn, her baby's intake of nonessential pre-operative medicine will benefit her baby.

5. *The Pregnant Patient has the right*, prior to the administration of a drug or procedure, to be informed of the areas of uncertainty if there is *no* properly controlled follow-up research which has established the safety of the drug or procedure with regard to its direct and/or indirect effects on the physiological, mental and neurological development of the child exposed, via the mother, to the drug or procedure during pregnancy, labor, birth or lactation (this would apply to virtually all drugs and the vast majority of obstetric procedures).

6. *The Pregnant Patient has the right*, prior to the administration of any drug, to be informed of the brand name and generic name of the drug in order that she may advise the health professional of any past adverse reaction to the drug.

7. *The Pregnant Patient has the right* to determine for herself, without pressure from her attendant, whether she will accept the risks inherent in the proposed therapy or refuse a drug or procedure.

8. *The Pregnant Patient has the right* to know the name and qualifications of the individual administering a medication or procedure to her during labor or birth.

9. *The Pregnant Patient has the right* to be informed, prior to the administration of any procedure, whether that procedure is being administered to her for her or her baby's benefit (medically indicated) or as an elective procedure (for convenience, teaching purposes or research).

10. *The Pregnant Patient has the right* to be accompanied during the stress of labor and birth by someone she cares for, and to whom she looks for emotional comfort and encouragement.

11. *The Pregnant Patient has the right* after appropriate medical consultation to choose a position for labor and for birth which is least stressful to her baby and to herself.

12. *The Obstetric Patient has the right* to have her baby cared for at her bedside if her baby is normal, and to feed her baby according to her baby's needs rather than according to the hospital regimen.

13. *The Obstetric Patient has the right* to be informed in writing of the name of the person who actually delivered her baby and the professional qualifications of that person. This information should also be on the birth certificate.

14. *The Obstetric Patient has the right* to be informed if there is any known or

indicated aspect of her or her baby's care or condition which may cause her or her baby later difficulty or problems.

15. *The Obstetric Patient has the right* to have her and her baby's hospital medical records complete, accurate, and legible and to have their records, including Nurses' Notes, retained by the hospital until the child reaches at least the age of majority, or, alternatively, to have the records offered to her before they are destroyed.

16. *The Obstetric Patient*, both during and after her hospital stay, has the right to have access to her complete hospital medical records, including Nurses' Notes, and to receive a copy upon payment of a reasonable fee and without incurring the expense of retaining an attorney.

It is the obstetric patient and her baby, not the health professional, who must sustain any trauma or injury resulting from the use of a drug or obstetric procedure. The observation of the rights listed above will not only permit the obstetric patient to participate in the decisions involving her and her baby's health care, but will help to protect the health professional and the hospital against litigation arising from resentment or misunderstanding on the part of the mother.

Source: Reprinted by permission of Doris Haire, President, American Foundation for Maternal and Child Health; Consultant, International Childbirth Education Association.

Appendix 5 The Pregnant Patient's Responsibilities

In addition to understanding her rights the Pregnant Patient should also understand that she too has certain responsibilities. The Pregnant Patient's responsibilities include the following:

1. The Pregnant Patient is responsible for learning about the physical and psychological process of labor, birth, and postpartum recovery. The better informed expectant parents are the better they will be able to participate in decisions concerning the planning of their care.
2. The Pregnant Patient is responsible for learning what comprises good prenatal and intranatal care and for making an effort to obtain the best care possible.
3. Expectant parents are responsible for knowing about those hospital policies and regulations which will affect their birth and postpartum experience.
4. The Pregnant Patient is responsible for arranging for a companion or support person (husband, mother, sister, friend, etc.) who will share in her plans for birth and who will accompany her during her labor and birth experience.
5. The Pregnant Patient is responsible for making her preferences known clearly to the health professionals involved in her case in a courteous and cooperative manner and for making mutually agreed-upon arrangements regarding maternity care alternatives with her physician and hospital in advance of labor.
6. Expectant parents are responsible for listening to their chosen physician or midwife with an open mind, just as they expect him or her to listen openly to them.
7. Once they have agreed to a course of health care, expectant parents are responsible, to the best of their ability, for seeing that the program is carried out in consultation with others with whom they have made the agreement.
8. The Pregnant Patient is responsible for obtaining information in advance regarding the approximate cost of her obstetric and hospital care.
9. The Pregnant Patient who intends to change her physician or hospital is responsible for notifying all concerned, well in advance of the birth if possible, and for informing both of her reasons for changing.
10. In all their interactions with medical and nursing personnel, the expectant parents should behave towards those caring for them with the same respect and consideration they themselves would like.
11. During the mother's hospital stay the mother is responsible for learning about her and her baby's continuing care after discharge from the hospital.
12. After birth, the parents should put into writing constructive comments and feelings of satisfaction and/or dissatisfaction with the care (nursing, medical and personal) they received. Good service to families in the future will be facilitated by those parents who take the time and responsibility to write letters expressing their feelings about the maternity care they received.

All the previous statements assume a normal birth and postpartum experience. Expectant parents should realize that, if complications develop in their cases, there will be an increased need to trust the expertise of the physician and hospital staff they have chosen. However, if problems occur, the childbearing woman still retains her responsibility for making informed decisions about her care or treatment and that of her baby. If she is incapable of assuming that responsibility because of her physical condition, her previously authorized companion or support person should assume responsibility for making informed decisions on her behalf.

Source: Reprinted by permission of Doris Haire, President, American Foundation for Maternal and Child Health; Consultant, International Childbirth Education Association.

Glossary

Abdominal pregnancy   one in which the fetus is situated within the abdominal cavity but outside the uterus.

Abortus   fetus usually less than 21 weeks' gestational age and weighing less than 500 grams.

Abruptio placentae   premature separation, partially or totally, of a normally implanted placenta.

Acceleration   periodic increase in the baseline fetal heart rate.

Acini cells   secretory cells in the human breast that create milk from nutrients in the bloodstream.

Acme   peak or highest point; time of greatest intensity (of a uterine contraction).

Acrocyanosis   cyanosis of the extremities.

Acromion   projection of the spine of the scapula, which forms the point of the shoulder.

Adenomyoma   tumor that affects the glandular and smooth muscle tissue, such as the muscles of the uterus.

Adnexa   adjoining or accessory parts of a structure; the uterine adnexa are the ovaries and fallopian tubes.

Afibrinogenemia   absence of or decrease in fibrinogen in the blood plasma, so that the blood does not coagulate; this condition may be acquired or congenital and may result from such obstetric complications as abruptio placentae and retention of a dead fetus.

Afterbirth   placenta and membranes expelled after the birth or delivery of the child during the third stage of labor; also called secundines.

Afterpains   cramplike pains due to contractions of the uterus that occur after childbirth. They are more common in multiparas and tend to be most severe during nursing.

AGA   appropriate growth for gestational age.

Agalactia   absence or failure of the secretion of breast milk.

Agenesis   failure of an organ to develop.

Allantois   tubular diverticulum of the posterior part of the embryo's yolk sac that passes into the body stalk. The allantoic blood vessels develop into the umbilical vein and paired umbilical arteries.

Allele   one of a series of alternate genes at the same locus; one form of a gene.

Alveolus   air sac in the lung.

Ambient   completely surrounding; environment.

Amenorrhea   absence of menstruation.

Amnesia   lack or loss of memory.

Amniocentesis   procedure in which amniotic fluid is removed from the uterine cavity by insertion of a needle through the abdominal and uterine wall and into the amniotic sac.

701

Amniography   x-ray examination of the amniotic sac following the injection of radiopaque dye into the amniotic fluid.

Amnion   the inner of the two membranes that form the sac containing the fetus and the amniotic fluid.

Amnionitis   infection of the amniotic fluid.

Amniotic fluid   the liquid surrounding the fetus in utero. It absorbs shocks, permits fetal movements, and prevents heat loss.

Amniotic sac   the bag or sac formed by the amnion and containing the fetus.

Amniotomy   artificial rupture of the amniotic sac.

Anaerobic catabolism   the breakdown of organized substances into simple compounds in the absence of free oxygen, with the release of energy.

Androgen   substance producing male characteristics, such as the male hormone testosterone.

Android pelvis   male-type pelvis.

Anencephaly   congenital deformity in which the cerebrum, cerebellum, and flat bones of the skull are absent.

Anomaly   malformation; an organ or structure that is abnormal in position, structure, or form.

Anoxia   deficiency of oxygen.

Anteflexion   state of being bent forward.

Antenatal   occurring or formed before birth; antepartal, prenatal.

Anterior fontanelle   diamond-shaped area between the two frontal and two parietal bones just above the newborn's forehead.

Anteversion   state of being turned forward.

Anthropoid pelvis   pelvis in which the anteroposterior diameter is equal to or greater than the transverse diameter.

Apgar score   numeric expression of the condition of a newborn obtained by rapid assessment at 1, 5, and 15 minutes of age (developed by Dr. Virginia Apgar).

Apnea   condition that occurs when respirations cease for more than 10 seconds with generalized cyanosis.

Areola   the ring of pigment surrounding the nipple.

Artificial insemination   introduction of viable semen into the vagina by artificial means for the purpose of impregnation.

Asphyxia   anoxia and carbon dioxide retention resulting from failure of respiration.

Asynclitism   oblique presentation of the fetal head; the pelvic planes and those of the fetal head are not parallel.

Atelectasis   pulmonary pathosis involving alveolar collapse.

Atony   lack of normal muscle tone.

Atresia   congenital absence or pathologic closure of a normal anatomic opening.

Atrophy   shrinkage and degeneration of vital components, resulting in partial or total loss of function.

Attitude   assumed body posture.

Auscultation   process of listening for sounds produced within the body in order to detect abnormal conditions.

Autoimmunization   development of antibodies against constituents of one's own tissues.

Autosome   chromosome that is not a sex chromosome.

Azoospermic   absence of spermatozoa in the semen.

Babinski reflex   extension of the great toe when the lateral aspect of the sole is stroked sharply. Abnormal after infancy.

Bag of waters   lay term for the amniotic sac containing amniotic fluid and fetus.

Balanced translocation   rearrangement of chromosomal material in which a piece of one chromosome is broken off and joined to another chromosome. An individual with a balanced translocation has the normal amount of genetic material but it is arranged abnormally, and thus the individual is at risk for producing offspring with chromosomal abnormalities.

Ballottement   technique of palpation to detect or examine a floating object in the body. In obstetrics, the fetus, when pushed, floats away and then returns to touch the examiner's fingers.

Bandl's ring   thickened ridge of uterine musculature between the upper and lower segments that occurs following a mechanically obstructed labor, with the lower segment thinning abnormally.

Barr body   the deeply stainable chromatin mass located against the inner surface of the cell nucleus. Found only in normal females; also called sex chromatin.

Bartholin's glands   glands situated one on each side of the vaginal canal opening.

Basal temperature   the lowest sustained temperature maintained by a normal individual in the course of a typical 24-hour period; for practical purposes, the body temperature, determined orally or rectally, that is present on awakening after a normal night's sleep.

Battledore placenta   placenta in which the umbilical cord is inserted on the periphery rather than in the central portion of the uterus.

Bell's palsy   distortion of the face caused by damage to the facial nerve, resulting in peripheral facial paralysis.

Biliary atresia　absence of the bile duct.

Bilirubin　pigment produced by the breakdown of hemoglobin in the red blood cells.

Bimanual　with both hands; performed by both hands, especially pelvic examination with the fingers of one hand in the vagina and the other hand on the abdomen.

Biopsy　removal and microscopic examination of a small piece of tissue.

Birth rate　number of live births per 1,000 population.

Blastodermic vesicle　blastocyst; the stage in development of a fertilized ovum in which the morula acquires a fluid-filled internal cavity.

Bloody show　vaginal discharge that originates in the cervix and consists of blood and mucus; increases as cervix dilates during labor.

Born out of asepsis (BOA)　pertaining to birth without the use of sterile technique.

Brachial palsy　partial or complete paralysis of portions of the arm. Results from trauma to the brachial plexus during a difficult delivery.

Braxton Hicks' contractions　light, irregular, painless contractions of the uterus during pregnancy.

Breech presentation　presentation in which buttocks and/or feet are nearest the cervical opening and are born first. Complete breech: simultaneous presentation of buttocks, legs, and feet. Footling (incomplete) breech: presentation of one or both feet. Frank breech: presentation of buttocks, with hips flexed so that thighs are against abdomen.

Bregma　the point on the surface of the skull at the junction of the coronal and sagittal sutures.

Brown fat　fat deposits in neonates that provide greater heat-generating activity than ordinary fat. Found around the kidneys, adrenals, and neck, between the scapulas, and behind the sternum.

Bulla　a large blister of 1 centimeter or more in diameter.

Bullous　characterized by large blebs or blisters.

Café-au-lait spots　light brown (coffee-with-cream) marks that appear on the body. The presence of more than six such spots may be accompanied by a neurologic disorder.

Candida albicans　a fungus causing infections such as candidiasis (moniliasis) and thrush.

Candidiasis　a yeastlike fungus infection caused by *Candida albicans*.

Carrier　individual possessing an abnormal gene or chromosome who manifests no outward signs but who can pass the abnormality on to offspring.

Caudal anesthesia   regional anesthesia in which the anesthetic agent is injected into the caudal area of the spinal canal through the sacral hiatus, affecting the caudal nerve roots and thereby anesthetizing the cervix, vagina, and perineum. Medication does not mix with cerebrospinal fluid (CSF).

Caul   portion of the fetal membranes covering the fetal head after the head has been delivered.

Cephalhematoma   accumulation of blood under the periostium of any of the cranial bones; usually induced by the trauma of birth.

Cephalic presentation   delivery in which the fetal head is presenting against the cervix.

Cephalopelvic disproportion (CPD)   condition in which the infant's head is of such a shape, size, or position that it cannot pass through the mother's pelvis.

Cerclage   the operative procedure of encircling the cervix with a ligature to prevent its premature dilatation.

Cerebral edema   swelling of the brain, especially of the cerebral hemispheres.

Cervical erosion   alteration of the epithelium of the cervix caused by chronic irritation or infection.

Cervical os   the opening of the cervix.

Cervical polyp   small tumor on a stem (pedicle) attached inside the cervix.

Cervical stenosis   narrowing of the canal between the body of the uterus and the cervical os.

Cesarean hysterectomy   removal of the uterus immediately after the cesarean delivery of an infant.

Cesarean operation   the operation consisting of cutting through the abdominal and uterine walls and delivering the fetus.

Chadwick's sign   violet color of the vaginal mucous membrane during pregnancy.

Chloasma   increased pigmentation over the bridge of the nose and cheeks of pregnant women and some women taking oral contraceptives; also known as mask of pregnancy.

Choanal atresia   congenital obstruction of the posterior cavity of the nares.

Chorioamnionitis   an inflammation of the amniotic membranes stimulated by organisms in the amniotic fluid, which then becomes infiltrated with polymorphonuclear leukocytes.

Chorion   the outer of the two membranes forming the sac that encloses the fetus in the uterus.

Chorionic villi   threadlike projections growing in tufts on the external chorionic surface.

Chvostek sign   a sign of facial nerve hyperirritability in which tapping of the face in front of the ear produces spasm of the ipsilateral muscles; an important sign in tetany and hypocalcemic states.

Cilia   hairlike processes that project from epithelial cells and that serve to propel mucus, pus, and dust particles.

Circumcision   the removal of the end of the prepuce or foreskin of the penis.

Circumoral cyanosis   bluish appearance around the mouth.

Cleft lip   incomplete closure of the lip; harelip.

Cleft palate   congenital deformity caused by the failure of the bones of the roof of the mouth to fuse in the midline.

Coloboma   a defect in development of closure of some portion of the eye or its lid.

Colostrum   secretion from the breast before the onset of true lactation; contains mainly serum and white blood corpuscles. It has a high protein content and provides some immune properties.

Colpotomy   any surgical cutting operation upon the vagina.

Complete dilatation   the state that occurs when the cervix is sufficiently dilated for the baby to pass through; usually 10 centimeters or five "fingers."

Compliance, lung   degree of distensibility of the lung's elastic tissue.

Condom   mechanical barrier worn on the penis for contraception; "rubber."

Condyloma   wartlike growth of the skin, usually seen on the external genitals or anus. There are two types, a pointed variety and a broad, flat form usually found with syphilis.

Consanguinity   blood relationship by descent from a common ancestor.

Contraction   tightening and shortening of the uterine muscles during labor, causing effacement and dilatation of the cervix; contributes to the downward and outward descent of the fetus.

Coombs' test   indirect: determination of Rh-positive antibodies in maternal blood; direct: determination of maternal Rh-positive antibodies in fetal cord blood. A positive test result indicates the presence of antibodies.

Coronal radiata   ring of elongated cells surrounding the zona pellucida.

Coronal suture   the suture between the frontal and parietal bones.

Corpus   the body.

Corpus luteum   a small yellow body that develops within a ruptured ovarian follicle; it secretes progesterone in the second half of the menstrual cycle and atrophies about 3 days before the beginning of menstrual flow. If pregnancy occurs, it continues to produce progesterone until the placenta takes over this function.

Cotyledon   one of the 15 to 28 visible segments of the placenta on the maternal surface, each made up of fetal vessels, chorionic villi, and an intervillous space.

Couvade in some cultures, the male's observance of certain rituals and taboos to signify the transition to fatherhood.

Couvelaire uterus uterus with blood forced within the uterine walls between the muscle fibers. May occur in premature separation of the placenta. Uterus may be atonic.

CPAP continuous positive airway pressure.

Craniotabes localized softening of cranial bones.

Credé's prophylaxis instillation of 1% silver nitrate solution into the conjunctival sacs of a newborn for the purpose of preventing gonorrheal ophthalmia.

Crepitus sound produced when pressure is applied to tissues containing abnormal amounts of air.

Crowning stage of delivery when the top of the fetal head can be seen at the vaginal orifice.

Cul-de-sac of Douglas the lowermost posterior portion of the peritoneal cavity, lying between the rectum and uterus in proximity to the posterior vaginal fornix.

Curettage scraping of the endometrium lining of the uterus with a curet to remove the contents of the uterus (as is done after an inevitable or incomplete abortion) or to obtain specimens for diagnostic purposes.

Cyanosis blueness of the skin due to insufficient oxygenation of the blood.

Cystocele hernial protrusion of the urinary bladder into the vagina.

Deceleration periodic decrease in the baseline fetal heart rate.

Decidua endometrium or mucous membrane lining of the uterus in pregnancy. It is shed after birth.

Decidua basalis the part of the decidua under the embryo that unites with the chorion to form the placenta.

Decidua capsularis the part of the decidua surrounding the chorionic sac.

Decidua vera nonplacental decidua lining the uterus.

Deletion loss of a piece of a chromosome that has broken off.

Desquamation shedding of epithelial cells of the skin and mucous membranes.

Diagonal conjugate distance from the lower posterior border of the symphysis pubis to the sacral promontory; may be obtained by manual measurement.

Diaphragmatic hernia congenital malformation of diaphragm that allows displacement of the abdominal organs into the thoracic cavity.

Diastasis recti abdominis separation of the two rectus muscles along the median line of the abdominal wall. This is often seen in women with repeated childbirths or with a multiple gestation.

DIC disseminated intravascular coagulation.

Dilatation and curettage (D&C)   vaginal operation in which the cervical canal is stretched enough to admit passage of an instrument called a curet. The endometrium of the uterus is then scraped with the curet to obtain tissue for examination or to remove the endometrial lining.

Diploid   containing a set of maternal and a set of paternal chromosomes. In humans the diploid number of chromosomes is 46.

Dizygotic   derived from two fertilized cells.

Dizygotic twins   fetuses that develop from two fertilized ova; also called fraternal twins.

Doderlein's bacillus   gram-positive bacterium occurring in normal vaginal secretions.

Dominant trait   gene that is expressed whenever it is present in the heterozygous state (e.g., brown eyes are dominant over blue).

Down's syndrome   an abnormality resulting from the presence of an extra chromosome number 21 (trisomy 21); characteristics include mental retardation and altered physical appearance. Formerly called mongolism.

Dry labor   lay term referring to labor in which amniotic fluid has already escaped. A "dry birth" does not exist.

Dubowitz assessment   estimation of gestational age of a newborn based on criteria developed for that purpose.

Ductus arteriosus   in fetal circulation, an anatomic shunt between the pulmonary artery and arch of the aorta. It is obliterated after birth by a rising PO_2 and change in intravascular pressures in the presence of normal pulmonary function.

Ductus venosus   in fetal circulation, a blood vessel carrying oxygenated blood between the umbilical vein and the inferior vena cava, bypassing the liver. It is obliterated and becomes a ligament after birth.

Duncan's mechanism   the presentation upon delivery of the maternal surface of the placenta rather than the shiny fetal surface.

Dysfunctional uterine bleeding   abnormal bleeding from the uterus for reasons that are not readily established.

Dysmenorrhea   difficult or painful menstruation.

Dyspareunia   painful coitus or intercourse.

Dystocia   prolonged, painful, or otherwise difficult delivery or birth because of mechanical factors produced by either the passenger (the fetus) or the passage (the pelvis of the mother) or because of inadequate powers (uterine and other muscular activity).

Ecchymosis   bruise; bleeding into tissue caused by direct trauma, serious infection, or bleeding.

Eclampsia acute "toxemia of pregnancy" characterized by convulsions and coma which may occur during pregnancy, labor, or the puerperium.

Ectoderm outer layer of embryonic tissue giving rise to skin, nails, and hair.

Ectopic pregnancy implantation of the fertilized ovum outside the uterine' cavity; common sites are the fallopian tubes, ovaries, and abdomen.

EDC expected date of confinement; "due date."

Edema excessive accumulation of fluid in tissues.

Effacement thinning and shortening of the cervix.

Effleurage gentle stroking of the abdomen, used during labor in the Lamaze method of childbirth.

Embolus any undissolved matter (solid, liquid, or gaseous) that is carried by the blood to another part of the body and obstructs a blood vessel.

Embryo the developing organism in its earliest stage; in humans, the period to 8 weeks' gestation, characterized by cellular differentiation.

Endocervical pertaining to the interior of the canal of the cervix.

Endometriosis tissue closely resembling endometrial tissue is aberrantly located outside the uterus, usually in the pelvic cavity.

Endometritis inflammation of the endometrium.

Endometrium the mucous membrane that lines the uterus.

En face an assumed position in which one person looks at another and maintains his or her face in the same vertical plane as that of the other.

Engagement the entrance of the presenting part into the pelvic inlet and the beginning of the descent through the pelvic canal.

Engorgement an exaggeration of normal venous and lymph stasis of the breasts.

Engrossment sustained involvement of a parent with an infant.

Entoderm the innermost layer of cells of the primitive embryo.

Epicanthus a fold of skin that extends from the top of the nose to the median end of the eyebrow, covering the inner canthus.

Episiotomy surgical incision of the perineum toward the end of second stage of labor to facilitate delivery and avoid laceration.

Epispadias defect in which the urethral canal opens on the dorsum of penis.

Epstein's pearls small, white blebs found along the gum margins and at the junction of the soft and hard palates.

Epulis tumorlike benign lesion of the gingiva seen in pregnant women.

Erb's palsy paralysis of the arm and chest wall as a result of a birth injury to the brachial plexus or a subsequent injury to the 5th and 6th cervical nerves.

Erectile tissue   tissue containing specialized blood vessels, which, when engorged with blood, cause the tissue to stand up or away from surrounding nonerectile tissue.

Ergot   a drug that stimulates the smooth muscles of blood vessels and the uterus, causing vasoconstriction and uterine contractions.

Erythema   redness, usually due to capillary dilatation.

Erythema toxicum   innocuous pink papular rash of unknown cause with super-imposed vesicles that appears within 24 to 48 hours after birth and resolves spontaneously within a few days.

Erythroblastosis fetalis   hemolytic anemia of the fetus and newborn occurring when the red blood cells of the fetus contain an antigen lacking in the mother's red blood cells, stimulating maternal antibody formation against the infant's erythrocytes.

Esophageal atresia   malformation in which the esophagus ends in a blind pouch or narrows into a thin cord, failing to form a passage to the stomach.

Estriol   major metabolite of estrogen that increases during the second half of pregnancy with an intact fetoplacental unit (normal placenta, normal fetal liver and adrenals) and normal maternal renal function.

Etiologic   pertaining to the cause of disease.

Exchange transfusion   replacement of 75 to 85 percent of circulating blood by withdrawing the recipient's blood and injecting a donor's blood in equal amounts, the purposes of which are to prevent an accumulation of bilirubin in the blood above a dangerous level, to prevent the accumulation of other by-products of hemolysis in hemolytic disease, and to correct anemia.

Expiratory grunt   a sign of respiratory distress indicative of the baby's attempt to hold air in the alveoli for better gaseous exchange.

Expulsion   driving or forcing out; tending to dispel.

Extraperitoneal   situated or occurring outside the peritoneal cavity.

Extrauterine   outside the uterus.

False labor   contractions of the uterus, regular or irregular, that may be strong enough to be interpreted as true labor but that do not dilate the cervix.

Ferguson's reflex   contractions of the uterus after stimulation of the cervix.

Fertility   the ability to produce offspring; power of reproduction.

Fertilization   union of an ovum and a sperm.

Fetal alcohol syndrome (FAS)   syndrome caused by maternal alcohol ingestion and characterized by microcephaly, intrauterine growth retardation, short palpebral fissures, and maxillary hypoplasia.

Fetal heart rate   the number of times the fetal heart beats per minute; normal range is 120 to 160 beats per minute.

Fetal lie   relationship of the long axis of the fetus to the long axis of the mother.

Fetus   the child in utero from the ninth week of gestation until birth.

Fibrinogen   a normal blood constituent necessary for the formation of clots.

Fibroid   fibrous, encapsulated connective-tissue tumor, especially of the uterus.

Fimbria   structure resembling a fringe, particularly the fringelike end of the fallopian tube.

FiO₂ (fraction of inspired oxygen)   percentage of oxygen a person is receiving.

First stage of labor   period of time extending from the onset of regular contractions to the complete dilatation of the cervix.

Fistula   abnormal passage that forms between two normal cavities, possibly congenital or caused by trauma, abscesses, or inflammatory processes.

Flaccid   characterized by complete relaxation or lack of tone.

Flaring of nostrils   widening of nostrils during inspiration in the presence of air hunger; a sign of respiratory distress.

Fontanelle   broad area, or soft spot, consisting of a strong band of connective tissue contiguous with cranial bones and located at the junctions of the bones.

Footling   a breech presentation in which one or both feet present.

Foramen ovale   opening between the atria of the fetal heart. It normally closes shortly after birth, but occasionally remains open or "persistent."

Foreskin   the prepuce, the fold of skin covering the glans penis.

Fornix   the blind inner termination of the vagina, divided by the cervix into anterior, posterior, and lateral fornices.

Fourchette   transverse fold of mucous membranes at the posterior angle of the vagina that connects the posterior ends of the labia minora.

Fraternal twins   nonidentical twins that come from two separate fertilized ova.

Friedman graph   a method of describing and recording labor progress.

Fundus   the upper rounded portion of the uterus between the points of insertion of the fallopian tubes.

Funic souffle   a soft, blowing sound produced in the umbilical cord.

Gamete   mature male or female germ cell; the mature sperm or ovum.

Glycosuria   the presence of glucose in the urine.

Goodell's sign   softening of the cervix, a presumptive sign of pregnancy.

Graafian follicles or vesicles   small spherical bodies in the ovaries, each containing an ovum.

Gravid   pregnant; with child; containing a fetus.

Gravida   a pregnant woman.

Gynecoid pelvis   typical female pelvis in which the inlet is round instead of oval.

Harlequin sign   rare color change of no pathologic significance occurring between the longitudinal halves of the neonate's body. When the infant is placed on one side, the dependent half is noticeably pinker than the superior half.

Hegar's sign   softening of the lower uterine segment that is classified as a probable sign of pregnancy and that may be present during the second and third months of pregnancy.

Hematoma   collection of blood in a tissue; a bruise or blood tumor.

Hemoconcentration   increase in the number of red blood cells resulting from either a decrease in plasma volume or increased erythropoiesis.

Hemorrhagic disease of newborn   bleeding disorder during first few days of life based on a deficiency of vitamin K.

Hemorrhoids   varicose veins of the rectum; may be external or internal.

Hirsutism   condition characterized by the excessive growth of hair or the growth of hair in unusual places.

Homan's sign   early sign of phlebothrombosis of the deep veins of the calf in which there are complaints of pain when the leg is in extension and the foot is dorsiflexed.

Hydatidiform mole   cystic proliferation of chorionic villi, resembling a bunch of grapes.

Hydramnios   an excessive amount of amniotic fluid.

Hydrocele   collection of fluid in a saclike cavity, especially in the sac that surrounds the testis, causing the scrotum to swell.

Hydrocephalus   excessive amount of cerebrospinal fluid in the brain cavities, surrounding the brain, or both.

Hydrops fetalis   massive edema (anasarca) of a fetus or newborn, usually due to Rh incompatibility (erythroblastosis).

Hymenal tag   normally occurring redundant hymenal tissue protruding from the floor of the vagina. It disappears spontaneously in a few weeks after birth.

Hyperbilirubinemia   excess bilirubin in the blood.

Hypercapnia   excessive arterial PCO_2 caused by inadequate ventilation.

Hyperemesis gravidarum   excessive vomiting during pregnancy, leading to starvation and dehydration.

Hyperreflexia   exaggeration of reflexes.

Hypertrophy   enlargement, or increase in size, of existing cells.

Hypocalcemia   diminished calcium in the blood.

Hypofibrinogenemia   deficiency of fibrinogen in the blood.

Hypospadias   anomalous positioning of the male urinary meatus on the under-surface of the penis.

Hypoxemia   low oxygen tension in arterial blood.

Hypoxia   insufficient oxygen to support normal metabolic requirements.

Hysterotomy   surgical incision into the uterus.

Iatrogenic   caused by a physician's words, actions, or treatment.

Icterus neonatorum   jaundice in the newborn.

IDM   infant of a diabetic mother.

Imperforate anus   congenital anomaly in which there is no anal opening.

Impetigo   a skin disease caused by staphylococci and characterized by pustules.

Implantation   embedding of the fertilized ovum in the uterine mucosa 6 or 7 days after fertilization; also called nidation.

Inborn error of metabolism   hereditary deficiency of a specific enzyme needed for normal metabolism of specific chemicals (e.g., deficiency of phenylalanine hydroxylase results in phenylketonuria [PKU]; a deficiency of hexosaminidase results in Tay-Sachs disease).

Incompetent cervix   a mechanical defect in the cervix making it unable to remain closed throughout pregnancy; produces dilatation and effacement leading to spontaneous abortion, usually during the second trimester or early third trimester.

Increment   increase or addition; to build up, as of a contraction.

Induction   the process of causing or initiating labor by use of medication or rupture of membranes.

Inertia   the absence or weakness of uterine contractions during labor.

Infant death rate   number of deaths of infants under 1 year of age per 1,000 live births in a given population per year.

Infantile uterus   failure of the uterus to attain adult characteristics.

Infertility   diminished ability to conceive.

Intertuberous diameter   distance between ischial tuberosities; measured to determine dimension of pelvic outlet.

Intervillous spaces   irregular spaces in the maternal portion of the placenta that are filled with maternal blood and serve as sites of maternal-fetal gas, nutrient, and waste exchange.

Intrapartal   occurring during birth or delivery; broadly, during delivery.

Intrathecal   within the subarachnoid space.

Intrauterine growth retardation (IUGR)   fetal undergrowth due to etiology such as intrauterine infection, deficient nutrient supply, or congenital malformation.

Introitus   the opening of the vagina.

Inverted nipple   congenital or acquired deformity of the nipple which prevents the projection of the bulk of the nipple above the surface of the breast.

Involution   the return of the pelvic organs to the nonpregnant state after the termination of pregnancy.

Ischemia   local diminution in the blood supply due to obstruction in the supply or to vasoconstriction.

Isoimmunization   development of antibodies in a species of animal with antigens from the same species (e.g., development of anti-Rh antibodies in an Rh-negative person).

Isolette   trade name for a self-contained incubator.

Jaundice   yellowness of the skin, eyes, and secretions due to the presence of bile pigments in the blood.

Kernicterus   an encephalopathy caused by deposition of unconjugated bilirubin in brain cells; may result in impaired brain function or death.

Kernig's sign   nuchal rigidity; stiffness of the neck.

Ketosis   increase in ketone bodies (acetone) from incomplete metabolism of fatty acids.

Klinefelter's syndrome   a chromosomal abnormality caused by the presence of an extra X chromosome in the male.

Labor   the physiologic process by which the fetus and the associated placenta and membranes are expelled from the body.

Laceration   irregular tear of wounded tissue; in obstetrics it usually refers to a tear in the perineum, vagina, or cervix caused by childbirth.

Lactation   the time or period of secreting milk.

Lactiferous ducts   tiny tubes within the breast that conduct milk from the acini cells to the nipple.

Lactogenic   stimulating the production of milk.

Laminaria tent   a cone made of dried seaweed which swells when in contact with moisture; used to dilate the cervix.

Lanugo   the fine hair on the body of the fetus; the fine, downy hair found on nearly all parts of the body except the palms of the hands and the soles of the feet.

Large for gestational age (LGA)   characterized by excessive growth in relation to the gestational time period.

Lecithin   a phospholipid that decreases surface tension; surfactant.

Leopold's maneuvers   series of four maneuvers designed to provide a systematic approach for determining fetal presentation and position.

Let-down reflex   oxytocin-induced flow of milk from the alveoli of the breasts into the milk ducts.

Leukorrhea   mucous discharge from the vagina or cervical canal.

Lie   relationship existing between the long axis of the fetus and the long axis of the mother; in a longitudinal lie the fetus is lying lengthwise or vertically, whereas in a transverse lie the fetus is lying crosswise or horizontally in the mother's uterus.

Lightening   the sensation produced by the descent of the presenting part into the pelvic cavity prior to labor.

Linea nigra   line of darker pigmentation seen in pregnant women during the latter part of term. It appears on the middle of the abdomen and extends from the symphysis pubis toward the umbilicus.

Linea terminalis   line dividing the upper (false) pelvis from the lower (true) pelvis.

Liquor amnii   amniotic fluid; fluid surrounding the embryo or fetus in utero.

Lithotomy position   position in which the woman lies on her back with her knees flexed and abducted thighs drawn up toward her chest.

Live birth   birth in which the neonate, regardless of gestational age, manifests any heartbeat, breathes, or displays voluntary movement.

Lochia   the vaginal (uterine) discharge present for several weeks after delivery.

Lochia alba   white vaginal discharge that follows lochia serosa and that lasts from about the 10th to 21st day following delivery.

Lochia rubra   red, blood-tinged vaginal discharge that occurs following delivery and lasts 2 to 4 days.

Lochia serosa   pink, serous, and blood-tinged vaginal discharge that follows lochia rubra and lasts until the 7th to 10th day after delivery.

L/S ratio   the ratio of the phospholipids lecithin and sphingomyelin produced by the fetal lungs; useful in assessing fetal lung maturity.

Lunar   pertaining to the moon; 1 month; 28 days; 4 weeks.

Luteinizing hormone (LH)   anterior pituitary hormone responsible for stimulating ovulation and for development of the corpus luteum.

Macerate   to waste away; to soften by steeping in a liquid.

Macroglossia   hypertrophy of the tongue.

Macrosomia   condition characterized by large body size and high birth weight; seen in infants born of prediabetic and diabetic mothers.

Macule   flat, discolored skin lesion, less than 1 centimeter in diameter.

Malpresentation   faulty, abnormal, or untoward fetal presentation.

Mastalgia   breast pain or tenderness.

Mastitis   inflammation or infection of the breast.

Maternal mortality rate   number of deaths from any cause during the pregnancy cycle per 100,000 live births.

Meconium   the fecal matter discharged by the newborn; a dark green substance, consisting of mucus, bile, and epithelial shreds.

Meconium-stained fluid   amniotic fluid that contains meconium because fetal distress has caused relaxing of the fetus's anal sphincter.

Menarche   beginning of menstrual and reproductive function in the female.

Meningomyelocele   a defect in the spinal column with resulting protrusion of the spinal cord and membranes.

Menopause   the period at which menstruation ceases; the "change of life."

Menorrhagia   an abnormally profuse menstrual flow.

Mentum   the chin.

Mesoderm   the middle of the three layers of the primitive embryo.

Metritis   inflammation of the endometrium and myometrium.

Metrorrhagia   abnormal uterine bleeding.

Microcephalic   having an abnormally small head in relation to total body size.

Micrognathia   abnormal smallness of the lower jaw.

Milia   tiny white papules appearing on the face of a neonate as a result of unopened sebaceous glands; they disappear spontaneously within a few weeks.

Milk leg   phlebitis and thrombosis of the femoral vein, resulting in venous obstruction and edema of the affected leg.

Miscarriage   spontaneous abortion.

Molding   the shaping of the baby's head to adjust itself to the size and shape of the birth canal.

Mongolian spot   dark flat pigmentation of the lower back and buttocks noted at birth in some infants.

Moniliasis   yeastlike fungus infection caused by *Candida albicans*.

Monitrice   an individual specifically trained to support women in labor using a psychoprophylactic method.

Monozygotic   derived from one fertilized cell.

Montgomery's tubercles   small, nodular follicles or glands on the areolae around the nipples.

Morula   the solid mass of cells formed by the division and redivisions of the fertilized ovum.

Mosaicism   condition in which some somatic cells are normal while others show chromosomal aberrations.

Mottling discoloration of the skin in irregular areas; may be seen with chilling, poor perfusion, or hypoxia.

Mucous plug a collection of thick mucus that blocks the cervical canal during pregnancy.

Multipara women who has borne two or more children; loosely, any pregnant woman who has had a child.

Multiple pregnancy pregnancy in which there is more than one fetus in the uterus at the same time.

Mutagen environmental agent, either physical, chemical, or biologic, capable of inducing mutation.

Mutation change or alteration in gene or chromosome structure that may be transmitted to offspring.

Nagele's rule method of determining the estimated date of confinement (EDC): after obtaining the first day of the last menstrual period, subtract 3 months and add 7 days.

Narcosis state of profound unconsciousness produced by a drug.

Natal pertaining to birth.

Neonatal mortality rate number of deaths of infants in the first 28 days after birth per 1,000 live births.

Neonate infant from birth through the first 28 days of life.

Neonatology study of the neonate.

Nevus mole, blemish, or mark.

Nidation implantation of the fertilized ovum in the endometrium of the uterus.

Nondisjunction failure of paired chromosomes to separate during cell division.

Nonstress test (NST) evaluation of fetal response (fetal heart rate) to an increase in fetal activity.

Nosocomial pertaining to a hospital.

Nulligravida female who has never been pregnant.

Nullipara woman who has not yet carried a pregnancy to viability.

Occiput posterior part of the skull.

Oligohydramnios deficiency of amniotic fluid.

Omphalic concerning the umbilicus.

Omphalitis infection of the umbilicus.

Omphalocele congenital defect resulting from failure of closure of the abdominal wall or muscles and leading to hernia of abdominal contents through the navel.

Oophorectomy surgical removal of the ovary.

Ophthalmia neonatorum   acute purulent conjunctivitis of the newborn usually due to gonorrheal infection.

Opisthotonos   tetanic spasm resulting in an arched, hyperextended position of the body.

Ossification   mineralization of fetal bones.

Oxygen toxicity   oxygen overdosage that results in pathologic tissue changes (e.g., retrolental fibroplasia, bronchopulmonary dysplasia).

Oxytocin   hormone released by the posterior pituitary that stimulates uterine contractions and the release of milk in the mammary gland (let-down reflex).

Oxytocin challenge test (OCT)   test designed to evaluate the fetoplacental unit to determine the ability of the fetus to withstand the stress of labor. While uterine contractions and FHR are externally monitored, oxytocin is administered to stimulate contractions. The FHR pattern is then assessed for evidence of a late deceleration pattern. The test is negative when there are three contractions in a 10-minute period without late deceleration.

$PaCO_2$ partial pressure of carbon dioxide in arterial blood.

PaO_2   partial pressure of oxygen in arterial blood.

Papule   an elevated area of skin less than 1 centimeter in diameter.

Parabiotic syndrome   anomaly occurring in a small percentage of identical twins in which one twin is anemic and the second suffers polycythemia as a result of a fetofetal blood transfer via placental vascular anastomoses.

Parametritis   inflammation of the parametrial layer of the uterus.

Parametrium   the fibrous subserous coat of the supravaginal portion of the uterus, extending laterally between the layers of the broad ligaments.

Parturition   the act or process of giving birth to a child.

Pathologic jaundice   jaundice that occurs within 24 hours of birth, secondary to an abnormal condition such as ABO or Rh incompatibility.

Perinatal mortality   number of deaths of fetuses or infants weighing 1,000 grams or over that occur between 28 weeks of gestation and 4 weeks of age (neonatal period).

Perinatal period   the time frame extending from the 28th week after conception to the 28th day after birth.

Perinatologist   physician specializing in fetal and neonatal care.

Perineum   the area between the vagina and the rectum.

Periodic breathing   sporadic episodes of cessation of respirations for periods of 10 seconds or less not associated with cyanosis and commonly noted in premature infants.

Petechia   small punctate red flecks in the skin that do not blanch when pressed.

Phenylalanine a naturally occurring amino acid essential for optimal growth and nitrogen balance in humans.

Phenylketonuria (PKU) a recessive hereditary metabolic error that causes the buildup of phenylalanine, leading to mental retardation, brain damage, light pigmentation, and other characteristics; can be treated with a low-phenylalanine diet.

Phimosis tightness of the foreskin.

Phlebitis inflammation of a vein.

Phlebothrombosis presence of a clot within a vein without associated symptoms of vein inflammation.

Phototherapy treatment of disease by light rays; used in the neonate to aid in bilirubin clearance.

Pica craving for unnatural articles of food; ingestion of nonnutritive substances.

Pigeon chest chest deformity in which the sternum is prominent; transverse diameters may be shortened.

Pilonidal cyst a hair-containing cavity in the sacrococcygeal area.

Pinna the part of the ear that lies outside the skull.

Placenta accreta abnormal adherence of the placenta to the uterine wall.

Placental dysfunction placental insufficiency; the placenta fails to meet fetal requirements.

Placental souffle soft blowing sounds produced by blood coursing through the placenta; has the same rate as the maternal pulse.

Placenta previa abnormal implantation of the placenta in the lower uterine segment. Classification of type is based on proximity to the cervical os: total completely covers the os; partial covers a portion of the os; marginal is in close proximity to the os.

Platypelloid pelvis broad pelvis with a shortened anteroposterior diameter and a flattened, oval, transverse shape.

Pneumothorax air within the chest cavity between the lung tissue and chest wall, creating a positive pressure space instead of negative pressure.

Polycythemia abnormal increase in the erythrocyte count or in hemoglobin concentration.

Polydactyly excessive number of digits (fingers or toes).

Polygalactia excessive secretion of milk.

Position the relation of the direction of the presenting part of the fetus to the maternal pelvis.

Posterior fontanelle small triangular area between the occipital and parietal bones of the skull.

Postmature infant infant born at or after the beginning of the forty-third week of gestation and exhibiting signs of dysmaturity.

Postnatal occurring after birth; postpartal; postpartum.

Preeclampsia a disorder encountered during pregnancy or early in the puerperium, characterized by hypertension, edema, and albuminuria.

Prematurity state of being born before the usual or expected time; less than 37 weeks of gestation.

Presentation that part of the fetus nearest the internal os; or that part which is felt by the physician's examining finger when introduced into the cervix.

Primigravida a woman who is pregnant for the first time.

Primipara a woman who has given birth to her first child of viable gestational age.

Prodromal premonitory; indicating the approach of a disease.

Projectile vomiting extremely forceful, expulsive vomiting.

Prolapsed cord umbilical cord that is expelled beside or ahead of the presenting part.

Promontory of the sacrum projecting process of the sacrum at the junction of the sacrum and L5.

Pseudocyesis a condition in which the woman has symptoms of pregnancy but in which hormonal pregnancy tests are negative; false pregnancy.

Pseudomenstruation discharge of blood-tinged mucus from the vagina of newborn female infants; caused by withdrawal of maternal hormones that were present during pregnancy.

Psychoprophylaxis psychophysical training aimed at preparing the expectant parents to cope with the processes of labor and to avoid concentration on the discomforts associated with childbirth.

Ptyalism excessive secretion of saliva.

Pubiotomy the operation of cutting through the pubic bone lateral to the median line.

Pudendum the external genital parts of either sex, but especially of the female.

Puerperium the period elapsing between the termination of labor and the return of the uterus to its normal condition, about 6 weeks.

Pustule a small pus-containing vesicle.

Pyloric stenosis stenosis or narrowing of the orifice of the pylorus.

Pylorospasm spasm of the pylorus or of the pyloric portion of the stomach.

Quickening first fetal movements felt by the mother, usually between 16 and 18 weeks' gestation.

Radioimmunoassay a test for pregnancy based upon the antigen-antibody reaction and measured by sensitive radioisotope technique.

Rales   crackling sounds heard as air passes through the fluid present within the terminal bronchioles and alveoli.

Recessive trait   genetically determined characteristic that is expressed only when present in the homozygotic state.

Rectocele   herniation or protrusion of the rectum into the posterior vaginal wall.

Rectovaginal fistula   an opening between the rectum and vagina.

Relaxin   a water-soluble protein secreted by the corpus luteum that causes relaxation of the symphysis and cervical dilation.

Residual urine   urine left in the bladder after voiding.

Respiratory distress syndrome (RDS)   condition resulting from decreased pulmonary gas exchange, leading to retention of carbon dioxide (increase in arterial PCO_2). Most common neonatal causes are prematurity, perinatal asphyxia, maternal diabetes mellitus, and hyaline membrane disease (HMD).

Restitution   in obstetrics the turning of the fetal head to the left or right after it has completely emerged from the introitus as it assumes a normal alignment with the infant's shoulders.

Resuscitation   restoration of life or consciousness by means of artificial respiration and cardiac massage.

Retained placenta   retention of all or part of the placenta in the uterus after delivery.

Retroflexion of the uterus   the bending back of the body of the uterus toward the cervix, resulting in a sharp angle at the point of bending.

Retrolental fibroplasia   formation of fibriotic tissue behind the lens; associated with retinal detachment seen with hyperoxemia in premature infants.

Rh factor   inherited antigen present on erythrocytes. The individual with the factor is known as positive for the factor.

Rhonchi   coarse, snorelike sounds produced as air passes through the fluid in the large bronchi.

Rhythm method   the timing of sexual intercourse to avoid the fertile time associated with ovulation.

Ritgen's maneuver   method of control of fetal head during delivery by pressure through the mother's perineal tissue against fetal forehead and chin.

Rooming-in unit   hospital unit where the infant can reside in the same room with his mother after delivery and during their postpartal stay.

Rooting reflex   an infant's tendency to turn his head and open his lips to suck when one side of his mouth or his cheek is touched.

Rotation   in obstetrics, the turning of the fetal head as it follows the curves of the birth canal downward.

Rubin's test   tubal insufflation with a gas, usually carbon dioxide, to test the patency of the tubes or to clear small obstructions.

Rugae   folds of vaginal mucosa.

Saddle block anesthesia   sensory and motor anesthesia of the buttocks, perineum, and inner aspects of the thighs, produced by spinal or entrathecal injection of an anesthetic agent at approximately L3–L5.

Salpingo-oophorectomy   surgical removal of a fallopian tube and an ovary.

Scanzoni's maneuver   forceps rotation of the occiput to an anterior position from a posterior position.

Scarf sign   the position of the elbow when the hand of a supine infant is drawn across to the other shoulder until it meets resistance.

Schultze's mechanism   delivery of the placenta with the fetal surface outermost.

Sebaceous glands   oil-secreting glands in the skin.

Second stage of labor   stage lasting from complete dilatation of the cervix to expulsion of the fetus.

Secretory phase of menstrual cycle   postovulatory, luteal, progestational, premenstrual phase of menstrual cycle; 14 days in length.

Secundines   fetal membranes and placenta expelled after childbirth; afterbirth.

Semen   thick, white, viscid secretion discharged from the urethra of the male at orgasm; the transporting medium of the sperm.

Sensitization   development of antibodies to a specific antigen.

Sex-linked trait   a characteristic that is determined by genes on the X chromosome.

Show   popularly, the blood-tinged mucus discharged from the vagina before or during labor.

Simian line   a single palmar crease frequently found in children with Down's syndrome.

Skene's glands   two glands opening just within the meatus of the female urethra, regarded as homologues of the seminal vesicles.

Small for gestational age (SGA)   characterized by inadequate weight or growth for gestational age; birth weight below the 10th percentile.

Smegma   a thick, cheesy, ill-smelling secretion found under the prepuce and around the labia minora.

Somnolence   sleepiness; also unnatural drowsiness.

Spermatogenesis   process by which mature spermatozoa are formed during which chromosome number is reduced by half.

Spermatozoa   mature sperm cells of the male animal produced by the testes.

Spina bifida occulta   a defect in the vertebra of the spinal column without protrusion of neural components; may be completely asymptomatic.

Spinnbarkeit   formation of a stretchable thread of cervical mucus under estrogen influence at time of ovulation.

Spontaneous abortion   abortion that occurs naturally.

Square window   angle of wrist between hypothenar prominence and forearm; one criterion for estimating gestational age of neonate.

Station   relationship of the presenting fetal part to an imaginary line drawn between the ischial spines of the pelvis.

Strabismus   deviation of one or both eyes from a point of focus.

Striae gravidarum   stretch marks; shiny, reddish lines that appear on the abdomen, breasts, thighs, and buttocks of pregnant women as a result of stretching the skin.

Stridor   harsh, high-pitched sound during respiration.

Subinvolution   failure of a part to return to its normal size after functional enlargement, such as failure of the uterus to return to normal size after pregnancy.

Sucking reflex   the infant's tendency to suck on any object placed in his mouth.

Supine hypotension syndrome   symptoms of bradycardia and lowered blood pressure when in a supine position late in pregnancy; due to compression of the inferior vena cava by the gravid uterus.

Surfactant   a surface-active mixture of lipoproteins secreted in the alveoli and air passages that reduces surface tension of pulmonary fluids and contributes to the stabilization of alveolar sacs.

Superfetation   fertilization and development of an ovum while a developing fetus is already in the uterus.

Supernumerary nipples   excess number of nipples, varying from small pink spots to normal size and pigmentation, usually present along an imaginary line from midclavicle to groin.

Suture   junction of the adjoining bones of the skull.

Symphysis pubis   the junction of the pubic bones.

Syndactyly   malformation of the fingers or toes in which there may be webbing or complete fusion of two or more digits.

Tachypnea   excessively rapid respiratory rate (e.g., in neonates, respiratory rate of 60 breaths per minute or more).

Talipes equinovarus   congenital defect of the foot with changes in the ligament and tendons consisting chiefly of contractures and anomalous insertions. The forefoot is adducted and supine and there is inversion of the heel and fixed plantar flexion of the foot. Also known as club foot.

Telangiectatic nevi   small clusters of pink-red spots appearing on the nape of the neck and around the eyes of infants; localized areas of capillary dilatation. Also referred to as stork bites.

Teratogen   an agent causing damage in the developing embryo.

Term infant   live infant born between weeks 38 and 42 of gestation.

Tetralogy of Fallot   congenital cardiac malformation consisting of pulmonary stenosis, intraventricular septal defect, dextroposed aorta that receives blood from both ventricles, and hypertrophy of the right ventricle.

Third stage of labor   the period from delivery of the fetus to the time when the placenta has been completely expelled.

Threatened abortion   a condition in which discharge of the fertilized ovum is threatened by bleeding from the vagina, which may be accompanied by cervical dilatation.

Thrombocytopenic purpura   hematologic disorder characterized by prolonged bleeding time, decreased number of platelets, increased cell fragility, and purpura, which result in hemorrhages into the skin, mucous membranes, organs, and other tissue.

Thromboembolism   obstruction of a blood vessel by a clot that has become detached from its site of formation.

Thrombophlebitis   inflammation of a vein associated with thrombus formation.

Thrombus   blood clot obstructing a blood vessel that remains at the place it was formed.

Thrush   fungal infection of the mouth or throat characterized by the formation of white patches on a red, moist, inflamed mucous membrane and caused by *Candida albicans*.

Tocodynamometer   external device that can be used to estimate uterine contraction pressures during labor.

Tongue tie   abnormally short frenulum of the tongue that limits its motion.

Tonic neck reflex   postural reflex seen in the newborn. When the supine infant's head is turned to one side, the arm and leg on that side extend while the extremities on the opposite side flex; also called the fencing position.

Toxemia   term previously used for hypertensive disorders of pregnancy or early puerperium, now known as preeclampsia and eclampsia; characterized by one or all of the following: edema, hypertension, and proteinuria.

Tracheoesphageal fistula   a congenital anomaly in which there is a communication between the trachea and the esophagus.

Transition   last phase of first stage of labor; cervical dilatation of 8 to 10 centimeters.

Translocation   condition in which a chromosome breaks and all or part of that chromosome is transferred to a different part of the same chromosome or to another chromosome.

Trichomonas vaginalis   a protozoon that may cause inflammation of the vagina characterized by itching and burning of vulvar tissue and by white, frothy discharge.

Trimester   time period of 3 months.

Trisomy   the presence of three homologous chromosomes rather than the normal two.

Trophoblast   the outer layer of the blastoderm that will eventually establish the nutrient supply with the uterine endometrium.

Trousseau's sign   a sign of tetany in which carpal spasm can be elicited by compressing the upper arm.

Turner's syndrome   a number of anomalies that occur when a female has only one X chromosome.

Ultrasonography   use of high frequency sound waves to discern fetal heart rate, placental location, or fetal body parts.

Umbilical cord (funis)   structure connecting the placenta and fetus and containing two arteries and one vein encased in a tissue called Wharton's jelly.

Umbilical hernia   protrusion of the bowel or omentum at the navel.

Umbilical vasculitis   inflammation of the umbilical cord and its contents.

Uterine souffle   a sound made by the blood in the arteries of the gravid uterus; it is synchronous with the maternal heartbeat.

Uterine tetany   prolonged or continuous uterine contractions.

Uterus   hollow muscular organ in which the fertilized ovum is implanted and in which the developing fetus is nourished until birth.

Vagina   the musculomembranous tube or passageway located between the external genitals and the uterus of the female.

Varices (varicose veins)   swollen, distended, and twisted veins that may develop in almost any part of the body but are most commonly seen in the legs, vulva, and anus during pregnancy.

Vasectomy   ligation or removal of a segment of the vas deferens, usually done bilaterally to produce sterility in the male.

Vernix caseosa   a protective cheeselike whitish substance composed of sebum and desquamated epithelial cells present on the fetal skin.

Version   act of turning the fetus in the uterus to change the presenting part and facilitate delivery.

Vertex   the top or crown of the head.

Vesicular   composed of or relating to small saclike structures filled with fluid (less than 1 centimeter in diameter).

Vestibule   a triangular space between the labia minora; the urinary meatus and the vagina open into it.

Viability   state of development theoretically compatible with extrauterine survival.

Villus   a small vascular process or protrusion growing on a mucous surface, such as the chorionic villi seen in tufts on the chorion of the early embryo.

Wharton's jelly   yellow-white gelatinous material surrounding the vessels of the umbilical cord.

Witch's milk   a whitish fluid secreted from enlarged mammary tissue in the neonate, presumably resulting from maternal hormonal influences.

X-linkage   transmission by genes located on the X chromosome.

Y chromosome   sex-determining chromosome found in half of all sperm.

Zero population growth   condition that occurs when, in a given year, live births equal the number of deaths (i.e., no population increase for that year).

Zona pellucida   the transparent layer surrounding a discharged ovum.

Zygote   a fertilized ovum.

INDEX

Index